Clemente's
Anatomy
Dissector

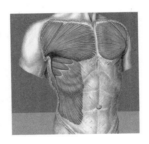

Guides to Individual Dissections in Human Anatomy With Brief Relevant Clinical Notes (Applicable for Most Curricula)

Benjamin Boyd, P.T.

Clemente's
Anatomy
Dissector

SECOND EDITION

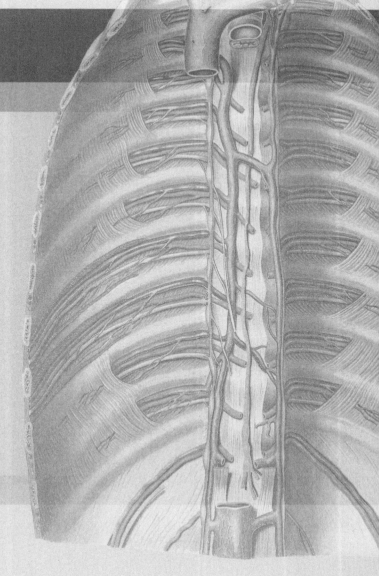

Carmine D. Clemente, PhD

Emeritus Professor of Anatomy and Neurobiology (Recalled)
UCLA School of Medicine
Professor of Surgical Anatomy,
Charles R. Drew University of Medicine and Science,
Los Angeles, California

 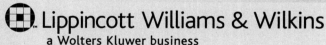

Lippincott Williams & Wilkins
a Wolters Kluwer business

Philadelphia · Baltimore · New York · London
Buenos Aires · Hong Kong · Sydney · Tokyo

Acquisitions Editor: Crystal Taylor
Managing Editor: Stacey L. Sebring
Marketing Manager: Valerie Shannahan
Production Editor: Jennifer P. Ajello
Designer: Risa J. Clow
Compositor: Maryland Composition, Inc.
Printer: Courier Corporation—Kendallville

351 West Camden Street
Baltimore, MD 21201

530 Walnut Street
Philadelphia, PA 19106

Printed in the United States of America

First Edition, 2002

Library of Congress Cataloging-in-Publication Data

Clemente, Carmine D.
   Clemente's dissector : guides to individual dissections in human anatomy with brief relevant clinical notes (applicable for most curricula) / Carmine D. Clemente.—2nd ed.
   p. cm.
Includes index.
ISBN 0-7817-6339-8
   1. Human dissections—Laboratory manuals. I. Title: Dissector. II. Title.

QM34.C545 2006
611.0078—dc22   2006040978

To purchase additional copies of this book, call our customer service department at **(800) 638-3030** or fax orders to **(301) 223-2320.** International customers should call **(301) 223-2300.**

Visit Lippincott Williams & Wilkins on the Internet: http://www.LWW.com. Lippincott Williams & Wilkins customer service representatives are available from 8:30 am to 6:00 pm, EST.

06 07 08 09 10
1 2 3 4 5 6 7 8 9 10

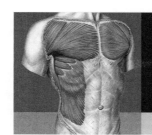

Preface to the first edition:

One of my objectives in writing this book was to combine a home study exercise with a laboratory dissection experience. Each chapter is a separate dissection and lesson. Indexed to Clemente's *Anatomy, A Regional Atlas of the Human Body* (4th Edition) with references to three other popular atlases (Grant's Atlas, 11th Edition; Netter's Atlas, 3rd Edition; and Rohen's Atlas, 5th Edition), the student learns the step-by-step dissection procedure for the laboratory along with relevant text information that enhances the laboratory work. At home, the learning process can be repeated by reading the text of each chapter and, following the dissection procedure, by simultaneously viewing the line drawings of this book and the relevant pages or plates in one of the referenced atlases.

The dissection directions are detailed beyond those of other currently used laboratory manuals, allowing students the opportunity to dissect on their own if they wish to do so, yet the text is brief and stresses essentials. Usually, each dissection will require one laboratory period of 2.5 to 3 hours. Exceptions to this may be the dissections of the pelvis and perineum, which may require some more time. The descriptions for these latter two dissections are similar in format. They include sections to be dissected similarly in both sexes and then special instructions required for individual dissections in male and female cadavers.

One need not defend again the value of dissecting the human body in schools of medicine and the other health professions. Experience through the centuries has proved its value in introducing the student to the study of medicine and its allied professions. Some have claimed that often "irrelevant" information was stressed in anatomy dissection courses. I have tried to select a dissection method that exposed essential structures in the most straightforward manner. No part of the body is summarily excluded, allowing the book to be of value for various types of curricula.

One departure from other dissection guides introduced in this book and suggested by my colleague, the late Professor David Maxwell, is the dissection of the posterior triangle of the neck immediately following that of the axilla but before the remainder of the upper limb. This allows the student to see the source of the neurovascular structures that supply the shoulder, arm, forearm, and hand.

In this book, significant attention is paid to *surface anatomy* in virtually every relevant dissection. This aspect of anatomy is of prime importance for its clinical implications.

Because the dissections are described in separate chapters, the study guide can be used in virtually any of the varied curricula and course sequences in our health science schools. The sequence of dissection chapters follows from the pectoral region to the upper limb, thorax, abdomen, pelvis and perineum, lower limb, back, neck, and head. Additionally, the separate dissection chapters and their subheadings can readily be selected to meet the needs of a systems curriculum or to a classical regional sequence that commences in parts of the body other than the pectoral and upper limb regions.

Many of the line drawings in this book were done by the artist Ms. Jill Penkhus in Los Angeles. Many others were produced under the direction of Professor Gene Colborn several years ago at the Medical College of Georgia for the Urban & Schwarzenberg Publishing Company. Still others were drawn by Ms. Patricia Vetter. I am most grateful to Ms. Penkhus, Ms. Vetter, and especially to Professor Colborn for their contributions. My appreciation is also extended to Mr. Timothy Satterfield and Ms. Susan Katz at Lippincott Williams & Wilkins for their patience as well as Ms. Ulita Lushycky for her most effective managing of the manuscript. Finally, but by no means least, I am most grateful to Julie, my wife, who has spent many hours at the computer during the development and eventual completion of the manuscript.

Los Angeles, 2002

Preface to the second edition:

My appreciation goes to the many faculty and students who have used the first edition of this dissector. Its wide acceptance not only in the United States but in foreign countries as well has been most gratifying. Several significant changes have been made. One is that in the first edition, dissection of the posterior triangle of the neck (which contains the neurovascular structures for the upper limb) was introduced just piror to dissections on the pectoral girdle and upper limb. In this edition, the posterior triangle of the neck has been shifted to the section on neck and head dissections (#29) just prior to the anterior triangle dissection. This change was made only because most courses use this latter dissection sequence and not because it especially makes better anatomic sense.

Since publication of the first edition of this dissector, new editions of the Grant, Netter, and Rohen atlases have appeared. Thus, this 2nd edition is now cross-referenced with the new 5th edition of the Clemente atlas, the 11th edition of the Grant atlas, the 3rd edition of Netter, and the 6th edition of Rohen. Many new figures have been introduced, several of which have come from the 30th American edition of *Gray's Anatomy,* which I edited and which appeared in 1985. Many positive comments have been received from course chairs that each dissection is a separate "chapter" in the book, making it easy in their assignments to the students. This format has also been appreciated by chairs whose courses do not include dissections of the entire body or, perhaps, even certain dissections within specific body regions.

I have also attempted to edit some descriptive material in the various dissections and have added paragraphs on clinical relevance. My appreciation again goes to Professor Gene Colborn for several drawings in this book, along with artists Jill Penkhus and Patricia Vetter. At Lippincott Williams & Wilkins, my appreciation is extended to Ms. Betty Sun and especially to Ms. Crystal Taylor and Ariel Winter. At UCLA my many thanks are exnteded to my Gross Anatomy colleagues Professors Shaleen Metten, Robin Fisher, Guido Zampighi, David Hovda, Charles Olmstead, Anna Taylor, Yau Shi Lin, Jayc Sedlmayer, and Francesco Chiappelli for their suggestions and for their use of this book in their courses.

Los Angeles, 2006

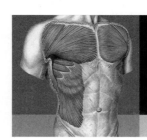

HOW TO USE THIS BOOK

This Dissector has been designed to assist students of medicine and health professions in performing comprehensive and efficient dissections. The text has the following features:

Each chapter can be used on its own, as a separate dissection and lesson, in the sequence most appropriate for any anatomy course. Therefore, the arrangement of the content makes this dissector applicable to varied curricula.

Basic information on surface anatomy and related preparatory techniques precedes the dissecting instructions. This text is printed in black on white background.

Dissection procedures are printed in black on a shaded red background.

Figure references are color-coded in red so the student can easily establish the connection between figures and dissecting steps.

Important structures are set in boldface in text. Some cautionary statements are set in capitalized letters.

References to Clemente's Atlas are embedded in the text. However, cross-references to other major atlases are placed in a shaded middle column next to the appropriate procedure. Red arrows clearly indicate to which column the references correspond.

The beginning of each dissection lists the referenced atlases, their corresponding edition numbers, and information indicating whether the numbers refer to plates or pages.

Clemente's Dissector is referenced to the following atlases:

Anatomy: A Regional Atlas of the Human Body, 5th edition
Carmine D. Clemente
Lippincott Williams & Wilkins, 2006

Grant's Atlas of Anatomy, 11th Edition
Ann M.R. Agur
Arthur F. Dalley II, Editors
Lippincott Williams & Wilkins, 2005

Netter's Atlas of Human Anatomy, 3rd Edition
John T. Hansen, Editor
Novartis Medical Education, 2003

Color Atlas of Anatomy: A Photographic Study of the Human Body, 5th Edition
Johannes W. Rohen
Chihiro Yokochi
Elke Lutjen-Drecoll
Lippincott Williams & Wilkins, 2002

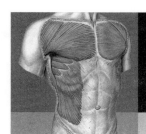

CONTENTS

Preface v

How to Use This Book vii

DISSECTION #1

Introductory Session and Surface Anatomy of the Thorax, Shoulder, and Upper Limb 1

   I. General Comments and Care of the Cadaver 1
   II. Dissection Instruments 1
   III. The Anatomic Position 1
   IV. Anatomic Planes 2
   V. Surface Anatomy of the Anterior Thorax, Shoulder, Axilla, and Upper Limb 2

DISSECTION #2

Mammary Gland and Pectoral Region 8

   I. Observe Other Cadavers 8
   II. Reflection of Skin 8
   III. Mammary Gland 9
   IV. Reflection of the Superficial Fascia 12
   V. Pectoral Muscles and Other Structures 13

DISSECTION #3

Deep Pectoral Region and Axilla 16

   I. Deep Pectoral Region 16
   II. Axilla 17

DISSECTION #4

Scapular and Deltoid Regions; Posterior Compartment of the Arm 23

   I. Surface Anatomy; Skin Incisions; Cutaneous Nerves 23
   II. Cut Scapular Attachments of Trapezius and Deltoid Muscles; The Supraspinous and Infraspinous Fossae 24
   III. Lateral Border of Scapula; Triangular and Quadrangular Spaces; Axillary Nerve and Deltoid Region 27
   IV. Anastomoses Around the Scapula 29
   V. Posterior (Extensor) Compartment of the Arm 30

DISSECTION #5

Anterior Brachial Region; Cubital Fossa; Anterior Forearm and Wrist 34

   I. Surface Anatomy; Skin Incisions; Superficial Veins and Nerves 34

   II. Anterior Compartment of the Arm: Muscles, Vessels, and Nerves 37
   III. The Cubital Fossa 40
   IV. Anterior Forearm Muscles, Vessels, and Nerves 40
   V. Tendons, Vessels, and Nerves on the Anterior Wrist 44

DISSECTION #6

Palmar Aspect of the Hand 46

   I. Surface Anatomy; Skin Incisions; The Palmar Aponeurosis and Digital Vessels and Nerves 46
   II. Ulnar Artery and Nerve; Fascial Spaces of the Hand 49
   III. Flexor Retinaculum; Flexor Tendons and Synovial and Fibrous Sheaths; Dissection of Middle Finger 50
   IV. Thenar Muscles; Movements of the Thumb; Dissection of the Distal Thumb; The Hypothenar Muscles 53
   V. Adductor Pollicis Muscle; Deep Palmar Arch; Deep Branch of the Ulnar Nerve; Interosseous Muscles 54

DISSECTION #7

Posterior Compartment of Forearm and Dorsum of Hand 56

   I. General Introduction 56
   II. Surface Anatomy; Removal of Skin; Superficial Veins and Nerves 56
   III. Muscles of the Extensor Compartment of the Forearm 58
   IV. Extensor Retinaculum; Extensor Synovial Sheaths; Structures Across the Dorsum of the Wrist 61
   V. Arteries and Nerves on Dorsum of Hand; Dorsal Interosseous Muscles 63

DISSECTION #8

Joints of the Upper Extremity 65

   I. Joints of the Shoulder Region 65
   II. Joints at the Elbow Region 68
   III. The Middle and Distal Radio-ulnar Joints 71
   IV. Joints at the Wrist 72
   V. Metacarpophalangeal and Interphalangeal Joints 74

DISSECTION #9

Thorax I: Anterior Thoracic Wall 76

   I. Surface Anatomy; Thoracic Vertebrae, Ribs, and Respiratory Movements; Projections of Heart and Lungs Onto the Thoracic Wall 76
   II. Anterior Thoracic Wall: Muscles, Vessels, and Nerves 82
   III. Removal of the Anterior Thoracic Wall 84
   IV. Pleura and Thoracic Viscera in Place; Removal of the Lungs 85

DISSECTION #**10**

Thorax II: Pleura and Lungs; Anterior Mediastinum; Middle Mediastinum and Pericardium; Removal of the Heart 88

  I. Pleural Reflections 88
  II. Lungs 89
  III. Mediastinum and Its Subdivisions; Anterior Mediastinum 93
  IV. Middle Mediastinum and Pericardium 94

DISSECTION #**11**

Thorax III: The Heart: Blood Circulation; Heart Surface Anatomy; Blood Supply, Chambers, and Conducting System of the Heart......................97

  I. Circulation of the Blood: General Comments 97
  II. Surface Anatomy of the Heart 97
  III. Arteries and Veins of the Heart 99
  IV. Chambers of the Heart 101
  V. Conducting System of the Heart 106

DISSECTION #**12**

Thorax IV: Posterior Mediastinum; Sympathetic Trunks; Diaphragm From Above; Superior Mediastinum 109

  I. Posterior Mediastinum 109
  II. Sympathetic Trunks and Splanchnic Nerves 112
  III. Diaphragm 113
  IV. Superior Mediastinum 113

DISSECTION #**13**

The Anterior Abdominal Wall 118

  I. Surface Anatomy of the Anterior Abdominal Wall 118
  II. Skin Incisions; Superficial Fascia; Cutaneous Vessels and Nerves 119
  III. Flat Muscles and Nerves of the Anterior Abdominal Wall 122
  IV. Rectus Abdominis Muscle and Sheath; Epigastric Anastomosis 124
  V. Inguinal Region 126
  VI. Scrotum; Spermatic Cord; Testis 128
  VII. Female Inguinal Canal, Round Ligament of the Uterus, and the Labia Majora 129

DISSECTION #**14**

Abdominal Cavity I: Topography of the Abdominal Viscera and Reflections of the Peritoneum......................131

  I. Exposure of Abdominal Cavity; Inner Surface of Abdominal Wall; Falciform and Round Ligaments 131

  II. Peritoneum and Abdominal Viscera *In Situ* 133
  III. Peritoneal Cavity; Greater and Lesser Peritoneal Sacs 137

DISSECTION #**15**

Abdominal Cavity II: Rotation of the Gut; Dissection of Stomach; Liver; Duodenum and Pancreas; Spleen 140

  I. Embryologic Events Related to the Development of the Gastrointestinal Tract 140
  II. Dissection of the Stomach, Liver and Gall Bladder, Duodenum and Pancreas, and Spleen 143

DISSECTION #**16**

Abdominal Cavity III: Intestinal Tract From Duodenojejunal Junction to Rectum 152

  I. Superior and Inferior Mesenteric Vessels 152
  II. Jejunum and Ileum 156
  III. Large Intestine 157

DISSECTION #**17**

Abdominal Cavity IV: Posterior Abdominal Wall 161

  I. Gonadal Vessels, Kidneys, Ureters, and Suprarenal Glands 161
  II. Muscles of the Posterior Abdominal Wall and the Lumbar Plexus 165
  III. The Diaphragm From the Abdominal Aspect 169
  IV. Abdominal Aorta; Inferior Vena Cava; Lumbar Sympathetic Chain 170

DISSECTION #**18**

The Pelvis: Male and Female 173

  I. General Features Found in Both the Male and Female Pelvis 173
  II. Male Pelvic Viscera: Urinary Bladder and Ureters; Seminal Vesicles and Ductus Deferens; Prostate Gland and Prostatic Urethra; Rectum 179
  III. Female Pelvic Organs: Urinary Bladder, Ureters, and Urethra; Ovaries and Uterine Tubes; Uterus and Vagina; Rectum 182
  IV. Lateral Pelvic Wall and Floor: Vessels, Nerves, and Muscles 185

DISSECTION #**19**

The Perineum: Male and Female 192

  I. General Information and Surface Anatomy 192
  II. Anal Triangle and Region 194
  III. Male Urogenital Triangle and Region 197
  IV. Female Urogenital Triangle and Region 203

DISSECTION #20

The Gluteal Region, Posterior Thigh, and Popliteal Fossa 209

   I. Surface Anatomy; Skin Incisions; Cutaneous Innervation   209
   II. Gluteal Region   212
   III. Posterior Compartment of the Thigh   216
   IV. Popliteal Fossa   220

DISSECTION #21

Anterior and Medial Compartments of the Thigh 223

   I. Surface Anatomy; Superficial Vessels and Nerves   223
   II. Femoral Triangle; Femoral Vessels and Their Branches; Adductor Canal; Femoral Nerve   226
   III. Quadriceps Femoris Muscle and Its Motor Nerves   228
   IV. The Medial (Adductor) Region of the Thigh   230

DISSECTION #22

Anterior and Lateral Compartments of the Leg and Dorsum of the Foot 234

   I. Surface Anatomy; Superficial Vessels and Nerves; Anterior Leg, Ankle, and Dorsum of the Foot   236
   II. Anterior Compartment of the Leg   239
   III. Lateral Compartment of the Leg   243
   IV. Ankle Region and Dorsum of the Foot   243

DISSECTION #23

The Posterior Leg and Sole of the Foot 248

   I. Surface Anatomy   248
   II. Incisions and Superficial Dissection of the Posterior Leg   249
   III. Posterior Compartment: Muscles, Vessels, and Nerves   249
   IV. Plantar Aspect of the Foot   253

DISSECTION #24

Joints of the Lower Limb 260

   I. Sacroiliac Joint   260
   II. Symphysis Pubis   263
   III. Hip Joint   264
   IV. Knee Joint   268
   V. Tibiofibular Joints   271
   VI. Ankle Joint (Talocrural Joint)   272
   VII. Joints Within the Foot   275

DISSECTION #25

Superficial and Deep Back; Spinal Cord 280

   I. Posterior Primary Rami; Trapezius and Latissimus Dorsi; Rhomboids and Levator Scapulae   280
   II. Intermediate Muscles of the Back   286

   III. Deep Muscles of the Back   287
   IV. Vertebral Canal and Spinal Cord   290

DISSECTION #26

Back of the Neck and the Suboccipital Region 297

   I. Posterior Skull and First Two Cervical Vertebrae   297
   II. Dorsal Rami of the Cervical Nerves   298
   III. Suboccipital Triangle   300
   IV. Vertebral Artery   300

DISSECTION #27

The Superficial Face and Anterior Scalp 303

   I. Bony Landmarks and Surface Anatomy of the Face and Forehead   303
   II. Skin Incisions; Reflections of Skin Flaps   304
   III. External Muscles of the Mouth   305
   IV. External Nose   306
   V. Anterior Orbital Region   307
   VI. Superficial Vessels and Nerves of the Face   309
   VII. Superficial Structures on the Lateral Face   312

DISSECTION #28

Temporal and Infratemporal Regions (Deep Face) 316

   I. Veins of the Temporal and Retromandibular Regions   316
   II. Masseter and Temporalis Muscles   318
   III. Infratemporal Fossa and Its Contents   319
   IV. Temporomandibular Joint   325

DISSECTION #29

Posterior Triangle of the Neck 328

   I. Boundaries of the Posterior Triangle; Skin Incisions   328
   II. Superficial Vessels and Nerves   330
   III. Omohyoid and Other Posterior Triangle Muscles   332
   IV. Expose the Subclavian Vessels and Brachial Plexus By Removing the Middle Third of the Clavicle   332
   V. Subclavian Vessels   332
   VI. Cervical Part of the Brachial Plexus   334

DISSECTION #30

Anterior Triangle of the Neck 337

   I. Surface Landmarks and Triangles of the Neck   337
   II. Superficial Anterior Cervical Structures   339
   III. Infrahyoid Strap Muscles; the Ansa Cervicalis   341
   IV. Thyroid Gland; Superior and Inferior Thyroid Arteries; Recurrent Laryngeal Nerves; Parathyroid Glands   343
   V. Structures Within or Adjacent to the Carotid Triangle   345
   VI. Suprahyoid Region   348
   VII. Deep Structures at the Root of the Neck   349

DISSECTION #31

**The Scalp; the Floor of the Cranial
Cavity; the Base of the Brain** 353

   I. The Scalp   353
   II. Removal of Skull Cap and Wedge of Occipital Bone   356
   III. Meninges; Removal of the Brain   357
   IV. Base of Skull: Bony Markings; Foramina   360
   V. Arterial Blood Supply to the Brain   362

DISSECTION #32

The Orbit: Superior and Anterior Dissections ..366

   I. The Bony Orbit   366
   II. The Orbit From Above   367
   III. The Orbit From the Anterior Approach   373

DISSECTION #33

**Craniovertebral Joints and
Prevertebral Region** 380

   I. Basilar Part of the Occipital Bone; the Atlas and Axis   380
   II. Median and Lateral Atlantoaxial Joints; Atlantooccipital Joints   381
   III. Separation of the Head and Cervical Viscera From the Vertebral Column   384
   IV. The Prevertebral Region   384

DISSECTION #34

**The Pharynx: External and
Internal Dissections** 386

   I. Structure and Relationships of the Pharynx; Vagus and Glossopharyngeal Nerves   386
   II. Pharyngeal Constrictor Muscles   388
   III. Interior of the Pharynx   390

DISSECTION #35

**The Nasal Cavity and Paranasal
Sinuses in the Bisected Head** 394

   I. Bisection of the Head   394
   II. Nasal Septum   395
   III. Roof and Floor of the Nasal Cavity   396
   IV. Lateral Wall of the Nasal Cavity   397
   V. Pterygopalatine Ganglion; Greater and Lesser Palatine Nerves and Vessels   399
   VI. Paranasal Sinuses   400

DISSECTION #36

**Nasopharynx; Oropharynx (Inner Wall);
Palate; Mouth and Tongue** 403

   I. Nasopharynx   403
   II. Soft Palate From Above: Levator and Tensor Palati Muscles   404
   III. Internal Structure of the Oropharynx   404
   IV. Hard Palate Dissected From Its Oral Surface   406
   V. Oral Cavity and Tongue   407

DISSECTION #37

The Larynx and Laryngopharynx 415

   I. The Skeleton of the Larynx   415
   II. Surface Anatomy of the Anterior Larynx   416
   III. The Posterior Larynx; the Laryngopharynx; the Lateral Laryngeal Muscles   418
   IV. The Interior of the Larynx   421

DISSECTION #38

**The External and Middle Ear and the
Semicircular Canals of the Inner Ear** 425

   I. The External Ear   425
   II. The Lateral (Mastoid) Approach to the Facial Nerve; Semicircular Canals; Tympanic Cavity   427
   III. The Superior (Cranial Cavity) Approach to the Middle Ear   430

INDEX   433

DISSECTION #1

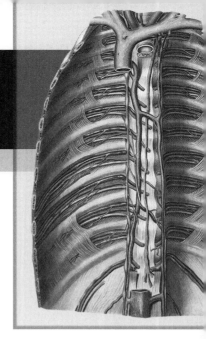

Introductory Session and Surface Anatomy of the Thorax, Shoulder, and Upper Limb

Atlas Key:

Clemente Atlas, 5th Edition = Atlas Plate #

Grant's Atlas, 11th Edition = Grant's Page #

Netter's Atlas, 3rd Edition = Netter's Plate #

Rohen Atlas, 6th Edition = Rohen Page #

I. General Comments and Care of the Cadaver

The first dissection period of a course in human anatomy proves to be a moving experience. It is inspiring simply to realize that the privilege exists to dissect the remains of another human being and that society today recognizes and approves the intrinsic value of human dissection in the education of the health professional. This was not always the case, and the history of anatomic dissection shows that a long struggle was waged through several centuries by courageous medical scientists to achieve our current state of enlightenment. It is important for the student to appreciate that the cadaver to be dissected was once a living person and that it commands both admiration and respect. Most bodies used for dissection in the United States and Canada are willed to medical schools by public-spirited citizens in the community.

Even properly embalmed cadavers require special attention. The hands, feet, and head of the cadaver must be wrapped in cloth (such as cheesecloth) that is liberally moistened with embalming fluid. This cloth should be moistened periodically. After each dissection period, the dissected regions should not be allowed to dry by remaining exposed to air.

The skin and superficial fascia are usually dissected as separate layers and will be retained as large tissue flaps to cover previously dissected regions. As dissection progresses, regions of the body already studied should be kept moistened so that they may be reviewed later.

II. Dissection Instruments (Figure 1-1)

Different types of dissection instruments are available.

Students should obtain the following instruments:

A. A **scalpel handle** that can receive detachable, large size #20 or #21, rounded contour blades.

B. **Two pairs of tissue forceps** (5½" to 6" in length): one with rounded blunt ends and the other with sharply ridged (rat-toothed) ends in order to grasp tissues securely.

C. **Two pairs of scissors:** one should be 5 to 6 inches in length and have either sharp ends or one sharp and one rounded end; the other should be a pair of fine dissection scissors with two sharp ends.

D. **A blunt inflexible metal dental probe.**

E. **A grease marking pencil** (one to a table) for outlining skin incisions.

III. The Anatomic Position

The anatomic position is the standard position of the body that is used universally to describe the location of anatomic structures. The body is in this position when the person is standing upright with the anterior surface

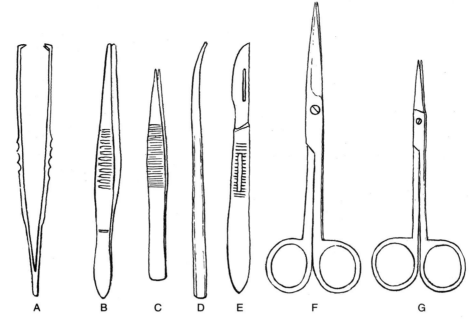

Figure 1-1. Dissection instruments to be used. A, B, and C, forceps; D, blunt probe; E, scalpel; F and G, scissors.

of the body facing forward, and the posterior surface oriented dorsally. The lower limbs and feet are together and oriented anteriorly. The upper limbs are by the side of the body with the palmar surface of the hands oriented anteriorly (**Figure 1-2**).

IV. Anatomic Planes

With the body in the anatomic position, structures and regions are often described in one or another plane. The **midsagittal (or median) plane** divides the body into right and left halves (**Figure 1-3A**). Planes parallel to the midsagittal plane are referred to as **parasagittal (paramedian) planes.** Vertical planes at right angles to the midsagittal plane are called **coronal planes.** A coronal plane down the middle of the body divides the body into anterior and posterior halves. **Transverse** or **horizontal planes** course across the body at right angles to the median and coronal planes (**Figure 1-3**).

V. Surface Anatomy of the Anterior Thorax, Shoulder, Axilla, and Upper Limb

During this first laboratory session, students should inspect and palpate structures on the surface of the body and identify certain bony landmarks and other anatomic features.

Clinical Relevance

It is important to have a thorough knowledge of the bony structures on the anterior thoracic wall because their locations can often be correlated to deeper structures and organs in the chest. Realize that descriptions of the incision sites through the chest wall to approach deeper structures or the identifications of surface lesions often use boney landmarks for precise communication.

One male student at each dissection table is to strip to the waist, so that the following surface structures can be identified:

A. Anterior Thorax.

1. **Jugular (or suprasternal) notch:** At the superior border of the sternum between the two clavicles (**ATLAS PLATES 101, 104, 105**).

2. **Sternal angle (of Louis):** A transverse ridge on the sternum approximately 4 to 5 cm (1.5 to 2 inches) inferior to the suprasternal notch where the manubrium and body of the sternum fuse (**ATLAS PLATES 104, 105**). Note that the 2nd ribs are attached to the sternum lateral to the sternal angle.

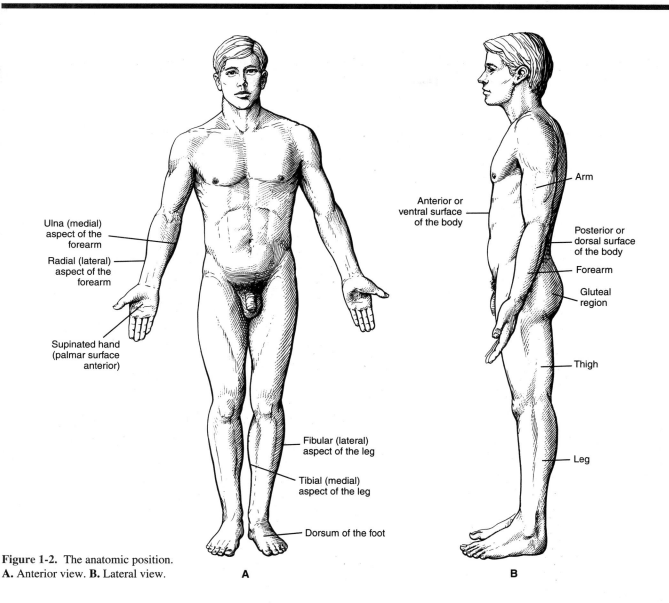

Ulna (medial)
aspect of the
forearm

Radial (lateral)
aspect of the
forearm

Supinated hand
(palmar surface
anterior)

Fibular (lateral)
aspect of the leg

Tibial (medial)
aspect of the leg

Dorsum of the foot

Arm

Anterior or
ventral surface
of the body

Posterior or
dorsal surface
of the body

Forearm

Gluteal
region

Thigh

Leg

Figure 1-2. The anatomic position.
A. Anterior view. **B.** Lateral view.

A

B

3. Manubrium of the sternum: Located between the suprasternal notch and the sternal angle (**ATLAS PLATES 104, 105**). Palpate the attachment of the clavicle to the manubrium at the sternoclavicular joint.

4. Body of sternum: Extends for about 10 cm (4 inches) inferior to the sternal angle. Note on a skeleton that ribs 3, 4, 5, and 6 attach to the body of the sternum (**ATLAS PLATE 105**).

5. Xiphoid process: Palpate the inferior extremity of the sternum in the midline for the xiphoid process. It attaches to the inferior border of the body of the sternum. The 7th ribs join the sternum at the xiphisternal junction (**ATLAS PLATE 105**).

◄
Grant's 2, 10, 12
Netter's 178, 179
Rohen 369, 372

6. Costal margins: Note on a skeleton that ribs 8, 9, and 10 join to form the cartilaginous lower costal margin of the rib cage (**ATLAS PLATES 4, 5**) and that ribs 11 and 12 do not attach to the sternum.

7. Infrasternal angle: The acute angle below the sternum between the costal margins.

8. Palpate the **clavicle** and the **sternoclavicular joint** (**ATLAS PLATES 79, 104**). Visualize several imaginary vertical lines on the chest wall (**Figure 1-4** and **ATLAS PLATE 2**).
  a. Midsternal line: Descends in the midline over the sternum.
  b. Parasternal line: Any line that descends parallel to the sternum.

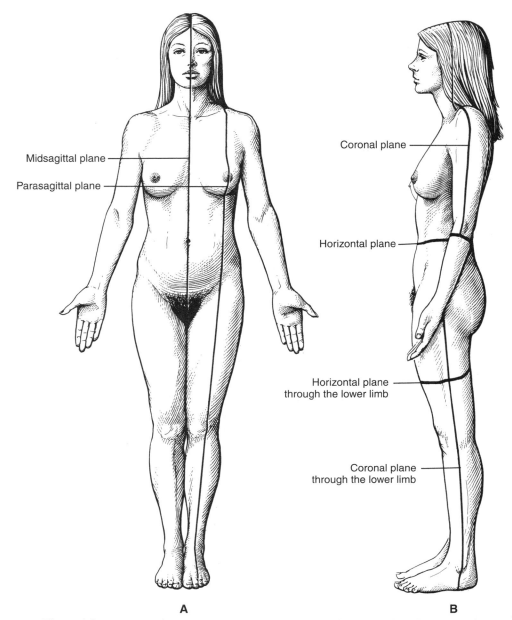

Figure 1-3. Planes used to define views of body structures. **A.** Frontal view. **B.** Lateral view.

c. **Midclavicular line:** Descends from the middle of the clavicle over the anterior thoracic wall. This line often courses near the nipple in the male or young female **(Figure 1-4)**.

d. **Midaxillary line:** A vertical line from the middle of the axillary fossa (armpit) down the lateral thorax.

9. Palpate the 2nd ribs through the skin. Feel the softer tissue in the 2nd intercostal space below the 2nd rib. Palpate the 3rd through the 7th ribs and intercostal spaces in this manner **(ATLAS PLATE 104)**.

10. Observe the **nipple**. In most men and young women it is located either over the 4th intercostal space or over the 5th rib **(Figure 1-4)**. The location of the nipple on the chest wall in older women may vary, because aging of connective tissue results in sagging of the breasts **(ATLAS PLATES 2–5)**.

B. Anterior and Lateral Shoulder and the Axilla.

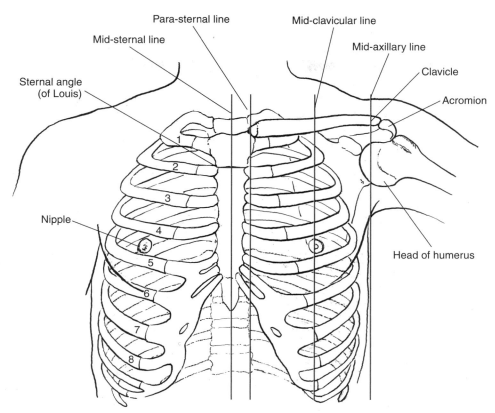

Figure 1-4. Imaginary vertical lines on skeleton of thoracic cage.

Clinical Relevance

Within the anterior and lateral shoulder region is located the glenohumeral (shoulder) joint. Additionally, anterior and posterior folds define a cone-shaped region called the axilla (armpit).

Located as a strut between the sternum and the acromion is the clavicle, one of the most frequently fractured bones in the body.

Dislocations of the humerus at the shoulder joint usually result from direct falls. Frequently the head of the humerus is dislocated through the joint capsule inferiorly and medially below the coracoid process. This painful injury also results in a loss of the normally smooth contour of the lateral shoulder.

1. At the jugular notch, palpate the **sternoclavicular joint** and follow the **clavicle** laterally to its articulation with the scapula called the **acromioclavicular joint** (**ATLAS PLATES 79–81**).

2. Palpate the rounded contour at the tip of the shoulder. The underlying bony structure is the **acromion** of the scapula (**ATLAS PLATES 28, 29, 82**).

◄
Grant's 10, 498, 475, 516
Netter's 178, 403–406
Rohen 368, 372

3. More difficult to feel is the **coracoid process.** Press inferior and slightly medial to the acromioclavicular joint (**ATLAS PLATES 79–81**) in a depression, the **infraclavicular fossa** (**Figure 1-5**).

4. With the upper limb abducted feel the hollow of the **axillary fossa** (armpit). Grasp the **anterior axillary fold**, consisting of the pectoralis major and minor muscles. Grasp the **posterior axillary fold,** formed by the subscapularis, teres major, and latissimus dorsi muscles (**ATLAS PLATE 28**).

5. Note the smooth contour of the shoulder formed by the **deltoid muscle** (**ATLAS PLATES 28, 29**). On a skeleton, find the **greater** and **lesser tubercles** on the head of the humerus. On your laboratory partner, palpate the **greater tubercle** deep to the soft tissue of the deltoid. Feel for the **lesser tubercle** on the anterior aspect of the humerus (**ATLAS PLATES 77, 79**). Between the two tubercles, palpate the **intertubercular (or bicipital) sulcus** containing the tendon of the long head of the biceps muscle.

C. The Arm and Forearm (**Figure 1-5**).

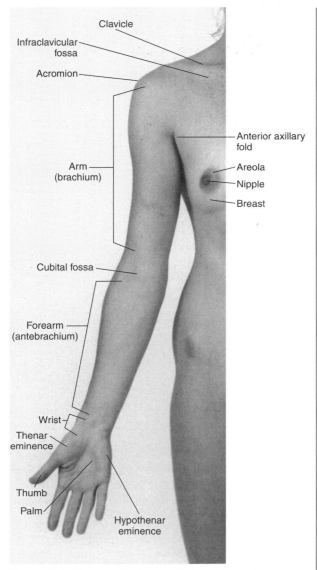

Clavicle
Infraclavicular fossa
Acromion
Anterior axillary fold
Arm (brachium)
Areola
Nipple
Breast
Cubital fossa
Forearm (antebrachium)
Wrist
Thenar eminence
Thumb
Palm
Hypothenar eminence

Figure 1-5. Photograph of upper limb and breast in a young woman.

▶
Grant's 476, 477, 538, 565, 569
Netter's 403, 404, 419, 423
Rohen 372–374

Clinical Relevance

Fractures of the humerus or of the radius or ulna frequently result from direct trauma or from falls. These fractures can injure or even sever large nerves, thereby disrupting neuromuscular functions. Fractures of the shaft of the humerus could injure the radial nerve, whereas fractures in the upper forearm can injure the ulnar nerve, especially near the posterior aspect of the elbow joint.

Blood is frequently drawn from veins (antecubital vein) on the anterior aspect of the elbow. Realize that deep to the superficial vein in the antecubital fossa are located the brachial artery and median nerve.

1. Between the elbow and shoulder joint is the **arm** (or brachium), and the **forearm** (or antebrachium) extends between the wrist and elbow (**ATLAS PLATE 1**). Flex the forearm and observe the belly of the **biceps brachii muscle.** This muscle is active both in **flexion** of the forearm and in **supination** (turning the hand over, so that the palmar surface lies anterior).

2. Note the bicipital furrows along the sides of the biceps muscle (**ATLAS PLATE 28**). Deep to the **furrow** course the brachial artery, its accompanying veins, and the median nerve. Feel for the arterial pulse through the skin. Identify the cephalic vein coursing along the lateral aspect of the arm (**ATLAS PLATES 27, 30**).

3. Palpate the triceps muscle on the posterior arm during extension of the forearm. At the elbow locate three bony structures posteriorly, the **olecranon** of the ulna, felt between the **medial** and **lateral epicondyles** of the humerus (**ATLAS PLATES 28, 29, 3**).

   With the forearm fully extended, note that the two condyles and the olecranon lie in a straight line. Flex the forearm to a right angle with the arm, and note that the olecranon lies distal to the two condyles. In full flexion, the olecranon lies anterior to the two condyles. These relationships are lost if the ulna is dislocated.

4. Feel the **ulnar nerve** behind the medial epicondyle (**ATLAS PLATE 42**). The sensation felt by palpating across this nerve will remind you of the "crazy bone" feeling in the hand when you bump your elbow.

5. In the supinated forearm position, palpate the **cubital fossa** anterior to the elbow joint (**ATLAS PLATE 27**). Feel the muscle mass bounding the fossa laterally. This consists of the brachioradialis muscle and the underlying extensor compartment muscles of the forearm (**ATLAS PLATE 54, 55**).

   Below the medial epicondyle, palpate the pronator teres muscle and the common origin of the flexor compartment muscles of the forearm. These form the medial boundary of the cubital fossa. Observe the **median cubital vein** superficially in the cubital fossa, and realize that the venous pattern is variable at this site (**ATLAS PLATE 27**).

   Deep to the median cubital vein, palpate the aponeurosis of biceps brachii muscle (**bicipital aponeurosis**). When the biceps muscle is tensed, this aponeurosis protects the underlying brachial artery and median nerve (**ATLAS PLATES 46, 50**).

6. Palpate the ulna from the olecranon distally to the wrist. When supinated, the ulna is the medial forearm bone at the wrist joint. Feel the **styloid process,** which is the distal end of the ulna. On the lateral side of the forearm, the radius lies deep to muscles, but the bone can be felt subcutaneously 4 inches above the wrist. Palpate the distal end of the radius, also called the **styloid process** (**ATLAS PLATES 84, 89**).

D. Wrist and Hand.

Clinical Relevance

Coursing into the palm deep to a strong ligament is the median nerve along with the tendons of the flexors digitorum superficialis and profundus within the carpal tunnel. Overuse of these tendons or the development of an inflammatory condition within this tunnel can cause pressure on the median nerve, resulting in weakness or loss of function of the thenar muscles of the thumb.

Perhaps the most important nerve in the hand is the recurrent branch of the median nerve. Feel at your wrist the most distal point of the radius. Project

▶
Grant's 498, 499, 538, 565, 569
Netter's 433, 434, 439
Rohen 375–377

distally into the hand a distance of about 1½ inches (or 4 cm) and realize that this nerve courses into the thumb muscles at that point. Injury of the nerve will impair functions of the thumb, especially in performing opposition to the other fingers.

1. Flex and extend the hand at the wrist. Note that you can bend your hand medially (ulnar flexion) and slightly laterally (radial flexion) at the wrist.

2. On a skeleton, observe the **8 carpal (wrist) bones, 5 metacarpal bones, and 14 phalanges** that form the bony structures of the wrist and hand (**ATLAS PLATES 90, 91**). Make a strong fist. This involves flexion at joints between the phalanges and between the metacarpal bones and the proximal phalanges of the fingers.

3. Place one of your hands alongside an articulated skeleton of a hand of the same side. Note that the transverse creases at the wrist, hand, and fingers are related to the joints. The three principal creases in the palm overlay the metacarpal bones (**Figure 1-6**).

Observe that the skin of the palm is taut and cannot be displaced across the underlying tissue. In contrast, note the "looseness" of the skin on the dorsum of the hand where the large veins of the upper limb commence.

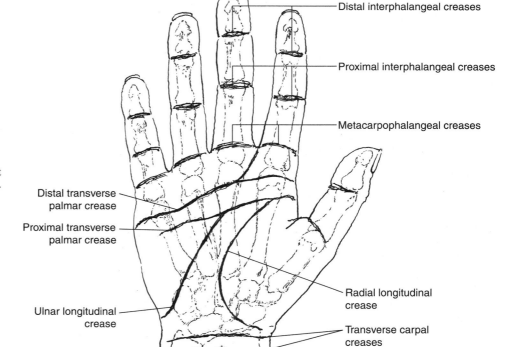

Figure 1-6. Palmar aspect of the right hand indicating longitudinal and transverse creases.

Distal interphalangeal creases

Proximal interphalangeal creases

Metacarpophalangeal creases

Distal transverse palmar crease

Proximal transverse palmar crease

Ulnar longitudinal crease

Radial longitudinal crease

Transverse carpal creases

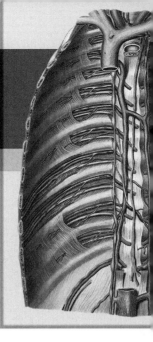

DISSECTION #2

Mammary Gland and Pectoral Region

OBJECTIVES

1. Remove the skin and superficial fascia from the pectoral region.

2. Dissect the nipple of the female mammary gland to see some of the lactiferous sinuses and ducts.

3. Study the blood supply and lymphatic drainage of the breast from figures in the Atlas.

4. Learn the course of a typical spinal nerve and learn how to dissect several lateral and anterior cutaneous branches.

5. Expose the pectoralis major muscle and the medial and lateral pectoral nerves that supply it.

6. Dissect the thoracoacromial artery and cephalic vein as they penetrate the clavipectoral fascia.

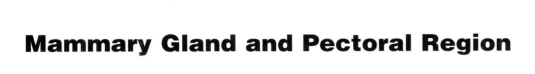

Atlas Key:

Clemente Atlas, 5th Edition = Atlas Plate #

Grant's Atlas, 11th Edition = Grant's Page #

Netter's Atlas, 3rd Edition = Netter's Plate #

Rohen Atlas, 6th Edition = Rohen Page #

I. Observe Other Cadavers

The primary objective of human dissection is to separate structures in the body and thereby observe their *three-dimensional relationships*. You must understand the meaning of terms such as **medial** and **lateral, superior** and **inferior, anterior** and **posterior** (dorsal and ventral), and **proximal** and **distal** because these are used to describe the relationships of structures to each other. Also, you must know what is meant by a **sagittal** or **median sagittal plane,** a **coronal plane,** and a **transverse plane.**

Take advantage of viewing the other cadavers in the laboratory. Because variation is a biologic constant, the precise location of structures as described in textbooks may not be duplicated in your cadaver. Vessels (and especially the superficial veins) are among the most variable of structures to be dissected. The large and important arteries are usually less variable than superficial veins, whereas the major nerve trunks, the muscles, and organs are typically similar from one body to the next. Size, body build, and gender account for certain differences in organ relationships. **Make it a habit to see and learn as much as you can in the dissection hall.**

II. Reflection of Skin

Before reflecting the skin of the anterior thorax, feel the **jugular** (suprasternal) **notch,** the **manubrium, body** and **xiphoid process of the sternum,** the **sternal angle,** the **acromion,** and the **clavicle.** Note also the position of the **nipple,** and in males (or young females), identify the rib or specific intercostal space on which the nipple is located.

> A. **Initial Incisions.** Make a midline incision (**Figure 2-1: A–C**) through the skin from the jugular notch to the xiphoid process. From this incision, make three other incisions laterally:
>
> 1. Between the upper border of the manubrium to the acromion (tip of the shoulder) along the clavicle (**Figure 2-1: A–D**). Extend this incision down the arm about 5 inches (**Figure 2-1: D–G**) and then around the arm (**Figure 2-1: G, H**).
>
> 2. From the midline laterally (encircling the pigmented areola) to the midaxillary line about 3 inches below the anterior axillary fold (**Figure 2-1: B–E**).
>
> 3. From the xiphisternal junction to the midaxillary line over the 6th rib (**Figure 2-1: C–F**).
>
> B. **Reflection of Skin.** Reflect the skin from the underlying superficial fascia. This is best done by beginning at the jugular notch (Point A in **Figure 2-1**) and proceeding laterally. Hold the scalpel edge at a slight angle to the underlying superficial fascia. Apply traction to the overlying skin by making an incision in the reflected skin through which the index finger of the free hand can be inserted as shown in **Figure 2-2**.
>
> When properly done, little or no fat will be adherent to the deep surface of the skin, which will show

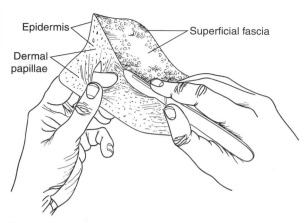

Figure 2-2. Suggested manual technique for dissecting the skin from the superficial fascia.

> many small pock marks, or pits, called **dermal papillae.** Keep the two skin flaps attached laterally. They will be replaced over the chest to prevent drying of the cadaver surface.
>
> Leave the nipple and areola attached to the underlying tissue. In males, note the location of the nipple on the anterior thoracic wall and proceed to reflect the superficial fascia (**ATLAS PLATES 2, 3**). Observe that the female breast lies completely in the superficial fascia. Any dissection of the mammary gland should be done **prior to the reflection of the superficial fascia.**

III. Mammary Gland (ATLAS PLATES 3–5)

The mammary gland, or breast, develops as a specialization of approximately 15 modified sweat glands, all of which open onto the surface of the nipple by way of the **lactiferous ducts.** Note that the fully formed breast extends between the lateral sternal line and the midaxillary or anterior axillary lines, and lies over the anterior chest wall between the 2nd and 6th ribs.

▶
Grant's 4–9
Netter's 175–177
Rohen 209, 290

> Dissect the breast by removing the fat that lies between several of the connective tissue septa called the suspensory ligaments of Cooper. Do this either with the handle of the scalpel or a large pair of forceps (**ATLAS PLATE 6 #6.1**). Note that these ligaments are attached to the skin superficially and to the deep fascia posterior to the breast.
>
> Dissect the deep surface of the **areola** and **nipple,** and identify one or more of the **lactiferous** ducts. These open on the nipple and are arranged in a radial pattern beneath the surface of the pigmented skin. Trace one duct more deeply where it enlarges to form **lactiferous sinuses** (**Figure 2-3**).

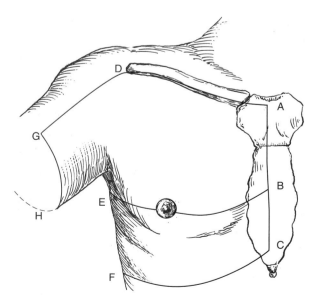

Figure 2-1. Incision lines for the pectoral region.

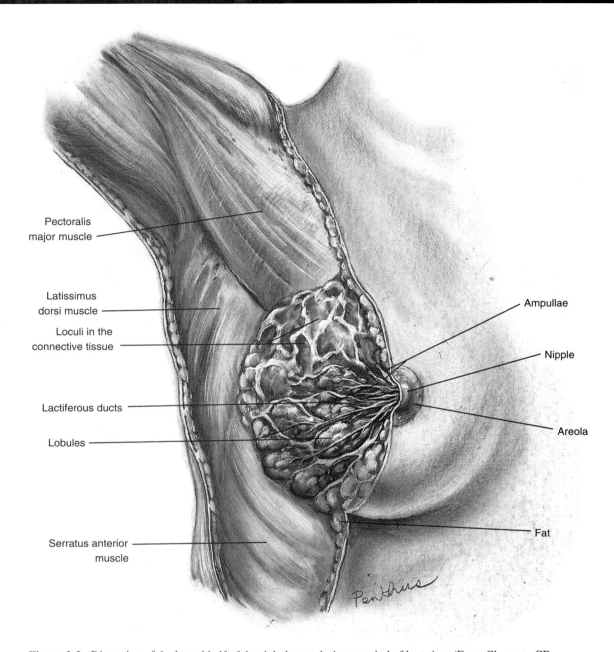

Pectoralis
major muscle

Latissimus
dorsi muscle

Loculi in the
connective tissue

Lactiferous ducts

Lobules

Serratus anterior
muscle

Ampullae

Nipple

Areola

Fat

Figure 2-3. Dissection of the lateral half of the right breast during a period of lactation. (From Clemente CD. Gray's Anatomy. 30th American Edition. 1985.)

Clinical Relevance

Pay particular attention to the blood supply (**Figure 2-4**) and the venous and lymphatic drainage (**Figure 2-5** and **ATLAS PLATES 3–5**) of the breast because of their importance as routes for the spread cancer cells.

The **arteries** that supply the breasts are derived from the axillary artery, the intercostal arteries, and the **internal thoracic artery.** The **lateral thoracic branch** of the axillary artery descends in the chest and gives off the **lateral mammary branches,** whereas medial mammary branches come from the internal thoracic artery as it descends just lateral to the sternum (see **Figure 2-4**). **Intercostal arteries** send **perforating branches** through the 2nd to the 5th intercostal spaces to supply blood to the deep regions of the breast.

Venous channels form an anastomotic ring around the nipple from which larger vessels are formed laterally and medially to drain into the **internal thoracic vein.** These vessels flow into the axillary and subclavian veins.

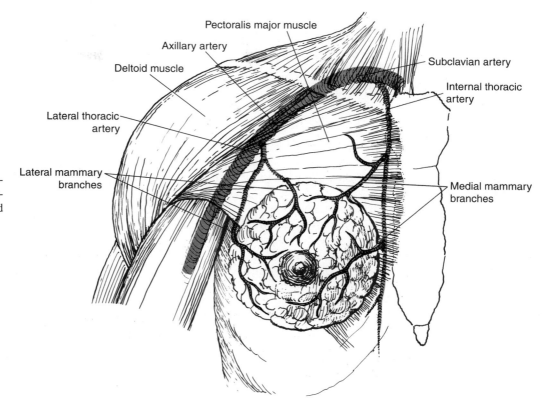

Figure 2-4. The lateral and medial mammary branches that supply the breast from the lateral and internal thoracic arteries.

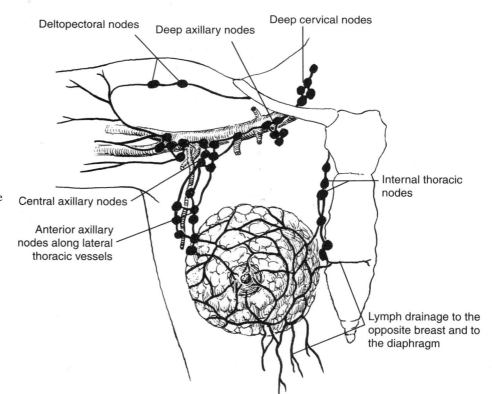

Figure 2-5. Lymphatic drainage from the right breast.

Lymphatic vessels from the mammary gland are numerous and of great clinical importance **(Figure 2-5)**. Channels from the deep regions of the gland course in the connective tissue between the glandular lobules and along the lactiferous ducts. From the central part of the gland and from the skin deep to the areola and nipple is the subareolar plexus. From these sources, collecting vessels course laterally and superiorly to the **anterior axillary** or **pectoral nodes** along the course of the lateral thoracic vessels and to the **central** and **deep** or **apical axillary nodes.**

Although most lymph drains superiorly and laterally, some channels drain medially along **parasternal or internal thoracic nodes (Figure 2-5)**. Lymph channels from the inferior and medial parts of the breast may communicate with diaphragmatic and abdominal vessels as well as with channels across the midline to the opposite breast.

IV. Reflection of the Superficial Fascia

The superficial fascia is to be reflected as a single layer, but **only after some of the anterior and lateral cutaneous branches of the spinal nerves are located.** Learn the general pattern and course of a typical spinal nerve **(Figure 2-6** and **ATLAS PLATE 8)**.

▶
Grant's 3, 20, 476
Netter's 182, 407,
412
Rohen 207, 208,
384, 408

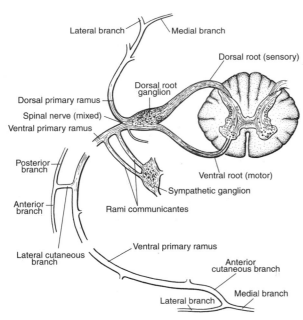

Figure 2-6. A typical spinal nerve and its branches.

With a probe and forceps, separate structures within the superficial fascia. Identify one or two **anterior and lateral cutaneous branches of the intercostal thoracic nerves** and the **supraclavicular nerves. (ATLAS PLATES 9, 12)**. Find these structures as follows:

A. **Anterior Cutaneous Branches.** Identify the 2nd, 3rd, and 4th ribs lateral to the sternum by probing through the fascia to the hard surface of the costal cartilages. In the 3rd intercostal space 1 cm lateral to the sternum, probe for the anterior cutaneous branch of the 3rd thoracic nerve usually accompanied by a small artery and vein **(ATLAS PLATE 9)**.

B. **Lateral Cutaneous Branches (Figure 2-7).** Palpate the 3rd and 4th ribs in the midaxillary line. In the 3rd intercostal space, dissect the lateral cutaneous branch of the 3rd intercostal nerve. Note other lateral cutaneous branches in the intercostal spaces inferiorly **(Figure 2-6)**. Larger than the anterior cutaneous branches, these nerves also are accompanied by lateral cutaneous branches of the intercostal vessels. Find the **intercostobrachial nerve** (T2), which emerges in the 2nd intercostal space and courses toward the axillary fossa and arm **(ATLAS PLATES 9, 20, 21)**.

C. **Supraclavicular Nerves (Figure 2-7).** Derived from the 3rd and 4th cervical nerves, these nerves descend in the superficial fascia and supply the skin over the clavicle and the first two intercostal spaces. To find them:

1. Make a 4-inch transverse incision through the superficial fascia **only,** commencing 1 inch lateral to the sternal angle. Cut only deep enough to see the deep fascia covering the darker muscle fibers of the pectoralis major.

2. Elevate the superficial fascia above the transverse cut, and identify strands of a thin sheet of muscle on the inner surface of the superficial fascia, called the platysma muscle **(ATLAS PLATES 472, 476)**.

3. Between this muscle and the deep fascia, locate at least one or more supraclavicular nerves **(ATLAS PLATES 9, 12)**.

muscles, the vessels and nerves that supply them, and the pectoral and clavipectoral fasciae.

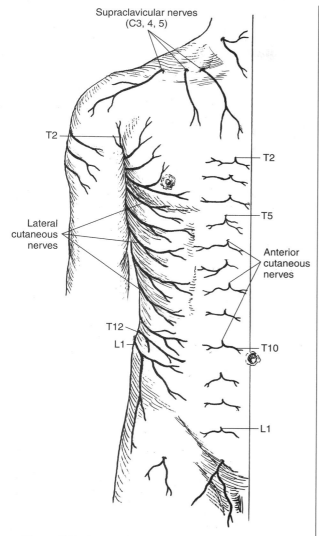

A. The Pectoralis Major Muscle. Clean the surface of the pectoralis major muscle and identify its clavicular, sternocostal, and abdominal parts (**ATLAS PLATE 10**). Within the groove that separates the pectoralis major from the deltoid muscle, find the **cephalic vein** (variable in size). This groove is the **deltopectoral triangle** (**ATLAS PLATE 13**), the three sides of which are the deltoid muscle, the pectoralis major muscle, and the clavicle. Its apex is directed inferiorly. Free the cephalic vein and note that it disappears deep to the pectoralis major muscle. Do not sever it at this time.

Locate the separation between the sternal and clavicular heads of the pectoralis major muscle. Widen this separation with a probe through the depth of the muscle to the underlying chest wall. Insert your index finger upward beneath the clavicular head, and carefully separate the clavicular head from the underlying clavipectoral fascia. Feel for the vessels and nerves that penetrate this fascia. These are branches of the **lateral pectoral nerve** and the pectoral branches of the **thoracoacromial artery and vein (ATLAS PLATE 15 #15.1)**.

Cut the clavicular head of the pectoralis major muscle close to its origin on the clavicle, and reflect it laterally (**Figure 2-8**). Observe the curved line of the attachment of the sternocostal and abdominal heads of the pectoralis major muscle (**ATLAS PLATE 13**). Feel for branches of the medial pectoral nerve penetrating through the pectoralis minor to enter the deep surface of the pectoralis major. Look for a branch of the lateral pectoral nerve entering the upper part of the sternocostal head.

Realize that the **lateral and medial pectoral nerves** are branches from the **lateral** and **medial** cords of the brachial plexus; hence, their names. Do not be disturbed that the medial pectoral nerve is located at a site on the anterior thoracic wall somewhat lateral to the lateral pectoral nerve. The lateral pectoral nerve supplies only the pectoralis major muscle, whereas the medial pectoral nerve supplies both the pectoralis major and minor muscles.

After freeing the pectoralis major muscle from its underlying fascial attachments, make a curved cut through it 1.5 inches from its sternal attachment

Figure 2-7. Cutaneous branches of spinal nerves supply.

▶
Grant's 3, 476
Netter's 182, 407, 412
Rohen 207, 208, 384, 408

D. On finding the cutaneous nerves, reflect the superficial fascia laterally. Make a longitudinal incision just lateral to the sternum through the superficial fascia and only as deep as the deep fascia covering the pectoralis major muscle. As you reflect the superficial fascia laterally, retain some of the cutaneous nerves for future review. Observe the fibers of the pectoralis major muscle beneath the layer of deep fascia over the muscle (pectoral fascia).

V. Pectoral Muscles and Other Structures

In addition to containing the mammary gland, the pectoral region contains the pectoralis major and minor

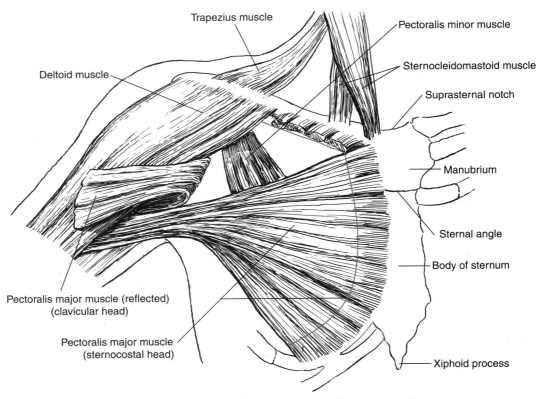

Trapezius muscle

Deltoid muscle

Pectoralis minor muscle

Sternocleidomastoid muscle

Suprasternal notch

Manubrium

Sternal angle

Body of sternum

Pectoralis major muscle (reflected) (clavicular head)

Pectoralis major muscle (sternocostal head)

Xiphoid process

Figure 2-8. The incision line for the pectoralis major muscle.

(Figure 2-8). Reflect the cut ends of the muscle and identify the branches of the nerves and of the **thoracoacromial artery** that supply the muscle (**ATLAS PLATES 15 #15.1, 16 #16.2, 21**).

B. Clavipectoral Fascia. Deep to the pectoralis major muscle, observe a broad sheet of deep fascia called the clavipectoral fascia (**Figure 2-9**). Extending down from the clavicle, it continues inferiorly to the axillary fascia. Observe that it encases the subclavius muscle, just below the clavicle, and the pectoralis minor muscle more laterally.

Identify the following structures penetrating the clavipectoral fascia:

1. The **cephalic vein** coursing into the axillary vein;

2. The **thoracoacromial artery;**

3. The **lateral pectoral nerve** and its branches.

◄
Grant's 480, 488
Netter's 182, 411
Rohen 208, 409

◄
Grant's 488
Netter's 411, 412
Rohen 208, 264, 385

C. The Pectoralis Minor Muscle. Note that the pectoralis minor attaches to the coracoid process of the scapula proximally and the 2nd, 3rd, 4th, and 5th ribs on the thorax distally (**ATLAS PLATE 15 #15.2**). Identify branches of the medial pectoral nerve that pierce the muscle from the underlying medial cord of the brachial plexus, thereby gaining access to the overlying pectoralis major.

Clinical Relevance

Sternal angle: The site of articulation of the manubrium and the body of the sternum has several important relationships.

a) At this site the second rib articulates with the sternum and that allows each of the lower ribs and intercostal spaces to be counted;

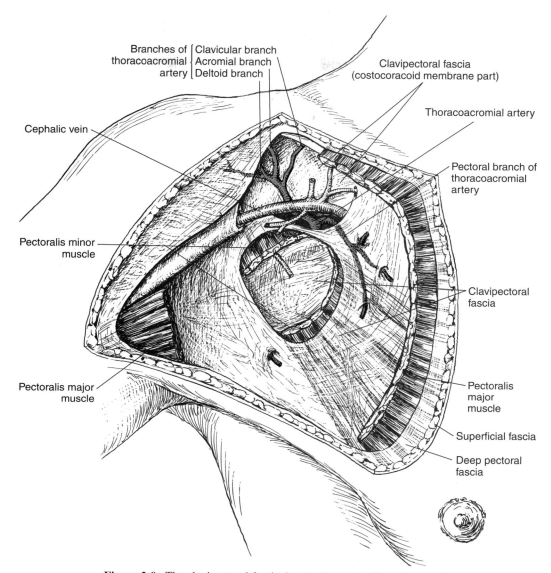

Branches of [Clavicular branch
thoracoacromial { Acromial branch
artery [Deltoid branch

Clavipectoral fascia
(costocoracoid membrane part)

Thoracoacromial artery

Cephalic vein

Pectoral branch of
thoracoacromial
artery

Pectoralis minor
muscle

Clavipectoral
fascia

Pectoralis major
muscle

Pectoralis
major
muscle

Superficial fascia

Deep pectoral
fascia

Figure 2-9. The clavipectoral fascia deep to the pectoralis major muscle.

b) A transverse plane at the sternal angle intersects the vertebral column between the 4th and 5th thoracic vertebrae. At this plane is the bifurcation of the trachea and the commencement of the ascending aorta from the left ventricle.

Thoracostomy by needle or tube through an intercostal space is often necessary for removal of air or fluids from the pleural cavity, thereby reducing a pneumothorax or hemothorax to restore breathing. **Bone marrow biopsy** is often achieved from the sternum, a bone that is rich in bone marrow and relatively easy to tap.

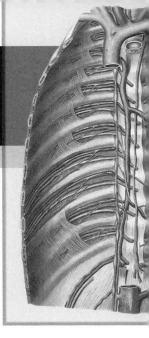

DISSECTION #3

Deep Pectoral Region and Axilla

OBJECTIVES

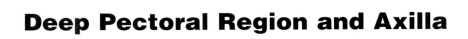

1 Identify the axillary vein and some of its tributaries.

2 Understand why the pectoralis minor is called the "key to the axilla."

3 Identify the branches of the axillary artery.

4 Find the **M** of the brachial plexus and dissect the cords of the plexus and its peripheral nerves.

5 Identify the subscapularis, latissimus dorsi, teres major, serratus anterior, coracobrachialis muscles, and the short head of the biceps brachii.

Atlas Key:

Clemente Atlas, 5th Edition = Atlas Plate #

Grant's Atlas, 11th Edition = Grant's Page #

Netter's Atlas, 3rd Edition = Netter's Plate #

Rohen Atlas, 6th Edition = Rohen Page #

I. Deep Pectoral Region

▶
Grant's 481, 483, 733
Netter's 182, 248, 411, 466
Rohen 170, 171, 398

Through the deep pectoral region and axilla course the nerves, arteries, and veins that supply the upper limb (**ATLAS PLATE 21**). Of additional importance are the lymphatic channels and nodes in these regions. They receive lymph from the upper extremity, but more significantly from the anterior thorax and—of special importance—from the mammary gland in women (**ATLAS PLATES 7, 14**). The axillary vein receives blood from the upper limb (including the shoulder) as well as from the pectoral region. It commences near the lower border of the teres major muscle at the junction of

▶
Grant's 480, 489
Netter's 410–412, 417
Rohen 208, 264, 409, 411–413

the basilic and brachial veins that ascend in the arm. The axillary vein becomes the subclavian vein as it ascends beneath the clavicle.

A. Axillary Vein. Abduct the upper limb of the cadaver nearly to a 45° angle. Remove fat lateral and medial to the pectoralis minor muscle and uncover the large axillary vein and the underlying axillary artery and cords of the brachial plexus (**ATLAS PLATES 21, 23, 36**). With your index finger, loosen the neurovascular structures deep to the pectoralis minor muscle. Trace the cephalic vein medial to the coracoid process and follow it to its junction with the axillary vein. Also identify the thoracoacromial branch of the axillary artery and the lateral pectoral nerve penetrating through the fascia from below (**ATLAS PLATE 15 #15.1**). Separate the axillary vein from the underlying axillary artery and cords of the brachial plexus.

Remove fat within the axilla down as far as the latissimus dorsi and teres major muscles. Because veins retain some coagulated blood after death, they

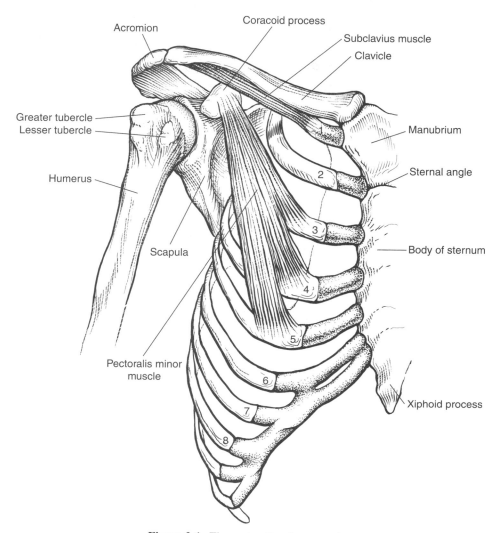

Figure 3-1. The pectoralis minor muscle.

often appear darker than the accompanying arteries. Cut away the smaller veins that flow into the axillary vein; however, do not cut the arteries that accompany these tributaries.

B. Reflect the Pectoralis Minor Muscle and Remove the Axillary Vein. Reflect the pectoralis minor muscle by severing its distal attachments to the 2nd, 3rd, 4th, and 5th ribs, but maintain its attachment to the coracoid process **(Figure 3-1)**. Relax the upper limb by slightly adducting it and dissect through the axillary fascia with a probe. This fascia partially surrounds the axillary vein but more completely envelops the axillary artery and cords of the brachial plexus.

Sever and remove the axillary vein and its tributaries from the clavicle to the tendons of the latissimus dorsi and teres major muscles. This will better expose the artery and nerves. **DO NOT CUT THE AXILLARY ARTERY, ANY OF ITS BRANCHES, OR THE CORDS OF THE BRACHIAL PLEXUS SURROUNDING THE AXILLARY ARTERY WHILE REMOVING THE VEINS.**

II. Axilla

The axilla is a cone-shaped or pyramidal region that lies deep to the pectoral muscles, superficial to the scapula and between the upper part of the brachium (arm) and the lateral chest wall. Its anterior wall is the pectoralis major and minor muscles and forms the anterior axillary fold; its posterior wall is formed by the teres major, latissimus dorsi, and subscapular muscles and

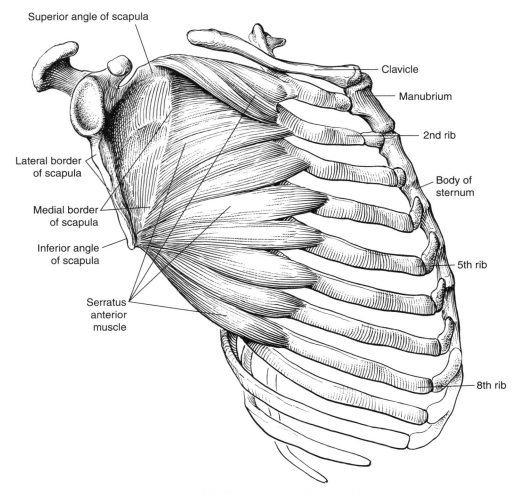

Superior angle of scapula

Clavicle

Manubrium

2nd rib

Body of
sternum

5th rib

Lateral border
of scapula

Medial border
of scapula

Inferior angle
of scapula

8th rib

Serratus
anterior
muscle

Figure 3-2. The serratus anterior muscle.

comprises the posterior axillary fold; its medial wall is the upper six ribs and intercostal spaces and is covered by the serratus anterior muscle (**ATLAS PLATE 15 #15.2**); and the lateral angle consists of the intertubercular groove or sulcus (bicipital groove) on the surgical neck of the humerus.

A. Identify the Following Muscles Associated With the Axillary Region.

1. **Pectoralis major and minor:** form the anterior axillary fold.

2. **Subscapularis:** occupies the subscapular fossa and inserts on the lesser tubercle of the humerus (**ATLAS PLATES 23 #23.1**).

3. **Latissimus dorsi:** ascends from the back of the trunk to attach on the medial lip of the bicipital groove of the humerus (**ATLAS PLATE 15 #15.2**).

◄
Grant's 489–491
Netter's 182, 407,
411, 412
Rohen 385, 386,
409, 415

4. **Teres major:** its tendon is located deep to that of the latissimus dorsi and with the subscapularis forms the posterior axillary fold (**ATLAS PLATES 36, 38**).

5. **Serratus anterior:** extends from the upper 8 or 9 ribs to the medial (or vertebral) border of the scapula (**Figure 3-2**). Probe its lateral surface longitudinally and find the **long thoracic nerve** (C5, C6, and C7).

6. **Short head of biceps brachii:** extends from the coracoid process and joins the long head of the biceps in the arm (**ATLAS PLATES 32, 34**).

7. **Coracobrachialis:** also arises from the coracoid process and inserts on the humerus (**ATLAS PLATES 32, 35**). **The musculocutaneous nerve usually pierces the coracobrachialis muscle** to enter the anterior arm region.

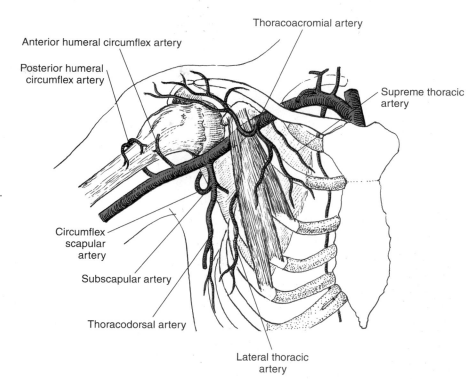

Figure 3-3. The axillary artery and its branches.

Anterior humeral circumflex artery

Thoracoacromial artery

Posterior humeral circumflex artery

Supreme thoracic artery

Circumflex scapular artery

Subscapular artery

Thoracodorsal artery

Lateral thoracic artery

B. Axillary Artery and Branches (Figure 3-3).

Replace the pectoralis minor and note that it divides the axillary artery into three parts (**ATLAS PLATE 16 #16.2**). The **first part** lies medial to the pectoralis minor and has one branch. The **second part** courses beneath the pectoralis minor muscle and has two branches, and the **third part** lies lateral to the pectoralis minor (as far as the lower margin of the teres major muscle) and has three branches. The axillary artery becomes the brachial artery below the teres major muscle. Realize that some variability in the pattern of these branches exists.

Find the branches of the axillary artery as follows (**Figure 3-3** and **ATLAS PLATE 16 #16.2**):

1. From the first part:
   a. **Superior (supreme) thoracic artery:** a small vessel arising just below the clavicle to supply the upper one or two intercostal spaces.
2. From the second part (**Figure 3-4**):
   a. **Thoracoacromial artery:** a short trunk that quickly divides into pectoral, acromial, clavicular, and deltoid branches. It frequently branches near the medial border of the pectoralis minor (**ATLAS PLATES 15 #15.1**).
   b. **Lateral thoracic artery:** in 30% of specimens it arises from the axillary artery near the lateral border of the pectoralis minor and

◄
Grant's 470, 488, 489
Netter's 176, 182, 410–412
Rohen 170, 396, 397, 411, 412

descends along the side of the chest (**ATLAS PLATES 20, 21**). In approximately 70% of specimens, it arises either from the thoracoacromial or the subscapular artery.

3. From the third part (**ATLAS PLATE 14 #23**):
   a. **Subscapular artery:** usually the largest branch from the axillary artery that is found on the anterior surface of the subscapularis muscle or near its axillary border. After 1½ inches, it divides into the **scapular circumflex branch** that courses around the lateral border of the scapula in the **triangular space,** and the **thoracodorsal artery** that descends to the latissimus dorsi muscle with the **thoracodorsal nerve.**

With a probe, pull the trunk of the axillary artery medially away from the humerus to see the following circumflex vessels:

   b. **Anterior humeral circumflex artery:** it is small and arises near the upper border of the teres major muscle. It passes anteriorly around the humerus.
   c. **Posterior humeral circumflex artery:** larger than the anterior, it passes posteriorly around the humerus. With a probe, trace the posterior humeral circumflex artery to the **quadrangular space,** through which it is accompanied by the **axillary nerve** to achieve the dorsal shoulder region. See **ATLAS**

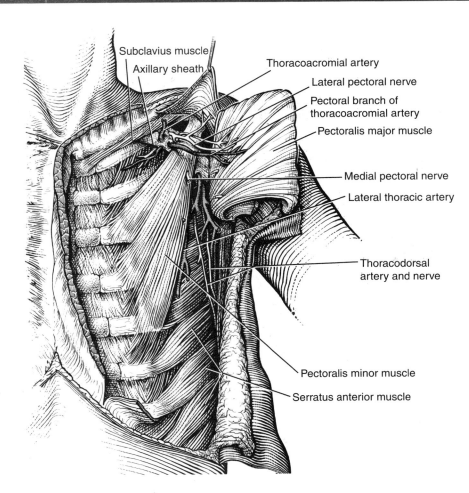

Subclavius muscle

Axillary sheath

Thoracoacromial artery

Lateral pectoral nerve

Pectoral branch of thoracoacromial artery

Pectoralis major muscle

Medial pectoral nerve

Lateral thoracic artery

Thoracodorsal artery and nerve

Pectoralis minor muscle

Serratus anterior muscle

Figure 3-4. The lateral pectoral nerve and some branches of the thoracoacromial artery coursing between the pectoralis major and minor muscles.

PLATES 24, 25 for triangular and quadrangular spaces.

C. Brachial Plexus and Its Branches (Figures 3-5 and 3-6).

Use **ATLAS PLATES 18, 19** to learn the general pattern of formation of the brachial plexus. This dissection is concerned with the infraclavicular (or axillary) part of the brachial plexus. This consists of the **lateral, medial,** and **posterior cords** of the plexus, and the terminal nerves that branch from them. The cervical portion of the brachial plexus will be studied with the posterior triangle of the neck.

1. Identify the **lateral cord** of the brachial plexus by finding the musculocutaneous nerve, which is the most lateral nerve of the plexus and the nerve that penetrates the coracobrachialis muscle (**ATLAS PLATES 36, 37**). Follow the musculocutaneous nerve proximally to its point of origin from the lateral cord. Also find

◀

Grant's 486, 488, 489
Netter's 176, 412, 413, 416
Rohen 186, 396, 409, 411, 415

the **lateral pectoral nerve,** which either comes off the lateral cord directly or arises higher in the axilla from divisions that form the lateral cord (**Figure 3-4**).

2. Note that the lateral cord contributes a large branch that helps form the median nerve.

3. Identify the median nerve and note that it receives another large contribution from the **medial cord.** Thus, the median nerve most often is formed by two large nerve trunks, one contributed from the lateral and the other from the medial cord.

4. From the medial cord, identify its other terminal branch, the **ulnar nerve.**

5. Place your index finger behind the musculocutaneous, median, and ulnar nerves and elevate them slightly from the axillary artery. Notice that their pattern resembles the letter **M** (**ATLAS PLATE 19**). Return to the me-

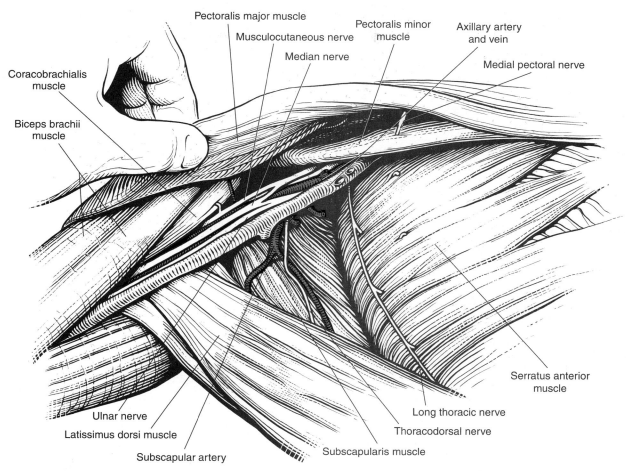

Figure 3-5. The axillary artery and vein and the musculocutaneous, median, and ulnar nerve branches from the medial and lateral cords of the brachial plexus.

dial cord and find three other nerves that arise from it above the origin of the ulnar nerve. These are:

a. the **medial antebrachial cutaneous nerve:** this large sensory nerve to the forearm is sometimes confused with the ulnar nerve.

b. the **medial brachial cutaneous nerve:** smaller than the preceding nerve, it arises slightly higher on the medial cord and often sends a communicating branch to the **intercostobrachial nerve** (T2) that passes through the 2nd intercostal space in the midaxillary line (**ATLAS PLATES 20, 21**).

c. the **medial pectoral nerve:** trace this nerve back to the medial cord from its site of penetration of the pectoralis minor muscle.

Clinical Relevance

Thoracic outlet syndrome: The apex of the cone-shaped axillary region is formed by three bones: the clavicle, scapula, and first rib. At this site the brachial vessels and the nerves of the brachial plexus might become compressed against the bones. Frequently this pressure results in symptoms related to spinal segments C7 and C8 (inferior trunk of the brachial plexus) and results in pain related to the distribution of the ulnar and medial antebrachial cutaneous nerves along the medial aspect of the forearm and hand.

Klumpke's paralysis: This syndrome is usually the result of a birth injury caused by the excessive abduction of the upper limb, which injures the C8 and T1 roots of the brachial plexus. The resulting deformity includes a "claw hand" owing to trauma to the inferior trunk of the brachial plexus (C8, T1) and consequent

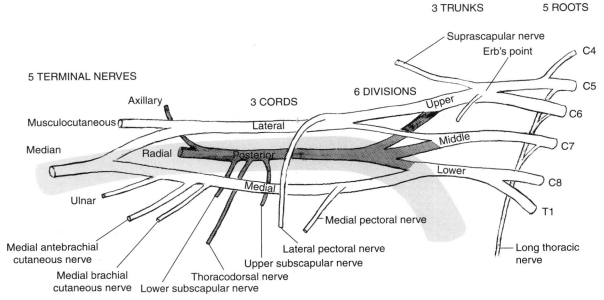

Figure 3-6. The roots, trunks, divisions, cords, and peripheral branches of the brachial plexus.

paralysis of muscles supplied by the ulnar nerve. Some flexion at the wrist occurs, but considerable flexion of the medial three fingers gives a clawlike appearance to the hand.

Winged scapula: Characteristic of this condition is the projection outward of the medial border of the scapula on the posterior chest wall in a manner that resembles a wing. This condition is caused by a weakness or paralysis of the serratus anterior muscle that holds the vertebral border of the scapula close to the posterior chest. At times when surgery is performed to remove lymph nodes along the course of the long thoracic nerve in women with breast cancer, inadvertent severance or trauma to this nerve on the lateral chest wall results in a winged scapula.

Erb-Duchenne paralysis: This syndrome is a partial paralysis of the brachial plexus that is usually the result of a birth injury. It involves the superior roots (or trunk) of the brachial plexus (C5, C6). The resultant deformity includes pronation of the forearm, extension at the elbow joint, and adduction of the upper limb. The pronated forearm and flexed hand projecting posteriorly is reminiscent of the hand of a waiter expecting a tip (waiter's tip position).

6. **Locate** the **posterior cord** of the brachial plexus behind the axillary artery. Identify its two terminal nerves, the large **radial nerve** and the **axillary nerve.** Trace the axillary nerve to

◄
Grant's 490
Netter's 413

the quadrangular space, which it traverses with the posterior humeral circumflex artery.

7. Higher on the posterior cord find three other nerves that course inferiorly. The upper subscapular nerve supplies the subscapularis muscle; the lower subscapular nerve supplies both the subscapularis and teres major muscles. Between these two nerves, locate the thoracodorsal nerve that descends with the thoracodorsal vessels to supply the latissimus dorsi muscle.

Clinical Relevance

Cervical rib: In 1 of 200 persons, an anomalous bony rib arises from the transverse process of the 7th cervical vertebra. Called a "cervical rib," it can cause pressure on the inferior trunk of the brachial plexus or the subclavian artery, resulting in a thoracic outlet syndrome.

Central venous line: Most often the right subclavian or right internal jugular vein is selected to place a catheter into the venous system. Visualized radiographically, the catheter is guided into the right brachiocephalic vein, then into the superior vena cava, and finally into the right atrium of the heart. A central venous line catheter is at times required to deliver therapeutic drugs or to measure venous pressure directly in the right atrium.

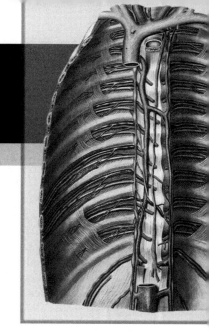

DISSECTION #4

Scapular and Deltoid Regions; Posterior Compartment of the Arm

OBJECTIVES

1 Study the surface anatomy of the upper back and posterior scapular region.

2 Detach the trapezius and the deltoid muscles from the spine of the scapula, expose the supraspinatus muscle, and locate the suprascapular vessels and nerve.

3 Dissect the infraspinatus muscle and identify the teres major and minor muscles.

4 Dissect the quadrangular and triangular spaces and find the axillary nerve, posterior humeral circumflex artery, and circumflex scapular artery.

5 Dissect the posterior compartment of the arm and expose the heads of the triceps muscle.

6 Separate the medial and lateral heads of the triceps brachii and follow the radial nerve and deep brachial artery around the shaft of the humerus.

Atlas Key:

Clemente Atlas 5th Edition = Atlas Plate #

Grant's Atlas 11th Edition = Grant's Page #

Netter's Atlas 3rd Edition = Netter's Plate #

Rohen Atlas 6th Edition = Rohen Page #

I. Surface Anatomy; Skin Incisions; Cutaneous Nerves

► Grant's 93, 282, 283, 591, 592
Netter's 8, 9, 167–169
Rohen 21, 29, 33, 192, 193

Place the cadaver face down (prone) and elevate the shoulders by means of a wooden block inserted under the anterior thorax. Partially abduct the upper limbs (to approximately 45°) and realize that the pectoral girdle is attached to the axial skeleton completely by muscles posteriorly and by muscles and one bony articulation anteriorly, the sternoclavicular joint.

A. Surface Anatomy and Bony Landmarks.

Before making the skin incision, review the surface anatomy of the back, and palpate the following several bony landmarks on one of your colleagues or on the cadaver or articulated skeleton.

1. **External occipital protuberance:** Found in the midline on the back of the skull (**ATLAS PLATES 328, 516**). Identify bony ridges, called **superior nuchal lines,** that extend laterally from the protuberance and its most central point, called the **inion.**

2. **Spinous process of the 7th cervical vertebra:** Pass your index finger in the midline down from the skull over the dorsal aspect of the cervical vertebrae. The first prominent bony process felt is the spinous process of the C7 vertebra, called the **vertebra prominens**

(**ATLAS PLATE 325 #325.2, 343 #343.1**). A fibroelastic membrane called the **ligamentum nuchae** covers the other cervical spines, making them less palpable.

3. Study the location of the **scapula** over the posterior thoracic wall on a skeleton (**ATLAS PLATE 105 #105.1**) and note its **superior, inferior,** and **medial angles.** Palpate the **spine of the scapula** and follow it laterally to the **acromion** (**ATLAS PLATE 325 #325.2**). Note that the **medial (vertebral) border** is parallel to the vertebral column and that the **lateral (axillary) border** is oriented toward the axillary fossa.

4. Palpate the posterior part of the **iliac crest,** a curved bony ridge below the waist (**ATLAS PLATES 265, 270 #270.2, 328**). It terminates at the **posterior superior iliac spine** on the surface of which is a dimple in the skin on each side.

B. Skin Incisions and Skin Reflection (Figure 4-1).

To dissect the posterior scapular region, remove the skin from the back of the neck and upper half of the back. Make an incision through the skin

►
Grant's 494, 496
Netter's 167, 407
Rohen 226, 227

►
Grant's 307
Netter's 170
Rohen 229, 234

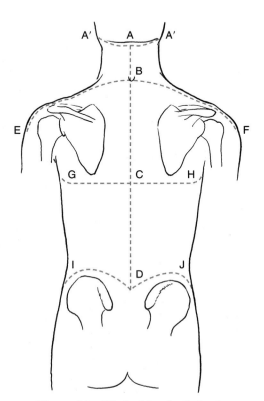

Figure 4-1. Skin incision for the back.

►
Grant's 496, 497,
506, 509
Netter's 167, 170,
407, 415
Rohen 226, 235,
405

along the posterior midline extending from the external occipital protuberance to 1 inch below the inferior angle of the scapula (**Figure 4-1 A to C**). Make two lateral incisions on each side at right angles to the midline cut as shown in **Figure 4-1, B to E and F and C to G and H.**

Initially, remove only the skin by reflecting it from the underlying superficial fascia in four flaps. Next, reflect the superficial fascia from the deep fascia that overlies the dark fibers of the **trapezius muscle** above and the **latissimus dorsi muscle** below (**ATLAS PLATE 328**) and look for branches of the **cutaneous nerves of the back** (**ATLAS PLATE 338**).

C. Cutaneous Nerves of Back (ATLAS PLATE 404, Figure 4-2).

Dissect several of the segmentally arranged **posterior primary rami** of the thoracic nerves. They are frequently accompanied by cutaneous blood vessels and they traverse the trapezius and latissimus dorsi muscles to become superficial, yet they **DO NOT** supply these muscles either with motor or sensory innervation. To locate these nerves, probe the fascia overlying the trapezius muscle 1 inch lateral to the spinous processes of the thoracic vertebrae. Realize that most of the thoracic nerves pierce the trapezius muscle, and, after becoming superficial, they course laterally in the superficial fascia across the back (**Figure 4-2**).

Now remove the superficial fascia over the scapular and deltoid regions, preserving short lengths of the dissected cutaneous nerves.

II. Cut Scapular Attachments of Trapezius and Deltoid Muscles; The Supraspinous and Infraspinous Fossae

To uncover the muscles within the fossae above and below the spine of the scapula, detach the trapezius and deltoid muscles but only from the acromion and spine of the scapula (**ATLAS PLATES 24, 328**).

A. Reflection of Trapezius and Deltoid Muscles.

Palpate the upper border of the trapezius and palpate the acromion and scapular spine. Cut the attachment of the trapezius along the medial margin of the acromion and along the superior aspect

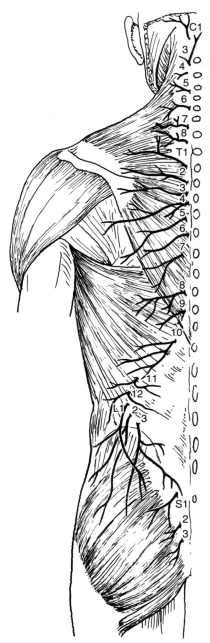

Figure 4-2. Cutaneous nerves of the back (posterior primary rami).

of the spine as far as its medial end. Using your finger, separate the trapezius from underlying structures. Cut those fibers attached to the clavicle, and reflect the trapezius medially to uncover the underlying **supraspinatus muscle** (see **ATLAS PLATE 38**).

Observe that the **deltoid muscle** attaches above to a bony arch formed by the clavicle anteriorly, the acromion laterally, and the spine of the scapula pos-

teriorly (**ATLAS PLATE 29 #29.1**). This muscle's fibers converge inferiorly to attach to the deltoid tuberosity. Cut the origin of the deltoid from the scapular spine and acromion and free its posterior border inferiorly to the deltoid tuberosity, leaving the clavicular origin intact. Reflect the deltoid anteriorly to uncover the underlying **infraspinatus** and **teres minor muscles** (**Figure 4-3** and **ATLAS PLATES 24, 38**).

B. Subacromial Bursa.

Deep to the deltoid muscle, identify the large **subacromial bursa** (**ATLAS PLATES 24, 82 #82.2**). Open it and, with your finger, explore its extensive sac. Note that it extends beneath the deltoid muscle (but superficial to the joint capsule) and is continued under the acromion and the coracoacromial ligament, superficial to the tendon of the supraspinatus (**ATLAS PLATES 82 #82.2, 78 #78.1**). When the bursa is inflamed, 90° abduction of the arm at the shoulder joint (using the supraspinatus and deltoid muscles) is painful because the entire bursa moves under the acromion.

C. Supraspinatus Fossa; Suprascapular Vessels and Nerve.

Remove the deep fascia overlying the **supraspinatus muscle**. Observe that it arises in the supraspinatus fossa, courses deep to the acromion, and inserts on the uppermost part of the greater tubercle of the humerus (**Figure 4-4**). Palpate the superior border of the scapula and locate the sharp edge of the **superior transverse scapular ligament** (**ATLAS PLATE 80**) where the suprascapular nerve and vessels pass into the supraspinatus fossa (**Figure 4-4**). Make a vertical cut across the supraspinatus muscle medial to the ligament, approximately $1\frac{1}{2}$ inches lateral to the vertebral border of the scapula. Reflect the lateral part of the muscle toward the humerus and note that the **suprascapular nerve** usually enters the fossa deep to the ligament and the **suprascapular vessels** pass superficial to the ligament (**ATLAS PLATE 25**, and **Figure 4-4**).

D. Infraspinatus Fossa.

Remove the deep fascia covering the **infraspinatus muscle** below the spine of the scapula. Observe that most of its fibers arise from the medial two-thirds of the infraspinatus fossa. From this origin, the muscle ascends over the fibrous capsule of the shoulder joint and termi-

► Grant's 512–514
Netter's 404, 414

► Grant's 493, 496, 497
Netter's 167, 186, 407–410, 460
Rohen 382, 383

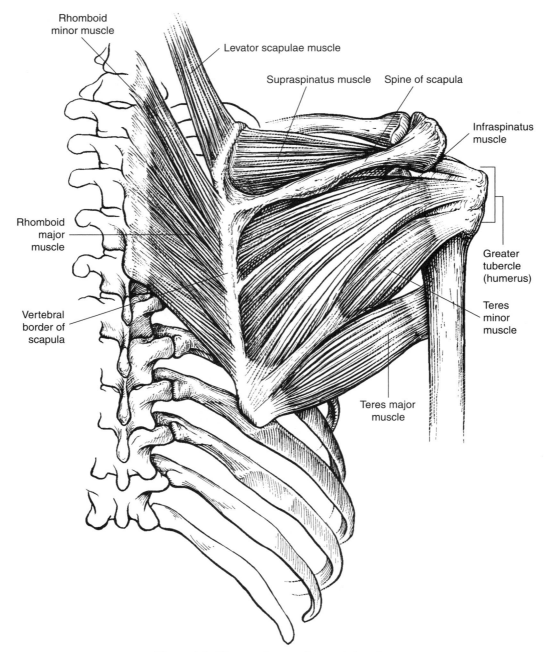

Figure 4-3. The scapular muscles, posterior view.

nates on the greater tubercle of the humerus below the supraspinatus muscle (**ATLAS PLATES 36, 408**).

Cut through the infraspinatus muscle vertically with a scalpel 2 inches lateral to the vertebral border of the scapula; reflect the lateral part of the muscle toward the humerus (**ATLAS PLATE 25**).

◄
Grant's 496, 497, 506
Netter's 167, 186, 407–410, 460
Rohen 382, 383, 405–407

25). Observe the suprascapular nerve and vessels passing into the infraspinatus fossa to supply this muscle by coursing through the **spinoglenoid notch** (greater scapular notch), located lateral to the free edge of the scapular spine (**Figure 4-4**). At times, a bursa is found between the infraspinatus tendon of the muscle and the capsule of the shoulder joint.

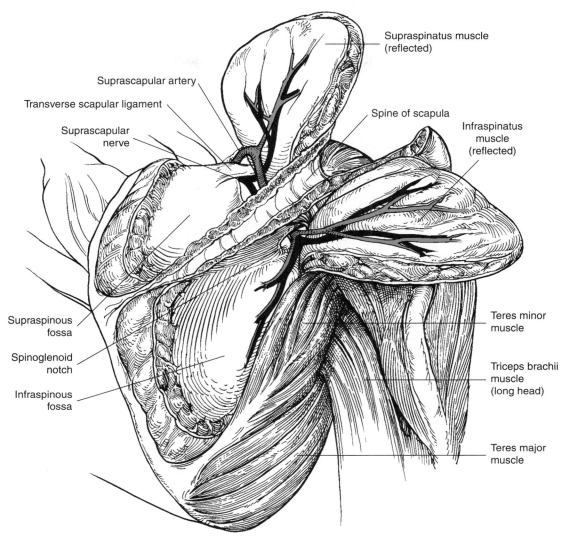

Figure 4-4. The suprascapular nerve and artery (posterior scapular view).

III. Lateral Border of Scapula; Triangular and Quadrangular Spaces; Axillary Nerve and Deltoid Region

The sharp lateral border of the scapula is thickly covered with muscles. These include the latissimus dorsi at the inferior angle and then the teres major, teres minor, and the long head of the triceps brachii attaching to the infraglenoid tubercle (**ATLAS PLATES 24, 38, 39**).

A. Lateral Border of the Scapula (Figure 4-3).

Clearly define the inferior border of the infraspinatus muscle and separate it from the **teres minor muscle,** which arises along the middle third of the

◄

Grant's 497,
504–506
Netter's 186,
407–410, 415, 460
Rohen 226, 382,
383, 405

lateral border of the scapula (**ATLAS PLATE 39**). Follow the teres minor muscle laterally and observe its insertion on the lower part of the greater tubercle of the humerus below the infraspinatus.

Find the **teres major muscle,** which arises from the lower one-third of the lateral border, as far as the inferior angle (**ATLAS PLATE 39**). Its fibers can be distinguished from those of the teres minor because they form a flat tendon (approximately 2 inches long) that courses to the anterior aspect of the humerus. The teres major muscle inserts along the medial lip of the intertubercular sulcus. At its insertion, the teres major tendon lies just behind that of the **latissimus dorsi muscle** (**ATLAS PLATE 32**).

Identify the **long head of the triceps brachii muscle** and observe its origin from the infraglenoid tubercle of the scapula (**ATLAS PLATES 38, 39, 41**). Follow the muscle inferiorly, and note that it passes between the teres major and minor muscles on the humerus.

As the long head of the triceps brachii muscle descends from the infraglenoid tubercle to the extensor aspect of the arm, it crosses a three-sided area bounded **above** by the lower border of the teres minor, **below** by the upper border of the teres major, and **laterally** by the surgical neck of the humerus. Two spaces are thereby formed from the three-sided area, one medial to the long head of the triceps, called the **triangular space,** and one lateral to the muscle, called the **quadrangular space** (**ATLAS PLATES 24, 38**).

B. Triangular and Quadrangular Spaces (Figure 4-5).

Find the long head of the triceps. Clean the lateral and medial borders of the muscle, and identify the **triangular space** bounded **laterally** by the long head of the triceps, **superiorly** by the teres minor muscle, and **inferiorly** by the teres major muscle (**ATLAS PLATE 38**). Find the **circumflex scapular branch** of the **subscapular artery** that

▶
Grant's 462, 490,
505, 506
Netter's 409, 460,
464
Rohen 400, 404,
407

◀
Grant's 505, 506
Netter's 409, 410
Rohen 403, 404

courses around the lateral border of the scapula and through the space from the axilla (**ATLAS PLATE 25**).

Similarly, identify the **quadrangular space** located lateral to the long head of the triceps muscle. Observe that it is bounded **superiorly** by the teres minor muscle, **inferiorly** by the teres major muscle, **laterally** by the neck of the humerus, and **medially** by the long head of the triceps. Probe for the **posterior humeral circumflex artery** and **axillary nerve** that pass through the quadrangular space from the axilla (**ATLAS PLATE 25, 43**).

C. Axillary Nerve.

Because the scapular origin of the deltoid muscle has already been detached, the muscle can be turned forward to demonstrate the axillary nerve that enters its deep surface (**ATLAS PLATE 43**). On its course through the quadrangular space, the axillary nerve gives sensory branches to the shoulder joint and supplies the teres minor muscle and the posterior part of the deltoid (**ATLAS PLATE 25**). This branch then becomes superficial over the deltoid muscle as the **upper lateral brachial cutaneous nerve** (**ATLAS PLATE**

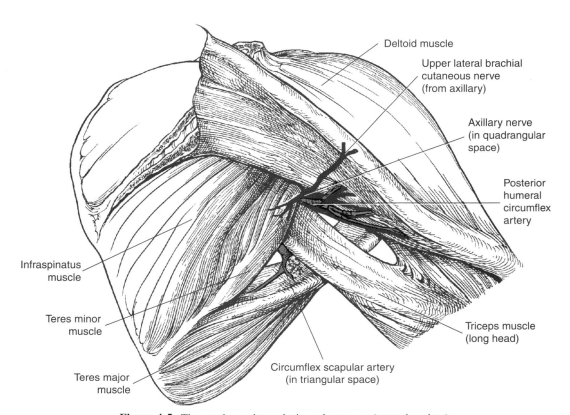

Figure 4-5. The quadrangular and triangular spaces (posterior view).

31). Another large branch continues around the humerus with the posterior humeral circumflex artery to supply parts of the deltoid attaching to the acromion and the clavicle.

Four structures are supplied by the axillary nerve: two muscles with motor innervation, the teres minor and deltoid; and two regions with sensory innervation, the shoulder joint and the cutaneous area covering the shoulder joint and deltoid.

Clinical Relevance

Axillary nerve injury. The axillary nerve branches from the posterior cord of the brachial plexus and traverses the quadrangular space to reach the posterolateral aspect of the shoulder. At this site it can be injured when the humeral head is dislocated or the surgical neck of the humerus is fractured, because that part of the humerus forms the lateral boundary of the quadrangular space. Resulting from this nerve lesion is the loss of innervation to the deltoid and teres minor muscles and a loss of sensory supply to the skin over the shoulder joint and, to some extent, the shoulder joint itself. Denervation of the deltoid muscle causes a loss of the smooth contour of the shoulder and a weakness or inability to abduct the upper limb beyond the first 20° still be performed by the intact supraspinatus muscle.

IV. Anastomoses Around the Scapula

The blood vessels in the scapular region participate in anastomoses that allow blood to reach the remainder of the upper limb should blockage occur between the first and third parts of the subclavian artery. The **transverse cervical artery** (with its descending branch coursing down the vertebral border of the scapula) and the **suprascapular artery** (which enters both the supraspinatus and infraspinatus fossae) both arise as branches off the thyrocervical trunk from the 1st part of the subclavian artery. These anastomose freely with the **circumflex scapular branch** of the **subscapular artery** and the **posterior humeral circumflex artery,** which arise from the 3rd part of the axillary artery (**Figure 4-6**).

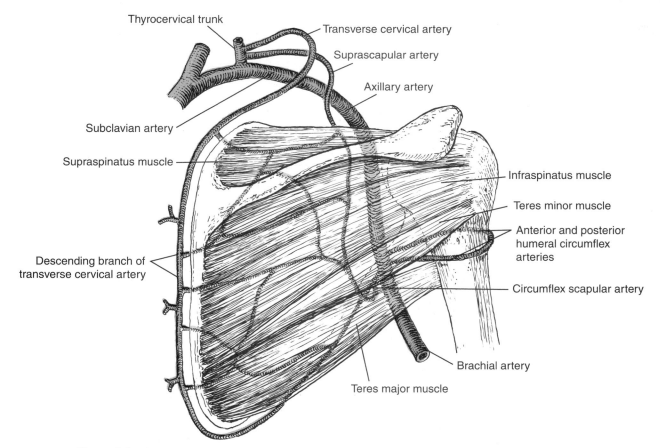

Figure 4-6. The scapular anastomosis on the posterior aspect of the shoulder. Note the descending branch of the transverse cervical artery, the suprascapular artery, circumflex scapular artery, and the two humeral circumflex arteries.

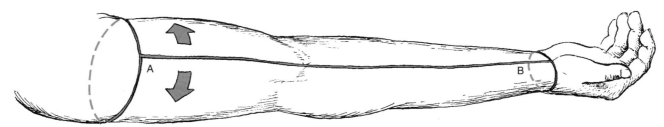

Figure 4-7. Skin incisions of arm and forearm.

V. Posterior (Extensor) Compartment of the Arm

The posterior compartment of the arm contains one large muscle with three heads—the **triceps brachii muscle**—and the important **radial nerve** with its accompanying **profunda brachii artery** (**ATLAS PLATES 40–43**). The principal function of the triceps is to extend the forearm at the elbow joint. However, because its long head arises from the infraglenoid tuberosity, the triceps also can extend the humerus at the shoulder joint.

Clinical Relevance

Suprascapular nerve injury. The suprascapular nerve runs laterally from the superior trunk of the brachial plexus and then courses deep to the supra-scapular ligament that overlies the suprascapular notch. It then enters the supraspinatus fossa where it supplies the supraspinatus muscle. Trauma to this nerve can occur in persons who have jobs that require carrying heavy objects, such as steel rods, or persons that ascend ladders with a V-shaped wooden container full of bricks (hod carrier). They begin to feel that something is wrong with their arm and, when told by their doctor to lift their upper limb, they bend the upper part of their body toward the side, gaining the first 20° of abduction of their arm, after which they easily raise their arm because the deltoid is intact. These patients are unable to initiate the first 20° of abduction because the supraspinatus muscle is denervated because of trauma to the suprascapular nerve.

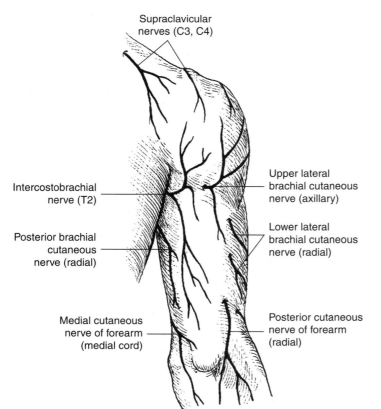

Supraclavicular nerves (C3, C4)

Intercostobrachial nerve (T2)

Posterior brachial cutaneous nerve (radial)

Medial cutaneous nerve of forearm (medial cord)

Upper lateral brachial cutaneous nerve (axillary)

Lower lateral brachial cutaneous nerve (radial)

Posterior cutaneous nerve of forearm (radial)

Figure 4-8. Cutaneous nerves of the arm (posterior view).

A. Superficial Nerves. From the circular incision through the skin around the upper part of the arm (**Figure 4-7**), incise the skin downward along the anterior surface of the arm and forearm to the wrist. Make another circular incision at the wrist (**Figure 4-7 A, B**).

Dissect the superficial fascia of the arm and find the **upper lateral brachial cutaneous nerve** from the axillary nerve over the deltoid muscle (described earlier). Find the **lower lateral brachial cutaneous nerve** (a branch of the radial nerve). It passes through the triceps muscle to become superficial just below the insertion of the deltoid muscle (**Figure 4-8**). More medially, find the **intercostobrachial nerve (T2)** extending through the 2nd intercostal space to supply the medial and posterior part of the arm (**ATLAS PLATE 30**).

B. Triceps Brachii Muscle. Remove the fascia completely and clean the three heads of the **triceps**. Trace the **long head** down from the scapula and follow it to the **lateral head** (**Figure 4-9**), which arises from the upper, posterior surface of the humerus above the spiral groove. Identify the **medial head** of the triceps arising from the posterior surface of the humerus below the insertion of the teres major muscle and just distal to the spiral groove (**ATLAS PLATE 41**).

Observe that the triceps tendon of insertion forms near the middle of the arm and inserts on the upper posterior part of the **olecranon** of the **ulna** (**ATLAS PLATES 40, 43**). Identify the small triangular **anconeus muscle** on the dorsal aspect of the elbow (**ATLAS PLATES 41, 42**).

C. Radial Nerve and Profunda Brachii Vessels (**Figure 4-10**). With the forearm extended, insert a probe deep to the lateral head of the triceps approximately 1 inch above its insertion (in the same direction as the spiral groove). Being certain that you do not sever the radial nerve and the profunda brachii artery, cut completely through the lateral head of the triceps and reflect its two ends (**ATLAS PLATE 43**). This will expose the radial nerve and its accompanying vessels within the spiral groove (see cross section (**ATLAS PLATE 94 #94.1**). Appreciate the vulnerability of these structures if the upper part of the shaft of the humerus is fractured.

Follow the main trunk of the radial nerve through the lateral intermuscular septum. Note that medially the brachialis muscle is found, and laterally the nerve is bounded by the brachioradi-

◄
Grant's 462, 463
Netter's 462, 464
Rohen 400–404

◄
Grant's 503–507, 522, 524, 578
Netter's 407, 415, 460
Rohen 382, 387, 404

◄
Grant's 470, 473, 485, 490
Netter's 415, 417, 460
Rohen 399, 403–405

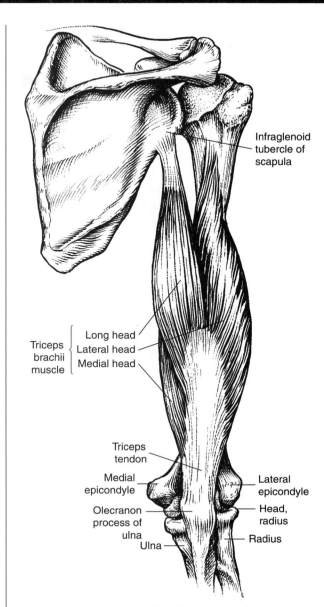

Figure 4-9. The triceps muscle.

Labels: Infraglenoid tubercle of scapula; Triceps brachii muscle — Long head, Lateral head, Medial head; Triceps tendon; Medial epicondyle; Olecranon process of ulna; Ulna; Lateral epicondyle; Head, radius; Radius

alis muscle and the extensor carpi radialis longus. Follow the nerve to the lateral epicondyle where it divides into superficial and deep branches, both of which enter the forearm.

In addition to the small cutaneous branches from the radial nerve that supply the posterior region of the arm, the larger **posterior cutaneous nerve of the forearm** is also derived from the radial nerve (**Figure 4-8** and **ATLAS PLATE 31**). This nerve traverses the lateral head of the triceps to become superficial 2 inches above the elbow. It then descends behind the lateral epicondyle to supply the skin on the dorsum of the forearm as far as the wrist (**ATLAS PLATE 45**).

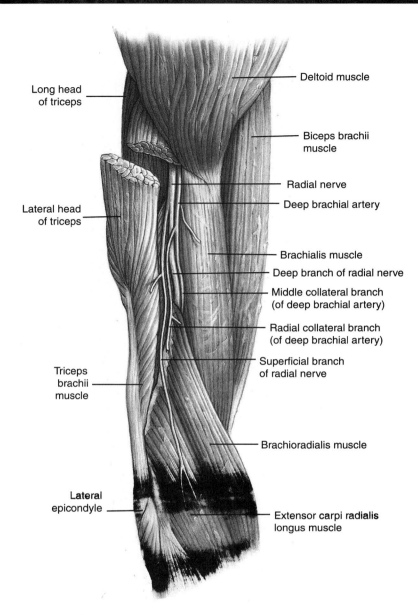

Long head of triceps

Deltoid muscle

Biceps brachii muscle

Radial nerve

Deep brachial artery

Lateral head of triceps

Brachialis muscle

Deep branch of radial nerve

Middle collateral branch (of deep brachial artery)

Radial collateral branch (of deep brachial artery)

Superficial branch of radial nerve

Triceps brachii muscle

Brachioradialis muscle

Lateral epicondyle

Extensor carpi radialis longus muscle

Figure 4-10. The radial nerve and profunda (deep) radial artery in the lateral brachial region.

Find the profunda, or deep brachial artery, coursing with the radial nerve in the spiral groove (**ATLAS PLATE 29 #29.1**). It branches from the brachial artery and courses laterally and posteriorly to join the nerve. Note that the vessel terminates by dividing into the **middle and radial collateral branches** (**ATLAS PLATE 29 #29.1**). These branches participate in the anastomosis around the lateral aspect of the elbow joint (**ATLAS PLATE 53 #53.3**). The middle collateral branch anastomoses with the interosseous recurrent artery (from the common interosseous artery), whereas the radial collateral branch anastomoses with the radial recurrent artery (from the radial artery) (**ATLAS PLATE 29 #29.1**).

◄
Grant's 470, 471
Netter's 417
Rohen 397

Clinical Relevance

Rotator cuff. This musculotendinous structure reinforces the capsule of the shoulder joint. It tends to retain the head of the humerus within the glenoid fossa. The cuff consists of the tendons of the supraspinatus, infraspinatus, teres minor, and subscapularis muscles. Tears in the rotator cuff frequently occur when dislocation of the humeral head occurs. The tendons reinforce the anterior, posterior, and superior aspects of the joint capsule, but not the inferior part. Consequently, these dislocations are most often inferior and medial to the joint. Rotator cuff injury frequently occurs in curveball pitchers when strong rotation of the upper limb is required to throw the ball.

Radial nerve injury. The course of the radial nerve (accompanied by the deep brachial artery) around the shaft of the humerus places the nerve vulnerable to injury or to severance in fractures of the humerus. The nerve can also be injured more proximally in the axilla by excessive pressure from the inept use of crutches or by the so-called "Saturday night palsy" when the arm or armpit of a drunken person is draped over a hard surface (such as the back of a chair) and the person falls asleep. Additionally, the nerve can be injured by an inferomedial dislocation of the humeral head. The resultant injury in the axilla paralyzes the triceps muscle and the posterior forearm muscles so that the person is unable to extend the forearm at the elbow joint, the hand at the wrist, and the fingers. "Wrist drop" (flexion of the hand) occurs because the flexor muscles of the forearm act unopposed. The flexed hand also reduces the strength of flexion of the fingers. Radial nerve lesions may result in some sensory loss along the middle of the posterior surface of the forearm and the lateral aspect of the dorsal hand.

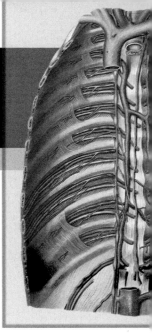

Anterior Brachial Region; Cubital Fossa; Anterior Forearm and Wrist

OBJECTIVES

1. Learn the surface anatomy and bony features of the arm and forearm.

2. Dissect the basilic vein and cutaneous nerves of the anterior arm and forearm.

3. Dissect the anterior compartment of the arm.

4. Dissect the structures in the cubital fossa.

5. Dissect the anterior compartment of the forearm.

6. Identify the tendons, vessels, and nerves at the anterior wrist.

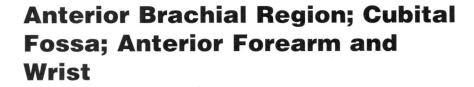

Atlas Key:

Clemente Atlas 5th Edition = Atlas Plate #

Grant's Atlas 11th Edition = Grant's Page #

Netter's Atlas 3rd Edition = Netter's Plate #

Rohen Atlas 6th Edition = Rohen Page #

I. Surface Anatomy; Skin Incisions; Superficial Veins and Nerves

Turn the cadaver onto its back and orient the upper limb anteriorly. Review several surface anatomy features of the anterior aspect of the upper limb introduced in the first Laboratory Session.

A. Surface Anatomy of the Arm and Forearm. Palpate the following structures on one of your dissection partners:

   1. **Greater and lesser tubercles; coracoid process; intertubercular (bicipital) sulcus.** The greater tubercle of the humerus is the most lateral bony structure felt when you palpate the

◄

Grant's 498, 512
Netter's 403
Rohen 373

►

Grant's 503, 578

rounded contour of the shoulder below the acromion (**ATLAS PLATE 79**). It moves with the humerus when the arm is rotated, but the acromion does not.

Feel a small depression, the **infraclavicular fossa,** just below the lateral end of the clavicle. Palpate the **coracoid process** of the scapula by pressing laterally and backward in the fossa.

The **lesser tubercle** of the humerus is oriented anteriorly and may be felt through the deltoid muscle 1 inch lateral and slightly below the coracoid process (**ATLAS PLATE 27**). On a skeleton, find the **intertubercular sulcus** between the two tubercles. On your arm, feel for the tendon of the long head of the biceps muscle within the sulcus.

   2. **Biceps brachii muscle; medial and lateral bicipital furrows.** The **biceps brachii muscle** is the rounded prominence on the anterior arm when the forearm is flexed.

Observe the **medial and lateral bicipital furrows** extending longitudinally on either side of the arm. Intermuscular septa project deeply from them and separate the flexor and extensor compartments of the arm (**ATLAS PLATES 28, 29 #29.1**). Deep to the medial furrow is a neurovascular compartment that contains the **brachial vessels,** the **basilic vein;** and the **median, medial antebrachial,** and **ulnar nerves** (**ATLAS PLATE 94**). Along the lateral furrow ascends the **cephalic vein** (**ATLAS PLATE 27**).

3. **Cubital fossa; median cubital vein; bicipital aponeurosis; brachial artery and median nerve.** The hollow in front of the elbow is called the **cubital fossa** (**ATLAS PLATE 30**). By applying pressure over the superficial veins above the elbow, the **median cubital vein** (used for venipuncture) becomes visible as it interconnects the **basilic vein** seen medially and the **cephalic vein** laterally (**ATLAS PLATE 44**).

   Have a lab partner flex the forearm against resistance, and feel the tendon of insertion of the biceps in the lateral part of the cubital region. Palpate the **bicipital aponeurosis** extending medially across the floor of the fossa (**ATLAS PLATE 32**).

   Feel the pulse of the **brachial artery** in the cubital fossa by pressing over the medial part of the cubital fossa with the forearm resting on a surface. At this site, the **median nerve** lies medial to the artery beneath the bicipital aponeurosis.

4. **Lateral and medial epicondyles; ulnar nerve; olecranon, shaft, and styloid process of the ulna.** With your left thumb and index finger, identify your right **lateral** and **medial epicondyles** by palpating the flexed lower end of the humerus. Feel for the ulnar nerve behind the medial epicondyle. Move laterally and feel the **olecranon** of the ulna and the tendon of the triceps at the back of the elbow (**ATLAS PLATES 38, 77**).

   From the olecranon, follow the sharp posterior border of the **shaft of the ulna** just deep to the skin to the wrist. At its distal end palpate the styloid process (**ATLAS PLATES 89–91**).

5. **Head and styloid process of radius; radial artery.** Feel the rounded **head of the radius** just below the lateral epicondyle of the humerus at the back of the elbow (**ATLAS PLATES 85–88**). Rotate the head of the radius by supinating and pronating the forearm.

▶
Grant's 498, 499, 538, 539
Netter's 422, 429, 435, 444
Rohen 374, 376, 423, 426

◀
Grant's 518–520
Netter's 414, 416, 462
Rohen 408, 419–423

◀
Grant's 522, 527, 531
Netter's 419, 422, 459
Rohen 374, 375, 399

▶
Grant's 462, 464, 508
Netter's 462–464
Rohen 398, 400, 419

The upper shaft of the radius is difficult to feel, but the lower 3 or more inches can be palpated. The distal extremity of the radius is also called the **styloid process,** and it extends $\frac{1}{2}$ inch below the ulna (**ATLAS PLATES 89, 90**). Feel the pulse of the **radial artery** above and medial to the styloid process on the anterior wrist (**ATLAS PLATES 89–91**).

B. **Skin Incisions. If not already done, make skin incisions as indicated in Figure 5-6 (A–B). Remove only the skin without cutting into the superficial fascia because the superficial veins and cutaneous nerves will be dissected before removing the fascia. The skin may be left attached at the dorsum of the wrist.**

   Two large superficial veins commence from venous plexuses on the radial and ulnar sides of the dorsal hand (**ATLAS PLATE 62 #62.1**). These are the **cephalic vein** laterally and the **basilic vein** medially. They ascend in the forearm to the cubital fossa where there is usually an interconnecting vein, the **median cubital vein**. The cephalic vein ascends to the deltopectoral triangle and enters the **axillary vein**. The basilic vein courses deep to the medial bicipital furrow and will join with the veins accompanying the brachial artery to form the axillary vein. In the lower arm, the basilic vein is accompanied by the **medial antebrachial cutaneous nerve**, and the cephalic vein lies adjacent to the **lateral antebrachial cutaneous nerve** at the cubital fossa.

C. **Superficial Veins and Cutaneous Nerves.** Isolate and clean the cephalic vein laterally in the arm (**ATLAS PLATES 30, 44**). On the medial side of the limb, clean the basilic vein in the superficial fascia. Follow it distally to the dorsal hand and proximally to the middle of the arm where it penetrates the deep fascia (**ATLAS PLATES 30, 44, 94**).

   Find the **medial antebrachial cutaneous nerve** (**Figure 6-2**) by probing the superficial fascia where the basilic vein penetrates the deep fascia. Follow the nerve distally, where it may divide in two or more branches (**ATLAS PLATES 30, 44**). Do not confuse this nerve with the ulnar nerve; both arise from the medial cord.

   Locate the **lateral antebrachial cutaneous nerve** (**Figures 5-1, 5-2**) by probing the fascia in the lateral part of the cubital fossa deep to the cephalic vein (**ATLAS PLATES 30, 44**). It is the continuation of the musculocutaneous nerve.

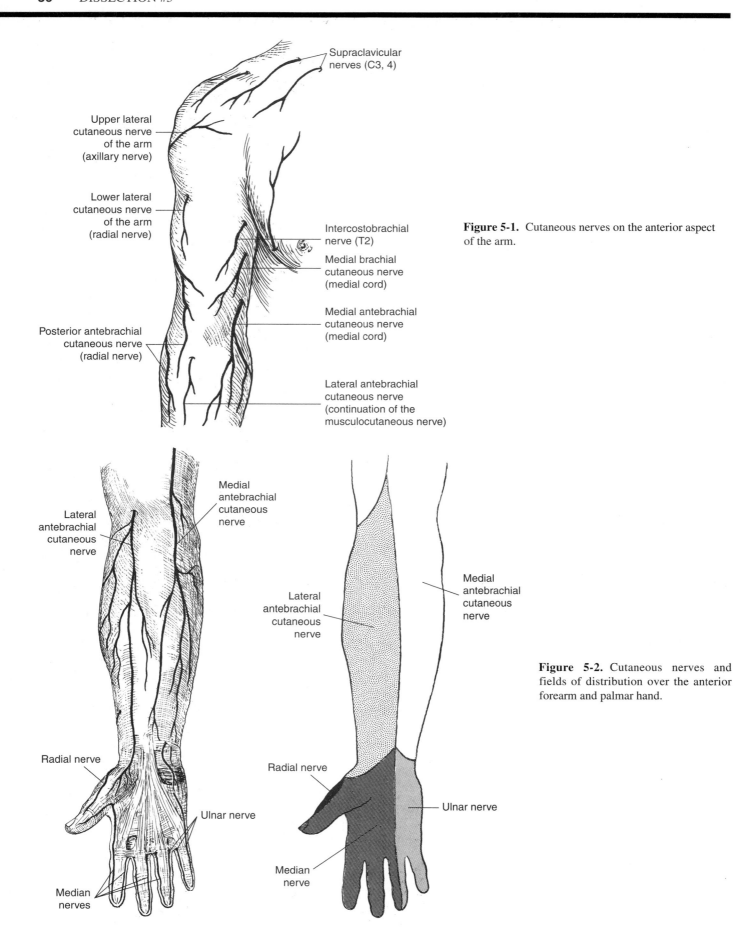

Figure 5-1. Cutaneous nerves on the anterior aspect of the arm.

Supraclavicular nerves (C3, 4)

Upper lateral cutaneous nerve of the arm (axillary nerve)

Lower lateral cutaneous nerve of the arm (radial nerve)

Intercostobrachial nerve (T2)

Medial brachial cutaneous nerve (medial cord)

Medial antebrachial cutaneous nerve (medial cord)

Posterior antebrachial cutaneous nerve (radial nerve)

Lateral antebrachial cutaneous nerve (continuation of the musculocutaneous nerve)

Lateral antebrachial cutaneous nerve

Medial antebrachial cutaneous nerve

Lateral antebrachial cutaneous nerve

Medial antebrachial cutaneous nerve

Radial nerve

Ulnar nerve

Radial nerve

Ulnar nerve

Median nerves

Median nerve

Figure 5-2. Cutaneous nerves and fields of distribution over the anterior forearm and palmar hand.

On the medial aspect of the brachium (arm), find the smaller **medial brachial cutaneous nerve (Figure 5-1, ATLAS PLATE 46).** This also arises from the medial cord of the brachial plexus above the origin of the medial antebrachial cutaneous nerve. It frequently communicates with the intercostobrachial nerve that emerges through the 2nd intercostal space to help supply the skin of the axilla and arm.

II. Anterior Compartment of the Arm: Muscles, Vessels, and Nerves

With the superficial fascia removed, observe that the deep fascia thickens laterally and medially to form the **lateral and medial intermuscular septa.** These descend to the lateral and medial epicondyles, and divide the arm into anterior (flexor) and posterior (extensor) compartments **(Figure 5-3A).**

A. Anterior Compartment Muscles and Musculocutaneous Nerve.

Identify the biceps brachii muscle and dissect its short head arising from the coracoid process adjacent to the origin of the **coracobrachialis muscle (ATLAS PLATE 34).** Observe that the short head joins the long head to form muscle mass of the biceps. The coracobrachialis descends to insert directly onto the medial aspect of the humerus **(Figure 5-4).**

Lift the lateral cord of the brachial plexus and find the musculocutaneous nerve. Follow its course through the substance of the coracobrachialis muscle, and then distally between the biceps and the underlying brachialis muscle. It supplies all three muscles **(ATLAS PLATES 36, 37).**

◄
Grant's 503, 507, 578
Netter's 414, 416
Rohen 386, 387, 415

Trace the tendon of the long head of the biceps superiorly to the **intertubercular sulcus,** where it is invested by a thin layer of synovial membrane extending down from the shoulder joint **(ATLAS PLATES 32, 34, 35).** Realize that the tendon arises from the **supraglenoid tubercle of the scapula (Figure 5-4A)** and descends within the capsule of the shoulder joint before it reaches the sulcus.

Separate the biceps from the underlying brachialis muscle, but do not cut the musculocutaneous nerve **(Figure 5-4B).** Sever the biceps muscle 2 inches above the cubital fossa, and reflect the distal part and its tendon to the cubital fossa. Identify the aponeurotic expansion from the tendon called the **bicipital aponeurosis,** which extends medially over the brachial vessels and median nerve **(ATLAS PLATES 34, 36).** Follow the tendon of insertion of the biceps to the **tuberosity of the radius (Figure 5-4A).**

Identify the **brachialis muscle** arising from the lower half of the anterior humerus **(ATLAS PLATE 35).** Follow its thick tendon of insertion to the **tuberosity of the ulna** and the anterior surface of the **coronoid process (Figure 5-4B).**

Dissect the musculocutaneous nerve distally to the lateral side of the biceps tendon of insertion just above the cubital fossa. Here it becomes the **lateral antebrachial cutaneous nerve (ATLAS PLATE 44).**

Review the muscles that insert on the upper half of the humerus **(Figure 5-5).** Identify the rotator cuff muscles: **supraspinatus, infraspinatus,** and **teres minor.** These insert on the posterior surface of the greater tubercle. More anteriorly, the **subscapularis** inserts on the lesser tubercle. Note that on the medial aspect of the intertubercular sulcus attach the **latissimus dorsi** and the **teres major,** while the **pectoralis major** inserts on the lateral lip of the sulcus.

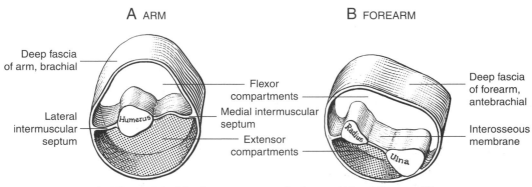

Figure 5-3. Muscle compartments in the arm **(A)** and forearm **(B).**

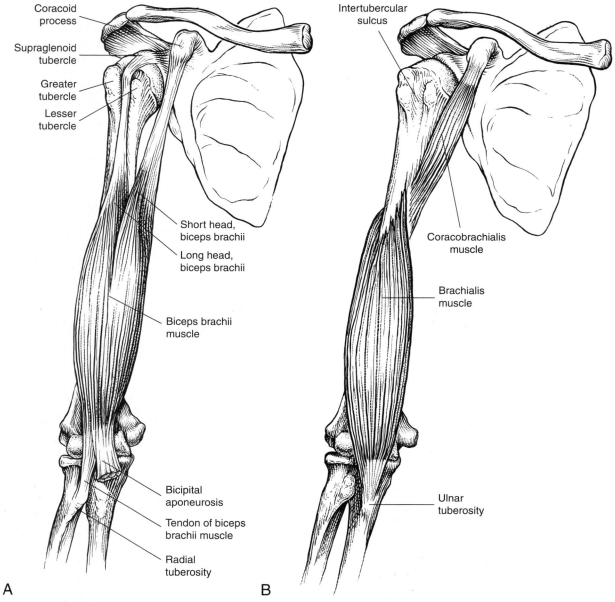

Figure 5-4. The muscles of the anterior (flexor) compartment of the arm: biceps brachii (**A**) and the brachialis and coracobrachialis (**B**).

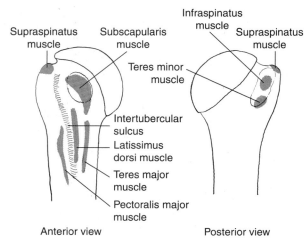

Figure 5-5. Insertions of muscles on the greater and lesser tubercles and neck of the humerus.

B. Anterior Compartment Vessels and Nerves.
Dissect along the medial bicipital furrow, and find the **brachial artery and veins** and the **median** and **ulnar nerves.** The brachial artery is the continuation of the axillary artery below the tendon of the teres major **(Figure 5-6)**. Clean the brachial artery and its accompanying veins distally to the cubital fossa **(ATLAS PLATES 36, 37)**. Just distal to the

◄
Grant's 503, 578
Netter's 416, 117, 456
Rohen 415

tendon of the teres major, find the site of branching of the **profunda** (deep) **brachii artery** from the main trunk of the brachial artery **(ATLAS PLATES 29 #29.2, 43)**. More inferiorly, find the **superior and inferior ulnar collateral branches,** which anastomose around the medial aspect of the elbow joint with **ulnar recurrent branches** from the **ulnar artery (ATLAS PLATE 29 #29.2)**.

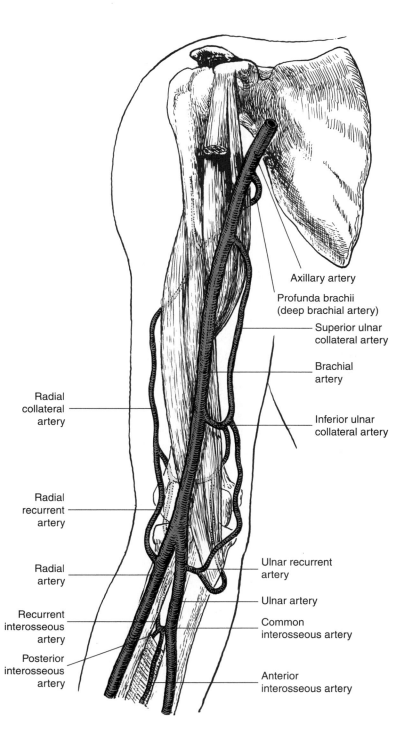

Figure 5-6. The brachial artery and its branches.

Axillary artery

Profunda brachii
(deep brachial artery)

Superior ulnar
collateral artery

Brachial
artery

Inferior ulnar
collateral artery

Radial
collateral
artery

Radial
recurrent
artery

Radial
artery

Recurrent
interosseous
artery

Posterior
interosseous
artery

Ulnar recurrent
artery

Ulnar artery

Common
interosseous artery

Anterior
interosseous artery

Trace the **median nerve** to the cubital fossa from the **lateral and medial cords** of the brachial plexus. Note that the median nerve accompanies the brachial artery. It courses anterior and lateral to the artery along the upper half of the arm but then passes over the artery to lie medial to the vessel in the cubital fossa (**ATLAS PLATES 36, 37**).

Find the **ulnar nerve** medial to the brachial artery, and follow it from the medial cord of the brachial plexus to the medial epicondyle accompanied by the **superior ulnar collateral artery.** Here, it lies superficial to the medial head of the triceps muscle (**ATLAS PLATES 37, 53 #53.1**).

III. The Cubital Fossa (Atlas Plate 28)

The cubital fossa is located in front of the elbow, and is bounded **above** by an imaginary line between the two epicondyles of the humerus; **medially,** by the **pronator teres muscle;** and **laterally,** by the **brachioradialis muscle.** The floor of the fossa is formed by the brachialis muscle and partially by the supinator, visible when the brachioradialis is pulled aside (**ATLAS PLATES 35, 37**).

Slightly flex the elbow to help identify the **bicipital aponeurosis (ATLAS PLATE 34)** deep to the **median cubital veins** and **superficial** to the brachial **vessels and median nerve.** Cut the bicipital aponeurosis and dissect the brachial artery as it divides into its **ulnar and radial branches (ATLAS PLATES 50, 51).** Note that the median nerve enters the forearm by coursing through the pronator teres muscle, i.e., between its superficial (**humeral**) and deep (**ulnar**) heads (**Figure 5-7**).

Separate the upper parts of the **brachioradialis** and **extensor carpi radialis longus muscles** from the brachialis muscle in order to expose the **radial nerve (ATLAS PLATE 52).** Verify that the radial nerve divides at this site into two terminal branches (**Figure 5-7**): the **superficial (cutaneous) branch,** which descends beneath the brachioradialis and the **deep radial nerve,** which **passes through the supinator muscle (ATLAS PLATE 60).**

Confirm that the cubital fossa contains **from medial to lateral** the median nerve, brachial artery, tendon of the biceps muscle, the deep radial nerve, and the superficial branch of the radial nerve (**ATLAS PLATE 52**).

◄
Grant's 518–520
Netter's 416, 417, 429, 430
Rohen 419–421

►
Grant's 534, 535
Netter's 423–426
Rohen 422, 423

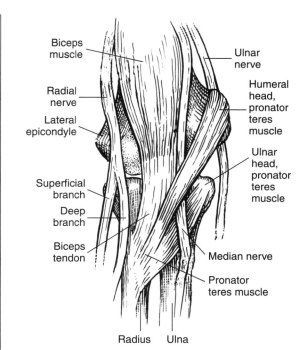

Figure 5-7. The location of the radial, median, and ulnar nerves as they enter the forearm.

IV. Anterior Forearm Muscles, Vessels, and Nerves (ATLAS PLATES 46–53, Figure 5-3B)

The anterior compartment of the forearm (**Figure 5-3B**) contains muscles that (1) flex the hand at the wrist, (2) flex the fingers at the interphalangeal and metacarpophalangeal joints, (3) pronate the hand and forearm, and (4) adduct (ulnar flexion) and abduct (radial flexion) the hand at the wrist. The muscles are arranged in three layers—superficial, intermediate, and deep. Two major arteries, the **radial** and **ulnar branches** of the **brachial artery,** descend in the anterior forearm, as do the **ulnar** and **median nerves.**

A. Anterior Forearm Muscles, Superficial Layer. Put your right thumb in your own left cubital fossa and palpate with your other four fingers the muscles below the lateral epicondyle. These are the brachioradialis and extensors carpi radialis longus and brevis muscles, and they will be studied with the extensor compartment muscles.

Now palpate the smaller flexor muscle mass medial to the cubital fossa and in front of the medial epicondyle. This mass consists of four **flexor-pronator muscles,** and they comprise the superficial anterior compartment layer. Arising from a common origin, the medial epicondyle and supracondylar ridge of the humerus, they include the **pronator teres,** the **flexor carpi radialis,** the **palmaris longus,** and the **flexor carpi ulnaris (ATLAS PLATES 46, 47).** The pronator teres and the flexor carpi ulnaris also have heads that arise from the ulna.

Remove the deep fascia from the front of the forearm and separate the four muscles of this superficial layer. Note how they fan out over the flexor surface (Figure 5-9A). Trace the tendons of the flexor carpi radialis, palmaris longus, and flexor carpi ulnaris to the wrist.

Do not cut the radial artery and the ulnar nerve and artery in this procedure (ATLAS PLATE 48). Dissect the most lateral muscle of this group, the pronator teres. **Being careful not to injure the median nerve** (which courses between its humeral and ulnar heads), follow the insertion of the pronator teres laterally to the radius. Then sever its humeral head near its middle to expose the median nerve (Figure 5-7).

At this point, it is important to trace the ulnar nerve, ulnar artery, radial artery, and the superficial branch of the radial nerve from the forearm to the wrist.

B. Ulnar Nerve and Artery; Radial Artery; Superficial Branch of Radial Nerve (Figure 5-8). Follow the **ulnar nerve** from its groove behind the medial epicondyle into the forearm. Passing **between the humeral and ulnar heads of the flexor carpi ulnaris, the ulnar nerve descends deep to the flexor carpi ulnaris muscle. Note that at the wrist the nerve lies just lateral to the tendon of this muscle (ATLAS PLATES 50, 52).**

Midway down the forearm find the ulnar artery at its origin. Follow it medially (deep to both the superficial layer of flexor muscles and the flexor digitorum superficialis) and dissect its distal half. The proximal part of the vessel is best seen after the flexor digitorum superficialis is cut **(ATLAS PLATE 52).**

Identify the **radial artery** at the wrist, where it lies just deep to the skin and fascia. During life, pulsations can easily be felt here because the vessel lies directly on the distal radius between the tendons of the brachioradialis laterally and the flexor carpi radialis medially (**ATLAS PLATE 50**). Dissect the artery distally as it courses backward to the dorsum of the hand (**ATLAS PLATE 63 #63.2**).

In the cubital fossa identify the **superficial branch of the radial nerve.** Dissect it distally

▶
Grant's 533–536
Netter's 422, 429, 430
Rohen 388, 421

◀
Grant's 535, 536
Netter's 430, 431, 456, 459
Rohen 423

▶
Grant's 530, 531, 536
Netter's 417, 430, 436
Rohen 398, 421, 423

deep to the brachioradialis muscle and, in the middle third of the forearm, find it just lateral to the radial artery (**ATLAS PLATES 50, 51**). Note that 3 inches above the wrist, the nerve leaves the vessel to descend over the radial side of the dorsal hand (**ATLAS PLATES 51, 62 #62.1**).

C. Flexor Digitorum Superficialis Muscle (Figure 5-9B) and the Median Nerve. Cut across the flexor carpi radialis and the palmaris longus muscle 5 inches below the medial epicondyle and reflect the severed ends. This exposes the flexor digitorum superficialis muscle, which comprises the intermediate layer of forearm muscles (**ATLAS PLATE 47, Figure 5-9B**). Note that from its origin on the common flexor tendon, as the muscle descends, it forms two more superficial and two deeper tendons. Pull on these tendons individually to verify that those going to the middle and ring fingers are more superficial and those going to the index and little fingers lie deeper.

With a scalpel, detach the flexor digitorum superficialis from its origin laterally on the radius (**ATLAS PLATE 51**). Turn the muscle medially to see the **median nerve** as it leaves the pronator teres. The nerve descends to the wrist along the deep surface of the superficialis (**ATLAS PLATE 52**). Two inches above the flexor retinaculum, the median nerve becomes more superficial and lies between the **tendons of the flexor carpi radialis and those of the flexor digitorum superficialis (ATLAS PLATE 50).** Detach the nerve from **the deep surface** of the flexor digitorum superficialis (**FDS**) and, **protecting the nerve,** cut across the belly of that muscle halfway down the forearm. Reflect the two ends of the FDS and expose the deep muscles of the forearm.

Find the **common interosseous branch of the ulnar artery** behind the ulnar head of the pronator teres. By dissecting distally, observe that this vessel branches into **anterior and posterior interosseous arteries,** which descend in front of and behind the interosseous membrane (**ATLAS PLATE 52**).

D. Anterior Forearm Muscles, Deep Layer (Figure 5-9C,D). Anterior Interosseous Artery and Nerve.

Deep to the flexor digitorum superficialis are located the **flexor pollicis longus** (laterally) and the **flexor digitorum profundus** muscles (Figure 5-9C,D, **ATLAS PLATE 48**). Deep to these, the four-sided pronator quadratus muscle is found (**ATLAS PLATE 67 #67.1**). Also descending in the forearm with these deep muscles

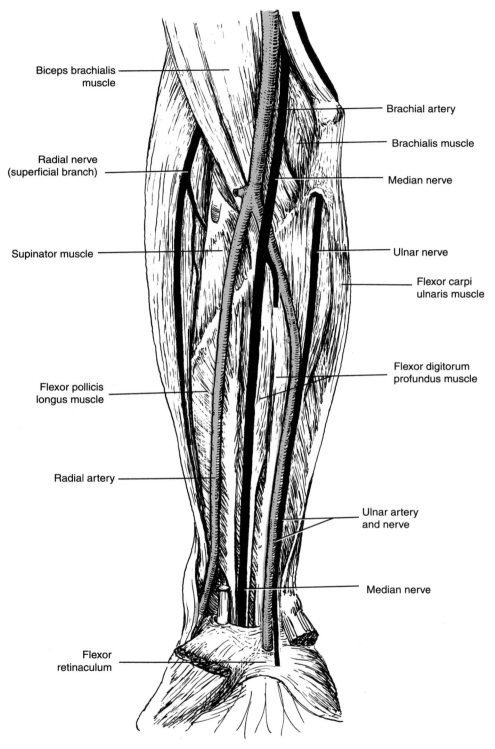

Biceps brachialis muscle

Radial nerve (superficial branch)

Supinator muscle

Flexor pollicis longus muscle

Radial artery

Flexor retinaculum

Brachial artery

Brachialis muscle

Median nerve

Ulnar nerve

Flexor carpi ulnaris muscle

Flexor digitorum profundus muscle

Ulnar artery and nerve

Median nerve

Figure 5-8. The arteries and nerves in the anterior forearm.

are the **anterior interosseous branch** of the **common interosseous artery** and the **anterior interosseous nerve,** a branch of the median nerve (**ATLAS PLATE 52**).

Turn back the ends of the flexor digitorum superficialis and identify the underlying **flexor digitorum profundus** and **flexor pollicis longus** (**ATLAS PLATE 48**). Pull on the tendons of these muscles near the wrist and note movements of the fingers and thumb on which these tendons insert. Now separate the tendons of the flexor digitorum profundus from the flexor pollicis longus, and expose the **in-**

◄
Grant's 533, 535–537
Netter's 426, 431, 456, 459
Rohen 389, 390, 398, 423

terosseous membrane (ATLAS PLATE 88 #88.1) along which descend the **anterior interosseous artery** and **nerve.** Follow the artery and nerve to the upper border of the transversely oriented **pronator quadratus muscle (Figure 5-9D).**

The median nerve supplies all of the anterior forearm muscles except the flexor carpi ulnaris and the medial half of the flexor digitorum profundus, which are supplied by the ulnar nerve. Note that the lateral half of the flexor digitorum, the flexor pollicis longus and the pronator quadratus all receive innervation from the median nerve by way of its anterior interosseous branch.

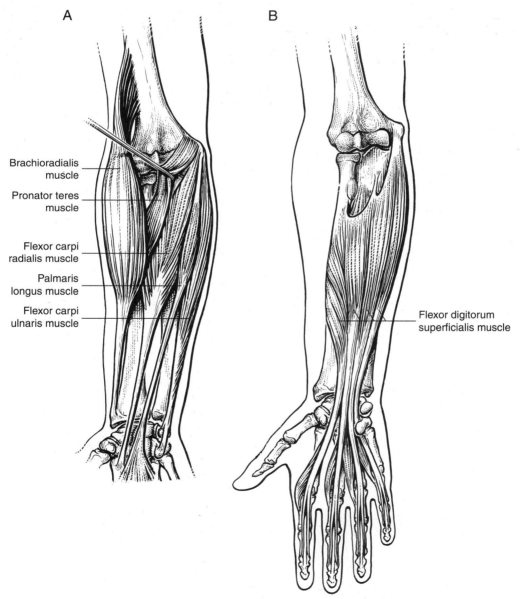

A   B

Brachioradialis muscle
Pronator teres muscle
Flexor carpi radialis muscle
Palmaris longus muscle
Flexor carpi ulnaris muscle

Flexor digitorum superficialis muscle

Figure 5-9. The muscles on the anterior aspect of the forearm: superficial muscles (**A**); Flexor digitorum superficialis (**B**).

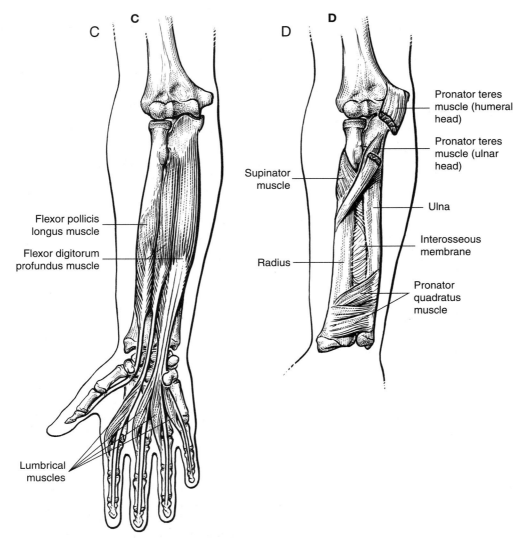

C

D

Pronator teres
muscle (humeral
head)

Pronator teres
muscle (ulnar
head)

Supinator
muscle

Ulna

Interosseous
membrane

Radius

Pronator
quadratus
muscle

Flexor pollicis
longus muscle

Flexor digitorum
profundus muscle

Lumbrical
muscles

Figure 5-9. The muscles on the anterior aspect of the forearm: Flexors digitorum profundus and pollicis longus (**C**); Pronator quadratus and interosseous membrane (**D**).

V. Tendons, Vessels, and Nerves on the Anterior Wrist

Before dissecting the palm of the hand, it is of important clinical value to be able to envision the sequential order of structures across the wrist anterior to the carpal bones.

Flex your hand and note the level of the most distal crease at the wrist. On the cadaver, cut away the skin of the wrist, but do not cut too deeply. Superficial to the fibrous flexor retinaculum, locate the tendons of the palmaris longus and flexor carpi ulnaris, the ulnar nerve and artery medially, and, if still intact, the superficial palmar branch of the radial artery laterally (**ATLAS PLATES 50, 70**).

Find the median nerve between the tendons of the flexor digitorum superficialis and flexor carpi radialis, and insert a probe into the carpal tunnel deep to the flexor retinaculum. Observe that, in addition to the median nerve, the tendons of the flexor digitorum profundus and the flexor pollicis longus also enter the palm by passing deep to this retinaculum (**ATLAS PLATE 70**).

Approximately 1 inch proximal to the carpal tunnel, identify **sequentially from the ulnar to the radial side** the following structure at the wrist (**ATLAS PLATE 70**):

A. Tendon of Flexor Carpi Ulnaris

B. Ulnar Nerve

C. Ulnar Artery

D. Four Tendons of the Flexor Digitorum Superficialis

E. Tendon of Palmaris Longus

F. Median Nerve

G. Tendon of Flexor Carpi Radialis

H. Radial Artery

Just beyond the lateral border of the radius are found more superficially:

I. Superficial Branch of the Radial Nerve

J. Cephalic Vein (near its commencement)

◄

Grant's 534, 538, 539, 550
Netter's 429, 442–445, 449
Rohen 388, 389, 428–430

Clinical Relevance

Bicipital tendinitis. Inflammation of the tendon of the biceps muscle occurs often following repeated direct trauma to the upper arm such as pushing your shoulder against a heavy door to open it. Within the bicipital sulcus on the anterior aspect of the humerus, the tendon is held securely within the sulcus by the transverse humeral ligament and overlying dense fascia. The inflamed, edematous tendon is tightly retained within the bicipital sulcus and it becomes painful without the opportunity to expand out of the sulcus.

Median nerve lesions. These lesions often occur in the arm as a result of a supracondylar fracture of the humerus, or in the lower forearm from wounds just above the wrist. Denervation of the muscles in the flexor compartments of the forearm and paralysis of the thenar muscles are debilitating. The thumb remains rotated laterally and adducted.

Supracondylar fracture (of the humerus). In a fracture of the humerus just above the elbow joint, the distal part of the humerus is pulled posteriorly because of the attached triceps muscle. If the brachial artery becomes displaced, the blood supply to the anterior forearm muscles could be compromised, resulting in an ischemia that causes severe contractures of the fingers or wrist (Volkmann's contracture).

Fracture of the head of the radius. This fracture occurs most often as a result of falling on the outstretched hand. The head of the radius articulates with both the ulna and the humerus, and the ascending force of the fall results in the head of the radius fracturing as it impacts the capitulum of the humerus. Often synovial fluid fills the synovial cavity, enhancing fat pads in the olecranon and coronoid fossae that become visible with a lateral radiograph.

DISSECTION #6

Palmar Aspect of the Hand

OBJECTIVES

1 Study the surface anatomy of the palm; visualize the recurrent branch of the median nerve.

2 Dissect the palmar aponeurosis; expose the digital vessels and nerves; and learn the cutaneous innervation of the hand.

3 Dissect the superficial palmar arch and the ulnar artery and nerve.

4 Open the carpal tunnel; dissect the flexor tendons and median nerve in the middle palmar compartment.

5 Dissect the middle finger: tendons, vessels, and nerves.

6 Dissect the thenar muscles and understand the movements of the thumb; dissect the hypothenar muscles.

7 Dissect the deep palmar arch, the deep branch of the ulnar nerve, and the interosseous muscles.

Atlas Key:

Clemente Atlas, 5th Edition = Atlas Plate #

Grant's Atlas, 11th Edition = Grant's Page #

Netter's Atlas, 3rd Edition = Netter's Plate #

Rohen Atlas, 6th Edition = Rohen Page #

The human hand is capable of performing many precise movements. It is the motor organ for grasping, and the richly innervated skin of the fingertips allows for fine tactile sensibility.

I. Surface Anatomy; Skin Incisions; The Palmar Aponeurosis and Digital Vessels and Nerves

A. Study the Surface Anatomy of the Palm. Flex your left hand and observe the creases at the wrist, palm, and fingers (**Figure 6-1**).

1. Realize that the **distal crease at the wrist** overlies the **flexor retinaculum**. This trans-

◄

Grant's 540, 541, 543, 548
Netter's 443, 444
Rohen 423, 426, 428

verse fibrous band converts the concave arch of the carpal bones into the **carpal tunnel.**

2. Observe that the **distal and proximal transverse palmar creases** cross the palm superficial to the metacarpal bones and that the distal crease crosses the palm proximal to the three medial fingers (**Figure 6-1**).

3. Note that the **thenar palmar crease** defines the muscles of the thumb that form the **thenar eminence.** Observe that the thumb can approximate the tip of each finger. Palpate the musculature on the medial side of the palm forming the **hypothenar eminence** (**Figure 6-1**).

4. Note the **metacarpophalangeal crease** located on each finger 1 cm distal to the metacarpophalangeal joint. The joints are found at the level of the knuckles on the dorsum of the hand. Observe that each of the four fingers has two **interphalangeal creases** but the thumb has only one.

5. With one of your thumbs, push across the palm of your other hand and try to displace the skin.

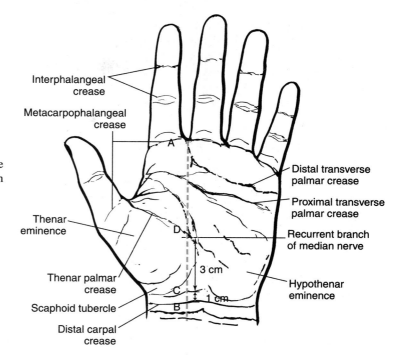

Figure 6-1. Surface anatomy of the palm. At point D along the dotted red line is the approximate site where the recurrent branch of the median nerve enters the thenar muscles.

Do the same on the dorsum of the hand. Note the looseness of the dorsal skin in contrast to that in the palm.

6. Envision a line on the palm from between the index and middle fingers to the distal crease at the wrist (**Figure 6-1A to B**). Along this line 1 cm distal to that crease, palpate the **tubercle of the scaphoid bone** (**Figure 6-1, at C**). Three cm distal to the tubercle along this line is the site where the important **recurrent branch of the median nerve** courses laterally and backward to supply the thenar muscles with motor innervation (**Figure 6-1, at D**). **This nerve is only a few millimeters deep to the skin at this point and is in a vulnerable position if the thenar eminence is injured.**

◀
Grant's 546, 547
Netter's 443

B. Skin Incisions and Reflection of the Skin. Make incisions in the palm only through the skin and not into the connective tissue. Palmar skin is especially adherent to the underlying **palmar aponeurosis.** Maintain your dissection plane between the skin and this aponeurosis.

Skin incisions on the palm and fingers are shown in **Figure 6-2.** Make two incisions from the midpoint of the distal crease of the wrist: one

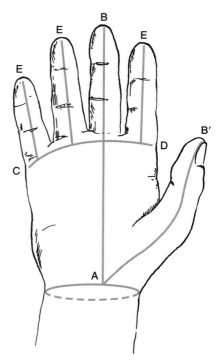

Figure 6-2. Lines of skin incisions on the palm, fingers, and thumb.

to the tip of the middle finger (**Figure 6-2 A to B**), and the other angled laterally to the tip of the thumb (**Figure 6-2 A to B′**). Make a transverse cut across the palm just proximal to the metacarpophalangeal crease (**Figure 6-2, C to D**) and additional incisions down the other three fingers.

Reflect the skin carefully. Start at the incision corners and skin the palm, thumb, and several fingers; also detach the skin from the dorsum of the hand.

With the palmar skin removed, note that the superficial fascia contains some fat and fibrous connective tissue that pad the palm. Deep to the superficial fascia is found a dense layer of deep fascia called the **palmar aponeurosis** (ATLAS PLATE 64). This tough fascia protects the underlying vessels and nerves from pressure and injury.

C. Palmar Aponeurosis; Digital Vessels and Nerves. Expose the palmar aponeurosis by re-

▶
Grant's 534, 541
Netter's 442
Rohen 422, 426

moving the superficial fascia. **Scrape away the fat** on the central palm with the scalpel edge until glistening longitudinal bands of the palmar aponeurosis become visible (**ATLAS PLATE 64**). Its fibers fan out distally from the flexor retinaculum as fibrous bands that extend to the proximal parts of the fingers. Probe between the margins of the aponeurosis in the webs of the fingers and identify the **common digital vessels and nerves. These divide into proper digital vessels and nerves,** which course distally along the fingers (**ATLAS PLATES 64, 70**).

On the lateral side of the palm, locate the **common digital branch of the ulnar nerve,** which divides between the ring and little fingers. Note that all of the other palmar digital nerves come from the median nerve (**Figures 6-3 and 6-4**). On the lateral sides of the four fingers, locate the delicate **lumbrical muscles** found deeper to the digital vessels and nerves (**ATLAS PLATE 65**).

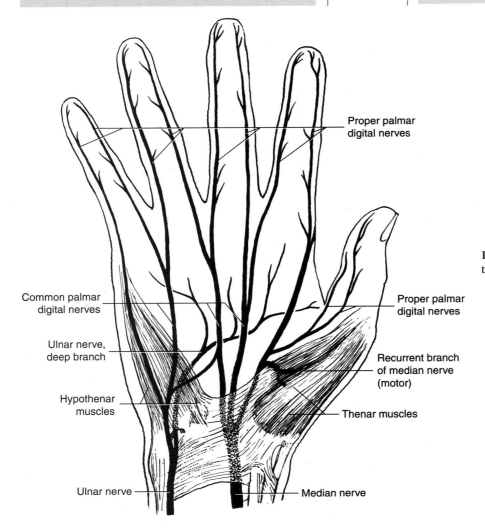

Proper palmar digital nerves

Common palmar digital nerves

Proper palmar digital nerves

Ulnar nerve, deep branch

Recurrent branch of median nerve (motor)

Hypothenar muscles

Thenar muscles

Ulnar nerve

Median nerve

Figure 6-3. The median and ulnar nerves and their branches.

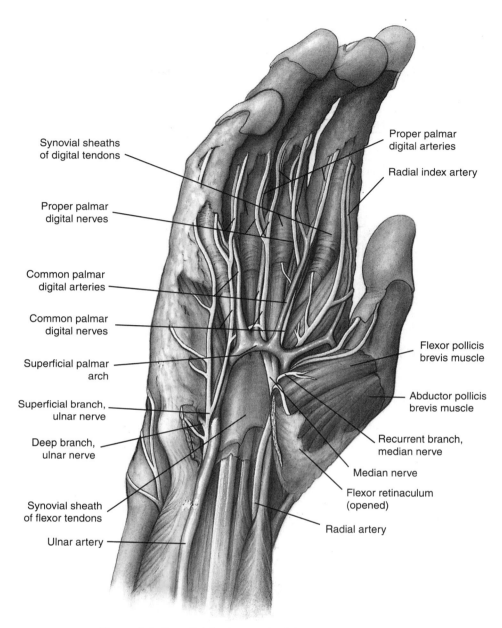

Figure 6-4. Superficial palmar arch; digital vessels and nerves.

II. Ulnar Artery and Nerve; Fascial Spaces of the Hand

The blood supply to the hand is derived from the ulnar and radial arteries. These vessels anastomose and form arterial arches called **superficial and deep palmar arches** (**ATLAS PLATES 70–73**).

A. The Ulnar Artery and Nerve. The **ulnar artery** is the principal contributor to the superficial arch, whereas the **radial artery** is the main vessel sending blood to the deep arch. The **ulnar nerve** sends a dorsal cuta-

▶
Grant's 534, 541, 546
Netter's 443, 444, 448, 449
Rohen 422, 423, 426

neous branch to the back of the hand (**ATLAS PLATE 62 #62.1**), but the main trunk of the nerve accompanies the ulnar artery superficial to the flexor retinaculum into the palm and divides into **superficial** and **deep (palmar) branches** (**ATLAS PLATE 70**).

Remove the superficial fat pad from the hypothenar eminence. On its deep surface may be found some transversely oriented fibers of the small **palmaris brevis muscle** coursing laterally from the palmar aponeurosis (**ATLAS PLATE 64**). Follow the ulnar nerve and artery into the palm and find where they send deep branches (not to be followed now) that penetrate the hypothenar muscles to get to deep palmar structures (**ATLAS PLATE 70**).

B. Fascial Spaces of the Hand (Figure 6-5). The palmar aponeurosis is fused laterally and medially to the fascial coverings over the thenar and hypothenar muscles. From these fusion sites, a septum passes into the palm to attach to deep fascia and metacarpal bones. Medially, the septum bounds the hypothenar muscles and attaches to the 5th metacarpal bone, enclosing the **hypothenar space (Figure 6-5)**. Laterally, the palmar septum penetrates deeply, medial to the thenar muscles, and then splits. One leaf courses laterally, attached to the 1st metacarpal bone, and encloses the **thenar spaces.** The other leaf continues medially, becomes fixed to the 3rd and 4th metacarpal bones, and helps enclose the **middle palmar space (Figure 6-5)**.

In the middle palmar space are the flexor tendons, the lumbrical muscles, branches of the median and ulnar nerves, and the superficial palmar arch and its branches (**ATLAS PLATE 98 #98.2**). Superficial to the adductor pollicis muscle is the **thenar space** into which infections can spread. Infections and edema can spread also to the middle palmar space deep to the flexor tendons. To dissect the middle palmar space, the palmar aponeurosis must be removed.

With forceps and scalpel, separate the palmar aponeurosis from underlying structures. Detach it from the flexor retinaculum and reflect it downward by cutting its lateral and medial fusions to the palmar septa.

▶
Grant's 546, 552
Netter's 443, 444, 449
Rohen 398, 422, 423, 426, 428, 429

◀
Grant's 584
Netter's 445

Dissect the superficial palmar arch and clean the common palmar digital arteries (usually three) that descend to the intervals between the fingers. Another branch also supplies the ulnar side of the little finger (**ATLAS PLATES 70, 72, 73**). Note where the ulnar artery in your cadaver is joined by a small **superficial branch of the radial artery.** Sometimes, the radial contribution may be difficult to find.

Identify the **ulnar** and **median nerves** found deep to the superficial palmar arch. Verify that they give rise to the common palmar digital nerves (**Figure 6-3**). Observe that the arteries are usually superficial to the nerves (**ATLAS PLATE 70**). Confirm that the median nerve supplies the lateral side of the palm, the thumb, the index and middle fingers, and, usually, the lateral half of the ring finger, whereas the ulnar nerve supplies the medial side of the palm, the little finger, and the medial half of the ring finger (see Figure 8-5).

Carefully remove the fascia over the thenar eminence and find the **recurrent branch of the median nerve** as it enters the thenar muscles approximately 3 cm below the scaphoid tubercle (**Figures 6-3, 6-4**).

III. Flexor Retinaculum; Flexor Tendons and Synovial and Fibrous Sheaths; Dissection of Middle Finger

A. Flexor Retinaculum. The flexor retinaculum is a strong, transversely oriented band of fibrous connective tissue measuring approximately 1 inch wide and 1 inch long (**Figure 6-8**). It bridges the carpal

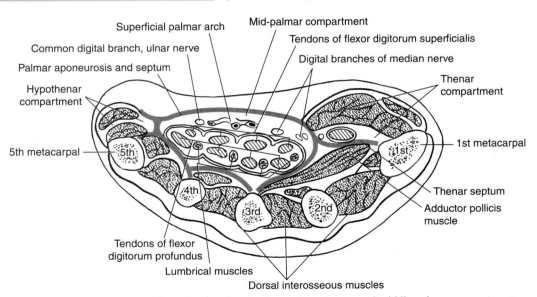

Figure 6-5. Cross section of the palm showing the thenar, hypothenar, and middle palmar compartments.

bones and transforms the concavity of these bones into the carpal tunnel (**ATLAS PLATES 65, 66**). The retinaculum attaches to the pisiform and hamate bones medially and the scaphoid and trapezium laterally. Through the tunnel descend the flexor tendons of the fingers and thumb, their synovial sheaths, and the median nerve (**ATLAS PLATE 70**).

Insert a probe directly behind the flexor retinaculum so that it enters the palm (**ATLAS PLATE 66**). Identify the main trunk of the median nerve both proximal to the retinaculum and then in the palm. **Be careful that the probe is located in front of the nerve and not behind it.** Cut through the flexor retinaculum but only as deeply as the probe, so that you do not injure the underlying structures. Flex the hand to release tension on the tendons, and separate the median nerve from the tendons.

Recognize that the median nerve and tendons lie in a restricted space between the flexor retinaculum and the carpal bones. Trauma that leads to fibrosis or any other

▶
Grant's 548
Netter's 444–446
Rohen 13, 393

▶
Grant's 536
Netter's 443, 445, 446
Rohen 389

◀
Grant's 547, 548
Netter's 443, 444
Rohen 423, 426, 428

condition that diminishes the size of the carpal tunnel could lead to motor and sensory loss caused by impairment of the nerve. This condition, called **carpal tunnel syndrome,** can be relieved surgically by severing part or all of the flexor retinaculum.

B. **Flexor Tendons and Synovial Sheaths (ATLAS PLATE 65).** As the tendons traverse the carpal tunnel, they are invaginated into glistening **synovial sheaths.** These tubular structures consist of tissue similar to that lining bursae, and each has an inner visceral layer adhering to the tendon and an outer parietal layer lining the osseous and fibrous canal. Between the layers is a small amount of lubricating fluid that allows the tendons to move freely.

Note that there are two synovial sheaths in the carpal tunnel: one surrounds the flexor pollicis longus, and the other, which is larger, surrounds all the tendons of the flexors digitorum superficialis and profundus. On **ATLAS PLATE 65,** observe that, distally, the sheath for the flexor digitorum tendons of the index, middle, and ring fingers ends as a blind pouch in the palm, but the sheath continues down the little finger. Individual synovial sheaths resume for the middle three fingers at the metacarpophalangeal joint and extend to the distal phalanx. Likewise, the synovial sheath for the flexor pollicis longus extends along the thumb to the distal phalanx.

Observe that in the carpal tunnel the superficialis tendons are arranged in pairs: tendons of the middle and ring fingers are anterior to those of the index and little fingers. The four profundus tendons lie behind the superficialis tendons and are all in the same plane (**ATLAS PLATE 67**). Separate the flexor tendons and turn them distally to the metacarpophalangeal joint.

Dissect the **lumbrical muscles** from their origin on the tendons of the flexor digitorum profundus to the lateral aspect of the metacarpophalangeal joints where they insert on the dorsal extensor tendon expansion (**ATLAS PLATES 67, 68 #68.1**).

C. **Fibrous Sheaths of Flexor Tendons; Dissect the Middle Finger.** The flexor tendons course along the palmar surface of each finger within fibrous-bony canals formed anteriorly and laterally by fibrous sheaths and dorsally by the phalangeal bones. Each fibrous sheath consists of strong bands of connective tissue that attach to both sides of the phalanges.

These become cruciform in shape and thin over the interphalangeal joints to permit free flexion (**Figure 6-6A**).

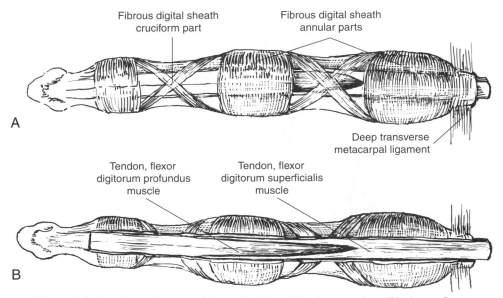

Figure 6-6. The fibrous flexor digital sheaths (**A**) and the flexor tendons (**B**) along a finger.

Surrounding the tendons **within the fibrous sheath** and lining the bony-fibrous canal is the digital synovial sheath (**ATLAS PLATES 65, 66**). The flexor retinaculum, palmar aponeurosis, and digital fibrous sheaths form a strong connective tissue binding, anterior to the flexor tendons, that maintains their position. This allows powerful flexor contraction of the fingers and hand without loss of strength owing to bowing of the tendons.

Clean the fascia from the anterior aspect of the middle finger and expose the **fibrous tendon sheath** anterior to the three phalanges (**Figure 6-6**). Dissect **only the middle finger; it serves as a model for all fingers** (**ATLAS PLATE 66**).

Slit the fibrous sheath longitudinally along the anterior midline of the middle finger (**Figure 6-6B**).

◀
Grant's 542, 545, 551
Netter's 443, 445–447, 454
Rohen 388, 389, 426, 428

Observe that the tendon of the flexor digitorum superficialis (FDS) lies anterior to the flexor digitorum profundus (FDP) tendon (**ATLAS PLATE 66**). Elevate the tendon of the superficialis and note that it flattens and then splits to form an opening through which the tendon of the FDP passes (**Figure 6-6**). See how the slips of the FDS tendon reunite, split again, and insert on the sides of the middle phalanx.

Follow the deep tendon to its insertion on the distal phalanx. Lift the superficialis tendon and find small folds of synovial membrane called **vincula** that allow minute blood vessels to enter the tendons (**Figure 6-7**). Dissect the proper digital arteries and nerves coursing distally along the lateral and medial aspects of the fibro-osseous canal (**ATLAS PLATE 71 #71.2**).

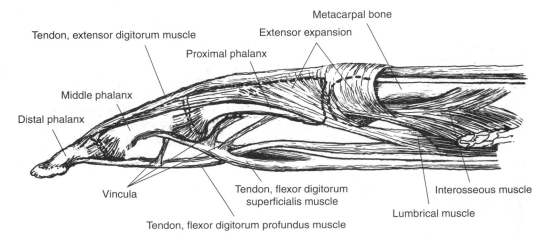

Figure 6-7. Lateral view of the flexor tendons along one finger showing how the lumbricals and interossei insert into the extensor expansions on the dorsum of the fingers.

IV. Thenar Muscles; Movements of the Thumb; Dissection of the Distal Thumb; The Hypothenar Muscles

A. Thenar Muscles (ATLAS PLATES 65–67, 89). Three superficial muscles of the thumb comprise the thenar eminence. These are the **abductor pollicis brevis,** the **flexor pollicis brevis,** and the **opponens pollicis,** and they are all supplied by the recurrent branch of the median nerve.

▶
Grant's 536, 544, 546–548
Netter's 443, 445, 448
Rohen 388, 392, 413, 414

Clinical Relevance

Recurrent branch of the median nerve. This nerve lies superficially along the medial surface of the thenar eminence about 4 cm distal to the end of the scaphoid process of the radius. Any small cut along the surface of the thumb could sever this nerve, resulting in a loss of the ability of the thumb to oppose the other fingers. This deficit seriously diminishes the use of the hand.

Identify and protect the recurrent branch of the median nerve (**Figures 6-3, 6-4**). Separate the most superficial layer of muscles (**abductor pollicis brevis laterally** and the adjacent **flexor pollicis brevis**) from the underlying **opponens pollicis** (**Figure 6-8**). Note that the fibers of the opponens are oriented more obliquely than those of the overlying muscles (**ATLAS PLATE 67**).

Find a cleavage line on the surface of the thenar eminence between the abductor brevis and the flexor brevis (**ATLAS PLATE 66**). Note that recurrent nerve branches cross over the belly of the flexor pollicis brevis. Cut the belly of the abductor pollicis brevis and reflect its ends to expose the opponens (**Figure 6-8**). Note that the thenar muscles arise from the trapezium and scaphoid bones and the flexor retinaculum. The abductor brevis and flexor brevis insert medially on the base of the proximal phalanx of the thumb, and the opponens pollicis inserts along the proximal anterior surface of the 1st metacarpal bone.

B.   Movements of the Thumb. Movements of the thumb are at right angles to those of the fingers. Flexion and extension are in the medial–lateral plane, and abduction and adduction occur in the anterior–posterior plane.

Extension–Flexion: Move your thumb to an outstretched position laterally, but in the same plane as the anterior surface of the palm. It is now fully

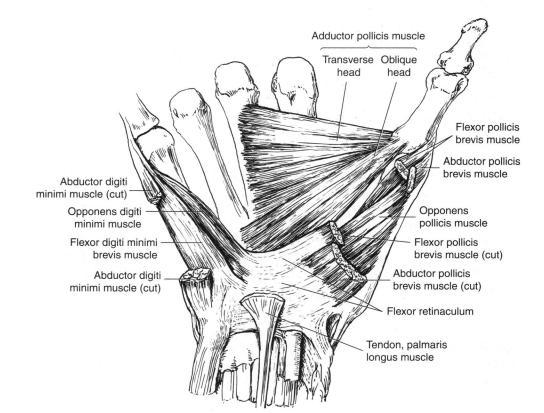

Figure 6-8. The thenar and hypothenar muscles.

Adductor pollicis muscle

Transverse head   Oblique head

Flexor pollicis brevis muscle

Abductor pollicis brevis muscle

Opponens pollicis muscle

Flexor pollicis brevis muscle (cut)

Abductor pollicis brevis muscle (cut)

Flexor retinaculum

Tendon, palmaris longus muscle

Abductor digiti minimi muscle (cut)

Opponens digiti minimi muscle

Flexor digiti minimi brevis muscle

Abductor digiti minimi muscle (cut)

extended. **Flex** your thumb by approximating the extended thumb to the radial border of the palm, and continue this action across the palm hugging closely the anterior surface of the palm until the tip of the thumb reaches the little finger. From this fully flexed position, **extend** your thumb by retracing this action until the thumb is once again outstretched laterally.

Abduction–Adduction: Abduct your thumb by pulling it forward at right angles anterior to the plane of the palm, and then **adduct** your thumb by moving it back to the anterior surface of the palm.

Opposition: Oppose your thumb by moving it across the palm and approximate its distal phalanx to the tip of any of the fingers.

C. **Dissection of the Distal Thumb.** The course of the tendons and nerves of the thumb is similar to that of the fingers, but the arterial source is principally from the radial artery.

Expose the fibrous sheath along the length of the thumb, but preserve the **proper palmar digital arteries and nerves.** Trace the two proper digital **nerves** back to the median nerve (**ATLAS PLATE 70**).

Find the two proper digital **arteries** of the thumb. See if they are derived from the **princeps pollicis artery** (**ATLAS PLATE 71**), which branches from the radial artery after that vessel enters the deep palm from the dorsum of the hand (**ATLAS PLATE 63 #63.1**). Open the fibrous sheath and dissect the tendon of the flexor pollicis longus and its synovial sheath to the distal phalanx.

D. **Hypothenar Eminence** (**ATLAS PLATES 65, 66**). The three muscles forming the hypothenar eminence correspond in name and mirror image to those seen in the thenar eminence. These include an **abductor,** a **flexor,** and an **opponens digiti minimi** (**Figure 6-8**). They arise from the pisiform and hamate bones and from the flexor retinaculum. The abductor and flexor digiti minimi insert into the base of the proximal phalanx of the little finger; the opponens is inserted along the shaft of the 5th metacarpal bone (**ATLAS PLATE 67**).

Separate and identify the hypothenar muscles. The abductor digiti minimi is the superficial muscle on the ulnar side. Separate it from the underlying flexor digiti minimi (**ATLAS PLATE 67 #67.1**). Cut the abductor pollicis brevis, reflect its ends and separate the flexor pollicis brevis from the opponens pollicis. Note that the fibers of the opponens are the most oblique of the hypothenar muscles (**Figure 6-8**). Identify the **deep**

▶
Grant's 544, 547, 550, 584
Netter's 445, 448
Rohen 393–394, 430

◀
Grant's 552
Netter's 449
Rohen 428, 429

▶
Grant's 530, 550, 552
Netter's 448, 449
Rohen 398, 428–430

◀
Grant's 536, 544
Netter's 443, 444, 448
Rohen 388, 422, 423, 426

branch of the ulnar nerve that supplies the hypothenar muscles as it courses between the abductor pollicis minimi and the flexor pollicis minimi. The nerve may be accompanied by a small branch of ulnar artery (**ATLAS PLATE 71 #71.1**).

V. Adductor Pollicis Muscle; Deep Palmar Arch; Deep Branch of the Ulnar Nerve; Interosseous Muscles

A. **Adductor Pollicis Muscle.** The adductor pollicis muscle and the other structures of the deep palm lie dorsal to the flexor tendons in the middle palmar space. Sometimes referred to as the adductor–interosseous space, this region contains the deep palmar arch, the deep branch of the ulnar nerve, and the interosseous muscles in addition to the adductor pollicis.

To approach the **adductor pollicis muscle,** cut the superficial palmar arch and reflect the tendons of the flexor digitorum superficialis down to the roots of the fingers. Sever the four tendons of the flexor digitorum profundus 2 inches above the flexor retinaculum, and also turn the distal ends of these tendons and their attached lumbrical muscles downward to the fingers. Note that the two medial lumbrical muscles receive innervation from the ulnar nerve (**ATLAS PLATE 71 #71.1**). Observe that the adductor pollicis has **transverse** and **oblique heads.** These converge to insert on the medial side of the first phalanx of the thumb (**Figure 6-8**).

B. **Deep Palmar Arch and Deep Branch of Ulnar Nerve.** Between the two heads of the adductor pollicis courses a branch of the radial artery (to help form the deep palmar arch) accompanied by the deep branch of the ulnar nerve.

Having the **deep palmar arch** now partially exposed, cut the origin of the oblique head of the adductor pollicis and reflect it to expose the radial artery as it enters the palm from the back of the hand (**ATLAS PLATES 63 #63.1, 71 #71.1**). Sever the opponens pollicis muscle, being careful to protect the ulnar nerve and artery that pierce the muscle before crossing the palm. Identify the **palmar metacarpal arteries** branching from the deep arch to join the common palmar digital arteries. On the radial side of the deep palm, again find the **princeps pollicis artery,** which supplies the thumb (**ATLAS PLATE 71 #71.1**), and the **radial indices artery,** which courses along the radial side of the index finger (**ATLAS PLATE 75**).

The **ulnar nerve** supplies the muscles of the hypothenar eminence, the medial two lumbricals, the adductor pollicis muscle and all of the interosseous muscles (and at times the deep head of the flexor pollicis brevis); the median nerve innervates the three thenar muscles and the lateral two lumbricals.

C. The Interosseous Muscles (Figures 6-9, 6-10). The muscles that lie between the metacarpal bones are the **palmar and dorsal interossei (ATLAS PLATE 68 #68.2, #68.3).** These muscles help flex the metacarpophalangeal joints and extend the interphalangeal joints. More important, the three palmar interosseous muscles **adduct** the fingers, and the four dorsal interossei **abduct** the fingers. These latter actions are considered in relationship to the middle finger, which serves as the longitudinal (median plane) axis of the hand (**Figure 6-9**).

The **palmar interossei** arise from the metacarpal bones of the index, ring, and little fingers (which they adduct) and insert onto the extensor surface of the corresponding fingers. Because the thumb and the little finger have their own abductors, the four **dorsal interossei** are inserted onto the index, middle, and ring fingers, the middle finger having two, one attached to

◄
Grant's 545, 549, 551
Netter's 447, 448, 453, 459
Rohen 394, 395, 427, 430

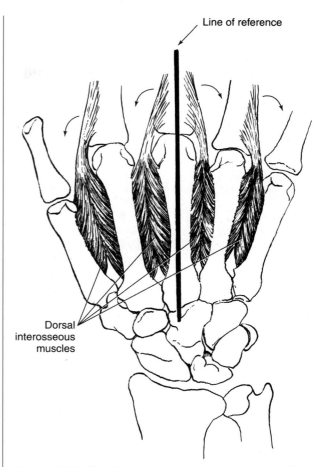

Figure 6-10. The four dorsal interosseous muscles. They **abduct** the fingers.

each side (**Figure 6-10**). These muscles move the fingers away from the long axis of the hand.

If time allows, try to identify some of the interosseous muscles in the deep palm and note that they are supplied by deep branches of the ulnar nerve (**ATLAS PLATE 71 #71.1**).

Clinical Relevance

Guyon's canal syndrome. The ulnar nerve at the wrist courses between the pisiform bone and the hamulus of the hamate bone. A ligament superficial to this site creates a canal within which the ulnar nerve may become compressed. The resulting syndrome includes a loss of sensory innervation to the ring and little fingers along with a weakness in movements because of the denervation of the interossei and hypothenar muscles.

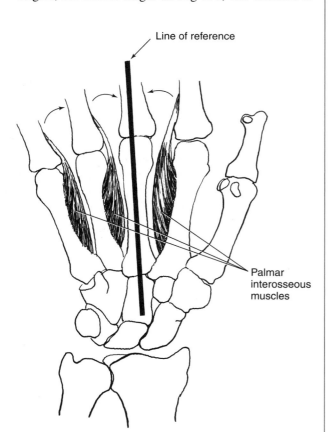

Figure 6-9. The three palmar interosseous muscles. They **adduct** the fingers.

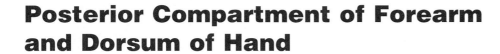

DISSECTION #7

Posterior Compartment of Forearm and Dorsum of Hand

OBJECTIVES

1. Learn the surface anatomy of posterior forearm and dorsum of hand.

2. Dissect the superficial nerves of the dorsal forearm and the venous plexus on the dorsum of the hand.

3. Dissect three superficial muscles in the extensor compartment on the lateral aspect of the forearm.

4. Dissect four superficial muscles on posterior aspect of the forearm.

5. Dissect five deep muscles of the posterior forearm.

6. Find the posterior interosseous nerve and artery.

7. Dissect the extensor retinaculum and identify the structures on the dorsal aspect of the wrist.

8. Dissect the dorsum of the hand and the dorsal interosseous muscles

Atlas Plate:
Clemente Atlas, 5th Edition = Atlas Plate #
Grant's Atlas, 11th Edition = Grant's Page #
Netter's Atlas, 3rd Edition = Netter's Plate #
Rohen Atlas, 5th Edition = Rohen Page #

I. General Introduction

The posterior compartment (**Figure 7-1**) of the forearm contains muscles that **extend** the hand at the wrist and the fingers and thumb at the metacarpophalangeal and interphalangeal joints. Certain posterior forearm muscles assist in abduction (radial flexion) and adduction of the hand at the wrist. The **brachioradialis** is an important flexor of the pronated forearm, while the **supinator**, as its name implies, supinates the forearm and the little **anconeus muscle** weakly assists the powerful triceps in extension of the forearm at the elbow.

Through the posterior forearm course the **deep branch of the radial nerve** and the **posterior interosseous artery** (**ATLAS PLATE 60**). Both the **cephalic** and **basilic veins** commence superficially on the dorsum of the wrist (**ATLAS PLATE 62 #62.1**). Cutaneous innervation of the extensor surface of the forearm is supplied by branches of the **radial nerve**, but the **lateral** and **medial antebrachial cutaneous nerves** supply its radial and ulnar borders (**ATLAS PLATES 26 #26.2, 27 #27.3**). Most of the dorsum of the hand is supplied by the **radial** and **ulnar** nerves, but the **median nerve** gives cutaneous innervation to the distal halves of the dorsal thumb, index finger, middle finger, and lateral half of the ring finger (**ATLAS PLATE 26**).

II. Surface Anatomy; Removal of Skin; Superficial Veins and Nerves

A. **Surface Anatomy.** Certain anatomical structures on the dorsal forearm and hand serve as important clinical landmarks in consideration of injuries or other conditions that require treatment.

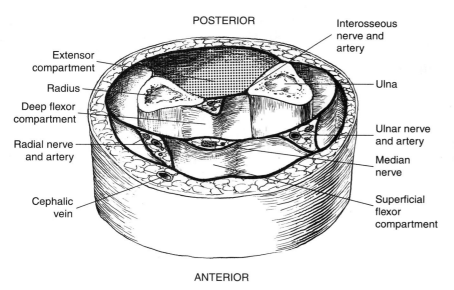

POSTERIOR

Extensor compartment

Radius

Deep flexor compartment

Radial nerve and artery

Cephalic vein

Interosseous nerve and artery

Ulna

Ulnar nerve and artery

Median nerve

Superficial flexor compartment

ANTERIOR

Figure 7-1. Cross section of the forearm showing the superficial and deep flexor compartments anteriorly and the extensor compartment posteriorly (stippled).

Identify the following bony structures on yourself or on your lab partner.

1. With the fingers of your right hand, follow the shaft of your left ulna (just deep to the skin) from the olecranon to the styloid process (**ATLAS PLATE 84 #84.1, #84.2**). Feel the head of the left radius below the lateral epicondyle. Palpate the shaft of the radius, deep to the muscle overlying it, down to the **styloid process** on the lateral aspect of its distal extremity (**ATLAS PLATE 84 #84.3, #84.4**).

   ◄ Grant's 498, 499, 524, 526, 527
   Netter's 419–422
   Rohen 374–381

2. Pronate your right hand and fully extend the thumb. Find the triangular depression 1 cm distal to the styloid process called the "anatomic snuff box." This small fossa lies between the prominent tendon of the extensor pollicis longus on the ulnar side of the fossa, and the tendons of the **extensor pollicis brevis** and **abductor pollicis longus** on the radial side of the fossa (**ATLAS PLATES 29 #29.1, 56, 58**). Know that the **radial artery** crosses the floor of the fossa deep to these three tendons (**ATLAS PLATE 63 #63.2**).

   ◄ Grant's 557, 564, 568
   Netter's 427, 450, 452, 453
   Rohen 394

3. Extend your right hand and fingers fully. With your left hand, palpate the extensor tendons leading down from the wrist and over the knuckles (which are the bases of the metacarpal bones) to the dorsal surfaces of the fingers. Proximal to the knuckles feel the **bodies of the metacarpal bones** and palpate the softer tissue (the **dorsal interosseous muscles**) between the bones (**ATLAS PLATE 63 #63.2**). The largest dorsal interosseous muscle forms the tissue

   ◄ Grant's 556, 562, 565
   Netter's 452, 453
   Rohen 389, 390, 418

between the index finger and the thumb (**ATLAS PLATE 62 #62.2**).

4. Note the looseness of the skin on the dorsum of the hand. This is why edema often occurs here even though an infection may be on the palmar aspect of the hand. Observe the prominent subcutaneous venous plexus, which is used at times for intravenous injections or catheters.

B. **Removal of Skin.** The cutaneous nerves of the forearm and hand are just deep to the skin, as are the basilic and cephalic veins (**ATLAS PLATE 62 #62.1**). Be aware of these on removal of the skin.

   Make an incision down the midline of the back of the hand to the root of the middle finger (**Figure 7-2, A to B**). Make transverse incisions across the knuckles to the lateral and medial margins of the hand (**Figure 7-2, B to C and B to D**) and turn back the two flaps. Remove the skin from the back of the thumb and fingers to the fingernails, but retain the dorsal digital nerves and vessels (**Figure 7-2, dashed lines**).

C. **Superficial Veins and Nerves.** Superficial digital veins on the palmar aspect of the hand drain into venous networks over the thenar and hypothenar muscles, and these drain dorsally. Digital veins on the dorsum of the fingers empty into venous channels on the dorsum of the thumb or on the hypothenar eminence.

   Dissect the superficial veins on the radial and ulnar sides of the dorsum of the hand in the superficial

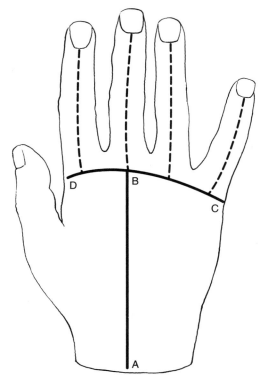

Figure 7-2. Skin incisions on the dorsum of the hand.

▶
Grant's 462, 558
Netter's 450–452
Rohen 399, 400,
416

◀
Grant's 464
Netter's 457, 463
Rohen 398, 416,
418

fascia and follow the formation of the **cephalic** and **basilic veins** (**ATLAS PLATES 43, 45, 62 #62.1**). Observe how the dorsal metacarpal veins on the ulnar side form the basilic vein, and the metacarpal veins of the thumb and index finger ascend into the cephalic vein.

The lateral and medial antebrachial cutaneous nerves course around the radial and ulnar sides of the forearm to supply the adjacent portions of the dorsal forearm. The skin of the middle region of the dorsal forearm between these two zones is supplied by the **posterior antebrachial cutaneous nerve** (**ATLAS PLATES 26 #26.2, 45**). The dorsum of the hand receives innervation from the ulnar, radial, and median nerves (**Figure 7-3**).

Identify and lift the brachioradialis muscle to uncover the radial nerve as it divides into its **posterior antebrachial cutaneous branch** (superficial branch) and its deep branch (**ATLAS PLATES 50–52**). Follow the posterior cutaneous branch down the forearm as it courses with the radial artery. Dissect the nerve distally and see how it divides into two or three branches that supply the dorsum of the hand. These **dorsal digital nerves** can be traced to the proximal halves of the thumb, index, and middle

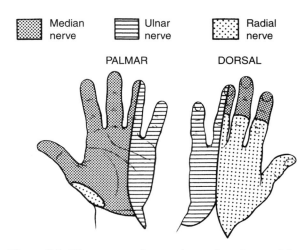

Figure 7-3. The cutaneous innervation on the palmar and dorsal surfaces of the hand.

fingers and the radial half of the ring finger (**ATLAS PLATES 61, 62 #62.1**).

Follow the ulnar nerve down the forearm and find its **dorsal branch** proximal to the wrist. Dissect this branch into the dorsum of the hand as it passes between the flexor carpi ulnaris and the ulna (**ATLAS PLATES 51, 52**). Find its two **dorsal digital branches** that supply the ulnar aspect of the little finger and the adjacent sides of the ring and little fingers (**ATLAS PLATE 62 #62.1**).

III. Muscles of the Extensor Compartment of the Forearm

The muscles of the extensor compartment of the forearm are divided into **superficial** and **deep layers.** The superficial layer contains three lateral muscles and four posterior muscles. The deep layer contains five muscles: three **"outcropping muscles"** of the thumb, which bound the "anatomic snuff box," plus the **extensor indicis** and the **supinator.**

A. Superficial Extensor Forearm Muscles, Lateral Group (Figure 7-4). Located on the radial side of the posterior forearm, these lateral muscles include the **brachioradialis** and the **extensor carpi radialis longus** and **brevis** (**ATLAS PLATE 55**).

Remove the superficial deep fascia covering the muscles of the posterior compartment as high in the forearm as possible and detach the cutaneous nerves and superficial veins. The **extensor retinaculum** located inferiorly should be left intact. Note how the retinaculum serves as a strong transverse band of

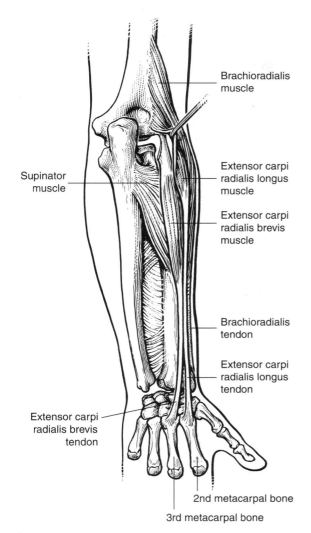

Figure 7-4. The three superficial lateral muscles plus the deeply located supinator muscle (dorsal/posterior view).

connective tissue that retains the tendons close to the wrist during extension of the hand (**ATLAS PLATES 54, 55**).

Separate the most superficial muscle of the lateral group, the **brachioradialis,** from the underlying **extensors carpi radialis longus** and **brevis.** Do not sever the **posterior antebrachial cutaneous nerve** that descends just deep to the brachioradialis. Observe the origin of the brachioradialis from the upper two-thirds of the **supracondylar ridge** above the lateral epicondyle of the humerus (**ATLAS PLATES 29 #29.1, 33, 55**). Follow its tendon of insertion to the lower end of the lateral radius where it attaches above the styloid process.

Separate the extensor carpi radialis longus away from the extensor carpi radialis brevis by following

▶
Grant's 556, 557
Netter's 424, 428
Rohen 390, 416

▶
Grant's 561–563
Netter's 424, 447
Rohen 390

◀
Grant's 556, 557
Netter's 424, 428
Rohen 389, 406, 416

▶
Grant's 556, 557
Netter's 424, 428
Rohen 390

their tendons upward from about 6 inches above the wrist to their muscle bellies. Note that the longus arises above the brevis from the lateral epicondyle (**ATLAS PLATES 29 #29.2, 55**). Follow the tendon of insertion of the longus onto the base of the 2nd metacarpal and the brevis onto the 3rd metacarpal (**Figure 7-4**). Observe that these two tendons course deep to the tendons of the abductor pollicis longus and the extensors pollicis longus and brevis (**ATLAS PLATES 58, 62 #62.2, 63 #63.2**).

B. **Superficial Extensor Forearm Muscles, Posterior Group** (**Figure 7-5A**). The muscles of the superficial posterior group include the **extensor digitorum, extensor digiti minimi, extensor carpi ulnaris,** and the small triangular **anconeus** muscle located behind the elbow (**ATLAS PLATE 54**).

Two inches above the extensor retinaculum identify and separate from lateral to medial the extensor digitorum, the extensor digiti minimi, and the extensor carpi ulnaris muscles and their tendons (**Figure 7-5A**). Observe that all three muscles arise from the common extensor origin on the lateral epicondyle of the humerus. Follow the tendons distally deep to the **extensor retinaculum** (**ATLAS PLATE 62 #62.2**).

On the dorsum of the hand, observe how the **extensor digitorum** becomes flattened and divides into four tendons. These diverge, and continue over the knuckles to reach the dorsum of each of the four fingers (**Figure 7-5A**). Note that the tendon to the index finger is accompanied by the tendon of the extensor indicis (one of the deep muscles). Follow the tendons distally where they spread over the dorsum of the fingers and are called **dorsal digital expansions.** Note that the expansions receive the insertions of the interosseous and lumbrical muscles (**ATLAS PLATE 69 #69.1**).

Identify the **extensor digiti minimi** medial to the extensor digitorum (**ATLAS PLATE 54**). Note that its tendon goes through a separate compartment of the extensor retinaculum (**ATLAS PLATE 56**). Follow the tendon to its insertion onto the dorsum of the little finger.

Follow the tendon of the **extensor carpi ulnaris** to its insertion on the ulnar side of the base of the 5th metacarpal bone (**ATLAS PLATE 56, 58**). If time permits, remove the deep fascia over the anconeus muscle, and uncover its attachments to the lateral epicondyle and the olecranon above and upper part of the ulna below (**ATLAS PLATES 56, 58**). This site becomes inflamed and edematous in the condition called "tennis elbow."

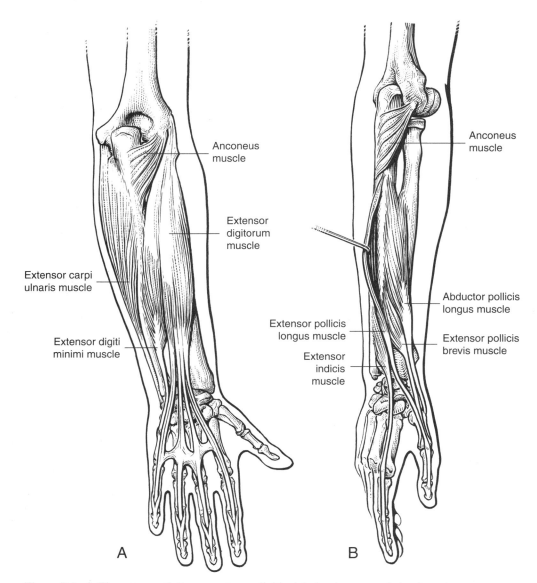

Figure 7-5. A. The extensor digitorum, extensor digiti minimi, extensor carpi ulnaris, and anconeus muscles (posterior view). **B.** The three outcropping muscles, and the extensor indicis and anconeus muscle (posterolateral view).

C. Deep Muscles of the Posterior Forearm (Figures 7-5B, 7-6). The deep muscles of the posterior forearm include the **supinator (Figure 7-4)**, the "outcropping" muscles of the thumb that bound the anatomic snuff box, i.e., the **abductor pollicis longus,** and **extensors pollicis brevis** and **longus,** and the **extensor indicis (ATLAS PLATE 58).**

To expose the **supinator muscle,** retract the brachioradialis and the extensors carpi radialis longus and brevis laterally (**ATLAS PLATES 58, 60**). Detach the lower end of their origins if necessary. Expose the remaining muscles of the posterior forearm

by cutting the extensor digitorum, extensor digiti minimi, and extensor carpi ulnaris 3 inches below the lateral epicondyle and then reflecting their bellies.

Identify the deep **branch of the radial nerve** as it enters the supinator muscle in front of the lateral epicondyle (**ATLAS PLATE 53 #53.2**). Find it again near the lower border of the supinator, where it is now called the **posterior interosseous nerve** and is joined by the **posterior interosseous branch of the common interosseous artery (ATLAS PLATE 60).**

Note that the **supinator muscle** arises from the lateral epicondyle of the humerus and the lateral

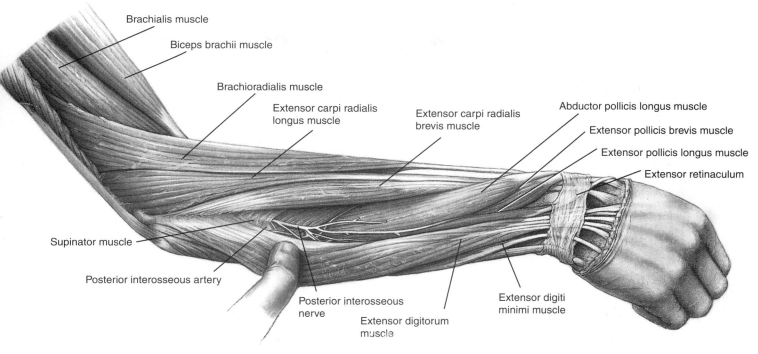

Figure 7-6. The posterior interosseous artery and nerve in the deep extensor forearm.

side of the upper ulna, and its fibers spiral around the forearm to insert on the upper radius (**ATLAS PLATE 58**). If the forearm is pronated, the fibers become more twisted. The action of this muscle results in untwisting its fibers, thereby **supinating the forearm.**

Below the supinator, find the **abductor pollicis longus** and follow its tendon down to the thumb where it inserts onto the 1st metacarpal (**ATLAS PLATE 75**). Below the abductor, identify the smallest of the outcropping muscles, the **extensor pollicis brevis.** Its tendon courses adjacent to that of the abductor to the proximal phalanx of the thumb where it inserts (**ATLAS PLATES 58, 75**).

Dissect the remaining two deep muscles, the **extensor pollicis longus** and the **extensor indicis,** both of which arise from the posterior ulna and the interosseous membrane. Observe that the **extensor pollicis longus** forms the lateral boundary of the "anatomic snuff box" and descends to the distal phalanx of the thumb (**ATLAS PLATES 58, 60**). Below the extensor pollicis longus in the forearm, find the **extensor indicis** and follow its tendon to the dorsal expansion hood of the index finger where it inserts (**ATLAS PLATE 58**).

◄
Grant's 556, 557
Netter's 424–428
Rohen 389, 390, 416

►
Grant's 561
Netter's 453
Rohen 390

IV. Extensor Retinaculum; Extensor Synovial Sheaths; Structures Across the Dorsum of the Wrist

The extensor retinaculum is an obliquely oriented band of deep fascia on the dorsal surface of the distal forearm (**ATLAS PLATES 62 #62.2, 63 #63.2**). It extends from the pisiform and triquetral bones medially to the antero-lateral border of the distal radius laterally. Connective tissue septa attach from the retinaculum to the underlying bone (**ATLAS PLATE 56**) and form six fibro-osseous compartments through which the extensor tendons and their synovial sheaths enter the hand (**ATLAS PLATES 62, #62.2, 98 #98.1**). The compartments are as follows (**Figure 7-7**):

1. The most lateral compartment contains the tendons of the abductor pollicis longus and the extensor pollicis brevis (**ATLAS PLATE 58**).
2. Deep to the "anatomic snuff box" is the compartment containing the tendons of the extensors carpi radialis longus and brevis (**ATLAS PLATE 98 #98.1**).
3. Next is a compartment that extends obliquely toward the thumb and contains the tendon of the extensor pollicis longus (**ATLAS PLATE 56**).
4. The tendons of the extensor digitorum and extensor indicis occupy a broad compartment over the middle part of the dorsal wrist (**ATLAS PLATE 56**).

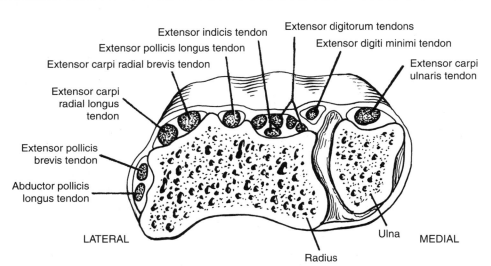

Figure 7-7. Cross section of the tendons and bones of the wrist showing the tendons in their compartments (anterior ventral view).

5. The fifth compartment lies over the distal radio-ulnar joint and contains the tendon of the extensor digiti minimi (**ATLAS PLATE 56**).

6. The most medial compartment lies over the distal ulna and contains the tendon of the extensor carpi ulnaris (**ATLAS PLATE 58**).

The synovial sheaths around these tendons commence proximal to the extensor retinaculum and terminate just distal to the retinaculum. All tendons have individual synovial sheaths, except for the abductor pollicis longus and flexor pollicis brevis, which share a common synovial sheath as do the extensor digitorum and extensor indicis tendons (**ATLAS PLATE 62 #62.2**).

Cut longitudinally through the extensor retinaculum along these extensor fibro-osseous compartments to expose the tendons and the synovial sheaths that they enclose (**ATLAS PLATES 56, 58**). Approximately 1 cm distal to the retinaculum, identify each of the following structures. (Vessels and nerves are listed in parentheses; tendons are numbered.) (**SEE ATLAS PLATES 56, 62 #62.2, 63 #63.2, 98 #98.1**).

1. Abductor pollicis longus tendon

2. Extensor pollicis brevis tendon
   (Cephalic vein)
   (Superficial branch of radial nerve)
   (Radial artery)

3. Extensor pollicis longus tendon

4. Extensor carpi radialis longus tendon

5. Extensor carpi radialis brevis tendon

◄
Grant's 556, 562
Netter's 452, 453
Rohen 416, 418

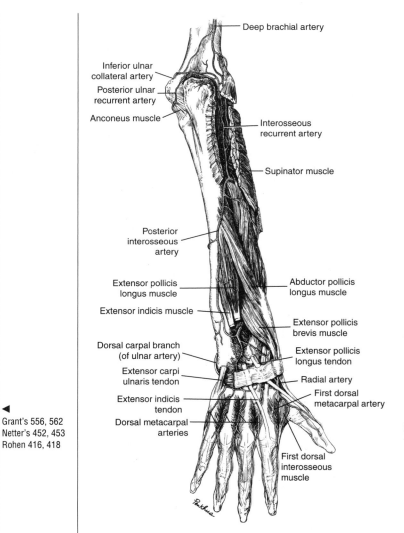

Figure 7-8. Arteries in the posterior forearm, wrist, and hand.

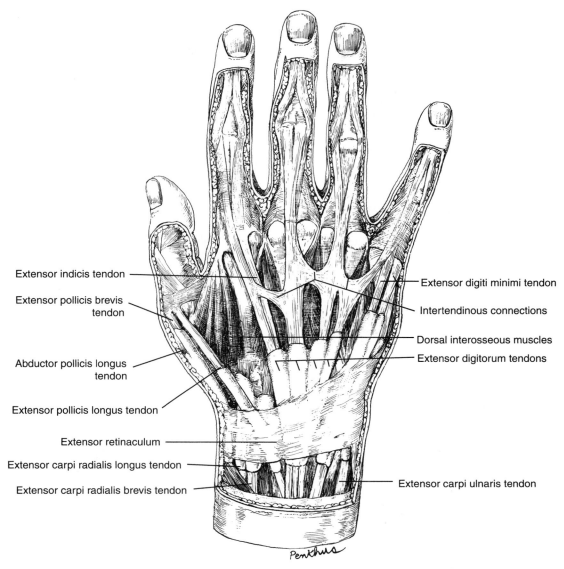

Extensor indicis tendon

Extensor pollicis brevis
tendon

Abductor pollicis longus
tendon

Extensor pollicis longus tendon

Extensor retinaculum

Extensor carpi radialis longus tendon

Extensor carpi radialis brevis tendon

Extensor digiti minimi tendon

Intertendinous connections

Dorsal interosseous muscles

Extensor digitorum tendons

Extensor carpi ulnaris tendon

Figure 7-9. Tendons and dorsal interosseous muscles on the posterior wrist and hand.

6. Extensor indicis tendon

7. Extensor digitorum tendon
   (Basilic vein)

8. Extensor digiti minimi tendon

9. Extensor carpi ulnaris tendon
   (Dorsal branch of ulnar nerve)

V. Arteries and Nerves on Dorsum of Hand; Dorsal Interosseous Muscles (Figs. 7-8, 7-9)

A. Arteries and Nerves on the Dorsum of the Hand.
The arterial supply to the dorsum of the hand is derived from **dorsal carpal branches of the ulnar and radial arteries** and terminal branches of the **anterior and posterior interosseous arteries** (**ATLAS PLATE 63 #63.1**). These vessels form an anastomosis called the **dorsal carpal network** that may appear as a **dorsal carpal arch.** From this network or arch descend **dorsal metacarpal arteries** that then divide into **dorsal digital arteries** (**ATLAS PLATE 63 #63.1**).

Cutaneous innervation on the dorsum of the hand (**Figure 7-3**) and the dorsum of the proximal half of the fingers is derived from the **superficial radial nerve** (thumb and radial $2\frac{1}{2}$ fingers) and from the **dorsal cutaneous branch** of the **ulnar nerve** (ulnar $1\frac{1}{2}$ fingers). Innervation of the distal half of the dorsum of the fingers comes to the dorsum from the median and ulnar **palmar** digital nerves (**ATLAS PLATES 26 #26.2, 27 #27.3**).

Dissect deep to the extensor tendons and identify dorsal carpal branches from the radial, ulnar, and interosseous arteries that join to form a delicate transversely oriented arch (**ATLAS PLATE 63 #63.1**). Find dorsal metacarpal arteries that descend from this network over the dorsal interosseous muscles. Follow one of the metacarpal arteries to the web between two fingers where it divides into dorsal digital arteries to supply their adjacent surfaces.

Find the radial artery as it passes from the floor of the "anatomic snuff box" through the two heads of the first dorsal interosseous muscle to enter the deep palm (**ATLAS PLATE 63**). It then gives off the **princeps pollicis** (**ATLAS PLATE 63 #63.1**) and **radial index** (**ATLAS PLATE 72**) **arteries** before continuing as the **deep palmar arch** (**ATLAS PLATE 68 #68.2**).

◄
Grant's 556, 557, 562
Netter's 450, 452, Rohen 399, 400, 416–418

B. Dorsal Interosseous Muscles. The four **dorsal interossei** abduct the fingers from the midline axis of the hand (**Figure 7-2**). The thumb and little finger have their own abductors. The dorsal interosseous muscles insert onto the ring and index fingers on the sides away from the midline axis. The middle finger has two dorsal interosseous muscles, one on each side, allowing it to be abducted both to the lateral or medial sides of the midline axis (**ATLAS PLATE 71 #71.1**).

Clean the fascia from the surfaces of the dorsal interosseous muscles in the intermetacarpal spaces. Observe that each dorsal interosseous muscle is bipennate and arises by two heads from the adjacent sides of two metacarpal bones (**ATLAS PLATE 68 #68.2**). Other delicate perforating arteries may be found between the heads of the 2nd, 3rd, and 4th dorsal interosseous muscles.

Dissect the tendons of insertion of the dorsal interosseous muscles distally to their attachments onto the extensor expansions of the index, middle, and ring fingers.

◄
Grant's 556, 584
Netter's 448, 452, 453
Rohen 389

Clinical Relevance

Tennis elbow. Tenderness and painful to pressure over the lateral epicondyle of the humerus is called "tennis elbow." It is caused by an overuse of the extensor muscles of the upper limb, usually in sports such as tennis or golf.

Bursitis at the olecranon. This inflammation occurs in the bursa that is located superficial to the olecranon of the ulna. It is usually caused by excessive or prolonged pressure on the posterior aspect of the elbow joint.

Wrist drop. This condition is caused by a radial nerve injury that results in paralysis of the extensor muscles in the forearm. The fingers are flexed as well, because the paralysis significantly reduces extension at the metacarpophalangeal and interphalangeal joints.

Synovial cysts at the wrist. These are usually small cysts filled with a semi-clear fluid, which occur dorsally on the wrist within or adjacent to the synovial tendon sheaths of the extensor muscles. Sometimes one is referred to as a "ganglion."

De Quervain's disease. This condition is caused by tenosynovitis of the common tendon sheath of the abductor pollicis longus and extensor pollicis brevis. Movements of the thumb are painful.

Colles' fracture. This is a fracture of the distal end of the radius (styloid process) caused by a fall on the outstretched hand. The distal fractured part is displaced dorsally and superiorly and usually results in a dorsal bump at the wrist.

Bennett's fracture. This is a fracture of the first metacarpal bone proximal to the phalanges of the thumb. Often this is caused by a direct force along the longitudinal axis of the thumb.

Metacarpal bone fracture. These long bones of the hand are usually fractured by a direct impact on the hand dorsally. At times it is caused by a clenched fist hitting a hard surface. Fracture of the two ulnar metacarpal bones (4th and 5th) is more common than fracture of the radial three metacarpal bones.

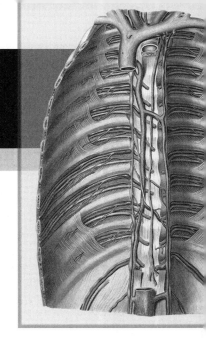

DISSECTION #8

Joints of the Upper Extremity

OBJECTIVES

1 Expose the acromioclavicular and coracoclavicular joints and dissect the glenohumeral (or shoulder) joint.

2 Dissect the elbow joint and open the proximal radio-ulnar joint.

3 Visualize the middle radio-ulnar joint and expose the distal radio-ulnar joint.

4 Open the radiocarpal joint and expose the distal row of carpal bones at the midcarpal joint.

5 Open the carpometacarpal, metacarpophalangeal, and interphalangeal joints of one finger.

Atlas Key:

Clemente Atlas 5th Edition = Atlas Plate #

Grant's Atlas 11th Edition = Grant's Page #

Netter's Atlas 3rd Edition = Netter's Plate #

Rohen Atlas 6th Edition = Rohen Page #

Dissect the joints of the upper extremity on **one limb only.** Save the soft tissues overlying the joints of the other limb for review.

I. Joints of the Shoulder Region

The clavicle participates in the formation of the **pectoral girdle** by attaching to the sternum medially and to the acromion of the scapula laterally. Note that the acromion and coracoid process of the scapula and the clavicle are bony structures that help protect the glenohumeral articulation, or **shoulder joint,** superiorly. The **acromioclavicular** and **coracoclavicular joints** are now to be dissected (**Figure 8-1**).

A. Acromioclavicular Joint. The acromioclavicular joint (**ATLAS PLATE 79**) is a synovial joint of the gliding or plane type, located between the lateral end of the clavicle and the medial border of the acromion (**Figure 8-1**).

> Elevate the shoulder by placing a wooden block under the upper back. Initially, the bony arch formed by the acromion, the clavicle, and their attached ligaments must be exposed. Palpate the acromion and lateral clavicle. Sever the deltoid muscle away from the clavicle anteriorly, the acromion laterally, and the scapula posteriorly (**SEE ATLAS PLATE 62**). Cut away the attachment of the trapezius muscle from the spine of the scapula.

Using a scalpel, scrape the soft tissue from the upper surface of the acromioclavicular joint. Note that the joint capsule consists of fibrous tissue comprising the **acromioclavicular ligament** (**Figure 8-1** and **ATLAS PLATE 80 #80.2**). Open the joint capsule by cutting close to the acromion. Determine whether a partial or complete fibrocartilaginous articular disc is present. Sometimes a disc divides the joint cavity into two separate synovial cavities.

◀
Grant's 508, 512
Netter's 408
Rohen 368, 372, 378

B. Coracoclavicular Joint. The coracoclavicular joint is the ligamentous union between the coracoid process of the scapula and the distal clavicle. It has no synovial cavity, but consists of interosseous ligaments between the two bones (a **syndesmosis**). The coracoclavicular ligament consists of two parts, the **trapezoid** and **conoid ligaments,** named because of their shapes (**ATLAS PLATES 80 #80.2, 81 #81.1**). These powerful ligaments support the lateral aspect of the scapula as it hangs from the clavicle (**Figure 8-1**).

By disarticulating the acromioclavicular joint, you will partly mobilize the distal end of the clavicle and expose the coracoclavicular ligaments. Elevate the clavicle and identify the **trapezoid ligament** between the clavicle and the coracoid process (**ATLAS**

▶
Grant's 493, 511, 515, 516
Netter's 406, 408, 414
Rohen 367

◀
Grant's 508, 512
Netter's 406, 408
Rohen 378

PLATE 80 #80.2). Define the borders of the **conoid ligament** posteromedial to the trapezoid ligament (**Figure 8-1**). Its shape resembles a cone with the base directed toward the clavicle and the apex toward the coracoid process.

The coracoclavicular ligaments provide stability to the acromioclavicular joint. They prevent the acromion from being dislocated medially under the clavicle after a fall on the outstretched hand. The force transmitted up the arm and then from the head of the humerus to the glenoid cavity is partially dissipated to the clavicle through the coracoclavicular ligaments (especially the trapezoid ligament).

The **coracoacromial ligament** is an intrinsic ligament of the scapula (**Figure 8-1**). This strong triangular band of fibrous tissue has its base attached to the coracoid process and its apex to the tip of the acromion (**ATLAS PLATE 81 #81.1**).

On disarticulating the acromioclavicular joint, identify the **coracoacromial ligament.** Note that, with the coracoid process and acromion, the ligament forms a fibro-osseous arch over the head of the humerus, protecting the shoulder joint from above. Note also that the subacromial bursa and supraspinatus muscle overlie the shoulder joint at this site (**ATLAS PLATES 82 #82.2**).

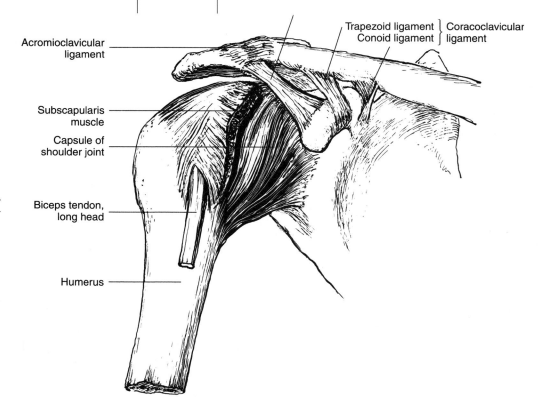

Figure 8-1. The acromioclavicular, coracoacromial, and coracoclavicular ligaments (anterior view).

Acromioclavicular ligament

Subscapularis muscle

Capsule of shoulder joint

Biceps tendon, long head

Humerus

Trapezoid ligament ⎫ Coracoclavicular
Conoid ligament ⎭ ligament

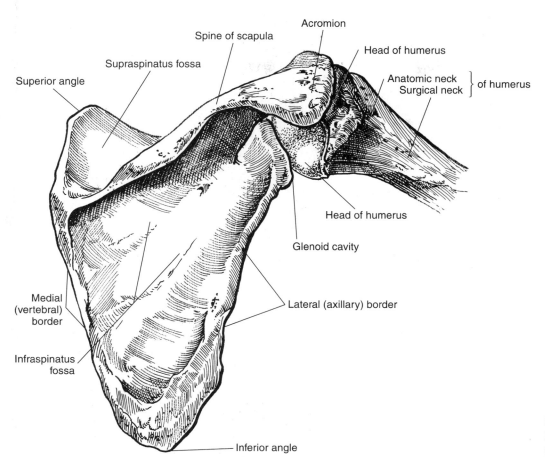

Superior angle

Supraspinatus fossa

Spine of scapula

Acromion

Head of humerus

Anatomic neck
Surgical neck } of humerus

Head of humerus

Glenoid cavity

Medial
(vertebral)
border

Lateral (axillary) border

Infraspinatus
fossa

Inferior angle

Figure 8-2. The scapula and humerus at the glenohumeral articulation (posterior view).

C. Glenohumeral (or Shoulder) Joint. The shoulder joint is a ball-and-socket type in which the head of the humerus is disproportionately large for the shallow glenoid cavity (**ATLAS PLATE 79, Figure 8-2**). This feature, combined with a loose articular capsule, allows freedom of movement, but at some expense to stability. Some protection against this weakness and tendency for dislocation is achieved superiorly by a fibro-osseous arch (see the previous discussion) and the clavicle and by muscles and their tendons around the joint. These muscles include the **deltoid** that surrounds the joint, the **subscapularis** anteriorly, the **supraspinatus** superiorly, the **infraspinatus** and **teres minor** posteriorly, and the **long head of the triceps** inferiorly (**ATLAS PLATES 32, 38**).

◄
Grant's 492, 493, 505, 506, 508
Netter's 406, 408, 409, 414
Rohen 383, 387

Dissection of the shoulder joint requires exposure of the articular capsule. If the **deltoid muscle** has not been reflected downward from the clavicle, acromion, and spine of the scapula, do it now. Cut the origins of the **coracobrachialis, short head of the biceps,** and **long head of the triceps** and reflect them downward. Cut the **subscapularis muscle** near its

insertion and reflect the muscle medially away from the joint. Posteriorly, sever the tendons of the **supraspinatus, infraspinatus,** and **teres minor** from their insertions on the greater tubercle and the joint capsule and reflect the muscle bellies medially (**ATLAS PLATE 81 #81.2**).

The articular capsule should now be exposed. Leave the teres major, latissimus dorsi, and pectoralis major muscles attached to the humerus so that the limb will not detach when the joint capsule is opened. Before opening the fibrous capsule, find the **coracohumeral ligament,** which is a wide fibrous band that strengthens the upper part of the joint capsule (**ATLAS PLATES 80 #80.3, 81 #81.1**). It extends over the shoulder joint from the lateral aspect of the coracoid process to the greater tubercle of the humerus.

Observe the attachments of the fibrous capsule to the margin of the glenoid cavity medially and the anatomic neck of the humerus laterally (**ATLAS PLATE 80 #80.3**).

The **superior, middle,** and **inferior glenohumeral ligaments** thicken the joint capsule and

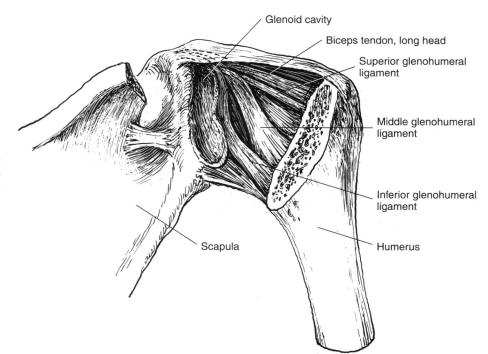

Figure 8-3. The interior of the shoulder joint opened from behind after the posterior part of the capsule has been removed and the head of the humerus cut away.

strengthen it anteriorly. They are best studied by opening the joint capsule from behind, removing the head of the humerus, and visualizing the inner surface of the anterior aspect of the joint capsule from this posterior view (**Figure 8-3**).

Make a longitudinal incision along the posterior aspect of the joint capsule. Make transverse cuts from the flaps so that the posterior parts of the capsule can be opened to expose the head of the humerus from behind (**ATLAS PLATE 79**). With a chisel and hammer, remove the head of the humerus by cutting through the anatomic neck just proximal to the tuberosities (**Figure 8-3**). Observe the fibrocartilaginous rim, called the **glenoid labrum,** around the circumference of the glenoid fossa. Note that it increases the depth of the glenoid cavity by approximately 5 millimeters.

At the uppermost part of the glenoid labrum, identify the **tendon of the long head of the biceps muscle** and the **superior glenohumeral ligament** (**Figure 8-3**). From the supraglenoid tubercle, the tendon passes across the joint cavity **anterior to the head of the humerus** (**ATLAS PLATE 79**). Observe that the narrow **superior glenohumeral ligament** also extends from the upper part of the glenoid cavity, but anterior to the origin of the biceps tendon. It courses laterally and helps form that part of the capsule attaching to the humerus just superior to the lesser tubercle.

▶
Grant 524, 526, 527
Netter's 419
Rohen 374, 375

◀
Grant's 511, 514
Netter's 406
Rohen 378

Identify the **middle** and **inferior glenohumeral ligaments** (sometimes seen as a single ligament). These also attach to the superior and anterior margins of the glenoid cavity and descend inferolaterally to strengthen the part of the capsule that attaches below the lesser tubercle (**Figure 8-3**).

II. Joints at the Elbow Region

There are two joints in the elbow region: (1) the **elbow joint,** which itself has two articulations, **humero-ulnar** and **humeroradial,** and (2) the **proximal radio-ulnar joint.**

A. Elbow Joint. Within a single articular capsule, the **capitulum of the humerus** articulates with the **head of the radius** as a gliding joint, and the **trochlea of the humerus** articulates with the **trochlear notch of the ulna** as a hinge joint (**Figure 8-4**). This is a compound synovial joint, and its synovial cavity is continuous with that of the proximal radio-ulnar joint (**ATLAS PLATE 87**).

Two inches above the antecubital fossa, sever the veins, nerves, and arteries, and turn their distal parts downward to expose the cubital fossa. Sever the main belly of the **biceps brachii muscle** and reflect the lower part to its insertion on the tuberosity of the

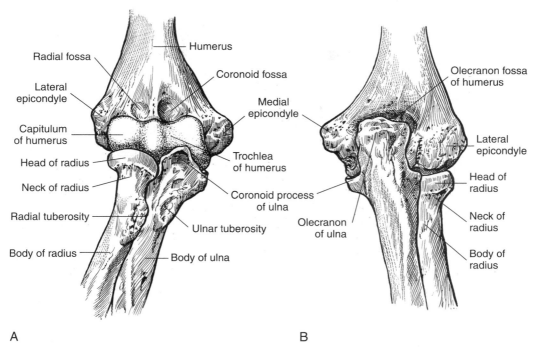

Figure 8-4. The humerus, radius, and ulna at the elbow joint. **A.** Anterior view. **B.** Posterior view.

radius. Cut the belly of the **brachialis muscle** in the lower arm and reflect the distal part downward away from the anterior aspect of the joint capsule. Cut the **triceps muscle** approximately 2 inches above the olecranon and reflect its lower part distally to its insertion without damaging the capsule.

Cut the origins of the **pronator teres, palmaris longus,** and **flexor carpi radialis** from the medial epicondyle. Remove the origins of the **flexor digitorum superficialis** and **flexor carpi ulnaris** and cut away the ulnar nerve. This exposes the medial aspect of the joint capsule and the **ulnar collateral ligament (Figure 8-5A).**

Laterally, sever the origins of the **brachioradialis** and **extensors carpi radialis longus and brevis** and reflect them downward. Cut and reflect upward the **extensor carpi ulnaris** and **extensor digitorum** in the posterior forearm and then sever their attachments on the humerus. This exposes the **supinator muscle.** Cut the attachments of the supinator muscle from the radius, ulna, and humerus, and remove the small **anconeus muscle.** This exposes the lateral aspect of the joint capsule and the **radial collateral ligament (Figure 8-5B).**

Note that the anterior part of the capsule also encloses the proximal radio-ulnar joint, and that superiorly, the capsule attaches to the medial epicondyle and shaft of the humerus (**ATLAS PLATE 86 #86.1**). Inferiorly, the capsule stretches to the coronoid process

▶
Grant's 526, 527
Netter's 421
Rohen 379

▶
Grant's 528
Netter's 421
Rohen 379

▶
Grant's 528, 529
Netter's 421
Rohen 379

of the ulna and blends with the **annular ligament.** Define the three bands of the **ulnar collateral ligament** (strong **anterior** and **posterior bands** and a thinner **oblique** or **middle band**). Note that they form three sides of a triangular ligament, the apex of which is the medial epicondyle (**Figure 8-5A**).

Laterally, observe that the articular capsule is reinforced by the **radial collateral ligament** (**ATLAS PLATE 86 #86.2**). This strong band, also triangular in shape, attaches superiorly to the lateral epicondyle and fans downward to blend with the annular ligament (**Figure 8-5B**).

Dissect the **annular ligament** and note that it attaches to both the anterior and posterior lips of the radial notch on the ulna, surrounding the head of the radius (**ATLAS PLATE 85, 87**). Verify by palpation that it forms a fibrous circular collar within which the head of the radius rotates.

Cut into the capsule of the elbow joint anteriorly and posteriorly by making transverse incisions **between** the ulnar and radial collateral ligaments (**Figure 8-6**). Leaving the ligaments intact, examine the synovial membrane lining the inner surface of the capsule as it extends over the fossae of the lower humerus. Note that the membrane attaches distally around the margin of the articular surface of the ulna and that the synovial cavity of the elbow joint is continuous with that of the proximal radioulnar joint.

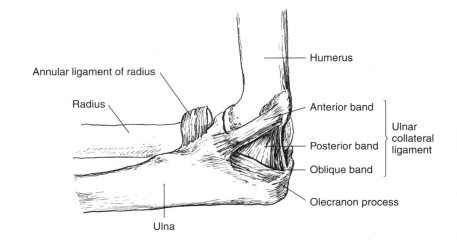

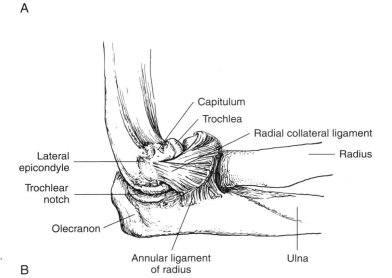

Figure 8-5. The ligaments of the elbow joint.
A. Medial view. **B.** Lateral view.

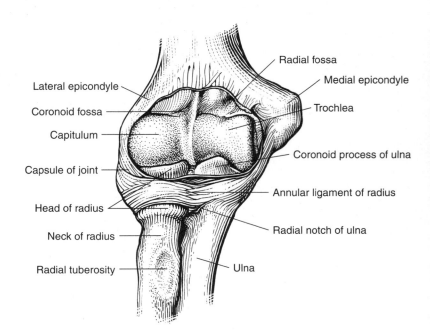

Figure 8-6. The elbow joint with the anterior part of the
capsule opened (anterior view).

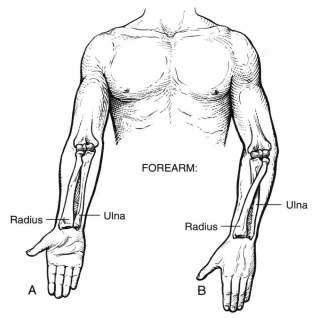

Figure 8-7. The bones of the forearm in the supinated (**A**) and (**B**) pronated positions.

B. Proximal Radio-ulnar Joint. The proximal radio-ulnar joint is a **single axis pivot joint** in which the head of the radius rotates within a fibro-osseous ring during supination and pronation (**Figure 8-7**). This ring is formed four-fifths by the annular ligament and one-fifth by the radial notch of the ulna.

▶
Grant's 528
Netter's 421
Rohen 379

Cut the annular ligament and observe that the synovial membrane lines the inner surface of the ligament and continues to attach to the neck and margin of the head of the radius (**ATLAS PLATE 88 #88.1**).

III. The Middle and Distal Radio-ulnar Joints

In addition to the proximal radio-ulnar joint, the radius and ulna are attached by an interosseous ligament (syndesmosis) between the shafts of the two bones that are called the **middle radio-ulnar joint,** and by a synovial joint (pivot) between the lower ends of the radius and ulna, the **distal radio-ulnar joint.**

A. Middle Radio-ulnar Joint. The interosseous borders of the shafts of the radius and ulna are joined by a strong fibrous interosseous membrane (**ATLAS PLATE 88 #88.1**). It provides a surface for the attachment of deep forearm muscles and assists in transmitting sudden forces from the hand and radius at the wrist (such as in falling), to the ulna along its shaft, and then to the humerus at the elbow.

On the flexor surface of the forearm, remove the flexor muscles and any other tissue necessary to expose the anterior surface of the interosseous

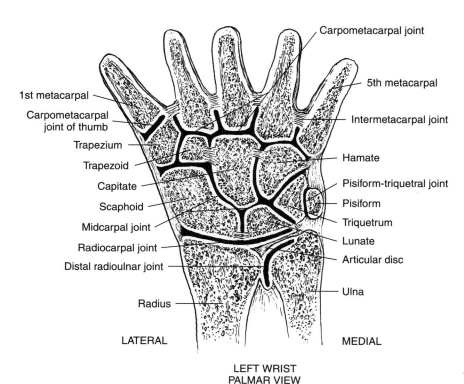

Figure 8-8. Coronal section through the left wrist showing the distal radio-ulnar joint, the radiocarpal joint, the midcarpal joint, the intercarpal joints, and the carpometacarpal joints.

membrane. Observe that its fibers course obliquely downward and medially from the border of the radius to the ulna (**ATLAS PLATE 88 #88.1**). Find the **posterior interosseous vessels** as they enter (leave) the extensor compartment through a gap just below the **oblique cord** (**ATLAS PLATE 88 #88.1**), which extends opposite in direction to the fibers in the interosseous membrane.

B. **Distal Radio-ulnar Joint.** The distal radio-ulnar joint interconnects the delicate head of the ulna and the **ulnar notch** on the medial surface of the distal radius (**ATLAS PLATE 88 #88.1**). Distal to the ulna is located a triangular **fibrocartilaginous disc** between the ulna and the carpal bones (**Figure 8-8**).

Clean the loose and weak capsule of the distal radio-ulnar joint (**ATLAS PLATE 92**). Open and reflect the capsule by making anterior and posterior longitudinal incisions. Probe the synovial cavity. Note that it extends between the disc and the ulna, and that it continues proximally between the radius and ulna. If the joint is cut longitudinally, the cavity appears L-shaped (**ATLAS PLATE 93 #93.3**).

IV. Joints at the Wrist

Below the distal radio-ulnar joint are the **radiocarpal joint** (or wrist joint proper), the **intercarpal joints** between the individual carpal bones, and the **carpometacarpal joints** that interconnect the distal row of four carpal bones with the five metacarpal bones (**ATLAS PLATE 93 #93.3**). The fibrous capsules of these joints blend to form a single continuous covering. The inner surface of the capsule is lined by the **synovial membranes** that bound the various joint cavities. These include a) a single synovial cavity for the radiocarpal joint, b) a single irregularly shaped cavity for the intercarpal joints, c) a separate small synovial cavity between the pisiform and triquetral bones, and d) a single synovial cavity between the distal row of carpal bones and the heads of the four digital metacarpal bones, which also extends between the heads of the metacarpal bones (**Figure 8-8**). A separate synovial cavity between the trapezium and the 1st metacarpal bone forms the carpometacarpal joint of the thumb (**ATLAS PLATE 93 #93.3**).

A. **Radiocarpal Joint.** This condyloid synovial joint lies between the radius and the articular disc adjacent to the ulna proximally and the **scaphoid, lunate,** and **triquetral bones** distally (**ATLAS PLATE 93**

◄
Grant's 525, 531
Netter's 422
Rohen 381

►
Grant's 571–573
Netter's 437, 438
Rohen 380, 381

◄
Grant's 571, 572
Netter's 437, 438
Rohen 380, 381

►
Grant's 570, 573, 574
Netter's 438
Rohen 380, 381

◄
Grant's 568, 569
Netter's 435, 436
Rohen 375–377

#93.3). The articular surface formed by the disc and the radius is concave and it receives the convex surface of the three carpal bones (**Figure 8-8**).

Laterally and medially observe the longitudinally oriented **ulnar** and **radial collateral ligaments of the wrist joint.** Note that on the ulnar side, the ligament attaches above to the styloid process of the ulna and below to the triquetral and pisiform bones. On the radial side, the ligament stretches from the styloid process of the radius to the scaphoid and trapezium. Also see how the fibrous capsule is reinforced by obliquely oriented thickenings anteriorly called the **palmar radiocarpal** and **palmar ulnocarpal ligaments** and posteriorly by the **dorsal radiocarpal ligament** (**ATLAS PLATE 92**).

Open the joint dorsally by making a transverse incision through the capsule between the articular disc and radius above and the scaphoid, lunate, and triquetral bones below (**ATLAS PLATE 93 #93.3**). Slightly flex the hand and identify the scaphoid bone below the radius, the smaller lunate bone between the radius and the articular disc, and the triquetral bone on the ulnar side of the lunate (**ATLAS PLATES 89, 93 #93.3**).

B. **Intercarpal Joints.** The intercarpal joints include joints between the individual carpal bones of both the proximal and distal rows, and a more extensive **midcarpal joint** between the two rows of carpal bones (**Figures 8-8, 8-9**). Individual bones in the two rows are interconnected by narrow fibrous **interosseous ligaments** that allow little movement. All of the intercarpal joints share a single irregularly shaped but continuous synovial cavity (**ATLAS PLATE 93 #93.3**). On the ulnar side, the **pisiform-triquetral joint** has its own synovial cavity (**Figure 8-8**).

Make another incision across the dorsal wrist capsule at the level between the proximal and distal rows of carpal bones (**ATLAS PLATE 93 #93.3**). Flex the hand and open the synovial cavity of the intercarpal joints. Identify the four distal carpal bones from ulnar to radial sides: the **hamate, capitate, trapezoid,** and **trapezium.** Note that the trapezium is opposite the base of the metacarpal bone of the thumb (**Figure 8-9**).

C. **Carpometacarpal Joints.** These are plane joints between the distal row of carpal bones and the four metacarpal bones of the fingers (**ATLAS PLATE 93 #93.3**). **The carpometacarpal joint of the thumb is**

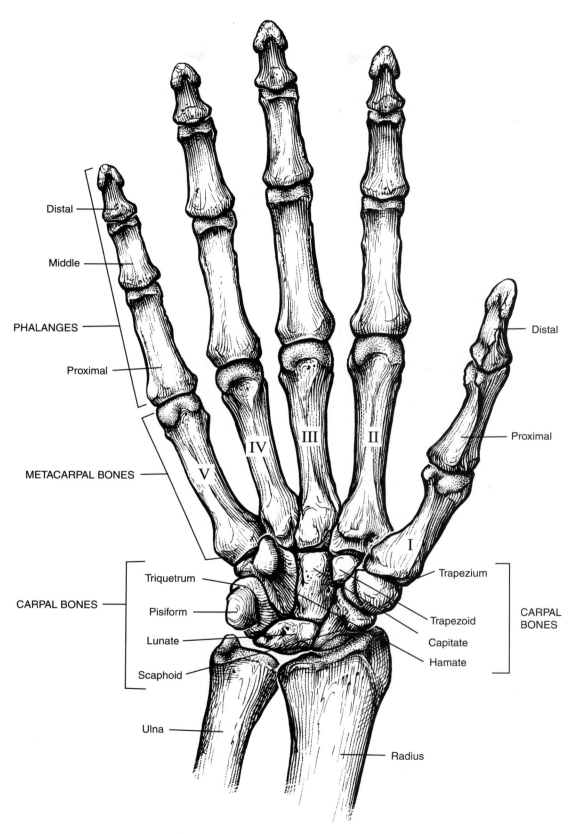

Figure 8-9. Bones at the wrist and in the hand.

a saddle-shaped joint between the first metacarpal bone and the trapezium (**Figures 8-8, 8-9**).

The capsules of the carpometacarpal joints are strengthened by carpometacarpal ligaments and the bases of the metacarpal bones are bound by strong transverse interosseous ligaments (**ATLAS PLATE 92**). On the palmar surface, the **radiate carpal ligament** extends from the capitate bone to the bases of the 2nd, 3rd, and 4th metacarpal bones (**ATLAS PLATE 92 #92.2**). The fibrous capsule of the carpometacarpal joint of the thumb is strong but loose and allows great mobility.

The carpometacarpal joints of the fingers are lined by a synovial membrane that forms a single synovial cavity. The capsule of the carpometacarpal joint of the thumb is lined by its own synovial membrane (**ATLAS PLATE 93 #93.3**).

◄ Grant's 568, 569
Netter's 435,436
Rohen 376, 377

Make a transverse incision across the capsule on the dorsum of the wrist between the distal row of carpal bones and bases of the four metacarpal bones (**ATLAS PLATE 93 #93.3**). Palpate the base of the metacarpal bone of the thumb and cut across the capsule between it and the trapezium. Flex the hand and the thumb and observe the synovial cavities of the carpometacarpal joint of the fingers and of the thumb. Note how the **hamate, capitate, and trapezoid** articulate with the four metacarpal bones of the fingers and that the thumb interconnects with its own carpal bone, the **trapezium** (**Figures 8-8, 8-9**).

V. Metacarpophalangeal and Interphalangeal Joints

The five condyloid **metacarpophalangeal joints** are each surrounded by a capsule lined by a synovial membrane (**ATLAS PLATES 92 #92.1, 93 #93.2**). They allow flexion, extension, abduction, and adduction. In contrast, the **interphalangeal joints** are uni-axial hinge joints that do not allow lateral or medial movements; these also are surrounded by fibrous capsules lined by synovial membranes (**ATLAS PLATE 93 #93.2**).

A. Metacarpophalangeal Joints. These joints interconnect the heads of the metacarpal bones within shallow concavities on the proximal phalanges (**ATLAS PLATES 89, 92 #92.1**). Strong **collateral ligaments**

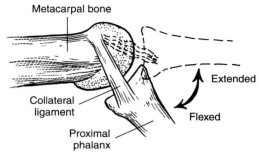

Figure 8-10. The collateral ligament at the metacarpophalangeal joint. Note that this ligament attaches proximally on the dorsal surface of the metacarpal bone but distally on the palmar surface of the proximal phalanx.

are found on the sides of the joint capsules. These ligaments attach to the **dorsal** tubercles of the metacarpal heads, cross the side of the joint obliquely, and attach distally onto the **palmar** aspect of the proximal phalanx (**Figure 8-10**). The capsules are covered dorsally by the extensor expansions, and on their palmar surface are found fibrocartilaginous plates that blend with the **deep transverse metacarpal ligaments** (**ATLAS PLATES 92 #92.2**).

◄ Grant's 551, 570, 573, 574
Netter's 437, 438, 441
Rohen 380, 381

► Grant's 569, 570
Netter's 441
Rohen 381

Dissect either the index or ring finger. Remove the tendons and soft tissues from both palmar and dorsal surfaces and expose the fibrous capsule of the metacarpophalangeal joint (**ATLAS PLATE 92 #92.1**). Dissect the obliquely coursing collateral ligaments on the sides of the joint. Note how they become more taut during flexion than extension (**Figure 8-10**).

B. Interphalangeal Joints. There are nine interphalangeal joints in each hand, two on each finger and one in the thumb. These uni-axial hinge joints allow only flexion and extension. Each joint has two collateral ligaments and a fibrous capsule that is lined by a synovial membrane.

Expose the fibrous capsules of the two interphalangeal joints. Find the collateral ligaments that function similar to those of the metacarpophalangeal joints. Dorsally cut across the capsules, flex the finger, and examine the synovial cavities (**ATLAS PLATE 93 #93.2**).

Clinical Relevance

Shoulder separation. This is a frequent sports injury most often happening in football. It involves the dislocation of the acromion of the scapula, which is thrust beneath the lateral end of the clavicle.

Avulsion of the greater tubercle. This involves the pulling away of the greater tubercle of the humerus from the humeral head, and it often occurs when a person falls on the acromion of the shoulder. It also can occur from a fall on the outstretched abducted hand.

Dislocation of the sternoclavicular joint. This dislocation can be either anterior or posterior; however, it rarely occurs because the clavicle often fractures before the joint dislocates due to the strong sternoclavicular ligaments. When it does occur and the dislocation is posterior, pressure may result on one or more of the large vessels in the superior mediastinum.

Monteggia's fracture. This fracture involves the proximal part of the ulna with the head of the radius dislocated anteriorly at the elbow joint.

Fractured elbow. This is actually a fracture of the olecranon of the ulna and is usually caused by a direct fall on the elbow. The fractured portion of the olecranon is then pulled away from the rest of the ulna by the pull of the triceps muscle.

Elbow dislocation. These dislocations of the ulna are usually posterior at the elbow joint and often result from falling on the outstretched hand. The ulnar collateral ligament is often torn, and fracture of the coronoid process or olecranon may occur.

Fracture of the scaphoid bone. These fractures result in tenderness and pain in the "anatomic snuff box" on the dorsal hand. The proximal fragment of the bone can lose its arterial blood supply that leads to an avascular necrosis after the fracture, because the sole blood supply to the bone enters the distal portion of the bone.

Dislocation of the lunate bone. This injury can be caused by the excessive dorsiflexion of the hand at the wrist joint. The lunate becomes displaced anteriorly and can put pressure on the median nerve within the carpal tunnel.

Thorax I: Anterior Thoracic Wall

OBJECTIVES

1. Review the surface anatomy and bony features of the thoracic wall and visualize the surface projection of the heart, lungs, and reflections of the pleura.

2. Dissect a typical intercostal space—its muscles, vessels, and nerve—and the internal thoracic vessels.

3. Remove much of the anterior thoracic wall as a single plate of bone and muscle, thereby opening the thorax.

4. Understand the pleural reflections and remove the lungs from the thorax.

Atlas Key:

Clemente Atlas 5th Edition = Atlas Plate #

Grant's Atlas 11th Edition = Grant's Page #

Netter's Atlas 3rd Edition = Netter's Plate #

Rohen Atlas 6th Edition = Rohen Page #

The thorax extends between the neck and abdomen. It contains, among other structures, the two lungs enclosed by a membranous sac called the **pleura** (**ATLAS PLATES 114–116**). The lungs are separated on their medial surfaces by a region called the **mediastinum,** within which is found the **heart** and its attached **great vessels** of Posteriorly, the mediastinum also contains the airway to the lungs (**trachea** and **bronchi**) and the **esophagus** leading to the stomach. Also located in the mediastinum are the **thoracic duct,** certain veins (**azygos** and **hemiazygos**), nerves (**vagus** and **splanchnic**), and several lymph nodes (**ATLAS PLATES 126, 128, 170, 171**).

In shape, the bony thorax resembles a truncated cone (**Figure 9-1**). Narrow superiorly at the root of the neck, it expands inferiorly to overlie the abdominal cavity, extending further posteriorly than anteriorly (**ATLAS**

► Grant's 12, 16
Netter's 178, 179, 231
Rohen 192

PLATE 154). Laterally, the rounded thorax follows the curvature of the ribs, and posteriorly it is flattened and overlain by the scapula, muscles of the shoulder, and the vertebral column.

I. Surface Anatomy; Thoracic Vertebrae, Ribs, and Respiratory Movements; Projections of Heart and Lungs Onto the Thoracic Wall

A. **Surface Anatomy and Anterior Thoracic Skeleton.** Because the skin and fascia (including the female breast) have been removed, and the pectoral muscles dissected, focus your review on the surface anatomy of the chest and on the bony thoracic wall. Before proceeding with the dissection, do the following:

1. On an articulated skeleton palpate or identify the following structures (**Figure 9-1**):
   Jugular (suprasternal) Notch
   Manubrium, Body, and Xiphoid Process of the Sternum
   Sternal Angle (of Louis)
   Second Rib and Costal Cartilage
   Infrasternal Angle
   Costal Margin of the Ribs

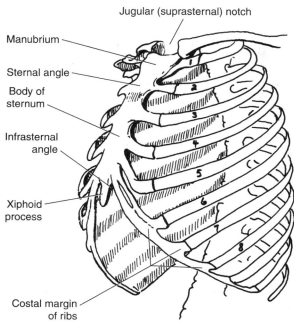

Figure 9-1. The thoracic skeleton: Anterolateral view.

Labels on Figure 9-1:
- Jugular (suprasternal) notch
- Manubrium
- Sternal angle
- Body of sternum
- Infrasternal angle
- Xiphoid process
- Costal margin of ribs

► Grant's 10, 22 Netter's 182, 183 Rohen 192 196, 208

► Grant's 10, 11 Netter's 178 Rohen 188, 189

► Grant's 10, 22 Netter's 178, 179, 183 Rohen 189, 192

◄ Netter's 260 Rohen 217

2. On the cadaver, visualize the following clinically useful imaginary lines (**Figure 9-2**; **ATLAS PLATE 2 #2.1**):
Mid-sternal Line
Lateral Sternal Line and Parasternal Line
Mid-clavicular Line
Anterior and Posterior Axillary Lines
Mid-axillary Line

3. Palpate the 2nd rib from its articulation on the sternum at the sternal angle to the anterior axillary line; then, count the ribs and intercostal spaces down to the 9th or 10th rib. **Realize that the intercostal space is numbered similar to the rib just above it (ATLAS PLATE 102).**

4. On an articulated skeleton, observe that the highly curved first ribs articulate with the vertebral column posteriorly and the manubrium of the sternum anteriorly, outlining the narrow **superior aperture of the thorax (ATLAS PLATES 104, 105)**. Note that the ribs become longer as does the width and cross-sectional area of the thorax (**Figure 9-1**).

5. Note that below the 6th rib the thorax continues to increase in width to its inferior aperture where the diaphragm separates the thorax from the abdomen (**ATLAS PLATE 154**).

6. Observe on **ATLAS PLATE 104 #104.1** that the costal margins, the 12th ribs, and the 12th thoracic vertebra outline the inferior aperture, and that the diaphragm closes this aperture as shown in mid-sagittal section (**ATLAS PLATE 173 #173.1**) and frontal section (**ATLAS PLATE 154**). Through the diaphragm course structures that pass between the mediastinum and the abdomen.

B. **Thoracic Vertebrae, Ribs, and Respiratory Movements.** The ribs and sternum afford some protection to the vital organs within the thorax, but

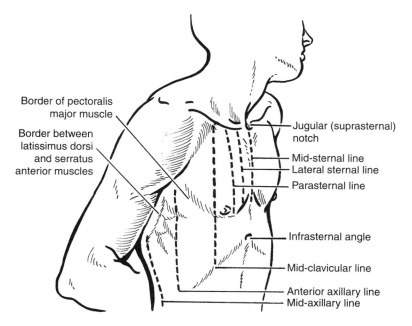

Labels on Figure 9-2:
- Border of pectoralis major muscle
- Border between latissimus dorsi and serratus anterior muscles
- Jugular (suprasternal) notch
- Mid-sternal line
- Lateral sternal line
- Parasternal line
- Infrasternal angle
- Mid-clavicular line
- Anterior axillary line
- Mid-axillary line

Figure 9-2. Imaginary longitudinal lines on the anterior surface of the thorax.

the principal active function of the ribs relates to the movements of the thorax during breathing. These movements increase intrathoracic volume during **inspiration** when air is pulled into the lungs, and the diaphragm descends as it contracts. During **expiration,** the ribs decrease intrathoracic volume, the diaphragm ascends as it relaxes, and air is expelled from the lungs.

1. **Thoracic vertebrae and ribs.** The heads of the ribs articulate with the thoracic vertebrae posteriorly.

▶
Grant's 10, 11
Netter's 178
Rohen 188, 189,
192

On an articulated skeleton, study the manner by which the thoracic vertebrae articulate with the head and neck of the ribs (**ATLAS PLATES 347 #347.5, 348, 349**).

▶
Grant's 11
Netter's 178, 179
Rohen 189, 192

On a thoracic vertebra, identify the flat weight-bearing vertebral body that is continuous on each side by way of **pedicles** to the **transverse processes.** Note that the transverse processes are continuous with the **laminae of the vertebral arch** and these join the long triangular **spinous process** posteriorly. These bony structures surround the vertebral canal wherein is located the spinal cord (**ATLAS PLATE 347 #347.1–347.5**).

◀
Grant's 286, 287
Netter's 147, 180
Rohen 192, 197

Study also a typical thoracic rib (such as the 8th rib) shown in **ATLAS PLATE 106.** Identify its **head, neck,** and **tubercle.** Note how the **body** of the rib bends ventrally at the angle and becomes twisted on its long axis.

a. On the lateral aspect of the vertebral body, find two articular facets (**ATLAS PLATE 347 #347.3**) that accommodate the **head of the rib** and the single facet on the transverse process (**ATLAS PLATE 347 #347.1, #347.3**) that articulates with the tubercle of the rib.

▶
Netter's 191
Rohen 196

b. Turn to **ATLAS PLATE 349 #349.1** and observe how the articular facets on the head of the rib articulate with **two** adjacent vertebral bodies, one facet on each body. These form the synovial **joints of the head of the rib.**

c. Still visualizing a thoracic vertebra and a rib, observe in **ATLAS PLATE 348 #348.1** how the tubercle of the neck of the rib articulates with the transverse process of the thoracic vertebra, forming the synovial lined **costotransverse joint.** Collectively, the **joints of the head of the ribs** and the **costotransverse joints** are called the **costovertebral joints.**

◀
Grant's 10, 11,
13–15
Netter's 178, 179
Rohen 188, 190,
192, 197

d. Observe that an articulated thorax consists of the 12 thoracic vertebrae posteriorly and the sternum anteriorly. These vertically oriented structures are interconnected by 10 pairs of ribs, with two pairs of floating ribs attached only to the vertebral column (**ATLAS PLATES 104, 105**). Observe that the bony ribs continue anteriorly as costal cartilages. The costal cartilages of the upper seven pairs of ribs attach directly onto the sternum (**ATLAS PLATE 105 #105.2, #105.3**).

e. Note that the first pair of ribs attaches to the upper lateral aspect of the manubrium; the 2nd at the **sternal angle** (junction of the manubrium and body of the sternum); the 3rd, 4th, 5th, and 6th attach to the body of the sternum; and the 7th to the articulation between the body of the sternum and the xiphoid process. The costal cartilages of the 8th, 9th, and 10th ribs ascend anteriorly and join to form the **costal margin,** which attaches to the lower border of the costal cartilage of the 7th rib (**ATLAS PLATE 104 #104.1**). The 11th and 12th ribs articulate only posteriorly on the 11th and 12th thoracic vertebrae and are known as "floating ribs."

f. Note the downward slope of the ribs from the vertebrae posteriorly (**ATLAS PLATES, 103, 105**). On an articulated skeleton, observe that a plane projected backward from the sternal angle passes between the 4th and 5th thoracic vertebrae posteriorly.

2. **Respiratory movements.** Contraction and relaxation of the diaphragm, the intercostal muscles, and the accessory muscles of respiration move the ribs during respiration. Because the anterior ends of the ribs are lower than the posterior portions, when the shafts of the ribs are elevated and the diaphragm descends during inspiration, the anterior parts of the ribs and sternum are elevated in a forward direction (**Figure 9-3**). The shafts of the ribs are depressed backward during expiration. This up and down movement is the so-called **"pump handle movement"** that increases the anterior posterior diameter of the thorax in inspiration and decreases the diameter in expiration.

Simultaneously, the transverse diameter of the thorax is increased during inspiration as the ribs rotate at the costovertebral joints, elevating their most lateral portions. This is especially true for the 7th, 8th, 9th, and 10th ribs. Sometimes called the "bucket handle movement," the action resembles the lifting and lowering of the semicircular handle often seen at the top of a bucket (**Figure 9-4**).

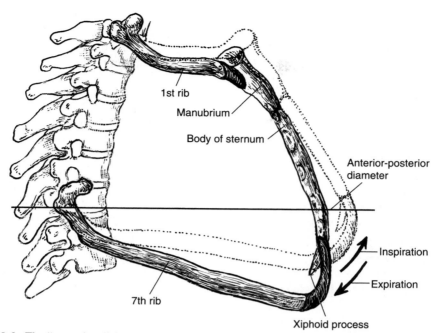

Figure 9-3. The "pump handle" movement of the sternum and ribs that increases and decreases the anterior–posterior diameter of the thorax during breathing (lateral view).

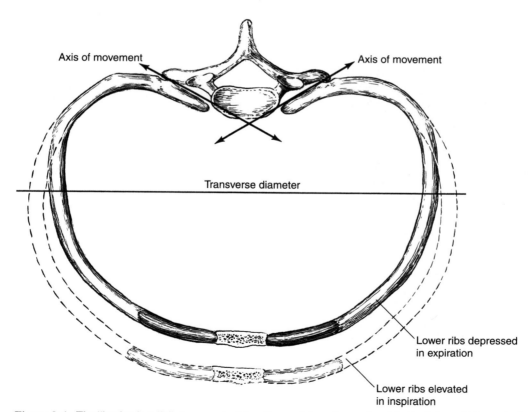

Figure 9-4. The "bucket handle" movement of the rib cage takes place only with ribs 8, 9, and 10 attached to the costal margin. In full inspiration, the transverse diameter of the rib cage is increased because of the elevation of the lower ribs; during expiration, it is decreased in a manner similar to lifting and dropping the handle of a bucket.

C. Projections of the Heart, Great Vessels, Pleura, and Lungs Onto the Anterior Thoracic Wall. The **heart** is centrally positioned in the thorax within the **middle mediastinum.** It is clinically valuable to be able to visualize on the surface of the thoracic wall the approximate location of the heart. Several key points on the chest allow you to project the position of the heart in the thorax (**Figure 9-5**).

◄
Grant's 26, 44, 48, 92
Netter's 278
Rohen 252

1. Projection of the heart (ATLAS PLATES 129, 131 #131.1).

Use a marking pencil on the cadaver (or on the thoracic wall of a friend) and locate the following:

a. A point 9 cm to the left of the midsternal line in the 5th intercostal space, the approximate site of the **apex of the heart.**

b. A point 2.5 cm lateral to the **left margin of the sternum** in the 2nd intercostal space. By inter-connecting this point with the apex, the **left margin** of the heart is outlined (**Figure 9-5**).

c. Draw a line from a point 1 cm lateral to the **right sternal margin** in the 2nd intercostal space to the 6th rib. This line defines the **right margin of the heart.**

d. Interconnect the right margin of the heart at the 6th rib and the apex of the heart through the xiphisternal junction. This defines the **lower border of the heart.**

e. Finally, interconnect the upper ends of the margins across the midline in the 2nd intercostal space. This represents the **base of the heart (Figure 9-5).**

►
Grant's 26, 30, 31
Netter's 192, 193
Rohen 248

2. Projection of the region containing the great vessels (ATLAS PLATE 129). It is of clinical importance, at times, to visualize the area on the

◄
Grant's 26, 48
Netter's 192
Rohen 252, 255

anterior thoracic wall where the great vessels (superior vena cava, aorta, pulmonary artery, and pulmonary veins) extend from the base of the heart.

Extend the right and left margins of the heart upward by **2 inches** beyond the transverse 2nd intercostal space line. Draw another transverse line across the sternum between these extended margins. This outlines an area approximately 2 inches (5 cm) square that reaches the upper border of the manubrium superiorly. Deep to this site are located the great vessels within the superior mediastinum.

3. Projections of parietal pleura and lungs (ATLAS PLATE 114 #114.1). Reflection lines of the lungs and parietal pleura may also be drawn on the surface of the thorax.

a. **Projection of parietal pleura (Figure 9-6).** Outline the parietal pleura on the **right side.**

1) Commence 2.5 cm (1 inch) above the right clavicle in the neck 4 cm (1½ inches) lateral to the right sterno-clavicular joint where the **cupula of the pleura** extends.

2) Carry the line downward and medially to the sternal angle in the midsternal line.

3) Continue the line down the middle of the sternum to the xiphisternal junction.

4) Direct the line laterally to the right along the border of the costal margin to the **mid-clavicular line** (at the level of the 8th rib), the **mid-axillary line** (10th rib), and the **vertebral column** posteriorly (12th rib).

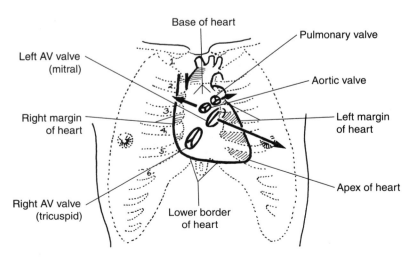

Figure 9-5. Projection of the heart and its valves onto the anterior surface of the rib cage. AV, atrioventricular.

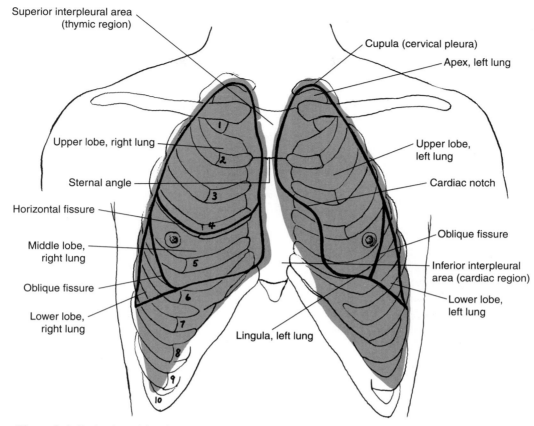

Figure 9-6. Projection of the pleural cavity and lungs onto the anterior surface of the rib cage. The pleural cavity is shown in red. The lungs extend to ribs 6, 8, and 10, whereas the pleura extends to ribs 8, 10, and 12 in the midclavicular, midaxillary, and posterior lines.

5) On the **left side,** draw the pleura comparably to the right. From the cupula anteriorly descend to approximately the 4th rib where the pleura curves laterally away from the midline to form a notch of 2 inches in diameter for the pericardium.

6) Continue the line along the costal margin around to the posterior chest at the same levels as on the right side (**ATLAS PLATES 114–116**).

b. Projection of the lungs (Figure 9-6).

1) As with the pleura, commence in the neck 2.5 cm above the clavicle and 4 cm lateral to the sternoclavicular joints where the apex of each lung occupies the cupula of the pleural sac (**ATLAS PLATE 114 #114.1**).

2) From this site draw the anterior borders of the two lungs just lateral to the midsternal lines taken by the pleura.

◄
Grant's 30, 31
Netter's 192, 193, 196
Rohen 247, 248

3) On the right side, draw the anterior border downward to the xiphisternal junction.

4) On the left side, draw a notch in the anterior margin of the left lung at the level of the 4th rib that deviates 5 cm (2 inches) to the left (**Figure 9-6**).

5) Draw the inferior borders of the lungs two ribs above the lines of the parietal pleura: the **6th rib** at the **midclavicular line,** the **8th rib** in the **midaxillary** line, and the **10th rib** in the **midportion of the back** (**ATLAS PLATES 114–116**).

The notch on the left side accommodates the heart and pericardium where it lies directly under the thoracic wall uncovered by lung tissue. Upon percussion here, a dull sound results rather than the resonant tone found over lung tissue containing air, and therefore, is called the area of **superficial cardiac dullness** (**ATLAS PLATES 113, 128, 129**).

II. Anterior Thoracic Wall: Muscles, Vessels, and Nerves

A. **Muscles of the Anterior Thoracic Wall.** In addition to the **pectoralis major** and **minor** that overlie the ribs, the **serratus anterior** arises laterally from the upper eight or nine ribs. Extending between the ribs are the **external, internal,** and **innermost intercostal muscles (ATLAS PLATES 110, 111).** Other neck muscles attaching to the clavicle or upper ribs (**scalene, infrahyoid, sternocleidomastoid,** and **subclavius**) will not be considered now. The **transverse thoracis muscle** will be seen on the inner surface of the anterior thoracic wall after the chest plate is removed (**ATLAS PLATE 110**).

> Cut away any remnants of the pectoralis major and minor muscles. More laterally, remove the fleshy digitations of the serratus anterior muscle that attach to the 3rd, 4th, and 5th ribs (**ATLAS PLATE 102**). Try to retain the lateral cutaneous branches of the intercostal nerves as they emerge between the ribs in the midaxillary line.

B. **Intercostal Muscles, Nerves, and Vessels.** The **external, internal,** and **innermost** intercostal muscles within the intercostal spaces are joined by the intercostal artery, vein, and nerve. The nerve and vessels course between the internal intercostal muscle and the innermost layer (**Figure 9-7**).

> Dissect at least one intercostal space and others, if necessary, to see the important intercostal structures. There are 11 intercostal spaces on each side and, therefore, 22 **external intercostal muscles.** Dissect an external intercostal muscle for 3 or 4 inches between the midaxillary and midclavicular lines. Note that their fibers course inferomedially, in the same direction as putting your hands in your pockets. Each external intercostal muscle commences posteriorly at the tubercle of the rib. Note that the muscular tissue is replaced by the glistening **external intercostal membrane** anteriorly (**ATLAS PLATE 102**).
>
> Sever the external intercostal membrane and its muscle along the upper border of the rib below, and reflect the membrane and muscle fibers superiorly. This will expose the **internal intercostal muscle** whose fibers course inferolaterally at right angles to those of the external intercostal muscles.

There are also 22 internal intercostal muscles, and they extend between the sternum anteriorly and the angle of the rib posteriorly. Between the angle of the

▶
Grant's 17–20, 476
Netter's 182, 183, 187
Rohen 196, 207–209, 397

◀
Grant's 22
Netter's 182, 183, 185
Rohen 208–211

▶
Grant's 20, 94
Netter's 184, 249, 250
Rohen 115, 214, 206

◀
Grant's 20–23
Netter's 183, 184
Rohen 196, 208–211

rib and the vertebral column, the muscle tissue continues as the thin **internal intercostal membranes** (**ATLAS PLATE 162**). The posterior portions of the intercostal spaces will be seen within the thorax after the lungs and heart have been removed (**ATLAS PLATE 335**).

> Identify the **lateral cutaneous branch** of an intercostal nerve coursing through its intercostal space in the midaxillary line (**Figure 9-7**). Trace the branch back through the intercostal muscles to the main trunk of the **intercostal nerve** located deep to the internal intercostal muscle along the lower border of the rib. **By carefully dissecting away the lower part of the rib along its margin with a pair of rongeurs or bone cutters,** find the intercostal artery and vein. Note that these vessels course around the thorax deep to the rib but slightly superior to the intercostal nerve. Confirm that the vein is superior and the nerve inferior, and that between these the intercostal artery is located (**Figure 9-8**). Clinically, it is safe to introduce a needle or a trochar into the thorax immediately above the **upper border** of a rib. You should avoid the lower rib borders along which the neurovascular structures course (**Figure 9-8**).

The eleven intercostal nerves are formed by the anterior primary rami of the T1 to T11 spinal nerves. The 12th thoracic nerve is the **subcostal nerve** and courses below the 12th rib. The typical spinal nerve is **mixed,** containing both sensory and motor fibers, and it is formed by the junction of dorsal and ventral roots from a single spinal cord segment. Immediately after the roots are joined, the spinal nerve divides into a **posterior primary ramus** and an **anterior primary ramus.**

The **posterior primary ramus** courses dorsally to supply the deep musculature of the back. It then pierces the superficial muscles (which it does not supply) to become cutaneous. The **anterior primary ramus** sends communicating branches with the **sympathetic nerve trunk (ATLAS PLATES 8 #8.1, 162, 255**) and enters the intercostal space accompanied by an **intercostal artery** off the aorta and **an intercostal vein (Figure 9-7**).

In the midaxillary line, **lateral cutaneous branches** of the nerve, artery, and vein course through the intercostal muscles to become superficial. The main trunks of the intercostal nerve and vessels continue around the intercostal space to the lateral border of the sternum where their **anterior cutaneous branches** become superficial (**ATLAS PLATE 8 #8.1; Figure 9-9**).

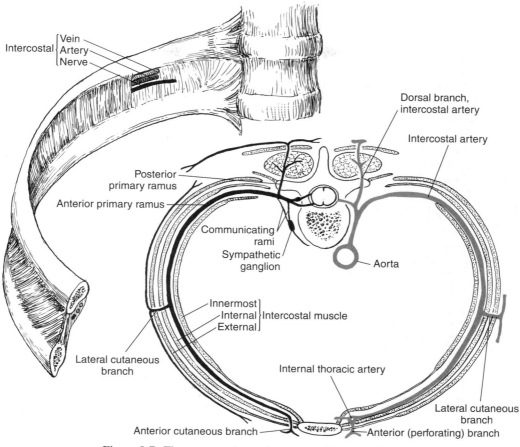

Figure 9-7. The nerves and vessels in a typical intercostal space.

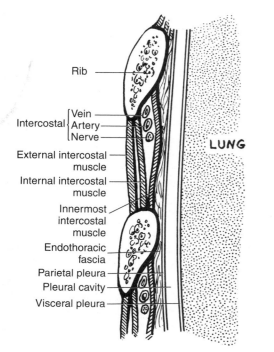

Figure 9-8. Vertical section through an intercostal space.

▶
Grant's 8, 20, 22
Netter's 183, 187,
247, 248
Rohen 209, 214,
215

C. Internal Thoracic Vessels. The **internal thoracic artery** arises from the first part of the subclavian artery, and descends on the inner surface of the anterior thoracic wall, $\frac{1}{2}$ inch lateral to the border of the sternum (**ATLAS PLATE 16 #16.2**). Below the 6th costal cartilage, it divides into the **musculophrenic** and **superior epigastric arteries** (**ATLAS PLATE 111**). As the internal thoracic artery descends, it sends **anterior intercostal branches** that anastomose in the anterior part of the intercostal spaces with the intercostal arteries coursing around the thoracic wall (**ATLAS PLATE 111**). In women the internal thoracic artery gives off (internal) **mammary branches** that help supply the breast. The artery is accompanied by paired **internal thoracic veins** and an important chain of parasternal lymph nodes that help drain the breast.

At the lateral border of the sternum, remove the intercostal muscles and membranes for a distance of approximately 3 inches from the anterior parts of the

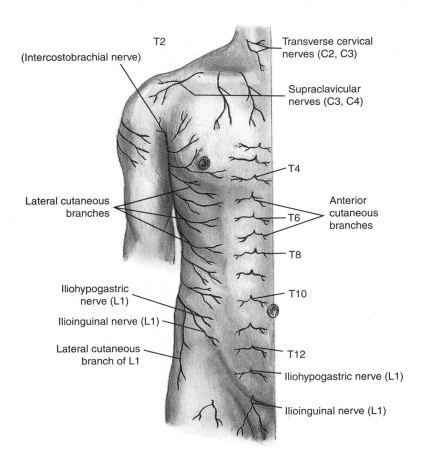

T2
(Intercostobrachial nerve)

Transverse cervical
nerves (C2, C3)

Supraclavicular
nerves (C3, C4)

T4

Lateral cutaneous
branches

Anterior
cutaneous
branches

T6

T8

Iliohypogastric
nerve (L1)

T10

Ilioinguinal nerve (L1)

Lateral cutaneous
branch of L1

T12

Iliohypogastric nerve (L1)

Ilioinguinal nerve (L1)

Figure 9-9. Spinal nerves on the lateral and anterior thoracic (and abdominal) wall.

4th, 5th, and 6th intercostal spaces. Dissect free the internal thoracic vessels descending 1/2 inch lateral to the sternum (**ATLAS PLATES 9, 16 #16.2, 111**). Behind the 5th and 6th intercostal spaces, look for the division of the artery into its two terminal branches (see above). On the inner surface of the anterior thoracic wall, identify the parietal pleura laterally and (on the left side) the external surface of the pericardium.

III. Removal of the Anterior Thoracic Wall

To enter the thoracic cavity, it is necessary to remove much of the anterior thoracic wall. This is done in one piece (**Figure 9-10**).

Expose the parietal pleura that lies deep to the ribs (costal pleura) by removing the muscles and membranes from several intercostal spaces. Moisten the pleura with a small amount of water and, with your gloved fingers, gently push the parietal pleura away

◄
Grant's 23, 26, 30
Netter's 184, 192, 194
Rohen 206, 264, 265

from the inner surface of the ribs. Continue this procedure medially and separate the pleura from the deep surface of the sternum.

Using a hand saw, cut across the manubrium of the sternum between the attachments of the 1st and 2nd pairs of ribs. Try not to tear the underlying pleura as you separate it from the inner rib surface (**Figure 9-10**). Sever the 2nd through the 6th ribs on both sides along the anterior axillary line with bone cutters. Divide the sternum just below the attachments of the 6th ribs. Sever the soft tissues across the 1st and 6th intercostal spaces on both sides and remove the bony plate by separating it from the parietal pleura attached to its inner surface (**Figure 9-10**). **BE CAREFUL NOT TO CUT YOUR FINGERS ON THE SHARP EDGES OF THE SEVERED RIBS.**

On the inner surface of the bony plate, identify the five or six muscle fascicles that comprise the **transverse thoracis muscle** (**ATLAS PLATE 111**). Note also the cut internal thoracic vessels descending on the inner aspect of the anterior thoracic wall.

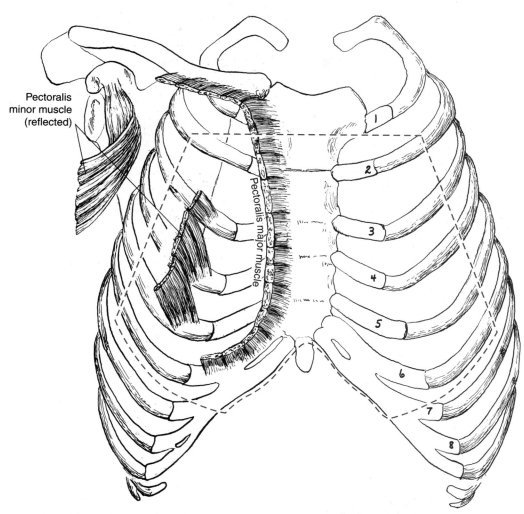

Pectoralis
minor muscle
(reflected)

Pectoralis major muscle

Figure 9-10. Anterior chest wall to be removed to gain access to thoracic viscera.

IV. Pleura and Thoracic Viscera in Place; Removal of the Lungs

Before removing the lungs, consider the relationships of the viscera in the undisturbed chest (**ATLAS PLATE 113**). A detailed examination of the pleura will be made on removal of the lungs.

> Observe that the lungs, surrounded by pleural sacs, occupy the two large lateral cavities of the thorax and between the cavities is a region called the **mediastinum** (**Figure 9-11**). From this anterior aspect, locate the superficial bare area of the pericardium not covered by lung tissue (**ATLAS PLATE 109**). Observe a small amount of fatty tissue, the remnant of the **thymus gland,** overlying the brachiocephalic veins and other great vessels in the **superior mediastinum** (**ATLAS PLATE 113**).

◄
Grant's 25, 30, 31, 64
Netter's 192–194
Rohen 243, 244, 248, 265–267

During development, the lungs invaginate the mesenchyme that occupies the thoracic cavities, and they become tightly and completely surrounded by a layer of mesenchymal cells, the **visceral pleura.** The walls of the thoracic cavities into which the lungs grow become lined by a layer of mesenchyme to form the **parietal pleura.**

The adult parietal pleura is a continuous sheet of mesothelial cells and has distinctive names depending on the surfaces to which it adheres. Covering the inner surface of the ribs is the **costal pleura.** Reflected over the organs between the lungs is the **mediastinal pleura,** and that applied to the diaphragm is called the **diaphragmatic pleura (ATLAS PLATES 114, 115).** An extension of the parietal pleura over the apex of the lung into the neck is the **cervical pleura** or **cupula** (**ATLAS PLATE 114 #114.**). The mediastinal part of the parietal pleura at the root of each lung becomes continuous with the visceral pleura that adheres snugly to the lungs. Pleura extending downward to the

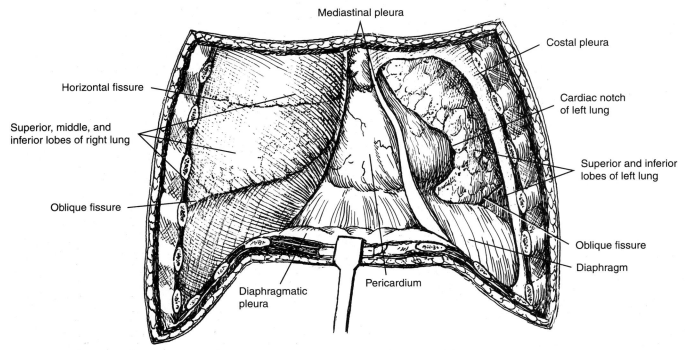

Figure 9-11. The inferior part of the opened thorax.

diaphragm from the root of the lung forms the two-layered **pulmonary ligament (ATLAS PLATE 108).**

On removal of the chest plate, most dissections will already have opened the pleural cavities **(Figure 9-11)**. With your gloved hand, explore the costal, mediastinal, and diaphragmatic reflections of the parietal pleura **(ATLAS PLATES 114–116)**.

Call an instructor for assistance if it is not possible for you to separate the parietal pleura from the visceral pleura and lung because of adhesions that occurred during life.

The **costomediastinal** and **costodiaphragmatic recesses** are extensions of the pleural cavities, which the lungs do not fill except at full inspiration. The costomediastinal recesses are located on each side along the anterior margins of the pleura **(ATLAS PLATES 114–116)**. The **costodiaphragmatic recesses** are found on each side along the lower margins of the pleura where the costal and diaphragmatic parts of the parietal pleura are continuous **(ATLAS PLATES 113–116)**.

Identify the left costomediastinal recess and palpate the anterior surface of the lungs downward until you reach the reflection of parietal pleura over the diaphragm **(ATLAS PLATES 101, 102)**. Explore this inferior margin in the costodiaphragmatic

◄
Grant's 65, 66
Netter's 192, 195,
226, 227
Rohen 249

▶
Grant's 48, 78,
65, 762
Netter's 170, 207,
208, 226, 227
Rohen 269–272,
275

◄
Grant's 28, 71, 155
Netter's 188, 192,
193, 542
Rohen 248, 255

recess as far laterally as the midaxillary line where the recess is deepest.

Pull the anterior margins of the lungs laterally and expose their medial surfaces and the roots of the lungs attached to the mediastinum **(ATLAS PLATE 101)**. Push the medial surfaces of the lungs laterally away from the mediastinum. Identify the **phrenic nerves** and **pericardiocophrenic vessels** that descend along the lateral surfaces of the pericardium **(ATLAS PLATES 130 #130.1, 134, 135)**. Avoid severing these nerves and vessels as you **transect the root of each lung with a scalpel close to the mediastinal surface.** Do not injure any mediastinal structure.

The lungs may now be removed from the chest by reaching around the lung to its posterior surface and pulling it forward. Place the organs in a plastic bag for study in the next dissection period.

Clinical Relevance

Dislocation of ribs. Usually this condition is the dislocation of the cartilaginous portion of the rib from the sternum at the sternocostal joint. Ribs 8, 9, and 10 form the smooth cartilaginous inferior border of the thoracic cage by articulating with the cartilage of the 7th rib. At these sites dislocation of the intercartilaginous joints could perforate the diaphragm and injure the underlying liver or spleen.

Rib fracture. Fracture of ribs is usually caused by severe trauma to the chest. Normally the first rib does not fracture; most frequently ribs 3 to 7 are the most vulnerable to fracture. The sharp edges of a fractured rib can penetrate the pleural cavity, causing a pneumothorax and injury to the lung. If the lower ribs fracture (ribs 10 to 12) the diaphragm may be torn even to the point of producing a diaphragmatic hernia.

Flail chest. This condition results from multiple rib fractures and can severely impair breathing. The fractured rib segments can move with inspiration and expiration. This painful condition usually requires surgical repair.

Pleural cavity. The pleural cavity normally is a potential space between the parietal and visceral pleural coverings of the lungs. If the cavity is perforated by a needle or trochar and air enters the pleural cavity, the lung collapses and a pneumothorax develops. If blood enters the pleural cavity from a traumatic injury, breathing can be compromised by a hemothorax.

Costochondritis. This inflammation occurs at the junction between the bony part of the rib and the cartilaginous portion of the rib. It can also develop between the cartilaginous part of the rib and the bony sternum.

Supraclavicular nerves. Supraclavicular nerves (C3, C4) descend over the clavicle to supply the skin of the first two intercostal spaces. Pain from gall-stones in the biliary tract can be referred to these cervical nerves and be perceived from the lateral sternal region to the acromion. Below the 2nd intercostal space segmental dermatomes supplied by nerves T2 to T12 innervate not only the intercostal muscles but also the sensory segmental fields. T4 or T5 supplies the region of the nipple, whereas T10 supplies the region of the umbilicus.

Apex of the lung. The apex of the lung extends above the first rib and the clavicle to lie in the root of the neck. Overlying the apex of the lung is the cervical dome of the pleura (sometimes called Sibson's fascia). Lesions at this site, such as stab wounds or needle punctures, can result in pneumothorax.

Intercostal space relationships. The intercostal nerves and vessels course close to the inferior border of the ribs or deep to the bone inferiorly. Thus, the superior border of the rib is safe being free of vessels and nerves; however, the inferior border is less safe. Intercostal nerve blocks to produce analgesia of the anterior or lateral chest wall should be done posterior to the midaxillary line before the lateral cutaneous nerve branches from the intercostal nerve.

Thoracocentesis or pleural tap. This procedure is done through an intercostal space to aspirate serous fluid or blood from the pleural cavity. Normally this is performed in the 6th to 8th intercostal spaces slightly posterior to the midaxillary line. Done at the superior border of the ribs avoids the intercostal vessels and nerve

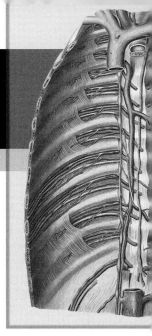

DISSECTION #10

Thorax II: Pleura and Lungs; Anterior Mediastinum; Middle Mediastinum and Pericardium; Removal of the Heart

OBJECTIVES

1 Understand the development of the pleural reflections.

2 Examine the anatomy of the two lungs and visualize their surfaces, borders, and fissures.

3 Study the hilum of each lung; expose the lobar and segmental bronchi and the pulmonary vessels at the hila.

4 Understand the subdivisions of the mediastinum.

5 Examine the anterior mediastinum.

6 Dissect the phrenic nerves and pericardiacophrenic vessels.

7 Open the pericardium; study the fibrous pericardium and understand the reflections of the serous pericardium.

8 Sever the great vessels and remove the heart from the pericardial sac.

I. Pleural Reflections

The pleurae are closed invaginated sacs consisting of serous membranes that cover the surface of the lungs (visceral layer). At the hilum the pleura reflects on itself and lines the inner surface of the corresponding half of the chest wall (parietal layer).

By visualizing the development of the lungs into the thoracic cavity, the formation of the parietal and visceral pleura and the pleural cavities between the layers can easily be understood (**Figure 10-1**). During the 4th prenatal week, the two lung buds grow laterally from the developing laryngotracheal tube into mesenchymal tissue within the thoracic cavities and form the two primary bronchi. During the 5th week, the buds enlarge and differentiate into two secondary bronchi on the left and three on the right and then into tertiary (segmental) bronchi. As each developing lung invaginates into the mesenchyme, it acquires a layer of mesenchymal cells that completely surrounds it, and this becomes the **visceral pleura (Figure 10-1A)**.

The growing lungs surrounded by visceral pleura fill the thoracic cavities and conform to their shape. The inner surfaces of these cavities, i.e., **costal** (deep to the ribs anteriorly, laterally, and posteriorly), **diaphragmatic** (inferiorly), **mediastinal** (medially), and **cervical** (superiorly, the **cupula**) become lined by somatic mesenchyme

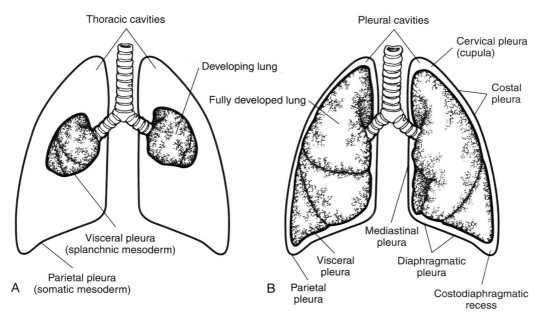

Figure 10-1. Diagrammatic schema of **(A)** the developing lungs and pleura, and **(B)** the adult lungs and pleura. Note how the developing lungs surrounded by visceral pleura eventually grow, thereby reducing the pleural cavity between visceral and parietal pleurae to a potential space.

to become the **parietal pleura (Figure 10-1B).** The mediastinal part forms a collar-like reflection around the structures at the root of the lung and becomes continuous with the visceral pleura that covers the lung. The visceral and parietal pleurae (continuous at the root of the lungs) are closely apposed elsewhere in the thoracic cavities. The potential space between them is moistened by tissue fluid and is called the **pleural cavity (Figure 10-1B).**

After removing the lungs, examine the reflections of the parietal pleura within the thoracic cage. Observe that the **costal pleura** completely lines the rib cage and sternum (**ATLAS PLATES 114–116**) and that it is thicker than the **mediastinal pleura** situated medially. Note on the dorsomedial wall that the costal pleura reflects anteriorly to become the mediastinal pleura.

Palpate the **diaphragmatic pleura** inferiorly as it covers much of the upper and lateral portions of the diaphragm (**ATLAS PLATES 113, 114**). Observe that it is continuous with the costal pleura and with the mediastinal pleura. Palpate the uppermost extent of the pleura, called the **cervical pleura or cupola,** as it projects upward above the clavicle into the root of the neck to overlie the apex of the lung (**ATLAS PLATES 114–116**).

Two points about the cervical pleura and the apex of the lung are important: (1) the cervical pleura is covered

◄
Grant's 26, 30, 64, 67
Netter's 192, 193, 195, 226, 227
Rohen 248, 264–266

◄
Grant's 64–67
Netter's 198, 200, 236, 237

by a layer of dense fascia that stretches between the 7th cervical vertebra and the first rib called the **suprapleural membrane** (or Sibson's fascia), AND (2) the arch of the subclavian artery (and vein) passes anterior to the suprapleural membrane, cervical pleura, and apex of the lung (**ATLAS PLATES 114–116**).

II. Lungs

Your study of the lungs should include (a) a visual inspection and palpation of the surfaces, borders, fissures and the impressions of other organs made on the surfaces of both lungs (**ATLAS PLATES 118, 120**) and (b) a dissection of the hilum (root) of both lungs.

The surface of the adult lung presents a mottled appearance with varying degrees of gray and black pigmentation from the carbon particles trapped within its phagocytes. The nondiseased lung is light, spongy, elastic, and crepitant to the touch because of air in the alveoli. The lungs are nearly conical in shape, but in the embalmed cadaver, they assume the shape of the pleural cavities. The right lung is generally slightly larger and heavier than the left.

A. Right Lung (ATLAS PLATES 118 #118.2, 120 #120.2). The right lung consists of three lobes. These are separated by an **oblique fissure** between the inferior and middle lobes and a **horizontal fissure** between the superior and middle lobes.

Hold the right lung over the right part of the thoracic cavity in its normal orientation, with the **anterior margin** oriented ventrally, the **apex** superiorly, and the **base** or **diaphragmatic surface** inferiorly. Identify the three lobes, superior, middle, and inferior. Separate the superior and middle lobes along the **horizontal fissure,** and probe the **oblique fissure** where it descends from the horizontal fissure to separate the middle and inferior lobes **(Figure 10-2).**

► Grant's 33, 34 Netter's 195, 197 Rohen 249, 251

Follow the oblique fissure medially and observe that it continues through the organ to the hilum **(ATLAS PLATE 120 #120.2).** Determine whether the horizontal fissure separates the middle and inferior lobes as far as the hilum. Note that it is incomplete in nearly two-thirds of the specimens.

◄ Grant's 25, 32 Netter's 192, 194 Rohen 243, 244, 249

Palpate the **costal surface** of the right lung. Note that its rounded contour comprises the area adjacent to the chest wall from the sternum to the vertebral column **(ATLAS PLATE 118 #118.2).** Examine the concave **diaphragmatic surface** at the base of the right lung and observe that it overlies the dome of the diaphragm **(ATLAS PLATE 120 #120.2).**

◄ Grant's 25, 30–32 Netter's 192–194, 197 Rohen 243, 249

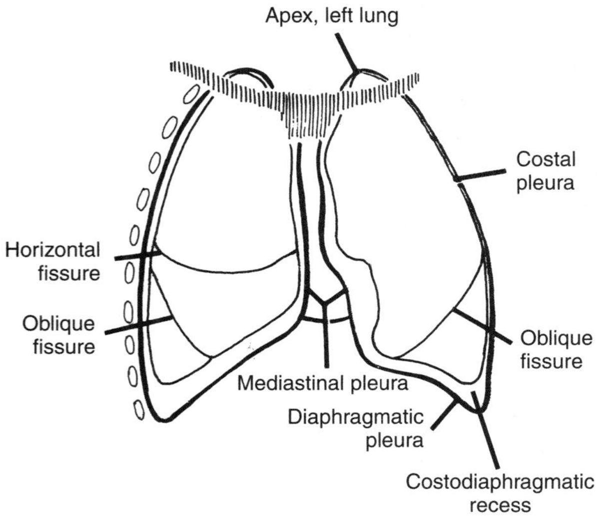

Turn to the **mediastinal surface** and note that it is slightly concave inferiorly to accommodate the heart and pericardium **(ATLAS PLATE 120 #120.2).** Posterior to the depression for the heart, identify the **hilum,** or **root,** of the lung within which is found the cut **right bronchus** and the **pulmonary artery** and **veins.** Just above the hilum can be found the arched sulcus made by the **azygos vein.** More difficult to see are the vertically oriented grooves

made by the superior vena cava and the right subclavian artery.

At the hilum of the right lung, find the bronchus located most dorsally **(Figure 10-3).** This can be distinguished from the blood vessels because of its position and because its cartilaginous wall is hard. Note that the right **primary bronchus** divides quickly into superior, middle, and inferior **lobar bronchi.** Locate the **pulmonary artery** just anterior to the bronchi. Note that the superior lobe bronchus lies *above the pulmonary artery* and is often called the **eparterial bronchus,** whereas the bronchus for the middle and inferior lobes branches *below the pulmonary artery* and is called the **hyparterial bronchus (ATLAS PLATE 120 #120.2).** Identify the **pulmonary veins.** These are usually located anterior and inferior to the other structures at the hilum **(Figure 10-3).**

B. Left Lung (Figures 10-2, 10-4). The left lung is divided into superior and inferior lobes by the **oblique fissure.** A small portion of the superior lobe at the lower border of the cardiac notch is called the **lingula** of the left upper lobe.

► Grant's 25, 26, 30–32 Netter's 190, 192–194 Rohen 249, 251

Examine the left lung by inspecting it in the same orientation as it exists in the left thoracic cavity during life. Position the **anterior margin** anteriorly with the **apex** of the lung directed superiorly and the **diaphragmatic surface** inferiorly **(ATLAS PLATE 118 #118.1).** Separate the superior and (the larger) inferior lobes by probing along the **oblique fissure,** which courses to the costal surface above and below the hilum of the left lung **(ATLAS PLATE 120 #120.2).** Also observe this fissure on the costal surface as it passes anteroinferiorly to the **base** of the lung. Note that the **apex** of the left lung and the **anterior border** are parts of the superior lobe, but the **base** (or diaphragmatic surface) is part of the inferior lobe **(ATLAS PLATES 118 #118.1, 120 #120.1).**

Palpate the smooth **costal surface** and the **diaphragmatic surface,** or **base,** of the left lung. Similar to the right lung, it is deeply concave and overlies the convexity of the diaphragm **(ATLAS PLATE 120 #120.1).**

Realize that the diaphragm extends higher on the **right** than on the left because the right lobe of the liver lies directly inferior to the diaphragm in the upper right abdomen **(ATLAS PLATE 154).** The diaphragm separates the base of the **left** lung from the left lobe of the liver, the fundus of the stomach, and more laterally, the spleen.

Figure 10-2. The lungs and pleura within the thoracic cavity. Observe the fissures of the lungs and the reflections of pleura.

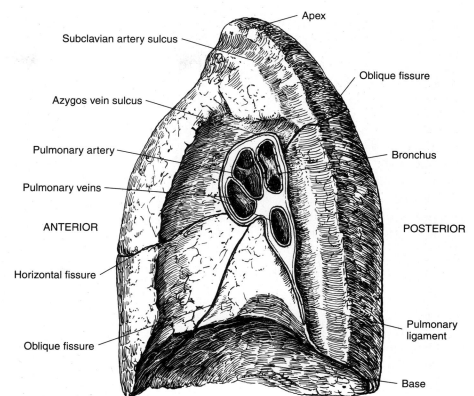

Figure 10-3. The medial surface and hilum of the right lung.

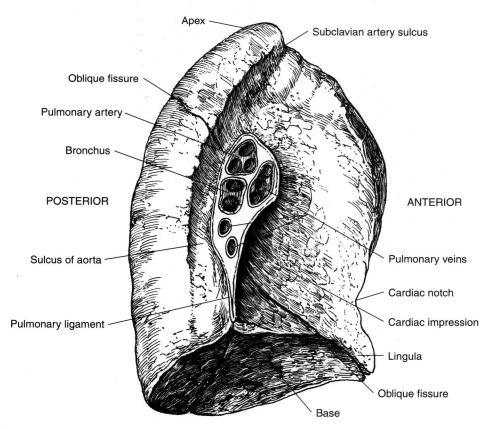

Figure 10-4. The medial surface and hilum of the left lung.

Examine the **posterior border** and **mediastinal surface** of the left lung. Between the posterior border and the root of the lung, identify the longitudinal groove made by the **descending aorta** (**ATLAS PLATE 120 #120.2**). Follow this groove superiorly where it curves over the hilum to accommodate the **aortic arch.** See if two or more grooves can be seen ascending from this arch for the left subclavian and left common carotid arteries. Observe also the large concavity anterior and inferior to the hilum in which the heart and pericardium extend.

Examine the hilum and identify the **left bronchus** posteriorly, the **pulmonary veins** anteriorly and inferiorly, and the **pulmonary artery** somewhat between the bronchus and veins (**Figure 10-4; ATLAS PLATES 120 #120.1, 121 #121.1**).

◄
Grant's 35
Netter's 195
Rohen 249, 251

►
Grant's 33, 36–40
Netter's 196–199
Rohen 250, 251

Place the lung, with the hilum exposed, on a flat surface. Identify the primary bronchus in the left lung or the eparterial and hyparterial bronchi in the **right lung.** With probe and forceps, pick away piecemeal the soft lung tissue surrounding the stiff bronchus at the hilum, thereby exposing the secondary and then tertiary, or segmental, bronchi. Observe comparable subdivisions of the pulmonary artery and vein that accompany the segmental bronchus. Note that together a single segmental bronchus and a segmental artery and vein supply portions of lung called bronchopulmonary segments.

1. **Bronchopulmonary segments of the RIGHT LUNG (Figure 10-5).** Start with the right superior or eparterial bronchus for the upper lobe, and probe its division into three segmental bronchi, the apical, posterior, and anterior segments (**ATLAS PLATES 119 #119.2, 121 #121.2**). Find the segmental arteries and veins that accompany the segmental bronchi.

OPTIONAL DISSECTION

C. **Bronchopulmonary Segments.** Structures enter and leave the lungs at the pulmonary hila. If time permits, the objective is to dissect the primary bronchi that divide into lobar bronchi and their subsequent subdivisions into tertiary **segmental bronchi** (**ATLAS PLATE 117**). Similarly, the pulmonary arteries and veins are to be found dividing into their lobar and segmental branches.

Usually, the **segmental pulmonary arteries** are centrally placed with the bronchi and distributed in close proximity to the segmental bronchi (often on their posterior surfaces). The **segmental vein** typically does not accompany the segmental bronchus in the center of the segment, but, superficially, it is found between segments. More deeply, they are located within the segment, anterior to the bronchus.

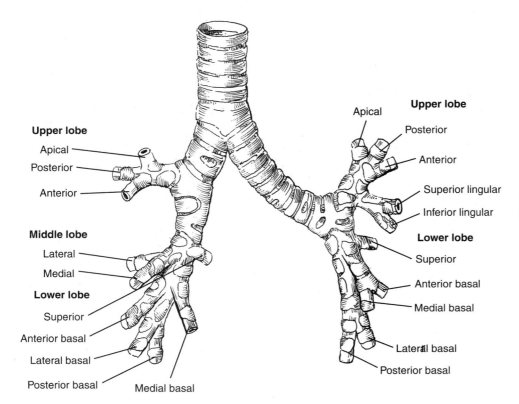

Figure 10-5. Segmental bronchi of both lungs.

Identify the **hyparterial bronchus** (for the middle and inferior lobes), and at the hilum separate it from the surrounding spongy lung tissue with forceps. Probe downward into the hyparterial bronchus until the right middle lobar bronchus is reached and seen to be branching laterally. Note that it divides into the **lateral and medial segmental bronchi** of the middle lobe. These two segments comprise the region between the horizontal and oblique fissures of the right lung (**ATLAS PLATES 119 #119.2, 117, 122**).

Probe the **inferior lobar bronchus** directly downward as a continuation of the hyparterial bronchus. Determine that the **superior segmental bronchus** of the lower lobe quickly branches from the lobar bronchus and courses upward to the highest segment of the inferior lobe. Probe the inferior lobar bronchus and identify the basal segmental bronchi that are oriented downward. Identify sequentially: the **medial basal, anterior basal, lateral basal,** and **posterior basal segmental bronchi** (**ATLAS PLATES 121 #121.2, 117, 122**).

2. **Bronchopulmonary segments of the LEFT LUNG (Figure 10-5).** Determine if the hilum was severed proximal or distal to the division of the primary bronchus into the two secondary lobar bronchi. Separate the primary bronchus (or the secondary bronchi) and the pulmonary artery and veins at the hilum from the surrounding lung tissue. Pick away soft lung tissue and follow the divisions of the hilar structures into the superior and inferior lobes. Identify blackened bronchopulmonary lymph nodes, often found at the hilum. Again, the **segmental arteries** are usually located posterior to the **segmental bronchi,** and the **segmental veins** typically course between two adjacent segments.

Probe the superior lobar bronchus. Note that it quickly subdivides into an ascending upper secondary bronchus and another secondary bronchus that courses laterally.

Note that these two secondary bronchi are comparable to the superior *and* middle **lobar** bronchi of the right lung. Thus, the left superior lobe consists of an upper part comparable to the superior lobe of the right lung and a more laterally located **lingular part** comparable to the middle lobe of the right lung.

Probe the ascending secondary bronchus to the left superior lobe and identify the **apicoposterior** and **anterior segmental bronchi** (**ATLAS PLATES 119 #119.1, 121 #121.1, 117, 122**). The left apicoposterior segment in the superior lobe corresponds to both

apical and posterior segments of the superior lobe in the right lung. The apicoposterior segment is directed superiorly and posteriorly in contrast to the anterior segment that occupies the anterior aspect of the right upper lobe. Probe the laterally oriented secondary bronchus of the superior lobe that courses to the lingular part of the left upper lobe. Note that it quickly divides into **superior lingular** and **inferior lingular segmental bronchi** (**ATLAS PLATES 117, 119 #119.1**).

Return to the hilum and identify the **inferior lobar bronchus,** which is directed downward. Observe that after approximately 2 centimeters, the **superior segmental bronchus** branches from the inferior lobar bronchus. It is directed superiorly and posteriorly in the inferior lobe. Continuing down the inferior lobar bronchus, probe the four basal segmental bronchi: the **medial basal, anterior basal, lateral basal,** and **posterior basal bronchopulmonary segments** (**ATLAS PLATES 119 #119.1, 121 #121.1, 122**). At one time the medial and anterior basal segments of the left lung were considered a single bronchopulmonary segment, but today they are considered separate segments.

Of importance clinically is the orientation of the **primary bronchi** from the **trachea.** The left primary bronchus is longer and courses more transversely than the right primary bronchus, which is oriented more vertically (**ATLAS PLATES 117, 122**). Because the right primary bronchus is more vertical (only 25° off vertical) than the left (45° off vertical), foreign bodies that are inadvertently swallowed are more likely to enter the right primary bronchus than the left.

III. Mediastinum and Its Subdivisions; Anterior Mediastinum

A. **General Comments and Definitions (Figure 10-6).** The **mediastinum** is the region of the thorax between the lungs, and it extends from the superior aperture of the thorax to the diaphragm. It is bounded posteriorly by the vertebral column and anteriorly by the sternum. A plane projecting backward from the sternal angle to the lower end of the T4 vertebra divides the mediastinum into the **superior mediastinum** above the plane and the **inferior mediastinum** inferior to the plane. The latter is further subdivided into **anterior, middle,** and **posterior mediastina.**

The **anterior mediastinum** lies between the body of the sternum and the pericardium. The **middle**

▶
Grant's 33, 36, 38
Netter's 198, 199
Rohen 246, 247, 251

◀
Grant's 33, 36, 40
Netter's 196–198
Rohen 250, 251

▶
Grant's 29
Rohen 243

◀
Grant's 33, 36, 37
Netter's 197–199
Rohen 251

mediastinum is the largest part of the inferior mediastinum and contains the **pericardium** and **heart** and the attachment of the great vessels to the heart. The **posterior mediastinum** lies behind the heart and pericardium and anterior to the vertebral column (**Figure 10-6**).

B. **Anterior Mediastinum.** In the adult, the anterior mediastinum contains only a small amount of fat, remnants of the lower part of the thymus, and the internal thoracic lymph nodes and channels. In the young child, the **thymus** is located in the superior mediastinum and extends into the anterior mediastinum to the level of the 4th costal cartilage (**ATLAS PLATES 112, 113**). The size of the thymus increases until puberty but then, through the process of fatty involution, the amount of functional thymic tissue diminishes. Some functioning tissue, however, remains throughout life.

◄
Grant's 64
Rohen 265, 266

Examine the fatty tissue anterior to the brachiocephalic veins and see if you can identify any glandular thymic tissue within it. Look for **thymic veins** that flow directly into the brachiocephalic veins. Then, remove the fat and any thymic remains and expose the right and left brachiocephalic veins that join to form the superior vena cava (**ATLAS PLATES 130 #130.1, 134**). Turn your attention to the pericardium that surrounds the heart.

IV. Middle Mediastinum and Pericardium

◄
Grant's 48
Netter's 207, 208, 226, 227
Rohen 269–272

The middle mediastinum contains the pericardial sac, the heart, the origins of the **great vessels** attached to the heart, the **phrenic nerves,** and **pericardiacophrenic vessels** (**ATLAS PLATE 130 #130.1**).

A. **Phrenic Nerves and Pericardiacophrenic Vessels.** The **phrenic nerves** (C3, C4, C5) and **pericardiacophrenic vessels** must be dissected **before the pericardium is opened.** The phrenic nerves descend from the neck (**Figure 10-7**) and are joined by the pericardiacophrenic artery, a branch of the internal thoracic artery. The pericardiacophrenic vein usually drains into the internal thoracic vein, but may drain into the brachiocephalic vein. The phrenic nerves are the only motor supply to the diaphragm, but they also contain sensory fibers from the diaphragm and from the pericardium and pleura. The pericardiacophrenic artery is a delicate and tortuous vessel that supplies the diaphragm, the pericardium, and pleura (**ATLAS PLATES 126, 127, 129, 134**).

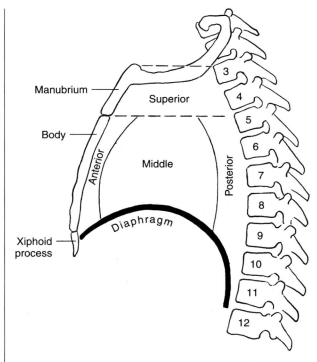

Figure 10-6. A midsagittal diagram showing the subdivisions of the mediastinum.

On both sides, remove the mediastinal pleura covering the **phrenic nerves** and **pericardiacophrenic vessels** on the lateral surface of the pericardium. Follow the **right** nerve and vessels upward into the superior mediastinum and observe that they lie lateral to the right brachiocephalic vein. Note that on the **left** side they course on the lateral surface of the aortic arch adjacent to the left common carotid and subclavian arteries (**ATLAS PLATES 127, 130**). Follow the nerves and vessels to the diaphragm.

B. **Opening of the Pericardial Sac.** The pericardium is a fibrous-serous sac that consists of an outer fibrous layer and an inner serous membrane. The inner serous membrane lines **the inner surface of the fibrous layer** and then is reflected over the **outer surface of the heart,** which it invests closely. The serous pericardium, thus, has **parietal** and **visceral layers,** similar to the pleura. To remove the heart, the pericardial sac must be opened.

Observe that the outer fibrous layer of pericardium forms a conical sac around the heart. Note how its upper part is fused at the base of the heart with the outer surface of the great vessels near their attachment to the heart (**ATLAS PLATES 130 #130.1**). Note the attachment of the pericardium inferiorly to the central tendon of the diaphragm.

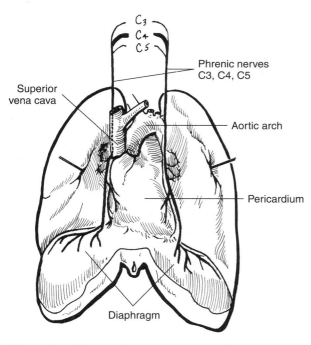

Figure 10-7. The phrenic nerves descending from the neck to the diaphragm. Note their relationship to the great vessels and the pericardium.

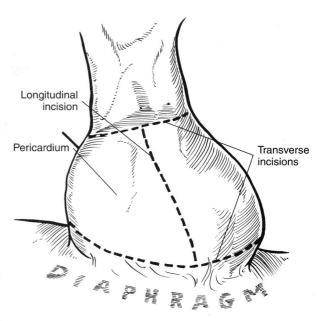

Figure 10-8. Incisions required to open the pericardial sac.

To open the pericardium, make one longitudinal and two transverse incisions as shown in **Figure 10-8.** Within the pericardial cavity find the **transverse** and **oblique pericardial sinuses.** Insert your index finger transversely within a cleft posterior to the **aorta** and **pulmonary artery,** but anterior to the **superior vena cava** and **pulmonary veins.** This cleft is the transverse pericardial sinus (**ATLAS PLATES 134, 135**).

Insert your hand within the pericardium in the recess behind the heart. This recess is the oblique pericardial sinus (**ATLAS PLATE 135**). Lift the apex of the heart and reach superiorly behind the heart. Feel how the serous pericardium reflects over the pulmonary veins and venae cavae to form a blind pouch that limits the sinus superiorly.

Carefully cut across the great vessels sequentially approximately 2.5 centimeters (1 inch) from their attachment to the heart. Cut the aorta, pulmonary artery, superior vena cava, and then the inferior vena cava just above the diaphragm. Finally, cut the four pulmonary veins and the serous pericardium between the transverse pericardial sinus and the oblique sinus (**ATLAS PLATE 135**).

◄
Grant's 25, 48, 49
Netter's 207, 208
Rohen 267–269

Clinical Relevance

Auscultation and percussion of the anterior chest wall. Auscultation of the lungs involves a stethoscope to hear sounds during breathing. Percussion is the technique of tapping fingers over the chest to detect the degree of resonance of the sounds. Use of the stethoscope detects the passage of air in the respiratory tract as well as heart valve sounds, while percussion can determine whether the lungs are clear or contain fluid or possibly a pathologic mass.

Resection of a lung lesion. To operate on the lungs for surgical removal of diseased regions, knowledge of the bronchopulmonary segments that comprise each of the lobes is vital to the surgeon. It is possible to remove only a bronchopulmonary segment for the diseased condition (segmentectomy) or it may require the removal of the whole lobe (lobectomy) or even the entire lung (pneumonectomy).

Swallowing of foreign objects. At times, children swallow coins or other small foreign objects that they put in their mouths, or dentists sometimes inadvertently allow filling material or pulled teeth to be aspirated by their patient. These objects, or even morsels of food, will tend to enter the trachea and then can descend into the right primary bronchus, which is wider and more vertical than the left.

Bronchoscopic examination. Lesions within the bronchial tree may require a physician to perform a bronchoscopic examination of the trachea and the primary bronchi. The bronchoscope is introduced orally or nasally and then directed to the nasopharynx, oropharynx, and through the larynx to the trachea. The carina is located at the site at which the trachea bifurcates into the two primary bronchi; it is located slightly to the left of the midline. Upon observing the bronchi, it might be necessary to take a small biopsy of their inner lining.

Cancer of the lung. Initial examination of persons suspected of having a lung tumor in the lung require that radiographs of the chest be taken. If any questionable lesion is visualized, the nature of the lesion must be assessed and computerized tomography (CT) or magnetic resonance imaging (MRI) may be done. Positron emission tomography (PET) studies using a radionuclide, such as fluorodeoxyglucose, can be used to determine potential sites in the lungs and also the locations of metastatic tumors that may have developed from the primary cancer. In these studies, cells of high metabolic activity (such as cancer cells) take up the gamma emitter, and this activity can be localized anatomically.

Emphysema. In this condition, the elasticity of the lungs is lost, and after inspiration, the lungs are less able to recoil and, thus, deflate. This causes an incomplete expiration which then must be helped by the accessory muscle of respiration. The most common cause of this condition is the long-term smoking of cigarettes in which the smoke is inhaled into the lungs.

Pulmonary embolism. If a blood clot obstructs a pulmonary artery or one of its branches, the condition is called a pulmonary embolism. Such clots most often develop after an operation in the lower body or after a severe injury, such as compound fractures of the tibia or femur. In these instances an embolus can enter the inferior vena cava and travel from the right ventricle to a pulmonary artery or one of its branches. If the embolus is large it will quickly cause acute respiratory distress and even death because blood returning to the right atrium accumulates on the venous side and cannot perfuse through the lungs. If the embolus is smaller, it might obstruct blood only to a bronchopulmonary segment, producing a pulmonary infarct.

The thymus. This important organ lies directly posterior to the manubrium of the sternum, but it can extend superiorly into the lower neck. It is large in children, but by the age of 25 years most of the thymic glandular tissue is replaced by fat, because its immunologic function is virtually complete. It does, however, continue to produce some T lymphocytes.

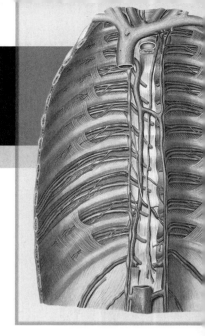

DISSECTION #11

Thorax III: The Heart: Blood Circulation; Heart Surface Anatomy; Blood Supply, Chambers, and Conducting System of the Heart

OBJECTIVES

1 Understand the structures that comprise the systemic and pulmonary circulations.

2 Visualize the external surface features of the heart.

3 Dissect the blood supply to the heart; open each of the four chambers and learn their internal structure.

4 Understand the conducting system of the heart.

Atlas Key:

Clemente Atlas, 5th Edition = Anatomy Plate #

Grant's Atlas, 11th Edition = Grant's Page #

Netter's Atlas, 3rd Edition = Netter's Plate #

Rohen Atlas, 6th Edition = Rohen Page #

I. Circulation of the Blood: General Comments

The heart is the principal muscular organ of the circulatory system. It consists of four chambers, two **atria,** and two **ventricles.** On contraction, the right and left halves of the heart simultaneously pump an equal amount of blood from their respective ventricle. **On the right side,** venous blood enters the right atrium from the two **venae cavae** and the **coronary sinus,** and it is projected through the right ventricle into the **pulmonary artery.**

On the left side, the **pulmonary veins** flow into the left atrium, and the left ventricle pumps its blood into the **aorta.** The right heart receives venous blood from the **systemic circulation** and delivers it into the **pulmonary circulation.** In contrast, the left atrium receives its blood from the **pulmonary circulation** and transmits it to the left ventricle, which pumps it into the **systemic circulation** by way of the aorta.

II. Surface Anatomy of the Heart

The heart and pericardium are located in the middle mediastinum. Covered by serous and fibrous pericardium, the heart is located obliquely behind the sternum with its base oriented upward, backward, and to the right. The heart is attached to the great vessels and its apex is directed downward, forward, and to the left (**ATLAS PLATES 108, 130**). The apex, normally located behind the 5th left intercostal space, is approximately 9 cm (3.5 in) lateral to the midline and just medial to the left

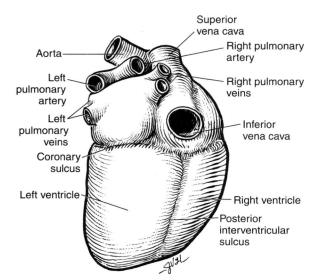

Figure 11-1. The base of the heart seen from its diaphragmatic surface.

mid-clavicular line, but its location changes with breathing (**ATLAS PLATE 129**).

A. Base of the Heart (Figure 11-1). Reposition the heart in its normal orientation within the pericardial sac to visualize its base, apex, surfaces, and borders. Observe that the **base** is formed by both atria and the vessels that attach to them. The four pulmonary veins open into the left atrium, and the superior and inferior venae cavae open into the right atrium (**ATLAS PLATE 137 #137.1**). Note that, in addition to the great veins, the base of the heart is attached to the pulmonary artery and aorta from the ventricles (**ATLAS PLATE 132**).

B. Apex of the Heart. Feel the **apex** of the heart and note that it normally lies deep to the anterior border of the left lung (**ATLAS PLATE 113**). Realize that the heart wall is thick at this site because the apex is a part of the left ventricle. Normally, the wall of the left ventricle is approximately three times the thickness of the right ventricle, 8 to 13 mm in contrast to 3 to 4 mm (**ATLAS PLATES 142, 144**). Also observe that the **anterior interventricular branch** of the **left coronary artery** and its accompanying **great cardiac vein** course along the anterior surface of the heart toward or near the apex (**ATLAS PLATE 132**).

Enlarged hearts, generally of older persons, are frequently encountered in the dissection laboratory. Often, these individuals had developed hypertension that resulted in muscular hypertrophy. The average normal human heart is approximately the size of that

▶
Grant's 46, 49
Netter's 208
Rohen 268, 270

◀
Grant's 50
Netter's 210, 211
Rohen 252

▶
Grant's 47, 50
Netter's 210
Rohen 252, 273

◀
Grant's 46
Netter's 208, 210
Rohen 252, 257,
258, 262

person's clenched fist. It might measure 11 to 12 cm (approximately 5 inches) from apex to base, 8 to 9 cm (approximately 3.5 inches) transversely at its widest point, and 6 to 7 cm (approximately 2.5 inches) thick anteroposteriorly. In males, the normal heart weighs an average of 300 grams, whereas in females it weighs approximately 50 grams less. Enlarged hearts can become enormous and weigh 2 to 3 times that of a normal heart.

C. Sternocostal Surface of the Heart. Palpate the convex **sternocostal** or **anterior surface.** Observe that it consists of a smaller atrial part, located above and to the right, and a larger ventricular part, located below the **coronary sulcus** that contains the right coronary artery and some fat (**Figure 11-2, ATLAS PLATE 132**). Note that this sulcus separates the atria above (largely hidden by the pulmonary trunk and ascending aorta) from the ventricles below. Follow the coronary sulcus around the right margin of the heart to the back of the heart, where it also separates the atria from the ventricles (**ATLAS PLATE 137 #137.1**). Examine the ventricular part of the sternocostal surface and realize that the left one-quarter (or more) of the anterior heart wall is left ventricle, while all of the remainder is right ventricular wall (**Figure 11-2**).

D. Diaphragmatic Surface of the Heart. Lift the apex of the heart and palpate its slightly convex **diaphragmatic surface,** formed principally by the left ventricle (**ATLAS PLATE 133**). Note that it rests on the central tendon of the diaphragm and

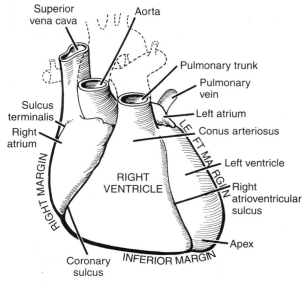

Figure 11-2. The sternocostal surface of the heart.

observe the following: 1) that the coronary sulcus, which contains the coronary sinus and continuations of both the right and left coronary arteries, separates most of the diaphragmatic surface (ventricles) from the atria; and 2) that the **posterior interventricular sulcus**, contains the **posterior interventricular branch** of the **right coronary artery** and the **middle cardiac vein** and these descend obliquely toward the apex (**ATLAS PLATES 133, 137 #137.1**).

E. **Left Margin of the Heart (Figure 11-2).** Examine the **left surface and margin of the heart.** Note that it is oriented obliquely to the left and consists almost entirely of left ventricle. The uppermost part, however, is formed by a portion of the left atrium and its auricular appendage (**ATLAS PLATE 134**). Note that the left surface is crossed by the coronary sulcus within which flows the **great cardiac vein** (as it becomes the coronary sinus) and the **circumflex branch of the left coronary artery** (**ATLAS PLATE 136 #136.1**).

◀

Grant's 46
Netter's 212
Rohen 252, 269

F. **Right Margin of the Heart (Figure 11-2).** Observe that the **right margin of the heart** is rounded and that its convexity consists essentially of the right atrial wall. Note also that the upper aspect of the right margin is formed by the wall of the **superior vena cava** as it enters the right atrium (**ATLAS PLATE 132**). Inferiorly, identify the short intrathoracic part of the **inferior vena cava** as it also enters the right atrium.

◀

Grant's 46
Netter's 208, 212
Rohen 252, 269

▶

Grant's 49, 52, 54
Netter's 212, 214
Rohen 255, 257,
262

G. **Inferior Margin of the Heart (Figure 11-2).** Palpate the inferior margin as it extends from the right margin nearly horizontally to the left as far as the apex of the heart. Frequently called the **acute margin of the heart,** note whether the marginal branch of the right coronary artery courses along this border in your cadaver (**AT-LAS PLATE 138 #138.1**).

◀

Grant's 46
Netter's 208
Rohen 252, 269

III. Arteries and Veins of the Heart (Figures 11-3 and 11-4)

The heart is supplied by the right and left coronary arteries, which arise from the ascending aorta just beyond its emergence from the left ventricle (**ATLAS PLATES 136 #136.2**). All the veins (except for the small venae minimi and anterior cardiac veins) that drain the heart enter the coronary sinus (**ATLAS PLATES 137**).

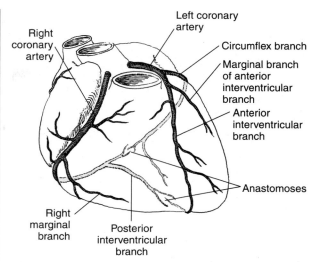

Figure 11-3. The coronary arteries (anterior view).

The coronary arteries branch from behind dilated pockets located between the semilunar cusps of the aortic valve and the wall of the aorta. These pockets are called the **aortic sinuses** and will be seen after the left ventricle is opened.

A. **Right Coronary Artery (Figure 11-3).** Dissect between the right auricular appendage and the pulmonary artery to find the origin of the **right coronary artery** from the aorta (**ATLAS PLATES 136 #136.2, 138 #138.1**). Remove the fat around the right coronary artery and follow the vessel across the heart in the coronary sulcus between the right atrium and right ventricle (**ATLAS PLATES 132, 136 #136.1**). Identify branches to the right atrium and ventricle and try to find the atrial branch that supplies the **sino-atrial node** by dissecting in the sulcus between the right auricular appendage and the aorta. This small **artery of the sinoatrial node** (approximately 1 mm in diameter) arises from the right coronary approximately two thirds of the time (**ATLAS PLATE 138 #138.1**). and from the circumflex branch of the left coronary artery in the other cadavers.

Variation in the pattern by which the arteries supply the heart is the general rule. Usually one or the other artery will be "dominant," i.e., will be the vessel that contributes the principal arteries to the posterior surface of the heart (**ATLAS PLATE 139**). Most frequently, the **posterior interventricular branch** is derived from the right coronary artery, but usually parallel branches from the left coronary artery also descend (**ATLAS PLATE 133**).

Find the **right marginal artery** coursing along the inferior border. This vessel usually branches from the right coronary just before it courses around the right border (**ATLAS PLATE 138 #138.1**). Follow the main stem around to the **posterior interventricular sulcus** and note that two or three posterior branches descend from the right coronary, but only one **posterior interventricular branch** descends in the sulcus.

◄
Grant's 52
Netter's 212, 214
Rohen 262

The posterior coronary artery anastomoses both with the circumflex branch of the left coronary on the posterior wall of the heart and with the anterior interventricular branch of the left coronary in the region of the cardiac apex.

B. Left Coronary Artery. Examine the **left coronary artery.** To find its origin, dissect on the sternocostal surface between the left auricular appendage and the pulmonary trunk. Observe that it arises from the aorta behind the left aortic cusp and sinus (**ATLAS PLATES 136 #136.1, 138 #138.1**). Follow the artery to the coronary sulcus, where it usually divides into two branches: the **anterior interventricular branch,** which descends in the anterior interventricular sulcus, and the **circumflex branch,** which passes to the back of the heart (**ATLAS PLATE 136 #136.2**). Note that the anterior interventricular branch may be embedded in fat and crossed by small fascicles of muscle. In its descent toward the apex, separate the artery from the **great cardiac vein** that accompanies it (**ATLAS PLATE 132**).

◄
Grant's 49, 52, 54
Netter's 212, 215
Rohen 257, 262, 270

Clean the circumflex branch as it curves to the left and is directed posteriorly. Separate the artery from the great cardiac vein, which then empties into the **coronary sinus** (**ATLAS PLATE 137**). Find the **left marginal branch** of the circumflex artery. In more than 80% of cases, it descends along the left border (margin) of the heart and it supplies the left ventricle nearly to the apex (**ATLAS PLATE 138 #138.1**).

On the posterior wall of the heart, identify one or more **posterior ventricular branches** (**ATLAS PLATE 133**). Determine if the **posterior interventricular artery** is derived from the right coronary or the circumflex branch of the left coronary artery.

►
Grant's 49, 50, 53
Netter's 210, 212
Rohen 262, 270

C. Venous Drainage of the Heart (**Figure 11-4**). Most of the venous blood from the heart drains into the right atrium via the **coronary sinus.** The major veins flow into the coronary sinus located

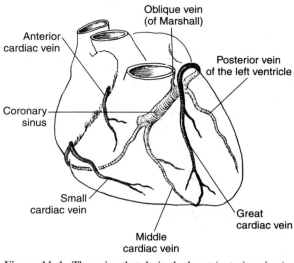

Figure 11-4. The veins that drain the heart (anterior view).

in the coronary sulcus on the posterior wall of the heart. Its largest tributaries are the **great cardiac vein** found along the anterior interventricular sulcus, the **middle cardiac vein** that ascends in the posterior interventricular sulcus, and the **small cardiac vein** that accompanies the right marginal artery (**Figure 11-4**). Additionally, there is a **small oblique vein** that drains into the coronary sinus from the posterior wall of the left atrium (**Figure 11-4**) and the **anterior cardiac veins** that drain directly into the right atrium. Small vessels called the **venae cordis minimae** (Thebesian veins) drain directly into the four heart chambers.

Dissect the **coronary sinus** on the posterior surface of the heart. It is often embedded in fat or muscle fibers along the groove of the coronary sulcus (**ATLAS PLATES 133, 137**). Follow the sinus along the posterior wall of the right atrium to its entrance into that chamber.

Identify the principal veins that flow into the coronary sinus. If not already dissected, find the **great cardiac vein** in the **anterior interventricular sulcus** with the anterior interventricular artery (**ATLAS PLATES 132, 136 #136.1**). Follow this vein upward and around the left margin of the heart where it is continuous with the coronary sinus. Dissect the **middle cardiac vein** as it ascends in the **posterior interventricular sulcus** and terminates in the coronary sinus (**ATLAS PLATES 133, 137**). Find the **small cardiac vein** that usually courses along the inferior border of the heart with the right marginal branch of the right coronary artery (**Figure 11-4**).

IV. Chambers of the Heart

The interior of the heart is to be dissected by opening each of the four chambers, examining the great vessels that are attached, and visualizing the valves that separate the chambers and guard their orifices. Dissect the chambers in the following sequence: right atrium, right ventricle and pulmonary artery, left atrium, left ventricle, and aorta.

A. Right Atrium (Figure 11-6). The **right atrium** receives the systemic blood by way of the superior vena cava superiorly and the inferior vena cava inferiorly. It also receives most of the venous blood from the heart muscle itself because the coronary sinus empties into it (**Figure 11-6**).

Identify the right atrial auricular appendage. It is the small pouch that overlies the right side of the ascending aorta. Make a transverse cut approximately 1 cm in length from the upper left part of the auricle across the atrium below the entrance of the superior vena cava to the right border of the heart (**Figure 11-5, A–B**). With scissors make a vertical cut downward along the right margin of the heart (**Figure 11-5, B–C**). Make another short transverse incision above the inferior vena cava to the coronary sulcus, but do not sever the vessels in the sulcus (**Figure 11-5, C–D**).

Open the atrial flap and with forceps remove the clotted blood from the right atrial cavity and auricle. Rinse the right atrium in running water so its inner wall can be studied. With a probe, examine the following structures:

1. the smooth posterior wall of the right atrium called the **sinus venarum (ATLAS PLATE 142)**. Identify the oval **orifice of the superior vena cava** oriented downward and forward toward the atrioventricular opening.

2. **the opening of the inferior vena cava** and the small semilunar, flap-like endocardial fold (valve) attached to its anterior margin (**Figure 11-6**). Note that this opening is directed superiorly and to the left toward the interatrial wall that is marked by an oval depression called the **fossa ovalis (Figure 11-6)**. Examine the superior and anterior rim of the fossa and see how it is encircled by a noticeable margin called the **limbus fossae ovalis.** With a probe examine the interatrial wall for a small opening into the left atrium that might persist beneath the upper part of the limbus. When present (25% of hearts), it is a vestige of the foramen ovale.

◄
Grant's 56
Netter's 216
Rohen 258

►
Grant's 56
Netter's 216
Rohen 258

►
Grant's 56
Netter's 216
◄
Grant's 56
Netter's 216
Rohen 258

1. ANTERIOR

2. POSTERIOR

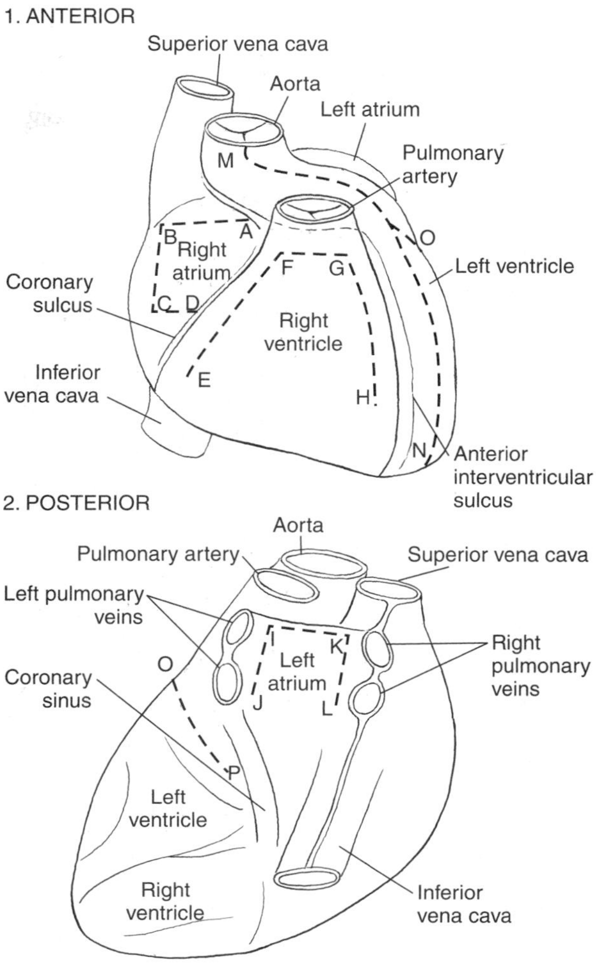

Figure 11-5. Incisions to open the atria and ventricles.

3. **the orifice of the coronary sinus (Figure 11-6),** located between the valve of the inferior vena cava and the atrioventricular opening. Insert a probe through the orifice and confirm that its tip has entered the coronary sinus. Observe the thin semilunar **valve of the coronary sinus** around the lower margin of the orifice.

4. **musculi pectinati** on the inner surface of the auricular appendage (**Figure 11-6**). Note that the muscular bundles are oriented in a parallel pattern and separated from the smooth part of the atrium by a vertical ridge called the **crista terminalis (ATLAS PLATE 142)**. Observe that this ridge corresponds in position to a groove called the **sulcus terminalis** on the external surface of the atrium between the right margins of the superior and inferior venae cavae (**ATLAS PLATES 133, 134, 137**).

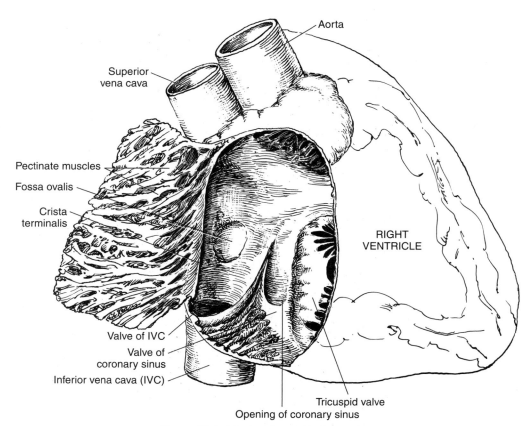

Figure 11-6. The interior of the right atrium.

5. the atrioventricular orifice. Look into the floor of the right atrium and note the oval-shaped opening between the right atrium and right ventricle. Place two fingers through the orifice and feel the fibrous annulus (or ring) of the **right atrioventricular valve** (tricuspid) to which the three cusps are attached (**ATLAS PLATES 142, 143**).

B. **Right Ventricle and Pulmonary Orifice and Valve (Figure 11-7, ATLAS PLATE 143).** The right ventricle forms most of the anterior surface of the heart. It receives blood through the tricuspid valve and sends it to the lungs through the pulmonary trunk.

Again insert two fingers through the right atrioventricular opening. With a pair of sharp-ended scissors in your other hand, penetrate one end of the scissors through the right ventricular wall approximately 1 cm below the atrioventricular sulcus and the right coronary artery. Cut through the right ventricular wall parallel to the sulcus as far as the right border of the heart (**Figure 11-5 E–F**). Place your index finger down the cut pulmonary trunk from above,

◄
Grant's 57, 60
Netter's 216, 218–220
Rohen 256, 258, 259, 261, 271

and note the level of the cusps of the pulmonary valve. Extend the incision upward toward the base of the pulmonary trunk to a point approximately 1 cm below these cusps (**Figure 11-5 E–F**).

Make a second cut (2 cm long) transversely across the ventricular wall 1 cm below the pulmonary cusps and extend it to a site approximately 2 cm from the anterior interventricular sulcus (**Figure 11-5 F–G**). Using scissors, make a third cut vertically from the left end of the second (transverse) cut parallel to the anterior interventricular sulcus, as far as the inferior border of the heart (**Figure 11-5 G–H**). Turn the three-sided flap downward and remove the clotted blood from the right ventricle. Rinse the right ventricle thoroughly in running cold water so that its interior can be studied.

The right ventricular cavity extends from the atrioventricular orifice to the inferior margin of the heart (**ATLAS PLATE 142**). Its outflow path ascends to the **conus arteriosus** and pulmonary orifice superiorly and to the left (**ATLAS PLATE 143**). Thus, blood from the right atrium initially flows inferiorly and to the left. It then courses superiorly and completes a U-shaped

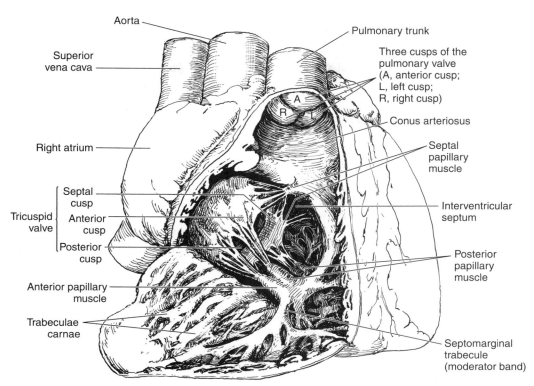

Figure 11-7. The interior of the right ventricle.

pattern to the **conus arteriosus** (or **infundibulum**) and the pulmonary orifice (**Figure 11-7**).

With a probe, examine the following:

1. **muscular ridges called trabeculae carnae** that characterize the inner wall of the right ventricle. Note that some are ridges and others bridge a small area of ventricular surface. Still others, the **papillary muscles,** are larger. These are attached at one end to the heart wall and at the other to glistening, string-like, inelastic cords, called **chordae tendinae** (**ATLAS PLATE 147 #147.1, 147.2**). Note that these cords attach to the cusps of the **tricuspid valve (Figure 11-8)**.

2. **right atrioventricular orifice** and the **three cusps of the tricuspid valve** (**ATLAS PLATE 143**). Identify the cusps as **septal** (oriented medially near the septum), **anterior,** and **posterior.** Confirm that the anterior cusp is usually the largest and the septal cusp smallest. Note that the fibrous ring to which the cusps are attached, the cusps, chordae tendinae, and papillary muscles form a functional unit (**Figure 11-8**). Attachment of the papillary muscles to the ventricular wall prevents the

▶
Grant's 57
Netter's 216, 219
Rohen 258

◀
Grant's 57
Netter's 216
Rohen 259

◀
Grant's 57
Netter's 213,
218–220
Rohen 255, 259,
261, 271

cusps from flapping into the atrium during ventricular contraction when pressure in the ventricle exceeds atrial pressure.

3. **septomarginal trabecula** (moderator band). Identify this ridge of muscle, which extends from the interventricular septum and attaches to the lower part of the ventricle at the base of the anterior papillary muscle (**Figure 11-7**). The septomarginal trabecula is important because it contains the right crus of the **atrioventricular bundle,** a part of the conducting system of the heart.

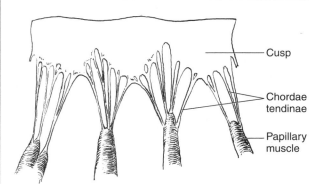

Figure 11-8. The chordae tendinae as they attach the papillary muscles to an atrioventricular valve cusp.

4. **conus arteriosus and pulmonary valve (Figure 11-7).** Open the pulmonary artery between two of its cusps (**ATLAS PLATE 144**). Observe the smooth funnel-shaped surface of the **conus arteriosus.** Place a finger behind one of the semilunar cusps into the pocket (or sinus) between the cusp and the arterial wall (**ATLAS PLATE 136 #136.2**). Observe that this is one of three **pulmonary sinuses.** Visualize how they become filled with blood and become apposed (thereby closing the pulmonary valve) when pressure in the pulmonary artery exceeds that in the right ventricle.

Palpate the free margin of the cusps and feel a small thickening or **nodule** at their centers, on both sides of which are thin crescenteric edges called **lunules.** Identify the anterior, right, and left cusps named according to their positions embryologically (**Figures 11-9, 11-12**).

C. Left Atrium (ATLAS PLATES 144, 148 #148.1).
Pulmonary veins return oxygenated blood from the lungs to the **left atrium.** This chamber extends behind the right atrium, but its small auricular appendage projects anteriorly around the left side of the pulmonary trunk and forms the uppermost part of the left border of the heart.

Turn the heart over and orient the left atrium so that the right pulmonary veins are to the right and the left veins to the left (**ATLAS PLATE 137 #137.1**). With scissors, make **two parallel incisions** adjacent to the two sets of pulmonary veins (**Figure 11-5, I–J and K–L**). Make a **third incision** interconnecting the upper ends of the first two cuts (**Figure 11-5, I–K**) and reflect the inverted U-shaped flap downward to open the left atrium. Remove the clotted

◄
Grant's 57
Netter's 216, 218, 220
Rohen 258, 259, 271

►
Grant's 62
Netter's 217, 220
Rohen 248, 251, 258, 261

►
Grant's 61
Netter's 217–220
Rohen 258, 259

blood and wash the left atrium in running water. Examine the following:

1. **the smooth-walled cavity of the left atrium (ATLAS PLATES 144, 148 #148.1).** Open the small tubular auricular appendage and note that the muscular ridges (musculi pectinati) are fewer than in the right atrium.

2. **the symmetrical orifices of the pulmonary veins.** Note that these are not guarded by valves and that the four pulmonary veins and the two venae cavae are surrounded by a sleeve of serous pericardium comparable to the one that envelopes the pulmonary artery and aorta.

3. **the interatrial septum from the left side (ATLAS PLATE 144).** Identify an oval-shaped depression in the interatrial septum. Note that this slight concavity coincides with the fossa ovalis of the right atrium.

4. **the left atrioventricular opening (ATLAS PLATE 144).** Insert a finger through the floor of the left atrium and palpate the left atrioventricular orifice. Observe that the opening is directed anteriorly and to the left and that the two cusps of the **mitral valve** attach to its fibrous rim.

D. Left Ventricle and the Aortic Orifice and Valve (Figure 11-10).
The left ventricle is located largely on the diaphragmatic surface of the heart and pumps oxygenated blood into the aorta for distribution throughout the body. Longer and more narrow than the right ventricle, its muscular wall is approximately three times as thick as the right ventricle (**ATLAS PLATE 143, 144**). The left ventricle receives blood through the **bicuspid** or **mitral valve.**

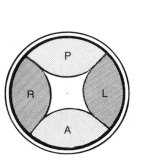
Truncus
arteriosus

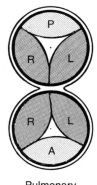
Pulmonary
artery

Aorta

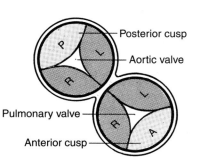
Posterior cusp
Aortic valve
Pulmonary valve
Anterior cusp

Figure 11-9. The names of the cusps of the aortic and pulmonary valves shown as the truncus arteriosus divides during development. R = right; L = left; P = posterior; A = anterior.

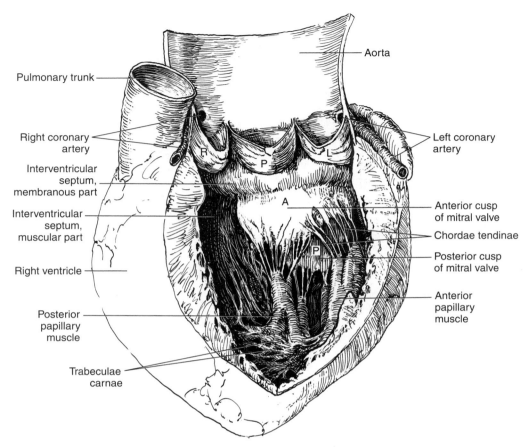

Pulmonary trunk

Aorta

Right coronary artery

Left coronary artery

Interventricular septum, membranous part

Anterior cusp of mitral valve

Interventricular septum, muscular part

Chordae tendinae

Right ventricle

Posterior cusp of mitral valve

Anterior papillary muscle

Posterior papillary muscle

Trabeculae carnae

Figure 11-10. The opened left ventricle and aorta.

With your fingers through the mitral valve from the left atrium, palpate the **interventricular septum.** Open the left ventricle below the coronary sinus by making an incision 1 cm to the left of, but parallel to, the septum (internally) and the interventricular groove (externally). Extend the incision down as far as the apex of the heart (**Figure 11-5, lower half of line M–N**). Palpate within the aorta from above and note the location of the right and left aortic sinuses (confirmed by the origins of the two coronary arteries). Extend the incision of the left ventricle superiorly through the aortic orifice between the right and left cusps of the aortic valve to the upper edge of the cut aorta (**Figure 11-5, upper half of line M–N**). In so doing, the circumflex artery and great cardiac vein will be severed.

From the longitudinal incision, make a transverse cut through the ventricular wall around toward the back of the heart below and parallel to the circumflex artery and/or coronary sinus (**Figure 11-5, O–P**). Open the left ventricle and ascending aorta, remove the blood clots, and wash the interior with tap water.

◄
Grant's 57, 59, 60
Netter's 216–218, 220
Rohen 256, 259
►
Grant's 61, 62
Netter's 217, 220
Rohen 256, 258

►
Grant's 61
Netter's 217–220
Rohen 258, 259

►
Grant's 59, 60
Netter's 218–220
Rohen 258, 259

Observe the following:

1. **the ventricular wall thickness** (8 to 13 mm or more); **the interventricular septum.** Note that the septum is so oriented within the thorax that the cavity of the left ventricle lies posterior to the septum and the right ventricular chamber is anterior to it.

2. **left atrioventricular (or mitral) valve** (**Figure 11-10**). Observe that the papillary muscles are attached to the **anterior** and **posterior cusps** of the bicuspid valve by **chordae tendinae** in a manner similar to that seen in the right ventricle. Note that the left ventricle contains a number of **trabeculae carnae.**

3. **aortic orifice and cusps of the aortic valve** (**Figure 11-10**). Palpate the three semilunar cusps of the aortic valve and observe that they are similar to the pulmonary cusps but thicker and somewhat stronger (**Figure 11-12**). Visualize how the aortic sinuses trap back-flowing blood to close the valve at the end of systole.

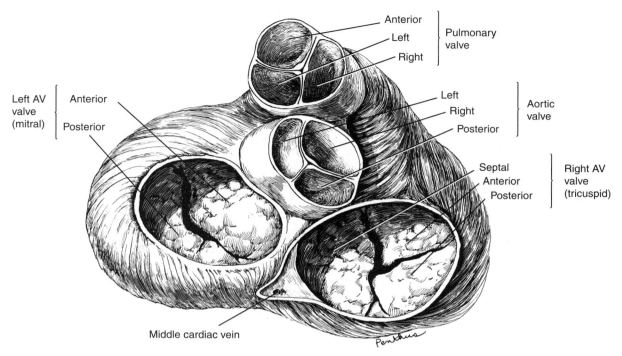

Figure 11-11. The valves of the heart and their cusps. AV, atrioventricular. (From Clemente CD. Gray's Anatomy. 30th American Edition 1985.)

Identify the **posterior, right,** and **left** cusps and probe the origins of the right and left coronary arteries **(Figures 11-11, 11-12).**

V. Conducting System of the Heart (Figure 11-13 and ATLAS PLATES 148, 149)

The conducting system of the heart is responsible for maintaining the rhythmicity of cardiac contraction. It is composed of specialized muscle fibers forming two nodes and a conducting pathway that excites the cardiac musculature in the ventricles. The **sinoatrial node** (SA node) in the right atrium initiates the impulse that results in the heartbeat. This node is called the "pacemaker" of the heart, and the impulse from this node spreads

◄
Grant's 62
Netter's 221
Rohen 261

through the musculature of both atria, causing them to contract. At some point, the impulse reaches the **atrioventricular node** (AV node, **ATLAS PLATE 148 #148.2**), where a brief atrioventricular conduction delay allows atrial contraction to complete. On increasing atrial contraction, atrial pressure supersedes that in the ventricles, thereby opening the two atrioventricular valves (tricuspid and mitral).

Extending into both ventricles from the AV node is the **atrioventricular bundle (ATLAS PLATES 148 #148.2, 149)**. This consists of fascicles of myocytes called **Purkinje fibers,** but these are not distinguishable in gross dissection. From the AV node, the bundle descends a few millimeters through the lower part of the interatrial septum to the level of the septal cusp of the tricuspid valve, where it divides into right and left branches **(Figure 11-13).**

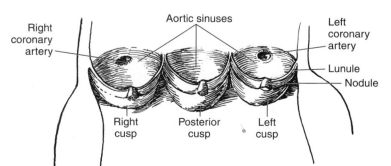

Figure 11-12. The opened aorta showing the cusps of the aortic valve and the aortic sinuses.

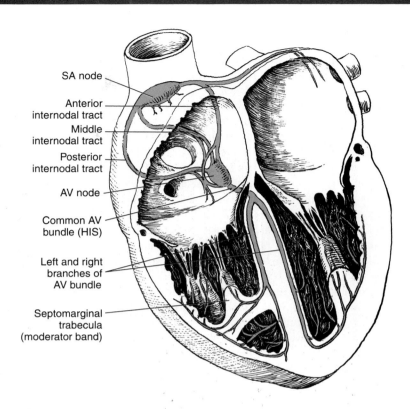

SA node

Anterior
internodal tract

Middle
internodal tract

Posterior
internodal tract

AV node

Common AV
bundle (HIS)

Left and right
branches of
AV bundle

Septomarginal
trabecula
(moderator band)

Figure 11-13. The conducting system of the heart.

Having reached the AV node, the impulse for contraction is then transmitted to both ventricles along the branches of the AV bundle, resulting in ventricular contraction. When pressure in the ventricles exceeds that in the atria, the tricuspid and mitral valves close, resulting in the **first of the two sounds of the heartbeat.** Ventricular pressure then exceeds that in the pulmonary artery and aorta, causing the pulmonary and aortic valves to open and allows blood into the two great arteries. Ventricular pressure quickly decreases. When pulmonary and aortic pressure exceeds that in the ventricles, blood attempts to rush back but becomes trapped in the pulmonary and aortic sinuses, thereby closing these valves. This produces the **second heart sound in the heartbeat.**

The SA and AV nodes are **not** to be dissected. These are microscopic in size; however, you should know their **approximate sites** in the heart wall.

Locate the site of the **SA node** in the wall of the right atrium at the upper end of the crista terminalis, anterior and to the right of entry of the superior vena cava (**ATLAS PLATE 148 #148.2; Figure 12-13**).

The **AV node.** Palpate the site of the AV node at the lower posterior part of the interatrial septum, near the attachment of the septal cusp of the tricuspid valve. It is located approximately 1 cm anterior to the opening of the coronary sinus (**ATLAS PLATE 148 #148.2**).

◄
Grant's 62
Netter's 221
Rohen 251

Clinical Relevance

Tetralogy of Fallot. This condition causes children to be cyanotic (blue baby), thereby limiting their physical activity. In this birth defect, four anomalies occur: a) a large ventricular septal defect; b) a narrowing or (stenosis) of the pulmonary trunk occurs; c) the aorta exits from the heart above the septal defect instead of the left ventricle; and d) a hypertrophy of the right ventricle develops because of the high blood pressure in that chamber.

Atrial septal defects. Prenatally the septum between the two atria contains an opening called the foramen ovale through which oxygenated blood passes from the right atrium directly into the left atrium. The opening normally closes after birth (although small remnants of the opening may persist). If, however, a large atrial-septal opening persists, then oxygenated blood in the left atrium will be shunted to the right atrium. In the newborn child this results in right atrial and ventricular hypertrophy and an overload of blood in the pulmonary system.

Ventricular septal defects. Formation of the interventricular septum occurs by a fusion of its membranous and muscular parts. Faulty development of the membranous part can result in a septal defect between the two ventricles. Although the size of the defect can vary, a large interventricular defect causes a significant left-to-right ventricular shunt of oxygenated blood, which increases pulmonary blood flow that causes pulmonary hypertension. This serious anomaly requires early surgical repair.

Angina pectoris. This pain originates in the heart and can be relatively mild or severe. It results from ischemia of the cardiac muscle that stimulates visceral afferent fibers that course through the sympathetic trunk to the upper four or five thoracic segments of the spinal cord. The pain is not perceived in the heart but is referred to the anterior chest wall. This pain can develop after strenuous exercise or after a large meal that deprives sufficient blood to the heart. The pain can be relieved by a nitroglycerin pill placed sublingually that dilates the arteries in the body along with those in the heart.

Coronary bypass operation. This procedure aims at increasing blood flow by grafting a segment of a vein or artery to the aorta and then attaching it to the distal end of the narrowed coronary artery. Vessels used for this procedure are segments of the saphenous vein

or a portion of the radial artery. Additionally, the proximal end of the internal thoracic artery (coursing anterior to the heart) can be attached to the distal end of an obstructed coronary artery, thereby bypassing the obstruction.

Coronary angioplasty. In this procedure surgeons use a catheter with a small balloon that can be inflated at the tip of the catheter. This catheter is passed through the femoral artery and advanced superiorly into the blocked coronary artery. When the obstruction is reached the balloon is inflated to enlarge the lumen of the vessel. At times, in using this technique, thrombokinase is released from the end of the catheter to dissolve the clot. After the vessel is opened an intravascular stent can be put in place to maintain the dilation of the artery.

Myocardial infarct. If an artery is occluded by an embolus, the region supplied by that vessel loses its blood supply, resulting in a myocardial infarct. The heart wall deprived of blood undergoes tissue death or necrosis.

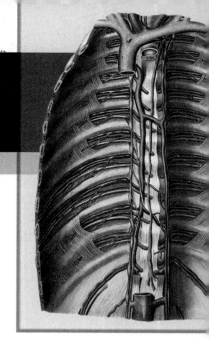

DISSECTION #12

Thorax IV: Posterior Mediastinum; Sympathetic Trunks; Diaphragm from Above; Superior Mediastinum

OBJECTIVES

1 Dissect the esophagus, the azygos system of veins, and the thoracic duct in the posterior mediastinum.

2 Study the thoracic aorta and dissect several posterior intercostal arteries.

3 Dissect the sympathetic trunks and splanchnic nerves.

4 Expose the diaphragm from above and identify the structures that traverse its openings.

5 Dissect the great veins and the arteries from the aortic arch in the superior mediastinum.

6 Find the phrenic, vagus, and recurrent laryngeal nerves.

7 Trace the trachea, esophagus, and thoracic duct through the superior mediastinum.

Atlas Key:

Clemente Atlas, 5th Edition = Atlas Plate #

Grant's Atlas, 11th Edition = Grant's Page #

Netter's Atlas, 3rd Edition = Netter's Plate #

Rohen Atlas, 6th Edition = Rohen Page #

I. Posterior Mediastinum

◄
Grant's 63, 72
Netter's 226–228
Rohen 273–276

The **posterior mediastinum** lies dorsal to the heart and pericardium and ventral to the lower eight thoracic vertebrae. It is bounded on both sides by **mediastinal pleura** and is an extension inferiorly from the dorsal part of the superior mediastinum. Several structures, such as the **esophagus, thoracic duct,** and **vagus nerves,** traverse both regions. The posterior mediastinum extends inferiorly to the 12th thoracic vertebra and continues behind the crura of the diaphragm. It contains the **trachea** at its bifurcation, the **primary bronchi,** the **azygos system of veins,** the **descending thoracic aorta,** and the **mediastinal lymph nodes** (**ATLAS PLATES 158–160**). The **splanchnic nerves** are also located within the posterior mediastinum, whereas the ganglionated **sympathetic trunks** course lateral to the bodies of the thoracic vertebrae and, strictly speaking, are not in the posterior mediastinum (**ATLAS PLATES 162, 163, 164 #164.1**).

A. The Esophagus (Figure 12-1). The **esophagus** is a 10-inch muscular tube that interconnects the pharynx to the stomach. It begins in the neck posterior to the cricoid cartilage of the larynx (C6 vertebral level) and descends through the superior and posterior mediastina to enter the abdomen through the esophageal hiatus of the diaphragm (**ATLAS PLATES 155–157**) (T10 vertebral level). Superiorly, the

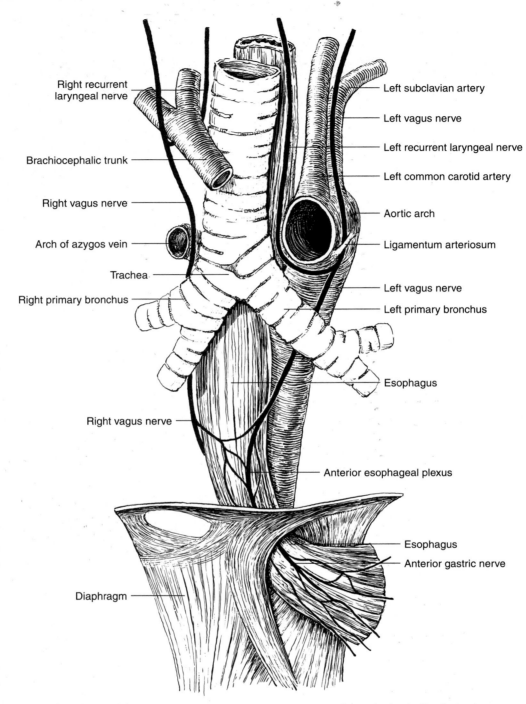

Figure 12-1. The trachea, esophagus, vagus nerves, and aorta in the mediastinum.

esophagus is located posterior to the trachea and anterior to the vertebral column, but below the tracheal bifurcation, it deviates to the left before penetrating the diaphragm (**Atlas Plate 155 #155.1**).

The esophagus receives its blood supply from three sources. Its **cervical part** is supplied by the **inferior thyroid branch of the thyrocervical trunk.** The **middle one-third** is supplied by esophageal branches from the thoracic aorta, and the **lower one-third** from esophageal branches of the **left gastric** and **left inferior phrenic arteries**. Its autonomic innervation comes from the two vagus nerves and the sympathetic trunks.

Incise the posterior part of the pericardial sac but save the phrenic nerves. Detach the pericardium from the diaphragm to expose the lower esophagus. Identify the **esophageal arteries** from the aorta (**ATLAS PLATE 156 #156.1**).

Find the **left and right vagus nerves** located behind the left and right primary bronchi (**ATLAS PLATE 162**). Follow the nerves to the esophagus and see how their branches join with fibers from the sympathetic trunk to form an **esophageal plexus (Figure 12-1)**. Note that the vagal fibers again form nerve trunks near the diaphragm on the anterior and posterior surfaces of the esophagus. Because of gut rotation during development, the fibers from the **left** vagus nerve regroup to form the **anterior vagal trunk,** and those of the **right** vagus course dorsally to form the **posterior vagal trunk.** At this site, they are often called the **anterior** and **posterior gastric nerves.**

B. Azygos System of Veins and the Thoracic Duct. The wall of the thorax and the posterior lumbar region are drained by the posterior intercostal and lumbar veins and these flow into the **azygos system of veins (Figure 12-2)**. This system consists of right and left vertically oriented veins that ascend in the posterior mediastinum adjacent to the bodies of the lower eight thoracic vertebrae. Usually, five terminal veins are in this system: the **azygos, hemiazygos, accessory hemiazygos,** and the **right** and **left superior intercostal veins** (**ATLAS PLATES 158, 159**).

The right ascending lumbar vein joins with the right subcostal vein to form the azygos vein. This ascends into the thorax through the aortic hiatus and receives the lower eight right posterior intercostal veins. Ascending posterior to the esophagus, the azygos vein is joined by the right superior intercostal vein and then curves anteriorly to enter the superior vena cava (**Figure 12-2**). In its ascent, it receives the hemiazygos veins from the left side as well as bronchial and esophageal veins.

On the left side, the **hemiazygos vein** receives the lowest four left posterior intercostal veins. The **accessory hemiazygos vein** receives the middle four left posterior intercostal veins, while the **left superior intercostal vein** receives the 2nd, 3rd, and 4th left intercostal veins. The latter vessel flows into the left brachiocephalic vein, and the hemiazygos and accessory hemiazygos veins both cross to the azygos vein.

The **thoracic duct** is a small diameter vessel that ascends in the posterior mediastinum posterior to the esophagus and between the azygos vein and aorta

◄
Grant's 72, 73, 75, 78
Netter's 226, 228, 233–236
Rohen 274–276, 279

◄
Grant's 73, 74, 76–78, 80, 81
Netter's 226, 234
Rohen 277, 279, 332

►
Grant's 73–76, 78, 80, 81
Netter's 202, 235
Rohen 18, 277, 279, 332

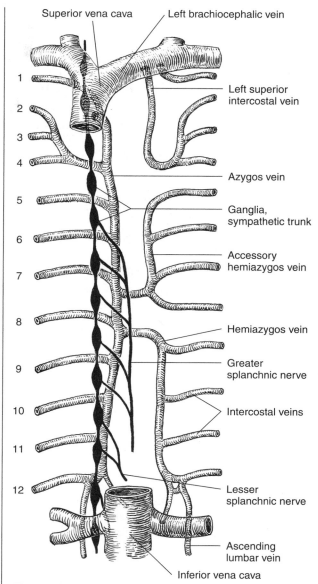

Figure 12-2. The sympathetic trunk, splanchnic nerves, and the azygos system of veins.

(**ATLAS PLATES 158, 159**). It returns lymph into the venous system and commences in the abdomen at the **cysterna chyli,** an elongated sac found anterior to the bodies of the first two lumbar vertebrae (**ATLAS PLATES 159, 168, 169**). It traverses the diaphragm through the aortic hiatus and ascends initially slightly to the right of the midline, but then at approximately the 5th thoracic vertebra, it inclines to the left (**ATLAS PLATE 168 #168.2**). In the root of the neck, the duct arches downward to enter the venous system at the junction of the **left subclavian** and **left internal jugular veins** (**ATLAS PLATES 168, 169**). The thoracic duct measures 33 to 40 cm (13 to 16 inches) in length and may easily be confused for a delicate vein.

Retract the esophagus to the left of the vertebral column to expose the **azygos vein.** Identify several **right posterior intercostal veins** that flow into it. Follow the azygos vein as it joins the superior vena cava (**ATLAS PLATE 159**). Note whether the right superior intercostal vein joins the azygos.

Now look for the **hemiazygos vein** on the left; note that it drains the lowest three or four left posterior intercostal veins. Identify the **accessory hemiazygos vein** and observe how it crosses the midline behind the aorta to flow into the azygos vein (**ATLAS PLATE 159**). Higher still, find the **left superior intercostal vein** as it drains into the left brachiocephalic vein.

Probe the fatty tissue behind the esophagus just above the diaphragm to find the thoracic duct in the posterior mediastinum between the aorta and the azygos vein. Note that the duct inclines to the left to ascend in the superior mediastinum posterior to the left margin of the esophagus (**ATLAS PLATES 158–160**).

C. **Descending Aorta.** The thoracic aorta descends from the aortic arch on the left side of the midline, but it gradually slants to the right and enters the abdomen in the midline between the crura of the diaphragm anterior to the 12th thoracic vertebra (**ATLAS PLATES 155 #155.2, 158**).

In the posterior mediastinum, the thoracic aorta gives off **visceral branches** to the pericardium, bronchi, and esophagus. Its **parietal branches** include nine pairs of **posterior intercostal arteries,** which enter the 3rd to the 11th intercostal spaces, and the **superior phrenic artery** to the diaphragm. The 12th pair of arteries course below the 12th rib and are called the **subcostal arteries.**

Clean the thoracic aorta and observe its gradual slant from left to right along its descent. Dissect several posterior intercostal arteries that arise from the **posterior surface** of the aorta. Note that the upper five or six **right** posterior intercostal arteries are longer than the left because they must cross the bodies of the vertebrae to reach the right intercostal spaces (**ATLAS PLATE 158**). Locate the bronchial and esophageal branches that arise from the **anterior** aspect of the aorta. Pull aside the lower esophagus and observe the aortic opening in the diaphragm (**ATLAS PLATE 155 #155.2**), two vertebral levels (T12) lower than the esophageal hiatus (T10).

▶
Grant's 17, 78–81
Netter's 205, 222, 226, 227, 236
Rohen 279–281

◀
Grant's 73, 74, 76–78, 80, 81
Netter's 202, 227–229, 233
Rohen 17, 18, 275–279, 281

▶
Grant's 75, 78–81
Netter's 205, 236
Rohen 15, 279–281

II. Sympathetic Trunks and Splanchnic Nerves (Figure 12-2)

The sympathetic division of the autonomic nervous system consists of **preganglionic** neurons, whose cell bodies lie in the thoracic and upper lumbar regions of the spinal cord, and **postganglionic** neurons, whose cell bodies are clustered in peripheral ganglia. The ganglia are located **paravertebrally** on both sides along the **sympathetic trunks** (**ATLAS PLATES 158, 162, 163**). Synapses between the preganglionic and postganglionic sympathetic neurons occur within all of these ganglia, but some preganglionic fibers pass through the sympathetic trunk to synapse in **prevertebral** (collateral) ganglia in the abdomen. These fibers form the **greater, lesser,** and **least thoracic splanchnic nerves,** which descend along the bodies of the lower thoracic vertebrae and pierce the crura of the diaphragm to enter the abdomen (**ATLAS PLATES 158, 159, 162**). To find the splanchnic nerves, it is best to dissect the sympathetic trunks first.

On the right side, strip the mediastinal and costal pleurae from the bodies of the thoracic vertebrae. Identify the **sympathetic trunk** coursing longitudinally along the inner surface of the posterior thoracic wall anterior to the ribs (**ATLAS PLATES 158, 162**).

Elevate parts of the sympathetic trunk with a probe to see the ganglia that form slight enlargements along the length of the trunk. Within several intercostal spaces, find the intercostal vessels and nerve. Dissect the delicate **communicating rami** that interconnect the sympathetic trunk with the thoracic intercostal nerves (**ATLAS PLATES 8 #8.1, 148, 163**).

The communicating branches are called **white** (myelinated) and **gray** (nonmyelinated) **rami communicantes.** White rami course from the intercostal nerves and carry myelinated **preganglionic** fibers to the sympathetic trunk and ganglia. They are located a bit lateral to the gray rami, which carry **postganglionic fibers** back to the intercostal nerve for distribution peripherally. You cannot distinguish between the white and gray rami by their color in the laboratory.

Next find the **splanchnic nerves.** Do this on the right side because of the aorta on the left. Note that branches emerge from the sympathetic trunk between the 5th to the 9th thoracic ganglia and cross anterior to the azygos and hemiazygos veins (**Figure 12-2**). They merge and descend through the diaphragm on each side as the **greater splanchnic nerve** (**ATLAS PLATE 158**). Find the **lesser splanchnic nerve** emerging from the 10th and 11th ganglia (**ATLAS PLATE 158**). The 12th thoracic ganglion sends a branch to form the **least splanchnic nerve,** but this is difficult to find. Observe that all of these nerves pierce the diaphragmatic crura to enter the abdomen where they join the preaortic ganglia.

III. Diaphragm (ATLAS PLATE 158)

The **adult diaphragm** is a dome-shaped sheet of muscle and tendon which separates the thorax from the abdomen. Muscular fibers radiate from the margin of the diaphragm into the central tendon; these are divided into **sternal, costal,** and **lumbar portions** (**ATLAS PLATES 158, 160 #160.2, 174**). The sternal fibers arise from the posterior part of the xiphoid process, and the costal part from the inner surfaces of the lower six ribs. The lumbar part attaches by strong tendons to the upper two or three lumbar vertebrae. They form the two **crura of the diaphragm** and, from their tendinous arches, the **medial** and **lateral arcuate ligaments** extend laterally on both sides. These thickenings arch over the upper parts of the **psoas major** (medial ligament) and **quadratus lumborum muscle** (lateral ligament) and will be seen from the abdominal side (**ATLAS PLATES 159, 250, 251**).

The diaphragm has three important apertures: the aortic, esophageal, and vena caval openings (**ATLAS PLATES 250, 252**). The **aortic opening** is in the midline at the **T12 level** and is bridged by the right and left crura. It transmits the aorta, the thoracic duct, and occasionally the azygos vein. The **esophageal opening** is located in the muscular part of the diaphragm at T10, approximately 2 cm to the left of the midline. Through this opening course the esophagus, the vagus nerves, and the esophageal branches of the left gastric vessels. The **vena caval opening** is found in the central tendon to the right of the midline at the **T8 level.** Smaller openings in each crus transmit the splanchnic nerves.

Observe the domelike contour of the diaphragm and remove any remaining pleura. Note that the right dome is higher than the left and that it rises as high as the 4th rib in forced expiration (**ATLAS PLATE 129 #129.3**). Observe that the central tendon receives muscle fibers around its entire periphery (**ATLAS PLATES 158, 160 #160.2**). Palpate the costal attachments of the diaphragm laterally and reach down into the **costodiaphragmatic recesses.** Visualize the

location of the liver, stomach, spleen, kidneys, and adrenal glands inferior to the diaphragm on the abdominal side (**ATLAS PLATES 154, 241**). Identify the vena caval, esophageal, and aortic openings. Dissect the phrenic nerves to their attachments on the diaphragm.

IV. Superior Mediastinum (Figure 12-3, ATLAS PLATES 134, 135, 158–160)

The superior mediastinum is that thoracic region between the manubrium of the sternum and the bodies of the upper four thoracic vertebrae (**ATLAS PLATES 130, 134**). It extends from the thoracic inlet to a transverse plane passing from the sternal angle to the body of the 4th thoracic vertebra. The superior mediastinum contains 1) the two **brachiocephalic veins,** the **superior vena cava** and **left superior intercostal vein;** 2) the **arch of the aorta** and its three large branches: the **brachiocephalic, left common carotid,** and **left subclavian arteries;** 3) the **vagus** and **phrenic nerves,** the **recurrent laryngeal branch of the left vagus,** and the **cardiac nerves** that descend to the cardiac plexus; 4) the **trachea** and **primary bronchi;** 5) the **esophagus;** and 6) the **thoracic duct.**

Posterior to the manubrium and anterior to the brachiocephalic veins are the fatty remnants of the **thymus** (**ATLAS PLATE 113**). To open the superior mediastinum, the manubrium and the attached medial one-third of both clavicles (with soft tissues) will be lifted as a block and folded upward over the neck.

With a handsaw, cut through both clavicles just lateral to the insertions of the clavicular heads of the sternocleidomastoid muscles. Divide the first ribs with bone cutters anterior to the subclavian vessels. Reflect the manubrium and the attached clavicles and first ribs upward. Remove the fatty remains of the thymus, but do not damage the underlying large brachiocephalic veins.

A. Great Blood Vessels in the Superior Mediastinum. The large veins and arteries in the superior mediastinum return blood to the heart or carry blood from the heart to the rest of the body.

  1. Great Veins. Identify the **right** and the more horizontally coursing **left brachiocephalic veins** (**ATLAS PLATES 134, 483**). Note their junction forms the **superior vena cava,**

► Grant's 65–67
Netter's 208, 226–228
Rohen 266–270

► Grant's 64, 66
Netter's 207
Rohen 265–268

◄ Grant's 71
Netter's 188
Rohen 283

► Grant's 64–66, 74
Netter's 207, 208
Rohen 265, 268, 269

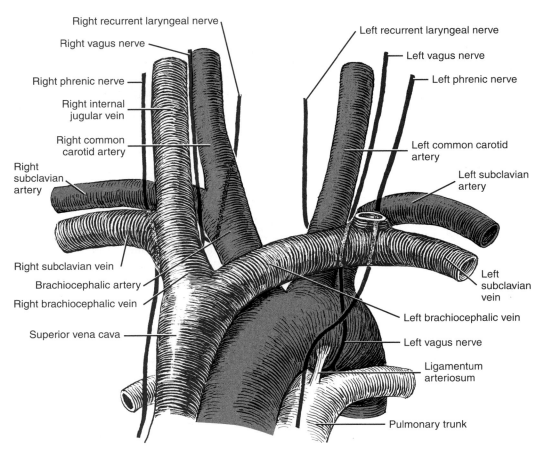

Right recurrent laryngeal nerve
Right vagus nerve
Right phrenic nerve
Right internal jugular vein
Right common carotid artery
Right subclavian artery
Right subclavian vein
Brachiocephalic artery
Right brachiocephalic vein
Superior vena cava

Left recurrent laryngeal nerve
Left vagus nerve
Left phrenic nerve
Left common carotid artery
Left subclavian artery
Left subclavian vein
Left brachiocephalic vein
Left vagus nerve
Ligamentum arteriosum
Pulmonary trunk

Figure 12-3. The great vessels and nerves in the superior mediastinum.

and each brachiocephalic vein is formed when the **internal jugular** and **subclavian veins** meet (**ATLAS PLATE 483**). Find the paired **internal thoracic veins,** each of which drains into its respective brachiocephalic vein, and identify the **inferior thyroid (ATLAS PLATE 483)** and **left superior intercostal veins (ATLAS PLATE 134),** which drain into the left brachiocephalic vein. Find the entrance of the azygos vein into the superior vena cava (**ATLAS PLATE 159**).

Find the **right phrenic nerve** that lies just lateral to the superior vena cava. Reflect the severed superior vena cava upward to study the underlying arch of the aorta and the major arteries that branch from it (**ATLAS PLATE 158**).

2. **Aortic Arch.** Note that the ascending aorta is 5 cm long and courses superiorly from the heart between the **superior vena cava** and the **pulmonary artery (ATLAS PLATE 134).** Observe that the aortic arch commences at the

◄
Grant's 65, 72
Netter's 208, 228, 262
Rohen 271, 279

level of the 2nd rib. Follow it posteriorly to the left of the trachea and esophagus. Identify its three large branches: the **brachiocephalic artery,** the **left common carotid artery,** and the **left subclavian artery (ATLAS PLATES 152, 155 #155.2).**

The **brachiocephalic artery** is the largest branch from the aortic arch, and it serves the right side of the head and the right upper extremity. It is approximately 5 cm long, courses upward and slightly to the right, and divides into the **right common carotid** and **right subclavian arteries** behind the right sternoclavicular joint (**ATLAS PLATES 483, 488**).

The **left common carotid artery** arises from the arch of the aorta to the left of the brachiocephalic artery. Ascending through the superior mediastinum, it enters the root of the neck behind the left sternoclavicular joint.

The **left subclavian artery** arises from the posterior part of the arch and ascends into the root of the neck behind the left clavicle. It arches to the left in the neck, deep to the anterior scalene muscle, and descends into the left axilla.

B. Phrenic, Vagus, and Recurrent Laryngeal Nerves (ATLAS PLATES 130, 134, 138). The **phrenic nerves** were dissected in the middle mediastinum coursing with the pericardiacophrenic vessels lateral to the pericardium (**ATLAS PLATE 134**). Arising from the C3, C4, and C5 segments, these nerves descend along the surface of the scalene muscles in the neck to enter the thorax.

> 1. **Phrenic Nerves.** Find the **left phrenic nerve** in the superior mediastinum lateral to the aortic arch between the left subclavian artery and vein (**ATLAS PLATE 135**). Follow its descent along the left side of the pericardium to the diaphragm (**ATLAS PLATE 134**). Identify the **right phrenic nerve** in the superior mediastinum posterior and lateral to the right brachiocephalic vein and then lateral to the superior vena cava.

The **vagus nerves** were visualized in the posterior mediastinum as they approached the esophagus to form the esophageal plexus. Most widely distributed of all the cranial nerves, they carry preganglionic parasympathetic nerve fibers to the viscera in the neck, thorax, and abdomen. As they descend through the superior mediastinum, their courses differ on the two sides (**ATLAS PLATE 162**).

> 2. **Right Vagus Nerve.** To find the **right vagus nerve** in the superior mediastinum, dissect behind the superior vena cava along the right margin of the trachea (**ATLAS PLATE 158, 162**). Follow the nerve to the posterior aspect of the hilum of the right lung, where it joins filaments from sympathetic ganglia to form the **right posterior pulmonary plexus.** From behind the right primary bronchus, follow branches to the **posterior surface** of the esophagus.

More superiorly is located the **recurrent laryngeal** branch of the right vagus. Too high to be dissected now, it winds around the first part of the subclavian artery and ascends in the neck on the right side of the trachea (**ATLAS PLATE 162**).

> 3. **Left Vagus Nerve.** To find the **left vagus nerve** in the superior mediastinum, dissect **slightly lateral** to the left common carotid artery (**ATLAS PLATES 130, 134, 162**). Follow the nerve to the left side of the aortic arch between

▶
Grant's 65, 66, 75, 79
Netter's 190, 205, 228, 236
Rohen 274, 276, 279

◀
Grant's 65, 78, 79
Netter's 207, 208, 210
Rohen 265, 271, 272

▶
Grant's 65–67, 72
Netter's 198, 204, 228
Rohen 275–278

◀
Grant's 65, 66, 78
Netter's 190, 205, 222, 236
Rohen 274, 276, 280

▶
Grant's 42, 66
Netter's 205, 222
Rohen 276, 278

the origins of the carotid and subclavian arteries and identify:

> a. the **left recurrent laryngeal** branch that courses under the aortic arch and the attachment of the **ligamentum arteriosum.** It ascends into the neck along a groove between the trachea and esophagus (**ATLAS PLATE 162**).
> b. delicate **cardiac branches** that descend to the deep part of the **cardiac plexus.**
> c. **pulmonary branches** that descend behind the root of the left lung that join sympathetic fibers to form the **left posterior pulmonary plexus;** follow branches from the hilum to the **anterior surface** of the esophagus (**ATLAS PLATE 162**).

C. Trachea, Primary Bronchi, Esophagus, and Thoracic Duct. The trachea begins in the neck at the lower end of the larynx at the C6 vertebral level. It is 4 inches long—2 inches in the neck and 2 inches the thorax—before it bifurcates at the lower level of the T4 vertebra (**ATLAS PLATES 122, 162**). The trachea lies deep to the manubrium in the superior mediastinum. Slightly lower, it lies posterior to the left brachiocephalic vein, arch of the aorta, and brachiocephalic and left common carotid arteries (**ATLAS PLATE 483**). Throughout its course, the trachea lies anterior to the esophagus, which separates it from the 7th cervical and upper four thoracic vertebrae.

> With the brachiocephalic veins reflected upward, study the relationships of the aortic arch, pulmonary arteries, and primary bronchi at the tracheal bifurcation. Observe that the **left primary bronchus** is more horizontal than the right and that it measures 5 cm before it divides into the secondary (lobar) bronchi (**Figure 12-4**). Note that the **right bronchus** is wider and more vertical than the left and is slightly more than 2.5 cm in length.

The larger width and more vertical course of the right primary bronchus explain why foreign bodies that are accidentally swallowed become lodged more frequently in the right primary bronchus than the left.

> Push the aortic arch to the left and expose the anterior aspect of the tracheal bifurcation. Identify vagal and sympathetic branches that join to form the **deep cardiac plexus,** usually located behind the aortic arch anterior to the tracheal bifurcation. Locate pigmented tracheobroncheal lymph nodes near the bifurcation

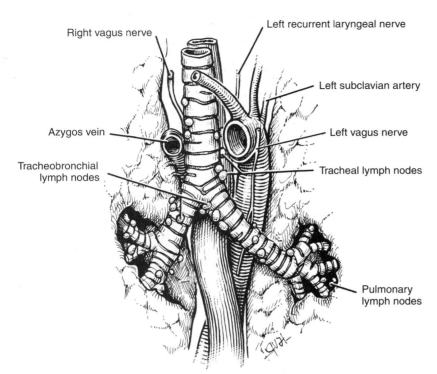

Right vagus nerve

Left recurrent laryngeal nerve

Left subclavian artery

Azygos vein

Left vagus nerve

Tracheobronchial lymph nodes

Tracheal lymph nodes

Pulmonary lymph nodes

Figure 12-4. The trachea and its bifurcation.

(Figure 12-4). Cut the bronchi longitudinally with scissors and visualize the interior of the tracheal bifurcation. On the posterior surface of the bifurcation, observe an internal cartilaginous ridge, the **carina,** and note that it is located slightly to the left of the midline.

In the superior mediastinum, the esophagus lies slightly to the left of the midline and descends between the trachea and the vertebral column **(Figures 12-5, 12-6)**. The thoracic duct ascends through the superior mediastinum and courses to the thoracic inlet posterior to the esophagus **(ATLAS PLATES 159, 168)**.

Displace the trachea to the right and observe the esophagus descending posteriorly **(ATLAS PLATES 155, 162)**. Identify the left recurrent laryngeal nerve ascending in a groove between the trachea and esophagus. Observe the left primary bronchus crossing anterior to the esophagus and the left border of the esophagus adjacent to the aortic arch. Displace the esophagus to the right, away from the midline. Probe longitudinally in the fat posterior to the esophagus for the thoracic duct. Observe that this small vein-like structure passes superiorly to the root of the neck on the left **(ATLAS PLATES 168, 159)**. Trace the duct to its termination at the junction of the left subclavian and internal jugular veins **(ATLAS PLATE 169)**.

◄
Grant's 65, 67, 72–75, 79
Netter's 202, 228, 233–236
Rohen 235, 274–279, 332

Clinical Relevance

Hiatas hernia. Hiatus hernia is the protrusion of a structure through the esophageal hiatus of the diaphragm. Most often, in this condition the upper part of the stomach (the esophageal-gastric junction or the fundus of the stomach) will protrude through the esophageal hiatus and lodge in the posterior mediastinum.

Gastroesophageal reflux. Regurgitation of the gastric contents into the esophagus is usually associated with hiatus hernia or peptic ulcer. Repeated injury to the esophageal mucosa can result in an esophageal carcinoma.

Esophageal varicosities. This condition is often caused by portal venous blood obstruction through the liver in patients who have cirrhosis of the liver. Blood in the portal vein seeks alternative routes in an attempt to return to the inferior vena cava and the right atrium. One of these routes involves anastomotic channels with veins in the lower one third of the esophagus. These veins then become greatly dilated, resulting in esophageal varicies on the internal surface of the mucosa where they are subject to hemorrhage.

Severance of the thoracic duct. The thoracic duct ascends anterior to the bodies of the thoracic vertebrae on its route to the left subclavian vein in the neck. It is a thin, veinlike structure and can easily be injured during posterior mediastinum operations. Lymph escaping from a severed duct accumulates in the pleural cavity and results in a chylothorax, a condition that requires attention.

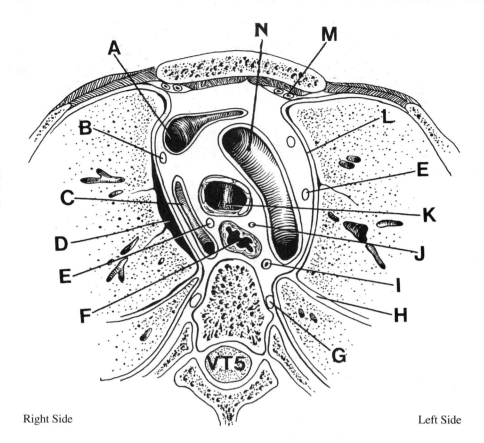

Figure 12-5. Transverse section of the thorax at the level of T-5. **A.** Superior vena cava. **B.** Phrenic nerve. **C.** Azygos vein. **D.** Pleural cavity. **E.** Right vagus nerve. **E.** Left vagus nerve. **F.** Esophagus. **G.** Sympathetic trunk. **H.** Oblique fissure. **I.** Thoracic duct. **J.** Recurrent laryngeal nerve. **K.** Bifurcation of the trachea. **L.** Mediastinal pleura. **M.** Internal thoracic vessels. **N.** Aorta.

Right Side   Left Side

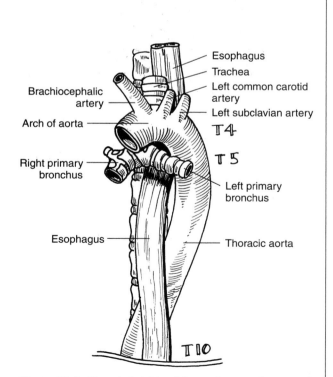

Figure 12-6. The relationship of the trachea, esophagus, and thoracic aorta.

Recurrent laryngeal nerve injury. The recurrent laryngeal nerve supplies all but one pair of intrinsic muscles in the larynx. Injury to this nerve can result from any operation in the superior mediastinum or in the neck where the nerve courses just lateral to the thyroid gland. Additionally, tumors of the esophagus or bronchi or even an aneurysm of the aorta can interrupt this nerve. Injury to one recurrent laryngeal nerve results in hoarseness of speech.

Coarctation of the aorta. This condition is a congenital narrowing of the aorta below the origin of the left subclavian artery. Because blood is somewhat impeded in the descending aorta, other vessels from the aorta become greatly enlarged (such as the intercostal arteries), and blood bypasses the constriction. The dilated intercostal arteries characteristically erode the lower borders of the ribs, thereby notching the ribs.

Patent ductus arteriosus. The ductus arteriosus is a fetal vessel that interconnects the aorta and the pulmonary artery so that maternally oxygenated blood can pass directly into the aortic systemic circulation and bypass the lungs. Normally, 2 or 3 weeks after birth the ductus arteriosus closes. If it does not close, aortic blood will flow into the pulmonary artery and result in pulmonary hypertension and hypertrophy of the right ventricle.

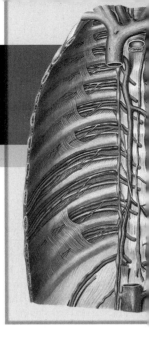

DISSECTION #13

The Anterior Abdominal Wall

OBJECTIVES

1 Learn the surface landmarks and the anatomic regions of the abdomen.

2 Dissect the superficial fascia and superficial vessels and nerves of the anterior abdominal wall.

3 Dissect the three flat abdominal wall muscles and their related vessels and nerves.

4 Dissect the rectus abdominis muscle and rectus sheath.

5 Dissect the inguinal region in males and understand the importance of the inguinal canal.

6 Understand indirect and direct inguinal hernias.

7 Dissect the scrotum, spermatic cord, and testes.

8 Dissect the female inguinal canal and visualize the round ligament of the uterus.

Atlas Key:

Clemente Atlas, 5th Edition = Atlas Plate #

Grant's Atlas, 11th Edition = Grant's Page #

Netter's Atlas, 3rd Edition = Netter's Plate #

Rohen Atlas, 6th Edition = Rohen Page #

The anterior abdominal wall overlies the viscera of the abdominal cavity. It extends from the **xiphoid process** to the **pubic symphysis.** Superiorly, it is bounded by the **costal margins** of the rib cage. Inferiorly, it extends to the crests of the ilia and the inguinal ligaments (**ATLAS PLATES 178, 179**).

▶
Grant's 96–99
Netter's 241–244
Rohen 207,
211–213

I. Surface Anatomy of the Anterior Abdominal Wall

Before dissecting the anterior abdominal wall, see some of its surface features and the subdivisions of the abdomen.

A. Surface Landmarks. Visualize or palpate the following anatomic features.

1. **Linea alba.** Median raphé between the xiphoid process and the symphysis pubis (**ATLAS PLATE 178**).

2. **Linea semilunaris.** Longitudinal curved lines that demarcate the two lateral borders of the

rectus abdominis muscle. Difficult to see in an obese cadaver, but when visible, they are concave medially and extend from the 9th costal cartilage to the symphysis pubis. Note that the point where the linea semilunaris crosses the right costal margin is the external landmark of the **gall bladder.**

3. **Pubic crest.** On a skeleton observe the rounded pubic crest on the anterosuperior border of the pubis, just lateral to the **symphysis pubis** (**ATLAS PLATES 268, 269**). Lateral to the pubic crest palpate the **pubic tubercle** where the medial end of the **inguinal ligament** attaches (**ATLAS PLATES 270, 271**).

4. **Iliac crests.** The bony upper borders of the ilium that can be felt on yourself at the lateral limits of your waist (**ATLAS PLATES 266, 267**). On a skeleton, follow the crest anteriorly to the **anterior superior iliac spine,** where the lateral end of the **inguinal ligament** attaches (**ATLAS PLATE 271 #271.1**). On the summit of the iliac crest, 5 cm posterior to the anterior superior iliac spine, locate the **tubercle of the iliac crest.**

B. **Anatomic Regions (Figure 13-1).** The anterior abdominal wall can be divided by two vertical and two horizontal planes into nine **regions.** The two vertical planes pass through the midpoints of the inguinal ligaments, and the two horizontal planes are the **transpyloric** and **transtubercular planes.**

These four lines form a grid of nine regions on the anterior abdominal wall (**Figure 13-1**). From above downward, the unpaired central regions are the **epigastric,** the **umbilical** (containing the umbilicus), and the **hypogastric regions.** The three paired regions from above downward are the **hypochondriac regions** (inferior to the

◄
Grant's 96
Netter's 260
Rohen 216

►
Rohen 217

◄
Grant's 102, 191
Netter's 251

◄
Grant's 186, 187, 291
Netter's 240, 468, 476
Rohen 189, 210, 439

costal margins), the **lumbar regions** (between the costal margins and iliac crests), and the **inguinal regions** (lateral to the hypogastric region above the inguinal ligaments).

The abdomen is also described as being divided into quadrants. Visualize a **vertical plane** passing through the umbilicus between the xiphoid process and the symphysis pubis and a **horizontal plane** also passing through the umbilicus across the abdomen. This topographic subdivision (often used by clinicians) results in **upper right** and **left quadrants** and **lower right** and **left quadrants.**

II. Skin Incisions; Superficial Fascia; Cutaneous Vessels and Nerves

The skin of the anterior abdominal wall is thin compared to skin on the back. Although surgical incisions should follow lines of cleavage in the skin (Langer's lines) to minimize scar tissue, incisions made for anatomic dissection need not conform to cleavage lines.

A. **Abdominal Skin Incisions (Figure 13-2).** Place the cadaver in the supine position (face up) and note any evidence of wounds or surgical scars visible on the abdominal surface.

Make a midline incision **through the skin only** (not into the superficial fascia) from the xiphoid process to the symphysis pubis. Leave the umbilicus intact by encircling it with the incision (**Figure 13-2, A to B**). Make cuts in both inguinal regions (again only through the skin), from the symphysis pubis laterally along the inguinal ligament to the anterior superior iliac spine (**Figure 13-2, B to C**). Continue these incisions posteriorly for 3 inches along the iliac crest. If not already done, make incisions laterally

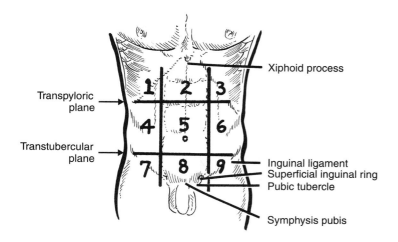

Figure 13-1. Anatomic regions of the abdomen: 1 and 3 = right and left hypochondriac regions; 4 and 6 = right and left lumbar regions; 7 and 9 = right and left inguinal regions; 2 = epigastric region; 5 = umbilical region; 8 = hypogastric region.

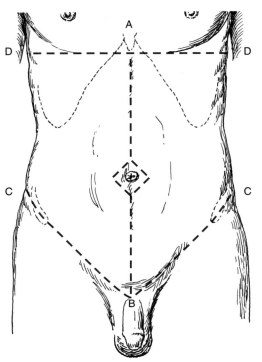

Figure 13-2. Abdominal skin incisions. These incisions are only skin deep.

from the xiphoid process to the mid-axillary lines on both sides (**Figure 13-2, A to D**).

Reflect the skin flaps laterally without cutting into the superficial fascia. You are dissecting in the correct plane if you can see the dermal papillae on the inner surface of the skin flaps.

B. Superficial Fascia (Figure 13-3). The superficial fascia over the anterior abdominal wall is different from other regions in that it can be dissected as two layers below the umbilicus but only as a single layer above. It contains a variable amount of fat and fibrous tissue, which combine in one layer above the umbilicus. Below the umbilicus, the superficial layer of superficial fascia is a layer of fat and is known as **Camper's fascia (Figure 13-3A).** Underlying this fatty layer is the deep layer of superficial fascia, called **Scarpa's fascia,** which is more membranous and contains many elastic fibers (**Figure 13-3A**). Separation of the two fascial layers is possible only in the region between the pubis and the umbilicus.

▶
Grant's 100, 104,
105
Netter's 241, 248,
360, 363

With the skin reflected, make a transverse incision midway between the umbilicus and symphysis pubis from a point 3 cm above the anterior superior iliac spine to the linea alba. Cut through both layers of superficial fascia to the fibers of the external oblique muscle and its glistening aponeurosis medially. Separate Scarpa's fascia from this aponeurosis and manually extend the separation inferiorly to the inguinal ligament. Observe the following:

1. How Scarpa's fascia fuses with the **fascia lata** (deep fascia) of the thigh (**Figure 13-3C**).

2. That you can insert your finger inferiorly into the scrotum along the path of the spermatic cord but not laterally into the thigh.

▶
Netter's 241, 251,
348
Rohen 212

3. That just above the symphysis pubis, you are unable to pass your finger across the midline

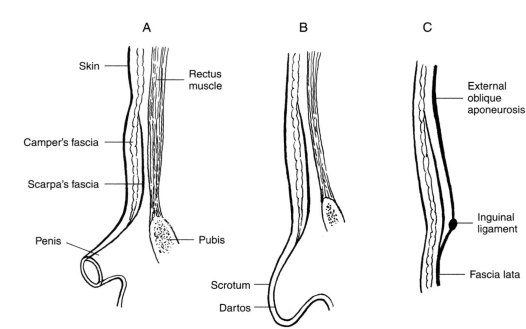

Figure 13-3. Diagram of superficial fascia over anterior abdominal wall. **A.** Longitudinal section near the midline over the penis. **B.** Section made more laterally over the scrotum. **C.** Section more laterally over the fascia lata of the thigh. (Redrawn after Hollinshead WH. Anatomy for Surgeons. 2nd Ed. New York: Hoeber-Harper, 3 vols., 1968.)

because of the attachment of the **fundiform ligament** of the penis or clitoris (**ATLAS PLATE 179 #179.1**).

4. That the aponeurosis of the external oblique muscle folds internally to form the **inguinal ligament.**

Scarpa's fascia continues into the scrotal sac, where it becomes the **dartos layer** (**Figure 13-3B**), and further into the perineum, where it is called **Colles' fascia.** If a rupture of the penile urethra occurs, extravasated urine will escape into the perineum and scrotum and spread deep to Colles' fascia and the dartos layer. It then continues upward on the anterior abdominal wall deep to Scarpa's fascia. Urine will **not spread** into the thighs because Scarpa's fascia terminates where it attaches to the fascia lata inferiorly (**Figure 13-3C**).

C. Superficial Vessels and Nerves (**ATLAS PLATE 176**). The cutaneous nerves are accompanied by superficial arteries and veins over the anterior abdominal wall. As in the thoracic wall, **lateral cutaneous branches** of the segmental nerves (T7–T12 and L1) pierce the soft tissues and emerge along the mid-axillary line, and **anterior cutaneous branches** become superficial just lateral to the linea alba (**ATLAS PLATE 176**).

In addition to the vessels that accompany the segmental nerves, the anterior abdominal wall receives blood from the more deeply coursing **superior** and **inferior epigastric arteries** and other arteries in the superficial inguinal region derived from the femoral artery (**ATLAS PLATES 9, 176**). Drainage is by segmental veins and by an anastomosing network of vessels around the umbilicus. Inferior to the umbilicus, veins drain into the **saphenous** and **femoral veins,** and superior to the umbilicus, venous blood drains into the **thoracoepigastric** and **axillary veins.**

1. **Superficial Vessels.** In the inguinal region, dissect the superficial fascia. Then, find the **superficial circumflex iliac** and **superficial epigastric arteries,** which often arise from a common branch of the femoral artery, and the **external pudendal artery,** which arises alone (**ATLAS PLATES 9, 368**).

   a. Dissect the **superficial circumflex iliac artery** as it courses laterally from the femoral artery 1 cm below the inguinal ligament upward toward the anterior superior iliac spine (**ATLAS PLATE 368**).

▶
Grant's 97
Netter's 247, 248
Rohen 209, 210,
214, 216
◀
Grant's 97–100,
107
Netter's 342–344
Rohen 213, 219,
445

▶
Grant's 94, 97
Netter's 249
Rohen 207

▶
Grant's 20, 97
Netter's 249, 250
Rohen 207, 214

   b. Find the **superficial epigastric artery,** which ascends over the inguinal ligament in an oblique course toward the umbilicus (**ATLAS PLATES 9, 176**).

   c. Locate the **external pudendal artery** (from the medial side of the femoral artery) coursing superiorly and medially above the symphysis pubis to supply the superficial inguinal region and lateral aspect of the scrotum (**ATLAS PLATES 188, 190**).

2. **Cutaneous Nerves.** Dissect one or more **anterior** and **lateral cutaneous** branches of the lower thoracic nerves (T7 to T12) and the **iliohypogastric** and **ilioinguinal** branches of the first lumbar nerve (**ATLAS PLATES 176, 190**).

   a. **Anterior Cutaneous Nerves** (**Figure 13-4**). Probe the superficial fascia 2 to 3 centimeters lateral to the linea alba, and find anterior cutaneous branches of the thoracic nerves piercing the sheath of the rectus abdominis (**ATLAS PLATE 9**). Find the

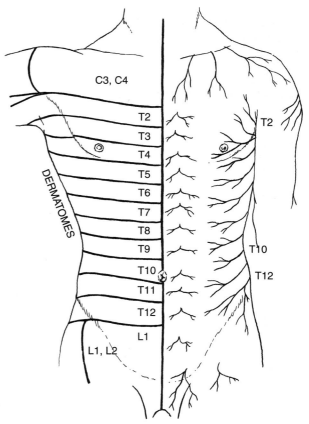

Figure 13-4. Cutaneous nerves and dermatomes of the anterior body wall. (Redrawn after Thorek P. Anatomy in Surgery. 2nd Ed. Philadelphia: J.B. Lippincott, 1962.)

T10 branch just near the umbilicus, the T7 nerve adjacent to the xiphoid process, and T12, approximately 3 centimeters below the umbilicus.

    b. Lateral Cutaneous Nerves (Figure 13-4). Dissect in the midaxillary line to find these nerves (T7 to T12). Identify the more superior ones (T7–9) emerging from the interdigitations of the serratus anterior and external oblique muscles (**ATLAS PLATES 9, 176**).

    c. Iliohypogastric Nerve. Dissect the superficial fascia 4 centimeters above the pubic crest and identify the **iliohypogastric nerve (L1)** (**ATLAS PLATES 176, 188**). Note that it courses between the transversus and internal oblique muscles (supplying both) and then perforates the aponeurosis of the external oblique to become sensory above the pubis.

    d. Ilioinguinal Nerve. Identify the **superficial inguinal ring,** which is a triangular opening in the aponeurosis of the external oblique, superior and lateral to the pubic crest. Find the **spermatic cord** and on its surface the ilioinguinal nerve (also L1) traversing the superficial inguinal ring (**ATLAS PLATES 176, 179, 188, 190**). It supplies the upper medial thigh and the upper part of the scrotum or labium majus.

    Reflect the superficial fascia from the anterior abdominal wall to study the muscles.

III. Flat Muscles and Nerves of the Anterior Abdominal Wall

The anterior abdominal wall contains three muscle layers. These enclose the abdominal cavity and: a) the direction of their fibers differ; b) they consist of muscle fibers laterally but form aponeuroses medially; and c) the aponeuroses of the three muscles fuse to form the **rectus sheath,** which encloses the longitudinally oriented **rectus abdominis muscle.** This muscle extends from the pubis to the thoracic cartilages on each side of the linea alba (**ATLAS PLATES 181, 183**).

    The three flat abdominal wall muscles stretch broadly from the flanks (or lumbar region) toward the midline. From superficial to deep, they are the **external oblique, internal oblique,** and **transversus abdominis muscles.** Between the latter two muscles is the neurovascular plane containing the lower six thoracic and first lumbar nerves along with their accompanying blood vessels (**ATLAS PLATE 8**).

◄
Grant's 20, 94, 97
Netter's 246, 249, 250
Rohen 205, 207, 214

◄
Grant's 98, 101, 104–106
Netter's 249, 259, 389
Rohen 212–214, 217

►
Grant's 98, 106, 101–103
Netter's 242, 244
Rohen 212, 213, 216, 217

►
Grant's 98, 102
Netter's 243, 244
Rohen 214, 215, 218

►
Grant's 100, 104, 353
Netter's 251
Rohen 211, 217, 220

◄
Grant's 94, 97
Netter's 241, 244
Rohen 205, 210, 211

►
Grant's 94, 97
Netter's 241
Rohen 210, 211

    A. External Oblique Muscle (Figure 13-5). The external oblique muscle arises by fleshy slips from the outer surface of the lower eight ribs, and its fibers course inferomedially in the same direction as putting one's hands in his or her side pockets (**ATLAS PLATE 178**). Its upper four slips of origin interdigitate with the serratus anterior muscle and its lower four with the latissimus dorsi. The most inferior fibers insert onto the iliac crest. Those from ribs 5 through 10 form a strong aponeurosis, which courses anterior to the rectus abdominis muscle, intersecting with fibers from the other side across the linea alba (**ATLAS PLATE 179**).

    B. Internal Oblique Muscle (Figure 13-6). The internal oblique arises from the lateral two-thirds of the inguinal ligament, the iliac crest, and the thoracolumbar fascia. Its fibers course superomedially at right angles to those of the external oblique, and then form an aponeurosis just lateral to the rectus abdominis and join the linea alba in the midline (**ATLAS PLATES 180–182**).

    C. Transverse Abdominis Muscle. The innermost muscular layer is the transversus abdominis muscle, and its fibers course transversely across the abdomen also ending in an aponeurosis (**ATLAS PLATE 183**). It arises from the lower margin of the rib cage, the lumbar fascia, iliac crest, and lateral third of the inguinal ligament. Most of its aponeurosis passes behind the rectus abdominis muscle and terminates in the linea alba (**ATLAS PLATE 177**). The lower aponeurotic fibers curve inferiorly and join with others from the internal oblique to form the **falx inguinalis** (conjoint tendon). This attaches to the pubic crest behind the superficial inguinal ring, and it strengthens a potentially weak part of the inguinal region (**ATLAS PLATES 177, 181**).

Having identified the superficial inguinal ring as a triangular opening in the external oblique aponeurosis, observe that its margins are the **medial crus** and **lateral crus.** These are strengthened by curved **intercrural fibers** that course around the lateral border of the ring (**ATLAS PLATE 179**). Before reflecting the external oblique muscle, it is important to determine its thickness.

    Use scissors and forceps to separate the fibers of the **external oblique** along their directional line for 5 centimeters below the 9th rib (**Figure 13-5, point A**). Identify the fibers of the underlying internal oblique coursing in the opposite direction. Being

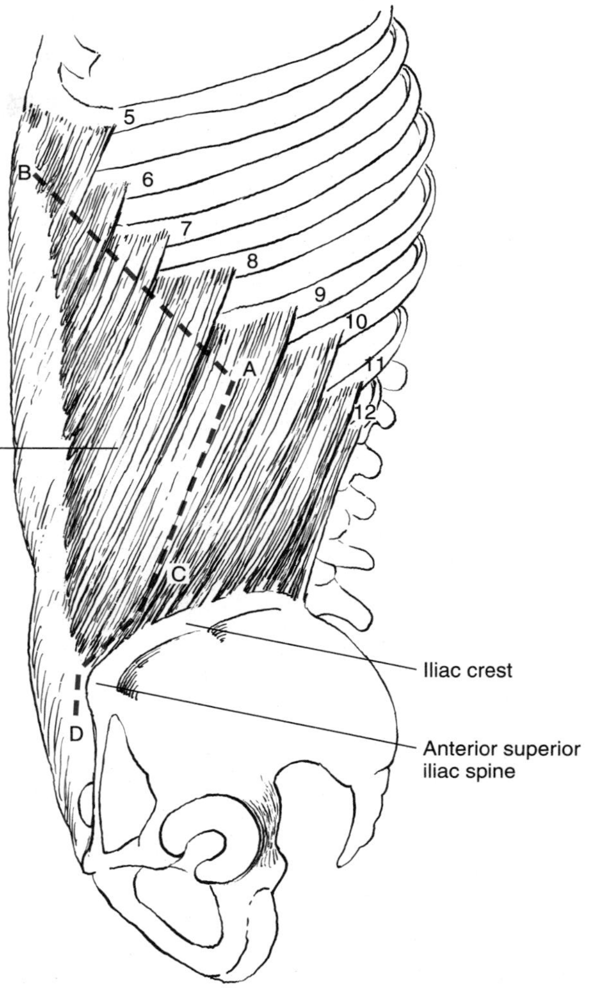

Figure 13-5. Incision lines for external oblique muscle (left lateral view).

certain of the correct plane, lengthen the scissors cut to the iliac crest (**Figure 13-5, point C**). Use your fingers to separate the two planes of muscle further.

Sever the external oblique muscle superiorly and medially to its attachment to the 5th rib (**Figure 13-5, A to B**). Extend the incision from point C anteriorly along the iliac crest to the anterior superior iliac spine (**Figure 13-5, C to D**). Reflect the external oblique flap medially to the lateral border of the rectus abdominis to expose the internal oblique muscle (**ATLAS PLATE 181**).

Clean the **internal oblique** and find the iliohypogastric and ilioinguinal branches of the L1 nerve approximately 3 to 5 cm medial to the anterior superior iliac spine (**ATLAS PLATES 9, 176**). Separate the fibers of the internal oblique for a short distance in a line approximately 2 cm below the costal margin. Determine the plane between the internal oblique and the underlying transversus abdominis (**Figure 13-6**).

◀
Grant's 98
Netter's 242
Rohen 212, 213

▶
Grant's 102, 105
Netter's 242, 243,
251
Rohen 218

Use your index finger to separate the two muscular planes but do not destroy the nerves and vessels that course between them. Lift the internal oblique and cut its attachment along the costal margin (**Figure 13-6, A to B**), then cut vertically from the 11th or 12th rib to the iliac crest (**Figure 13-6, B to C**). Sever the internal oblique attachment along the iliac crest to the anterior superior iliac spine and continue the cut along the inguinal ligament (**Figure 13-6, C to D**).

Lift the internal oblique and reflect it medially to the rectus sheath. In the inguinal region, identify the **falx inguinalis** (conjoint tendon), if present. This structure is a fused portion of the aponeuroses of the internus and transversus and inserts into the pubic crest and pectineal line. It forms the important **posterior wall** of the medial third of the inguinal canal (**ATLAS PLATES 177, 181**).

On male cadavers, identify the **cremaster muscle** as it extends from the lower border of the internal

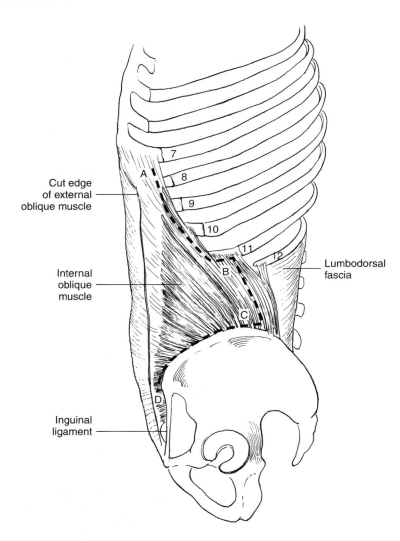

Cut edge
of external
oblique muscle

Internal
oblique
muscle

Inguinal
ligament

Lumbodorsal
fascia

Figure 13-6. Incision lines for internal oblique muscle (left lateral view).

oblique. Note that its fibers are arranged in loops on the surface of the spermatic cord (**ATLAS PLATE 192**). Find the delicate **genital branch of the genitofemoral nerve** (L1, L2) that supplies the cremaster muscle from its deep surface.

◄
Grant's 101, 102, 106, 107
Netter's 242, 251, 370
Rohen 246

In life, the cremaster muscle contracts reflexly on stimulation of the skin on the upper medial thigh. This initiates the **cremasteric reflex,** which results in an elevation of the testis.

►
Grant's 94
Netter's 249, 250
Rohen 207, 212, 215, 216

Identify the ascending branch of the **deep iliac circumflex artery** coursing vertically along the transversus muscle (**ATLAS PLATE 187**). It branches from the external iliac artery and anastomoses with lumbar and inferior epigastric arteries.

◄
Grant 's103, 106, 353
Netter's 247
Rohen 216, 480, 481

D. Nerves of the Anterior Abdominal Wall (ATLAS PLATES 8, 176). These nerves are the lateral and anterior branches of the lower six thoracic and 1st lumbar spinal nerves.

Identify the segmental nerves by using **T10** as a reference because it supplies the region around the umbilicus. Find the **T12 (subcostal) nerve** below the 12th rib and again the **iliohypogastric** and **ilioinguinal branches of the L-1 nerve.**

IV. Rectus Abdominis Muscle and Sheath; Epigastric Anastomosis

The **rectus abdominis** muscles are long and flat (**Figures 13-7, 13-8**), and they are separated in the midline by the linea alba. Each extends upward from the pubic crest to the 5th, 6th, and 7th costal cartilages on the anterior surface of the rib cage (**ATLAS PLATES**

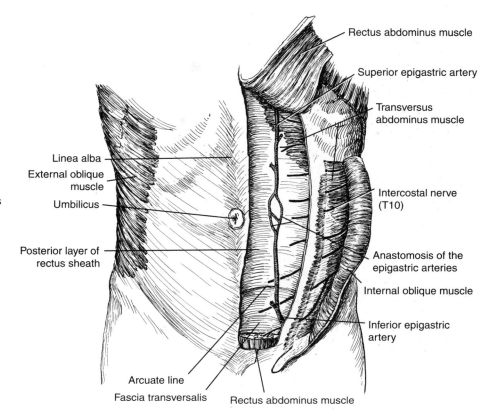

Figure 13-7. The epigastric anastomosis within the rectus abdominis muscle.

181–183). Its fibers are crossed by three or four **tendinous intersections,** which strengthen the muscle (**ATLAS PLATES 182, 183**).

On each side, the rectus abdominis is enclosed within a sheath formed by the aponeuroses of the flat abdominal muscles (**Figure 13-8**). At the lateral border of the rectus muscle, the aponeurosis of the internal oblique splits into two laminae (**ATLAS PLATE 186 #186.1**). One lamina courses posterior to the rectus muscle, blends with the aponeurosis of the transversus, and forms the **posterior layer of the rectus sheath**

◄
Grant's 92, 106
Netter's 242, 244
Rohen 210–216

◄
Grant's 98
Netter's 243, 245
Rohen 213, 216

(**ATLAS PLATES 177, 183**). The other lamina courses anterior to the rectus and blends with the aponeurosis of the external oblique to form the **anterior layer of the rectus sheath (Figure 13-8**).

Midway between the umbilicus and the symphysis pubis, the posterior layer of the sheath terminates (**ATLAS PLATES 177, 183**). Below this site, the aponeuroses of all three muscles course in front of the rectus abdominis muscle. The curved **arcuate line** marks the inferior margin of the posterior rectus sheath (**ATLAS PLATES 183**). Below the arcuate line, the rectus abdominis lacks a

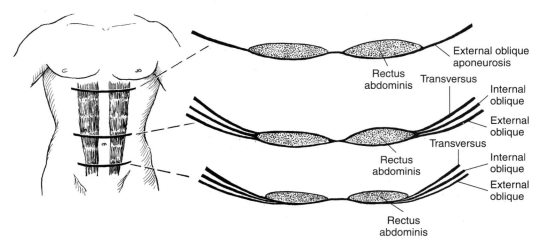

Figure 13-8. The rectus sheath.

posterior sheath and rests directly on the fascia transversalis (**ATLAS PLATE 186 #186.2**).

> Open the rectus sheaths of both muscles. Make longitudinal incisions in the sheaths from a point 2 cm lateral to the linea alba just below the xiphoid process to a site 1 cm lateral to the linea alba at the symphysis pubis (**ATLAS PLATE 181**). Cut any adhesions from the tendinous intersections that attach to the anterior layer of the sheath. Identify the thoracic nerves that penetrate the sheath laterally to supply the muscle with T10 at the level of the umbilicus.
>
> Cut the rectus abdominis transversely near its middle. Reflect its lower half and identify the curved arcuate line and the **inferior epigastric artery** that enters the rectus sheath at this line (**ATLAS PLATE 187**). Reflect the upper half of the rectus abdominis and find the **superior epigastric artery.** Note that the two epigastric vessels perforate the muscle and anastomose (**Figure 13-7, ATLAS PLATES 111, 187**).

Anastomosis of the epigastric veins provides a route for the return of venous blood to the heart in patients with an obstruction of the inferior vena cava. The epigastric arterial anastomosis allows a collateral route for arterial blood to flow downward in instances of aortic obstruction as occurs in congenital malformations such as coarctation of the aorta.

V. Inguinal Region

The inguinal region is important because it contains the inguinal canal that transmits the spermatic cord in males (**ATLAS PLATES 190, 192**). The inguinal canal also exists in women, but it contains the round ligament of the uterus, a structure of little importance (**ATLAS PLATE 188**). Because the canal passes through the flat muscles of the abdomen, its location weakens the lower medial part of the anterior abdominal wall and makes it subject to hernias. During development, the male inguinal canals form as pathways for the testes in their descent to the scrotal sac (**ATLAS PLATE 195 #195.2**). The ovaries also descend in females but only to the brim of the pelvis, but the round ligaments of the uterus course through the inguinal canals to terminate in the labia majora.

The inguinal canal commences at the **deep** (abdominal) **inguinal ring.** This is an opening in the transversalis fascia near the midpoint of the inguinal ligament under cover of the internal and external oblique muscles

▶ Grant's 101, 104, 353
Netter's 241, 242
Rohen 217–220

▶ Grant's 101–105
Netter's 242, 243, 245, 251
Rohen 217–241

▶ Grant's 353
Netter's 243, 252, 255

◀ Grant's 98, 106
Netter's 243, 245, 247
Rohen 212, 214, 216

▶ Netter's 245, 351

◀ Grant's 236, 237, 239, 241
Netter's 251, 254
Rohen 218, 220, 362

▶ Grant's 109
Rohen 219

◀ Grant's 102, 106
Netter's 245, 251
Rohen 219, 220

(**ATLAS PLATE 177**). The deep ring lies just lateral to the inferior epigastric artery and vein (**ATLAS PLATE 177**). From this site, the inguinal canal extends in an oblique inferomedial direction for 5 cm (or less) to the **superficial inguinal ring** (**Figures 13-9, 13-10**), already identified in the aponeurosis of the external oblique (**ATLAS PLATES 178, 179**).

The inguinal canal is bounded **anteriorly** by skin, superficial fascia, and the aponeurosis of the external oblique (**ATLAS PLATES 178, 179 #179.2**). Additionally, the lateral part of the canal is covered anteriorly by the internal oblique muscle (**ATLAS PLATES 180, 181**). **Posteriorly,** the wall of the inguinal canal is formed by the **transversalis fascia** throughout and more medially by the **inguinal falx** (conjoint tendon) as well as the **reflex inguinal ligament** (**Figure 13-9, ATLAS PLATE 181**). **Superiorly,** the inguinal canal is bound by the arching fibers of the internal oblique and transversus muscles, while **inferiorly** is found the transversalis fascia along its attachment to the **inguinal ligament** and, more medially, the **lacunar ligament** (**Figure 13-9**). This latter ligament is a crescent-shaped extension of the inguinal ligament that courses backward and slightly upward along the pectineal line of the pubis (**ATLAS PLATE 179 #179.2**). The continuation of the lacunar ligament along the **pectineal line** is called the **pectineal ligament of Cooper** (**Figure 13-9, ATLAS PLATES 252, 270 #270.2**).

The **inferior epigastric vessels** form the **lateral border** of the important **inguinal (Hesselbach's) triangle.** The **inferior border** of this triangle is the **inguinal ligament,** and **medially** the triangle is bounded by the **lateral border of the rectus abdominis muscle.** The triangle is clinically significant because it helps define the nature of inguinal hernias. An **indirect hernia** usually results from a congenital condition in which there is a retention of the peritoneal lining, called the **processus vaginalis.** This led from the abdomen to the scrotum along which the testis descended during development. Usually, this pathway becomes obliterated because the peritoneum of the processus vaginalis normally fuses, except for that part immediately around the testis, called the **tunica vaginalis** (**ATLAS PLATE 195 #195.2**). When fusion does not occur, an **indirect congenital inguinal hernia** may result, in which a loop of bowel (surrounded by a peritoneal sac) enters the inguinal canal at the abdominal inguinal ring and moves through the inguinal canal to the scrotum. Such a hernia commences lateral to the inferior epigastric artery and, therefore, **lateral to the inguinal triangle.**

In contrast, **direct inguinal hernias** result from a weakening in the anterior abdominal wall of the inguinal region, frequently of the conjoint tendon. These hernias are acquired and not congenital. A loop of bowel

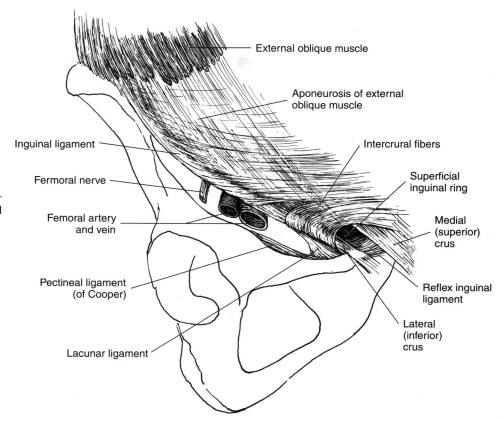

Figure 13-9. The inguinal, lacunar, and pectineal ligaments, and the superficial inguinal ring.

External oblique muscle

Aponeurosis of external oblique muscle

Inguinal ligament

Fermoral nerve

Femoral artery and vein

Pectineal ligament (of Cooper)

Lacunar ligament

Intercrural fibers

Superficial inguinal ring

Medial (superior) crus

Reflex inguinal ligament

Lateral (inferior) crus

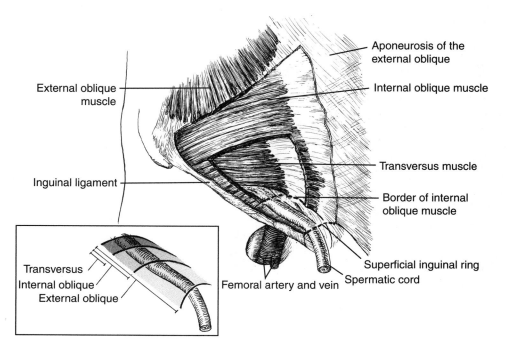

Figure 13-10. The spermatic cord within the inguinal canal.

External oblique muscle

Inguinal ligament

Transversus
Internal oblique
External oblique

Aponeurosis of the external oblique

Internal oblique muscle

Transversus muscle

Border of internal oblique muscle

Superficial inguinal ring

Spermatic cord

Femoral artery and vein

surrounded by a peritoneal sac pushes through the weakened site in the abdominal wall causing an enlargement of the superficial inguinal ring. The herniation can then continue into the scrotum. Direct hernias occur medial to the inferior epigastric artery and, therefore, lie **within the inguinal triangle.**

Dissection of the inguinal region should be done in both male and female cadavers. Regardless of which sex you are dissecting, you should study the inguinal region in a cadaver of the opposite sex.

The male inguinal canal transmits the **spermatic cord** (**Figure 13-10**) between the scrotum and the abdomen (**ATLAS PLATE 192**). The spermatic cord consists of the ductus (vas) deferens, the arteries, veins and lymphatics of the testis, and the fascial covering over these structures (**ATLAS PLATES 190, 192**). The female inguinal canal contains the round ligament of the uterus, which extends from the pelvis to the labium majus (**ATLAS PLATE 188**). The dissection procedures of the inguinal canal in the two sexes are somewhat comparable.

Replace the abdominal muscles to their original positions and find the superficial inguinal ring. Using scissors, cut the aponeurosis of the external oblique muscle from the lateral end of the superficial inguinal ring to the anterior superior iliac spine. Separate the two flaps of the aponeurosis and palpate the attached inferior flap from the anterior superior iliac spine to the pubic tubercle. This attached portion of the external oblique aponeurosis comprises the **inguinal ligament** (**Figure 13-9**).

In male cadavers, examine the inferior border of the internal oblique muscle and observe how the looping fibers of the cremaster muscle unite with areolar connective tissue to form the **cremasteric fascia** around the spermatic cord (**ATLAS PLATES 190, 192, 193 #193.3**). Elevate the spermatic cord and identify the conjoint tendon helping to form the posterior wall of the medial part of the inguinal canal. Behind the spermatic cord identify, if present, the **reflected inguinal ligament** (**Figure 13-9**).

The reflected inguinal ligament consists of fibers of the external oblique aponeurosis from the opposite side that decussate across the midline to terminate on the pubic tubercle (**ATLAS PLATE 181**). When present, these fibers also unite with the conjoint tendon and help strengthen the posterior wall of the inguinal canal.

► Grant's 107, 109, 111
Netter's 348, 370, 372
Rohen's 218, 341

◄ Grant's 97, 98, 102, 103, 106, 107
Netter's 241–243, 251–253
Rohen 217, 219

► Grant's 107, 110, 111
Netter's 247, 251, 381
Rohen 217, 219, 341, 348

Pull back the internal oblique muscle and identify the transversus muscle and the layer of transversalis fascia deep to the transversus (**ATLAS PLATES 183, 184, 186**). Find the deep inguinal ring and trace the spermatic cord laterally until it disappears into the abdominal cavity. Place your index finger within the deep inguinal ring and palpate on the inner surface of its medial margin for the **inferior epigastric vessels.** The ductus deferens courses around these vessels on its way to the posterior wall of the bladder (**ATLAS PLATES 191, 253**).

VI. Scrotum; Spermatic Cord; Testis (ATLAS PLATES 190–195)

The **scrotum** is a pouch composed of skin and superficial fascia that is divided into two compartments by a midline septum. Each compartment contains a testis, an epididymis, and the lower part of the spermatic cord and its coverings. The skin and subcutaneous tissue, called the **dartos,** is fat-free and contains smooth muscle fibers, which normally lend a creased or rugous character to the skin (**ATLAS PLATE 192**). Beneath the skin and dartos is a deeper layer of superficial fascia, called **Colles' fascia,** which is continuous with Scarpa's fascia over the anterior abdominal wall. Deep to Colles' fascia the scrotal wall contains three fascial layers, the **external spermatic fascia,** the **cremasteric fascia,** and the **internal spermatic fascia.** These surround the spermatic cord and are continuous with similar layers over the testis (**ATLAS PLATES 192–194**).

The testis is surrounded by the loose areolar external spermatic fascia, derived from the external oblique aponeurosis; the cremasteric fascia, containing fibers of the cremaster muscle; and the internal spermatic fascia, which comes from the transversalis fascia (**ATLAS PLATE 192**). Under normal circumstances, the spermatic cord contains only a delicate threadlike remnant of the peritoneum because the **processus vaginalis** fuses after testicular descent; however, the testis retains its peritoneal covering, called **tunica vaginalis.** Under its fascial coverings, the **spermatic cord** contains the following:

1. the **ductus (vas) deferens**, a duct continuous from the epididymis (**ATLAS PLATES 191, 192, 194 #194.1**).
2. the **artery of the ductus deferens**, usually a branch from the superior vesicular artery (**ATLAS PLATE 194 #194.1**).
3. the **testicular artery** that branches from the abdominal aorta (**ATLAS PLATES 192, 194 #194.2**).

4. the **cremasteric artery,** from the inferior epigastric artery.
5. the **pampiniform plexus of veins** that surrounds the ductus deferens and testicular artery and becomes the testicular vein (**ATLAS PLATES 192, 194 #194.2**).
6. ascending **lymphatic vessels** from the testis that convey lymph upward in the inguinal canal to pre-aortic lymph nodes.
7. **autonomic nerve fibers:** sympathetic fibers to the testicular artery and both sympathetic and parasympathetic fibers to the ductus deferens.

The testis is an oval organ 4 cm long and 2.5 cm wide (**ATLAS PLATES 192–194**). It is composed of many delicate **seminiferous tubules** that anastomose into a network called the **rete testis.** From the rete testis emerge 15 to 20 **efferent ductules** that initially are quite straight but become coiled to form the proximal **epididymis** (**ATLAS PLATE 194 #194.1**).

Observe that the skin of the scrotum often shows folds, or rugae. Make an incision from the superficial inguinal ring midway down the anterolateral aspect of the scrotum (**ATLAS PLATE 192**). Reflect the cut edge of the scrotal sac and dissect some of the skin away from the underlying dartos layer. On the deep surface of the dartos, note the loose areolar **external spermatic fascia.** Identify the underlying cremasteric muscle (fascia) along the spermatic cord. Free the spermatic cord and testis from the scrotal sac and cut the lowest attachment of the testis to the scrotum, the **gubernaculum testis.**

Dissect a part of the spermatic cord and free several centimeters of the ductus deferens. Observe the delicate **artery to the ductus deferens** that courses along the duct as far as the testis. Identify the larger **testicular artery,** which is surrounded by the tortuous **pampiniform plexus** of veins (**ATLAS PLATE 194 #194.2**). The spermatic cord also contains autonomic nerve fibers and lymphatics.

Dissect the testis by making a longitudinal slit through its peritoneal covering, the **tunica vaginalis testis** (**ATLAS PLATES 192, 193**). See that it reflects on itself so that both parietal and visceral layers around the testis enclose a sac between them. Laterally, identify a semilunar, longitudinally oriented recess, called the **sinus of the epididymis,** separating the body of the epididymis from the testis (**ATLAS PLATE 193 #193.3**). Dissect the peritoneal fold that attaches the sinus and locate several delicate **efferent ductules** that interconnect the upper pole of the testis and the **head of the epididymis.**

Trace the ductus deferens down to the **tail of the epididymis** and observe how the epididymis becomes tortuous and convoluted (**ATLAS PLATE 194 #194.1**). Cut through the fibrous capsule of the testis (the **tunica albuginea**) longitudinally along its medial border (**ATLAS PLATE 193 #193.2**). Continue the incision through the organ and fold open the two halves. Tease apart a few minute seminiferous tubules of which there are thought to be about 500 in each testis.

VII. Female Inguinal Canal, Round Ligament of the Uterus, and the Labia Majora (ATLAS PLATES 188, 189)

The anatomy of the inguinal canal and its coverings in females is essentially the same as in males, but it is smaller in diameter. It transmits the **round ligament of the uterus,** a narrow flat band that receives similar fascial coverings found around the spermatic cord. These layers are more delicate than in the male and are difficult to dissect.

The round ligament becomes fibrous strands that blend with the subcutaneous areolar tissue of the labia majora (**ATLAS PLATE 188**). The labia majora are longitudinally oriented cutaneous folds that contain subcutaneous connective tissue, a venous plexus, and a small quantity of smooth muscle. They are the homologous female structures to the two halves of the scrotum in males.

Dissect the anterior and posterior walls of the female inguinal canal as described above for the male. Find the round ligament of the uterus and the ilioinguinal nerve and trace them through the superficial inguinal ring into the labium majus (**ATLAS PLATES 188**).

▶
Grant's 104, 105
Rohen 210, 220, 351, 363
◀
Grant's 107, 109–111
Netter's 348, 370, 371
Rohen 336, 339, 341, 348

A persistent processus vaginalis in women can give rise to a congenital indirect inguinal hernia similar to that seen in men. This occurs much less frequently than in males, but it can result in a loop of bowel surrounded by a peritoneal hernial sac going through the superficial inguinal ring and reaching the labia.

Clinical Relevance

Surgical incisions. A long vertical incision in the midline from the xiphoid process to the symphysis pubis allows laparotomy of the abdominal cavity. Other smaller incisions generally follow the cleavage (Langer's) lines. Abdominal muscles are often split in the direction of their fibers, such as are currently popular to approach the appendix. Horizontal suprapubic incisions are used to approach pelvic organs or for cesarean sections. Endoscopic surgery now is minimally invasive and has replaced some former incisions.

Epigastric anastomosis. This is the anastomosis between the superior and inferior epigastric vessel within the sheath of the rectus abdominis muscle. The veins in this anastomosis form a collateral channel between the inferior and superior venae cavae. The anastomosis of the arteries provides an interconnection between the femoral artery and the subclavian artery.

Indirect inguinal hernias. These occur much more commonly in men than in women. This hernia results when a patent processus vaginalis remains from the formation of the inguinal canal and some protruding parietal peritoneum (and possibly a loop of bowel) enters the inguinal canal by passing through the abdominal inguinal ring. If the processus vaginalis is complete the hernia can extend all the way to the scrotum. These hernias are normally congenital.

Direct inguinal hernias. These hernias are acquired after birth and result from a weakness in the anterior abdominal wall within the inguinal triangle. A peritoneal sac and transversalis fascia pass into the inguinal canal, medial to the inferior epigastric vessels, and they traverse the inguinal canal, perhaps as far as the superficial inguinal ring.

Femoral hernias course through the femoral canal into the upper medial thigh and frequently occur in women who have just given birth. **Umbilical hernias,** common in newborn babies, result from the incomplete closure of the umbilicus. **Spigelian hernias** are hernias on the deep surface of the rectus abdominus muscle that enter the rectus sheath at the actuate line and pass upward posterior to the muscle. **Paraumbilical hernias** are bulges around the umbilicus.

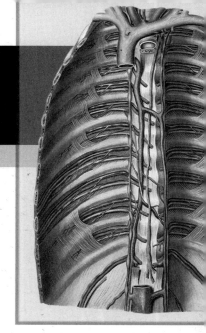

Abdominal Cavity I: Topography of the Abdominal Viscera and Reflections of the Peritoneum

OBJECTIVES

1 Expose the contents of the abdominal cavity.

2 Study the inner surface of the anterior abdominal wall and dissect the falciform and round ligaments of the liver.

3 Study the peritoneal reflections and relationships of the abdominal viscera in their normal positions.

4 Visualize the mesenteries and understand the formation of their roots.

5 Envision the greater and lesser peritoneal sacs and find their communication at the omental (epiploic) foramen.

Atlas Key:

Clemente Atlas, 5th Edition = Atlas Plate #

Grant's Atlas, 11th Edition = Grant's Page #

Netter's Atlas, 3rd Edition = Netter's Plate #

Rohen Atlas, 6th Edition = Rohen Page #

I. Exposure of Abdominal Cavity; Inner Surface of Abdominal Wall; Falciform and Round Ligaments

The anterior abdominal wall encloses the viscera of the abdomen. These include the stomach; small and large intestines; liver, gall bladder, and pancreas and their duct systems; spleen; kidneys and suprarenal glands; aorta and its branches; inferior vena cava and portal vein and their tributaries; cysterna chyli and its related lymphatic channels; and the visceral nerves and autonomic ganglia.

A. Incisions Through the Anterior Abdominal Wall.
To open the abdominal cavity, it is necessary to cut through the posterior layer of the rectus sheath, the transverse abdominis muscle, transversalis fascia, and peritoneum.

Using scissors:

1. Make two parallel vertical incisions, each 1 cm lateral to the midline, from the umbilicus to the xiphoid process (**Figure 14-1, A to B and A′ to B′**). These will cut through the posterior layer of the rectus sheath, the transversalis fascia, and peritoneum.

2. Make inferolateral incisions on each side from the umbilicus to the anterior superior iliac spine (**Figure 14-1, A to D and A′ to C**).

3. Interconnect these two incisions across the midline just below the umbilicus (**Figure 14-1, A to A′**).

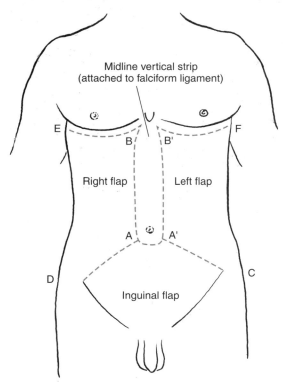

Midline vertical strip
(attached to falciform ligament)

E

F

B   B'

Right flap   Left flap

A   A'

D   C

Inguinal flap

Figure 14-1. Skin incisions on the anterior abdominal wall.

4. Make lateral incisions on both sides through the transversus abdominis (and other) muscles along the costal margins from the xiphoid process to the midaxillary line (**Figure 14-1, B′ to E and B to F**).

5. Reflect the three flaps (**Figure 14-1**) and lift the central 2 cm vertical strip noting that it is attached on its deep surface to the **falciform ligament** (**ATLAS PLATES 204, 212 #212.1**).

B. Inner Surface of Anterior Abdominal Wall. The inner surface of the anterior abdominal wall (**Figure 14-1**) is covered by a glistening layer of parietal peritoneum.

Reflect the lower flap (**Figure 14-1**) and note that three longitudinal ridges descend from the umbilicus toward the pelvis: one in the midline, called the **median umbilical fold,** and one at an angle on each side called the **medial umbilical folds** (**ATLAS PLATES 204, 242**). Probe through the peritoneal coverings of these folds and find a fibrous cord in each. These are remnants of structures that were functional in fetal life.

The **median** umbilical fold (**Figure 14-2**) consists of the fibrous **urachus** and an overlying layer of parietal peritoneum. Coursing from the apex of the bladder to the umbilicus (**ATLAS PLATE 264**), the urachus was a duct between the urinary bladder and the allantois during fetal life. The medial umbilical folds are fibrous remnants of the two **umbilical arteries,** and they are also covered by peritoneal reflections (**ATLAS PLATES 204, 264**). In fetal life, the umbilical arteries carried deoxygenated blood to the placenta for oxygenation.

More laterally, identify two other ridges on the inner surface of the anterior abdominal wall called the **lateral umbilical folds** (**ATLAS PLATE 204**). Probe through the overlying peritoneum of these folds and expose the inferior epigastric vessels, which are fully functional in the adult (**ATLAS PLATE 264**).

C. Falciform Ligament and Round Ligament of the Liver. The falciform ligament is a remnant of the **ventral mesogastrium (mesentery).** The early developing foregut is suspended to the abdominal wall both dorsally and ventrally by peritoneal attachments called **mesogastria** or **mesenteries** (**ATLAS PLATE 202 #202.1**). During the third prenatal week, the developing liver grows outward from the foregut and proliferates into the ventral mesogastrium. As the liver does this, the ventral mesogastrium is divided into two portions. One extends from the anterior body wall to the liver, which becomes the **falciform ligament,** and the other between the liver and the stomach, which becomes the **lesser omentum.** The latter consists of the **hepatogastric** and **hepatoduodenal ligaments.**

Within the falciform ligament is found the **round ligament of the liver.** This is the adult remnant of the fetal **left umbilical vein** (**ATLAS PLATE 202 #202.1**), which carried oxygenated blood from the placenta to the **ductus venosus** but which became a fibrous cord after birth.

Lift the midline vertical strip (**Figure 14-1**) and cut it free from the umbilicus. Observe that the anterior abdominal wall is attached to the anterior surface of the liver by a fold of peritoneum called the **falciform ligament** (**ATLAS PLATE 212 #212.1**). Dissect the midline vertical strip by cutting through its attachment to the ligament. Dissect the lower edge of the falciform ligament and find a cordlike structure called the **round ligament of the liver (ligamentum teres hepatis)** between the layers (**ATLAS PLATE 277 #217.1**).

▶
Grant's 113
Netter's 245, 266
Rohen 219, 293, 338

▶
Grant's 113, 128, 142, 144
Netter's 245, 267, 261, 279
Rohen 268, 298, 312

▶
Grant's 113, 128, 142, 144
Netter's 225, 245, 279
Rohen 298, 306, 312

◀
Grant's 113, 198, 225
Netter's 244, 245, 266
Rohen 219, 293, 338

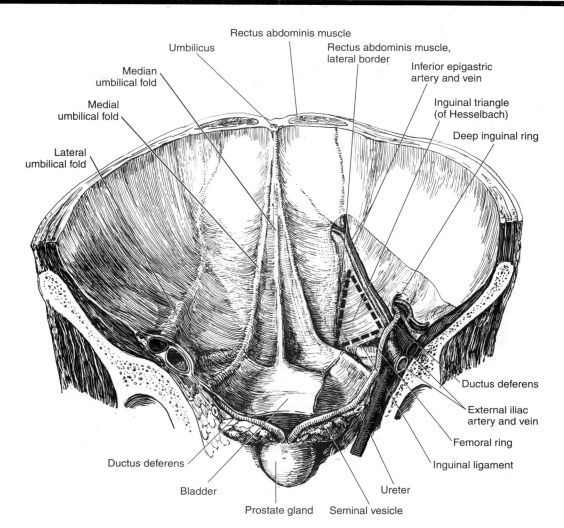

Figure 14-2. Umbilical folds on the inner surface of anterior abdominal wall.

Rectus abdominis muscle
Umbilicus
Rectus abdominis muscle, lateral border
Median umbilical fold
Inferior epigastric artery and vein
Medial umbilical fold
Inguinal triangle (of Hesselbach)
Deep inguinal ring
Lateral umbilical fold
Ductus deferens
External iliac artery and vein
Femoral ring
Inguinal ligament
Ductus deferens
Bladder
Prostate gland
Seminal vesicle
Ureter

II. Peritoneum and Abdominal Viscera *In Situ*

◄
Grant's 113
Netter's 261
Rohen 306, 307

Before dissecting the abdominal organs, inspect the viscera in their normal positions and **understand the reflections** of peritoneum.

A. Peritoneum. With the abdominal contents completely exposed anteriorly, understand the following statements about the peritoneum before manipulating the abdominal organs.

1. In the male, the peritoneum is a completely closed sac that lines the abdominal wall **(parietal layer)** and then becomes reflected around the organs of the abdomen **(visceral layer).** The same is true in females except the closed sac has opening into it the free ends of the uterine tubes. These communicate with the uterine cavity, and, through that, with the vagina and the exterior.

2. Areolar connective tissue (fat) is found between the abdominal wall and the parietal peritoneum that lines it. This extraperitoneal fat differs in amount in different regions, being sparse under the diaphragm but more abundant on the posterior abdominal wall, especially around the kidneys.

3. The visceral peritoneum is firmly adherent to the surfaces of the organs, to the inferior surface of the diaphragm, and to the inner surface of the linea alba. However, it is more loosely arranged at other sites such as the lower part of the anterior abdominal wall. This accommodates certain organs that change in size. For example, as the urinary bladder fills it distends upward from the pelvis and separates the loosely attached peritoneum from the inner surface of the lower anterior abdominal wall.

4. Only the anterior surface of some abdominal organs is covered by peritoneum. These organs are **retroperitoneal** and are fixed in position; they include the duodenum and pancreas, the kidneys, ureters and suprarenal glands, and the ascending and descending colons. In contrast, other organs become totally invested by peritoneum and are

therefore more mobile; these include the stomach, liver and gall bladder, spleen, jejunum and ileum, cecum and appendix, and the transverse and sigmoid colons.

5. The **omenta** are two-layered folds of peritoneum that attach along the borders of the stomach. The **lesser omentum** attaches along the lesser curvature of the stomach, and the **greater omentum** stretches along the greater curvature (**ATLAS PLATE 212 #212.1**).

6. Two-layered folds of peritoneum, called **mesenteries,** extend from the posterior abdominal wall and suspend regions of the intestines. There are three of these: one suspends the transverse colon and is called the **transverse mesocolon;** a second suspends the jejunum and ileum and is called the **mesentery of the small intestine;** and the third, called the **sigmoid mesocolon,** suspends the sigmoid colon from the posterior part of the left pelvic wall (**ATLAS PLATES 203 #203.1, 240**).

7. Coursing between the two peritoneal layers of the mesenteries are the arteries, veins, nerves, and lymphatics that supply the gastrointestinal tract (**ATLAS PLATE 235**). The mesenteries also

▶
Grant's 113, 116, 117, 123, 156
Netter's 261, 264, 265, 336
Rohen 298, 307, 311

◀
Grant's 113, 114, 116, 117
Netter's 261, 265, 267
Rohen 306, 322

◀
Grant's 132, 133, 140
Netter's 2s62, 263, 266
Rohen 308, 310, 313, 318

▶
Grant's 92, 113
Netter's 261
Rohen 306, 307

contain a variable amount of fat, which surrounds these neurovascular and lymphatic structures.

8. Other two-layered folds of peritoneum that connect an organ to the abdominal wall or that interconnect two organs are called **ligaments.** An example of the former is the **falciform ligament** of the liver (between the liver and the anterior abdominal wall), and of the latter, the **gastrosplenic ligament** (between the stomach and spleen).

9. The **peritoneal cavity** is the potential space enclosed between the parietal and visceral layers of peritoneum. It is not an actual cavity in the normal living subject. Instead, the peritoneal lining of the abdominal organs is in direct contact with the peritoneal lining of the abdominal wall. The only substance within the peritoneal cavity is a thin film of serous fluid that facilitates movement. The presence of disease may result in accumulations of blood or other substances within the peritoneal cavity.

B. Abdominal Viscera *In Situ* (Figure 14-3, ATLAS PLATE 198, 204, 205). Abdominal organs are to be

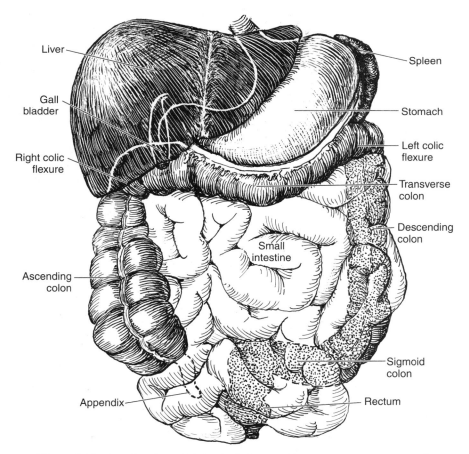

Figure 14-3. Anterior view of abdominal viscera with greater omentum removed.

dissected while the embalmed cadaver is supine (on its back). The relationships and positions of some organs in the living abdomen, however, are affected by posture and breathing.

1. **Identify** the following structures:
   a. the sharp **inferior border of the liver** in the upper right quadrant. Observe how the left lobe of the liver overlies the **stomach** along its **lesser curvature (ATLAS PLATE 212 #212.1).**
   b. the **gall bladder** projecting below the inferior border of the right lobe of the liver. A slight greenish discoloration in this region is caused by the diffusion of some residual bile through the wall of the gall bladder.

When projected onto the surface of the anterior abdominal wall, the gall bladder is found at the intersection between the lateral edge of the right rectus abdominis muscle and the right costal margin of the rib cage.

   c. the **stomach** and its **greater curvature.** Observe that the stomach normally projects below the left costal margin, inferior and somewhat to the left of the liver. Note that the greater curvature of the stomach is directed to the left and that along this border is attached the **greater omentum (ATLAS PLATE 206).** Observe that the greater omentum resembles an apron covering the intestines and that it attaches to the transverse colon just inferior to the stomach (**ATLAS PLATE 204, 206**).

2. Palpate the glistening anterior and diaphragmatic surfaces of the **liver.** With your hand reach upward and behind the right and left lobes and observe how the diaphragm forms a dome-like roof for the abdomen (**ATLAS PLATES 250–252**). At the upper lateral extremities of the liver, feel for the **left** and **right triangular ligaments.** These peritoneal ligaments help stabilize the liver by attaching it to the peritoneum covering the inferior surface of the diaphragm (**ATLAS PLATES 216, 217**).

The **triangular ligaments** are formed by the fusion of the anterior and posterior peritoneal leaves of the **coronary ligament** at their extreme right and left limits. The two layers of the coronary ligament nearly cover the entire liver, but dorsal to the right lobe is found a triangular area not covered by peritoneum. This is the **bare area of the liver** directly adjacent to the muscle fibers of the diaphragm (**ATLAS PLATES 216 #216.2, 217 #217.2**).

◀
Grant's 113
Netter's 261
Rohen 307,311

▶
Grant's 116–118,
123, 152, 156
Netter's 264–266,
289
Rohen 300, 311

◀
Grant's 113, 114
Netter's 261, 267
Rohen 311–314

▶
Grant's 114, 116,
117
Netter's 265, 267
Rohen 294, 295,
311, 312

◀
Grant's 142–144
Netter's 278–280
Rohen 298

▶
Netter's 267, 280
Rohen 312, 318

▶
Grant's 132, 133
Netter's 261
Rohen 308

The peritoneal attachments of the spleen include the **lienorenal** and **gastrosplenic ligaments** (**ATLAS PLATES 212 #212.2, 215, 235**). The lienorenal ligament is a double-layered fold of peritoneum extending from the left kidney to the hilum of the spleen and enclosing the tail of the pancreas. Between its two layers, the splenic vessels course. That portion of the dorsal mesogastrium between the greater curvature of the stomach and the hilum of the spleen persists as the gastrosplenic ligament (**Figure 14-4A**).

3. To palpate the spleen, stand on the right side of the cadaver and with your right hand reach across the abdomen to the left of the stomach and up under the left costal margin. Note that the spleen lies in contact with the diaphragm, deep to the 10th, 11th, and 12th ribs. Cup the spleen in the palm of your right hand and use two of your fingers to palpate the **lienorenal ligament** posterior to the spleen but anterior to the kidney. Using your thumb, feel for the **gastrosplenic ligament** anteriorly between the spleen and the greater curvature of the stomach (**Figure 14-4B**). With the hilum of the spleen between your thumb and fingers, palpate the splenic vessels.

4. Elevate the left lobe of the liver and simultaneously pull the stomach downward to see the **lesser curvature of the stomach** along which is attached the lesser omentum. Follow this two-layered peritoneal fold from the stomach and upper duodenum to the liver, and note that it surrounds the structures at the hilum of the liver (**ATLAS PLATE 212 #212.1**).

The portion of lesser omentum from the liver to the stomach is the **hepatogastric ligament** and that part between the liver and the duodenum is the **hepatoduodenal ligament.** The lesser omentum is composed of two layers derived from the prenatal **ventral mesogastrium,** as were the coronary and falciform ligaments. This explains why these layers are continuous with the two leaves of the coronary ligament and why these are continuous with the peritoneum forming the falciform ligament (**ATLAS PLATE 202 #202.2B**).

5. Reflect the **greater omentum** upward over the costal margin and separate any adhesions that exist between it and the viscera. Adhesions may develop because the omentum is capable of motility and responds to inflammatory processes by attempting to seal them off. Observe that the greater omentum descends from the greater curvature of the stomach over the anterior surface of the **transverse colon.** Once

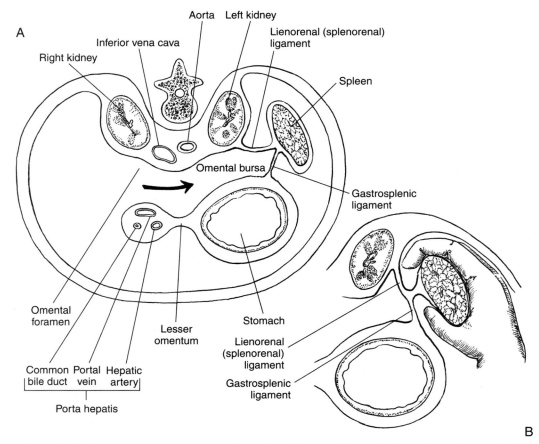

Figure 14-4. A. Peritoneum in transverse section of the abdomen at the level of the spleen and stomach with the lining removed. **B.** How to manipulate the spleen to feel the lienorenal and gastrosplenic ligaments.

the greater omentum has been turned upward, most of the transverse colon is exposed, as is much of the small intestine (**ATLAS PLATES 226, 228**).

The greater omentum is initially formed as two layers of peritoneum extending between the greater curvature of the stomach and the transverse colon. Below the transverse colon, these two layers are joined posteriorly by an inferior extension of the **transverse mesocolon,** resulting in the fusion of four layers as shown in **ATLAS PLATE 203.** The stages in its development and the formation of the **omental bursa** (or lesser peritoneal sac) are demonstrated in **ATLAS PLATE 203 #203.1 A–C.**

6. With the greater omentum still reflected upward, pull the mass of small intestine (the **jejunum** and **ileum**) to the left and find the junction of the distal ilium with the **cecum** (**ATLAS PLATE 226**). Find the **appendix** near the **ileocecal junction** and the **ascending colon** coursing superiorly upward from the cecum. Note that the appendix and cecum are mobile while the ascending colon is fixed to

▶
Grant's 132, 133, 140
Netter's 262, 263
Rohen 310

◀
Grant's 132, 135, 136, 140, 141
Netter's 263, 273, 276
Rohen 307, 310, 318

the posterior abdominal wall by peritoneum covering its anterior surface. Observe the ascending colon as it bends to the left just below the liver at the **right colic (or hepatic) flexure** to become the transverse colon

7. Pull the jejunum and ileum to the right and find the **duodenojejunal junction** (**ATLAS PLATE 228**). Note that at this site the small intestine acquires a mesentery and that certain peritoneal folds and fossae exist to the **left of the duodenojejunal junction.**

The paraduodenal and superior and inferior duodenal fossae (recesses) and the adjacent peritoneal folds are important because hernias of the small intestine can occur into these fossae. Behind the fossae is located the inferior mesenteric vein, which is in danger of becoming obstructed by such a hernia (Compare **ATLAS PLATES 228** for recesses **and 230** for vein.)

8. Identify the descending colon coursing inferiorly from the **left colic (or splenic) flexure** and note that it also is fixed to the posterior ab-

dominal wall by peritoneum. Follow the descending colon to the brim of the pelvis where it becomes the **sigmoid colon (ATLAS PLATE 228)**. Manipulate the sigmoid colon from the sigmoid flexure to the presacral region in the midline. Note that a mesentery, the **sigmoid mesocolon (ATLAS PLATE 235)**, gives it considerable motility. In the midline, observe that the sigmoid colon becomes the rectum by angling inferiorly into the pelvis, behind the bladder in males and behind the uterus in females (compare **ATLAS PLATES 274 and 305 #305.2**).

9. Understand the **roots** of the three principal mesenteries by studying **ATLAS PLATES 235 and 240**. From a site just below the right lobe of the liver to the spleen is the **root of the transverse mesocolon**. Below the root of the transverse mesocolon and to the left of the midline, find the duodenojejunal junction (**ATLAS PLATE 240**). Note that the **root of the mesentery of the small intestine** extends only approximately 6 inches in length to the ileocecal junction, and yet its two peritoneal layers encase more than 21 feet of jejunum and ileum. In the lower left quadrant, find the **root of the sigmoid mesocolon (ATLAS PLATE 240)**.

◀
Grant's 132, 138, 140, 141
Netter's 263, 276, 277
Rohen 310, 318

◀
Grant's 140, 154
Netter's 263, 266
Rohen 318, 319

▶
Grant's 116, 117
Netter's 264, 265, 336
Rohen 311–313, 322

III. Peritoneal Cavity; Greater and Lesser Peritoneal Sacs (Figure 14-5, ATLAS PLATE 203)

The **peritoneal cavity** is the potential space between the parietal and visceral layers of the peritoneum. Upon opening the anterior abdominal wall, the parietal peritoneum covering its inner surface was cut through, thereby opening the peritoneal cavity. During life, the surfaces of the organs (covered by visceral peritoneum) are in contact with the parietal peritoneum of the body wall, reducing the peritoneal cavity only to a potential space containing some serous fluid.

The **peritoneal cavity** consists of a large portion called the **greater sac** and a smaller part called the **omental bursa** (or lesser sac). The omental bursa forms as a diverticulum of the dorsal mesentery during the embryologic process of gut rotation and becomes situated posterior to the stomach and anterior to the pancreas. It is usually described as having a **superior recess** that lies behind the lesser omentum and liver and an **inferior recess** that lies behind the stomach and extending down into the greater omentum (**Figure 14-5**).

The omental bursa communicates with the greater sac only by way of the omental foramen or **epiploic foramen (of Winslow)**, a vertical opening 4 cm long behind the lesser omentum at the porta hepatis (**ATLAS PLATES 212 #212.1, 213 #213.1**). Because the lesser omentum surrounds the **hepatic artery, common bile**

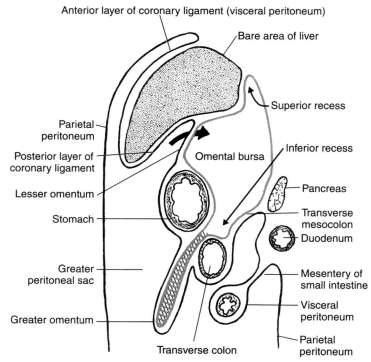

Figure 14-5. Reflections of peritoneum in a sagittal diagram of abdomen. The omental bursa shown in red.

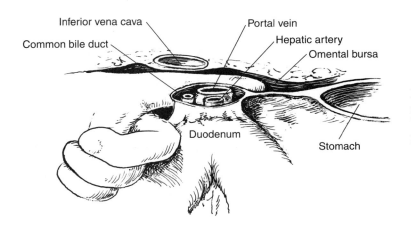

Figure 14-6. Placement of index finger into the omental foramen of Winslow behind the structures at the porta hepatis (after Thorek P. Anatomy in Surgery. 2nd Ed. Philadelphia: J.B. Lippincott, 1962).

duct, and **portal vein,** the omental foramen can be located behind these structures at the hilum of the liver.

A. Omental Foramen (Figure 14-6). Replace the greater omentum and the transverse colon to their normal locations below the stomach. Lift the lower border of the liver and follow the gall bladder upward to its neck adjacent to the structures of the porta hepatis. To enter the omental bursa, traverse the omental foramen by passing your index finger transversely from right to left behind the (**Figure 14-6**). Palpate between your thumb and index finger the **hepatic artery,** the **common bile duct,** and more posteriorly, adjacent to your index finger, the **portal vein (Figure 14-7).**

B. Omental Bursa. To explore the omental bursa, dissect through the lesser omentum attaching along the lesser curvature of the stomach. Insert the index and middle fingers of your left hand

► Grant's 116, 117
Netter's 264, 265, 267, 337
Rohen 311–313 322

◄ Grant's 114, 116–118
Netter's 264, 265, 267
Rohen 311, 312

through the opening into the omental bursa located behind the stomach. Reach transversely to the left as far as the boundary of the lesser sac formed by the peritoneal ligaments of the spleen (**Figure 14-4**). Reach into the **superior recess** of the omental bursa and feel the liver anterior to your fingers and the diaphragm posterior to them (**Figure 14-5**). Palpate the **inferior recess** by passing your fingers downward behind the stomach and anterior to the pancreas, and transverse colon into the upper part of the greater omentum.

Note that the lower limit of the inferior recess is variable because of differing levels of fusion of the peritoneum. Study **ATLAS PLATE 203** and observe the four layers of peritoneum that form the greater omentum. Note the inferior recess of the omental bursa (shown in black behind the stomach) extending to the level of the transverse colon.

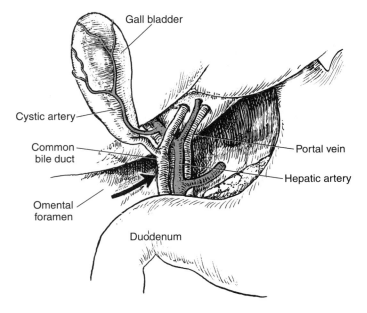

Figure 14-7. The structures at the porta hepatis. Arrow indicates omental foramen of Winslow.

Clinical Relevance

Topography of upper abdominal organs. The stomach, liver, and spleen project superiorly to lie under the domes of the diaphragm. Note that the falciform ligament attaches to the anterior abdominal wall and separates the liver into its left and right lobes.

Transpyloric line. This transverse line normally extends across the abdomen at the midpoint between the superior end of the sternum and the symphysis pubis. At this level the pyloric end of the stomach continues to the right to the first part of the duodenum. The transpyloric line projects posteriorly to the lower border of the L1 vertebra.

Surface projection of the gall bladder. The location of the gall bladder in the upper abdomen can be determined by noting the site where the lateral border of the rectus abdominis muscle intersects the costal margin of the thoracic cage.

McBurney's point. This site on the anterior abdominal wall has been used to identify the location of the underlying vermiform appendix when that structure descends over the pelvic brim. It is one third of the distance from the right anterior superior iliac spine along a line to the umbilicus.

Location of the vermiform appendix. The variable position of the appendix in the lower right quadrant must be considered in the diagnosis of appendicitis.

Its location may be posterior to the cecum (retrocecal). More frequently it descends over the pelvic brim to the upper part of the right pelvis. In instances of incomplete rotation of the gut the appendix can be located just below the liver in the right upper quadrant.

Root of the mesentery. The mesentery of the jejunum and ileum projects from the posterior abdominal wall as two peritoneal sheets that encase the small intestine from the duodenojejunal junction to the ilocolic opening. It allows free movement of the small intestine distal to the duodenum.

Location of the spleen. The spleen is normally located in the upper left quadrant of the abdomen and lies just inferior to the diaphragm opposite the 9th, 10th, and 11th ribs. It is surrounded by peritoneum, and its peritoneal attachments are to the left kidney (lienorenal ligament) and the stomach (gastrosplenic ligament). Because of these peritoneal attachments the spleen is easily movable and can be brought forward from its deep subdiaphragmatic location.

Superficial inguinal ring. This inferomedial end of the inguinal canal can be examined by invaginating the scrotum with the index finger. The finger is used to palpate the spermatic cord superolaterally and to determine whether the superficial ring is dilated. The patient is asked to cough, and if a hernia is present, a sudden pressure on the finger may indicate an inguinal hernia.

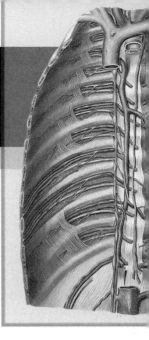

DISSECTION #15

Abdominal Cavity II: Rotation of the Gut; Dissection of Stomach; Liver; Duodenum and Pancreas; Spleen

OBJECTIVES

1 Understand certain embryologic events related to the development of the gastrointestinal tract.

2 Study and dissect the stomach, liver, gall bladder, and biliary ducts, as well as the duodenum, pancreas, and spleen.

3 Learn the blood supply and venous drainage of the upper abdominal organs.

I. Embryologic Events Related to the Development of the Gastrointestinal Tract

Studying the development of the gastrointestinal tract in an embryology textbook is important to understand the stages in the rotation of the gut. Use the following sequential statements to help guide your reading.

A. Before the 6th prenatal week, the primitive gut is a simple tube suspended by **dorsal and ventral mesenteries.**

B. The ventral mesentery of the midgut and hindgut disappears. The embryonic **liver** develops as an outgrowth from the foregut into the ventral mesentery **of the foregut** between the primitive **stomach** and the anterior abdominal wall (**ATLAS PLATE 202**

#202.1). This mesentery now is called the **ventral mesogastrium** because it attaches to the stomach. It forms the **falciform ligament,** the peritoneal ligaments of the liver (**coronary** and **triangular**), and the **lesser omentum.**

C. Derived from the dorsal mesentery are the **mesentery of the small intestine, the ligaments of the spleen** (gastrosplenic and splenorenal), the **greater omentum,** the **transverse mesocolon,** and the **sigmoid mesocolon** (**ATLAS PLATES 202, 203**).

D. In addition to the pharynx, esophagus, liver, and pancreas, the foregut gives rise to the stomach and to the duodenum as far distally as the entrance of the common bile duct. During the 5th prenatal week, the caudal part of the simple foregut tube dilates. Growth occurs faster along its dorsal border than the ventral to become the convex **greater curvature** of the stomach, while the ventral border becomes the concave **lesser curvature** (**Figure 15-1 A, A'**).

E. The liver grows and migrates to the right within the ventral mesogastrium. Simultaneously, the **stomach rotates 90° in a clockwise direction** and becomes displaced to the left (**Figure 15-1 B, B'**). The former ventral border of the stomach becomes the lesser curvature oriented superiorly and to the right, and the former dorsal border becomes the lesser curvature oriented inferiorly and to the left. The left side of the original simple tube becomes the anterior surface of the stomach, and the right side becomes posterior surface of the stomach. The **left vagus nerve** that coursed along the left side of the GI tube becomes the nerve of the anterior stomach wall, and the **right vagus** becomes the nerve of the posterior wall.

F. With rotation of the stomach, the dorsal mesentery invaginates to the left and folds on itself. It elongates inferiorly and descends with the transverse mesocolon to form the **greater omentum.** In this manner, a diverticulum of the greater peritoneal sac, or the **omental bursa,** is formed (**ATLAS PLATE 202 #202.2B**). The stomach has assumed its normal location as the remainder of the gastrointestinal tube develops.

G. The anterior abdominal wall grows more slowly than the liver and intestines, and by the end of the 5th week, the abdominal cavity is incapable of

containing the enlarging organs. A U-shaped loop of developing gut protrudes (herniates) into the umbilical cord. This loop comprises the **midgut,** and it gives rise to the small intestine (except the upper 10 cm of the duodenum) and the large intestine nearly to the splenic flexure.

H. The arteries that supply the gastrointestinal tract are three unpaired vessels derived from the aorta, all of which are retroperitoneal. The aortic branches are the **celiac, superior mesenteric,** and **inferior mesenteric arteries,** and they supply, in order, the foregut, midgut, and hindgut. These vessels and branches course from their retroperitoneal origins to organs they supply between the two leaves of the dorsal mesentery. When the midgut herniates into the umbilical cord, it takes with it the attached superior mesenteric artery.

I. The "herniated" loop is initially oriented in the median sagittal plane such that the **proximal part of the loop** is superior to the attachment of the superior mesenteric artery and the **distal part of the**

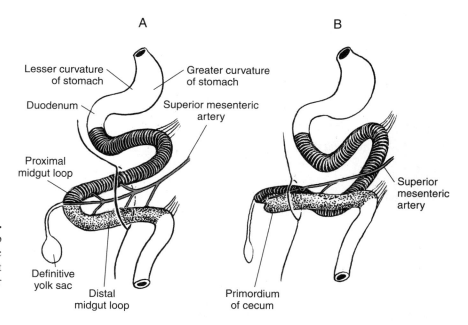

Figure 15-1. Stages in the rotation of the gut. **A.** Before rotation commences. Note the relationship of the midgut loops and the superior mesenteric artery seen in cross section in **A′. B** and **B′.** First stage of rotation, 90° counterclockwise (after Moore).

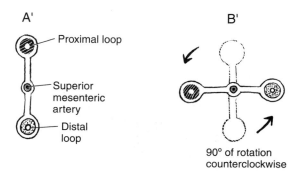

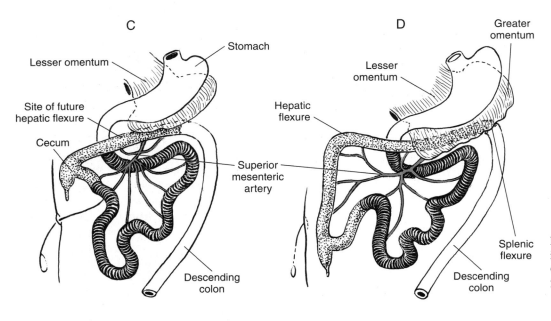

Figure 15-1 *(continued)*. Stages in the rotation of the gut. **C** and **C′**. 180° of rotation. **D** and **D′**. 270° of rotation (after Moore).

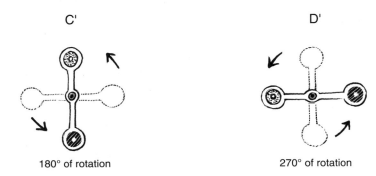

180° of rotation

270° of rotation

loop is inferior to the vessel (**Figure 15-1 A, A′**). The **vitelline duct** extends from the apex of the loop into the umbilical cord to the yolk sac.

J. By the time the midgut loop has fully entered the umbilical cord, it has **rotated 90° counterclockwise** around an axis formed by the **superior mesenteric artery.** The loop is now oriented in the transverse plane with the proximal part on the right side of the embryo and the distal part on the left (**Figure 15-1 B, B′**).

K. During the 10th week, the herniated loop returns to the abdomen. The coils of small intestine from the proximal part of the loop are withdrawn first. These pass behind the superior mesenteric artery and, by the time the distal part of the loop is withdrawn, **the counterclockwise rotation of the midgut progresses a second 90° to 180° (Figure 15-1 C, C′).** At this point, the derivatives from the distal part of the midgut loop (cecum and proximal large colon) are oriented superior and anterior to the derivatives of the proximal part (jejunum and

ileum), which are directed inferiorly. The **cecum** becomes located in the subhepatic region, close to the right lobe of the liver (**Fig. 15-1 C, C′**).

L. **The third and final 90° of counterclockwise midgut rotation** around the superior mesenteric artery occurs as the proximal part of the large colon lengthens and the cecum migrates to its definitive site in the right iliac fossa (**Fig. 15-1 D, D′**).

M. With the derivatives of the midgut in their final locations, the two leaves of mesocolon that surrounded the ascending colon become pressed posteriorly where they fuse to the body wall, leaving the ascending colon with peritoneum covering only its anterior surface (retroperitoneal).

N. As the midgut reenters the abdominal cavity, the **hindgut,** with its attached dorsal mesocolon, moves to the left and posteriorly from its original midline position. Its mesocolon fuses with the peritoneum of the dorsal abdominal wall, except at the brim of the pelvis where it remains as the **sigmoid mesocolon.** The descending colon becomes retroperitoneal and fixed to the posterior abdominal wall (similar to the ascending colon) by a single layer of peritoneum over its anterior surface.

II. Dissection of the Stomach, Liver and Gall Bladder, Duodenum and Pancreas, and Spleen

The most effective way to commence a study of the upper abdominal viscera is to learn and locate the main blood vessels that supply the region and then to observe the more significant anatomic features of each organ.

▶
Grant's 122, 123
Netter's 290, 291
Rohen 314

A. Celiac Artery and Its Branches; Porta Hepatis. The **celiac artery** is the principal vessel that supplies derivatives of the embryonic foregut. Its three branches are distributed to the lower esophagus, stomach, upper duodenum (to the entrance of the common bile duct), liver, spleen, and pancreas (**Figure 15-2**). The celiac artery is a short, thick trunk arising from the abdominal aorta between the right and left crura of the diaphragm and the right and left celiac ganglia. Also called the **celiac trunk,** it quickly divides into the **left gastric, hepatic,** and **splenic arteries** and often may give off one or both **inferior phrenic arteries.**

◀
Grant's 118, 122, 123, 127
Netter's 290–294
Rohen 314–318

Elevate the liver and retain the elevation by tying a string around the organ and attaching it to one of the ribs above or some other stable structure. Pull the stomach downward so that its lesser curvature and the porta hepatis, surrounded by lesser omentum, becomes exposed. Dissect the lesser omentum along the lesser curvature.

Probe the **left gastric artery and vein** along the esophageal (cardiac) end of the lesser curvature and the **right gastric artery and vein** along the pyloric end of the lesser curvature (**ATLAS PLATES 206, 208 #208.2**). Note that the right and left gastric vessels anastomose. Trace the right gastric artery to its origin (most arise from the common hepatic, proper hepatic, or gastroduodenal artery). Follow the left gastric artery branches back to a single stem from the celiac trunk (**ATLAS PLATE 207**). Note that the celiac trunk is surrounded by the celiac plexus of autonomic nerves. The plexus must be dissected through to expose the celiac artery and its branches (**ATLAS PLATES 242, 255**).

Place your index finger through the **omental foramen** behind the porta hepatis, and use a probe to dissect into the lesser omentum between the stomach and liver (**ATLAS PLATE 212 #212.1**).

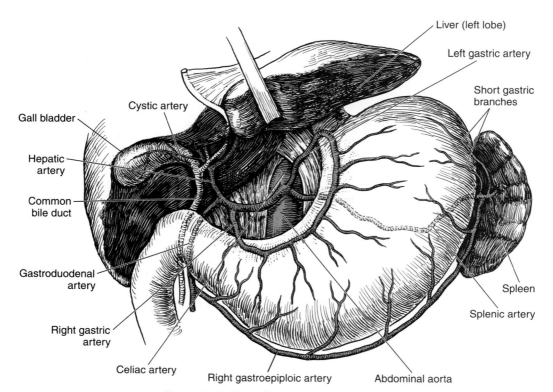

Figure 15-2. The celiac trunk and its branches.

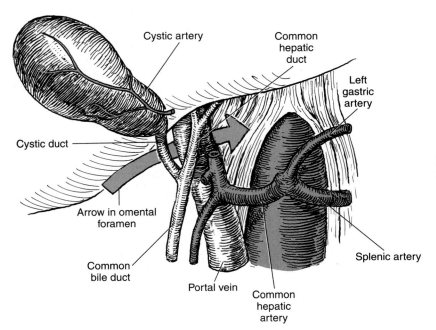

Figure 15-3. The porta hepatis and the omental foramen.

At the porta hepatis are located the hepatic artery, common bile duct, and portal vein (**Figure 15-3**). There also are lymph nodes and lymphatic channels (**ATLAS PLATE 215 #215.2**) and the hepatic plexus of autonomic nerves, but these are not to be dissected.

▶
Grant's 143,
148–150
Netter's 290, 292
Rohen 315, 317

> Dissect the **common hepatic artery** ascending toward the liver to the left of **common bile duct.** Trace the artery back to the celiac trunk and determine whether the right gastric artery arises from it or some other source. Find the **gastroduodenal branch** of the hepatic artery arising near the upper border of the duodenum. Trace the vessel downward behind the first part of the duodenum (**ATLAS PLATES 206, 207**). Follow the **proper hepatic artery** toward the liver and find its division into right and left hepatic branches.

◀
Grant's 122,123,
128, 143, 148–150
Netter's 290–292
Rohen 314, 315

In approximately 50% of cadavers, the right gastric artery arises from the common hepatic and from other vessels in the other 50%. Of the other vessels, the most common sources are the proper hepatic, gastroduodenal, and left hepatic arteries. In approximately 5% of cadavers, the hepatic artery arises from the superior mesenteric artery, not the celiac. More frequently, **accessory left** or **right hepatic arteries** may be found, and these may arise from the superior mesenteric or gastroduodenal arteries.

> Identify the **cystic artery,** which usually arises from the right hepatic to supply the **gall bladder** (**Figure 15-2, ATLAS PLATE 206**). Dissect the neck of the gall bladder and follow it to the **cystic duct.** Trace the cystic duct to its junction with the **common hepatic duct (ATLAS PLATE 221).** Follow the common hepatic duct upward to its formation by the junction of the **right** and **left hepatic ducts.** Find the junction of the cystic duct and common hepatic duct that forms the **common bile duct.** Follow the common bile duct inferiorly and note that it descends behind the first part of the duodenum (for variations see **ATLAS PLATE 221 #221.2**). Owing to variations, look at the vascular pattern at the porta hepatis in other cadavers.

Variation in the branching pattern of the cystic artery is common and is of significant surgical importance. In approximately 10% of cases, the cystic artery arises from some vessel other than the right hepatic, such as the left hepatic or the common hepatic. Another important variation is the relationship of the right hepatic artery (and its cystic branch) to the common hepatic duct. The right hepatic artery crosses posterior to the common hepatic duct in approximately 80% of cases and anterior to it in most remaining ones. Double cystic arteries are found in approximately 20% of cases.

The **portal vein** is a large vessel that carries blood to the liver from the gastrointestinal tract (lower esophagus to upper rectum), and from the spleen, pancreas, and gall bladder. It is 3 inches long and is formed by the junction of the **superior mesenteric** and **splenic veins** (ATLAS PLATES 207, 211 #211.A–F). The portal vein can best be observed in the dorsal part of the porta hepatis before it divides to flow into the liver.

Identify the large **portal vein** coursing between the duodenum and liver posterior to the hepatic artery and common bile duct (**Figure 15-3**). Note the tributaries draining into it, such as the left and right gastric veins (ATLAS PLATE 218, 219, 223 #223.2). Dissect the portal vein as it divides into left and right branches to enter the left and right halves of the liver.

The celiac artery also gives off the long and tortuous **splenic artery,** which courses to the left across the abdomen to the spleen. On its path, this vessel, accompanied by the splenic vein, sends **pancreatic branches** into the neck, body, and tail of the pancreas, as well as **short gastric branches** to the fundus of the stomach. At the splenic hilum, it gives off the **left gastroepiploic artery,** which courses around the greater curvature of the stomach.

Elevate the stomach and follow the **splenic artery** posterior to the stomach and omental bursa to the splenic hilum (ATLAS PLATES 207, 210). Inferior to the artery and adjacent to the pancreas, find the **splenic vein** (ATLAS PLATES 207). Identify pancreatic and short gastric branches from the artery. The vessel then passes between the leaves of the splenorenal ligament anterior to the left kidney to the splenic hilum. Clean the branches that enter the spleen and find the **left gastroepiploic branch,** which runs anteriorly within the gastrosplenic ligament to the greater curvature. Probe the greater omentum to expose the left gastroepiploic artery (and vein). Note how its straight branches help supply the stomach and the greater omentum (ATLAS PLATE 208 #208.2).

Elevate the pyloric end of the greater curvature and find the **gastroduodenal branch** of the common hepatic artery. Trace this vessel to its division into the **right gastroepiploic** and **superior pancreaticoduodenal arteries** (ATLAS PLATE 207).

From the pyloric end of the greater curvature, trace the right gastroepiploic vessels to their anastomosis with the left gastroepiploic vessels (ATLAS PLATE 208 #208.2). Follow the superior pancreaticoduodenal arteries downward, and observe the formation of arcades anterior and posterior to the head of the pancreas. Note that these anastomose with **inferior pancreaticoduodenal branches** ascending

Grant's 126
Netter's 291, 292, 294, 297
Rohen 316

Grant's 119, 152
Netter's 299–301
Rohen 300, 301, 303

Grant's 114, 121–124, 127
Netter's 265, 267–269
Rohen 294, 295, 311–314

Grant's 119, 122, 123, 127
Netter's 290–292
Rohen 314–317, 333

Grant's 818
Netter's 309–311
Rohen 279

Grant's 122, 123, 126, 127
Netter's 290, 291, 294, 297
Rohen 314–317

from the superior mesenteric artery (**Figure 15-4**). Understand that within the head of the pancreas and the duodenum, the celiac and the superior mesenteric circulations anastomose.

Veins draining the stomach, spleen, pancreas, duodenum, and gall bladder flow into the portal vein as do the superior and inferior mesenteric veins (**ATLAS PLATE 218, 218.2**). The liver receives all of the portal venous blood as well as arterial blood from the hepatic artery. Blood from these incoming sources drains into its **hepatic veins** that flow directly into the **inferior vena cava.**

B. **The Stomach.** The **stomach** is a dilated muscular bag situated between the lower end of the esophagus and the duodenum. From above downward, its parts include the **fundus, body, pyloric antrum,** and the thickened **pylorus** (ATLAS PLATE 208 #208.2).

Identify the esophageal end of the stomach and know that its opening, the **cardiac orifice,** is located to the left of the midline at the level of the 10th thoracic vertebra (ATLAS PLATES 155 #155.2). Above the cardiac end, note that the fundus of the stomach projects superiorly and contacts the left dome of the diaphragm. Follow the lesser curvature of the stomach from the esophagus to the horizontally oriented pyloric part (**Figure 15-5**). Look for the **incisura angularis** (angular notch) on the lesser curvature, marking the transition between the longitudinal part (fundus and body) and the horizontal pyloric part (pyloric antrum and pyloric canal).

Using your thumb and index finger, palpate the esophageal end of the stomach to feel the **vagus nerves** that enter the abdomen on the **anterior** and **posterior** esophageal surfaces (ATLAS PLATES 162). With a probe, stroke longitudinally along the anterior surface of the abdominal part of the esophagus to locate the (**anterior**) **left vagus** nerve. Similarly, identify the (**posterior**) **right vagus** on the dorsal side of the esophagus. Manipulate the pyloric end of the stomach and feel the thickened muscular wall formed by the pyloric sphincter that guards the pyloric orifice (ATLAS PLATE 209).

C. **Liver and Gall Bladder.** The **liver** is the largest gland in the body, and it participates in many functions. It metabolizes digested products such as proteins and carbohydrates, stores and releases glucose, synthesizes many proteins, detoxifies poisonous substances, and secretes bile, which is de-

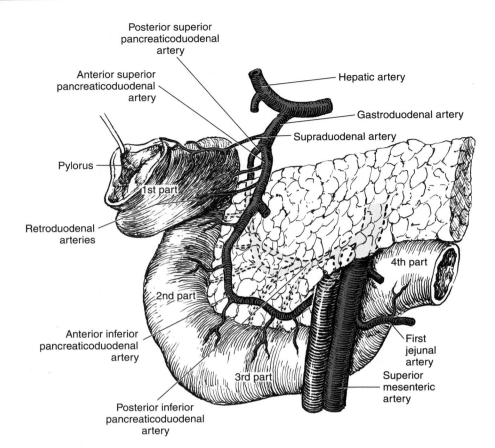

Figure 15-4. The pancreaticoduodenal arteries.

livered to the duodenum by way of the biliary duct system. In the adult, the liver weighs approximately 1500 grams (3.3 pounds) and even though it lies under protection of the rib cage (**ATLAS PLATE 216 #216.1**), it is easily injured. Its shape is largely determined by adjacent structures such as the diaphragm, right kidney, stomach, duodenum, gall bladder, and the right colic flexure. These

►
Grant's 113, 114, 142–144
Netter's 278, 279
Rohen 298, 299

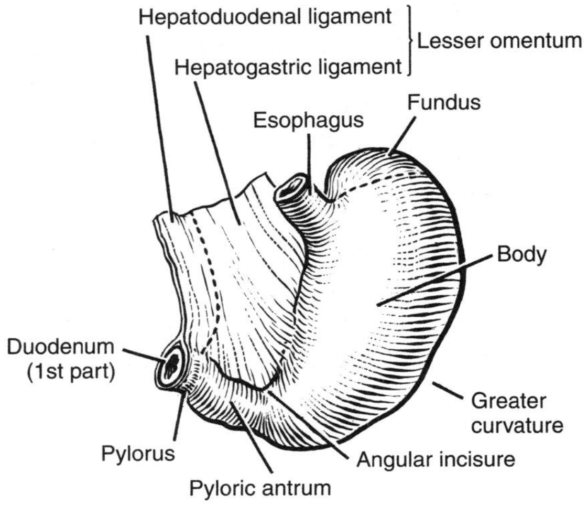

structures also help define its two principal surfaces: the **diaphragmatic surface** in contact with the diaphragm and anterior abdominal wall, and the **visceral surface** onto which the contours of adjacent organs are impressed (**ATLAS PLATE 217**).

The diaphragmatic surface has **anterior, superior, right,** and **posterior areas** (the latter includes the **bare area**) and is separated from the visceral surface by a sharp, lower border, called the **inferior margin** (**ATLAS PLATE 217 #217.1**). The visceral surface is marked by the **inferior vena cava** (into which the **hepatic veins** flow); the **porta hepatis** containing the **hepatic artery, hepatic duct,** and **portal vein;** and the **gall bladder.**

The peritoneal attachments of the liver must be severed to remove it from the right upper quadrant. The **falciform ligament** divides the liver into a large right and a considerably smaller left lobe (**ATLAS PLATE 212 #212.1**). Its attachment to the anterior abdominal wall commences at the diaphragm, where the anterior leaf of the **coronary ligament** covering the right lobe and that portion covering the left lobe meet at the midline (**ATLAS PLATES 216, 217**). Both anterior and posterior leaves of the coronary ligament adhere to the liver and cover both surfaces, except at the bare area.

Figure 15-5. The stomach and the lesser omentum.

►
Grant's 142–144
Netter's 279
Rohen 298, 299

The two leaves fuse at the extremity of the left lobe to form the **left triangular ligament.** This attaches the left lobe of the liver to the abdominal surface of the diaphragm; similarly, the smaller **right triangular ligament** attaches the right lobe to the diaphragm (**ATLAS PLATES 216, 217**).

The **gall bladder** is a pear-shaped sac located under the visceral surface of the right lobe of the liver (**ATLAS PLATES 221, 222**). It receives bile from the liver, and its **cystic duct** joins the **common hepatic duct** to form the **common bile duct.** The gall bladder has a capacity of 30 to 50 cc. Normally, its **fundus** projects downward beyond the lower border of the right hepatic lobe. The neck of the gall bladder and the cystic duct are marked by oblique ridges of mucosa that form **spiral valves.** The gall bladder usually receives a cystic branch from the right hepatic artery.

◄
Grant's 128, 130, 143, 144, 148–151
Netter's 279, 285–287, 291
Rohen 297, 299

►
Grant's 114, 143, 148
Netter's 276
Rohen 299

►
Netter's 225
Rohen 289

Examine the diaphragmatic surface of the liver by palpating the superior area of both the right and left lobes, noting that their summits fit into the domes of the diaphragm. Reach under the costal margin and palpate the limit of this superior area formed by the reflection line of the anterior leaf of the coronary ligament.

Remove the liver so that its visceral surface can be examined. Cut the falciform ligament away from its anterior abdominal wall attachment. Pull the liver downward and cut the **anterior leaf of the coronary ligament** and the attachments of the two triangular ligaments to the diaphragm.

Reach upward on the diaphragmatic surface beyond the cut coronary ligament and gently shell away the loose attachment of the bare area from the diaphragm. Identify the **inferior vena cava** located between the liver and the diaphragm. Sever the **hepatic veins** that enter the inferior vena cava just below the diaphragm, and then cut through the inferior vena cava before it ascends through the diaphragm (**ATLAS PLATE 216 #216.2, 218**).

Sever the **posterior leaf of the coronary ligament** under the right lobe. In some cadavers, the inferior vena cava is embedded in the liver. If this is the case in your dissection, cut the inferior vena cava and remove part of this large vein with the liver. Cut the hepatic artery, common bile duct, and portal vein in the lesser omentum and remove the liver and gall bladder.

Examine the visceral surface of the liver and the posterior area of the diaphragmatic surface. Expose the visceral surface by orienting the liver similar to that seen in **Figure 15-6** (showing that a segment of

◄
Grant's 142,143
Netter's 276
Rohen 298

►
Grant's 143, 144, 148
Netter's 276
Rohen 299

►
Grant's 143, 148, 149–151
Netter's 285, 286
Rohen 296, 297, 299, 317

◄
Grant's 143,144, 148
Netter's 276
Rohen 299

the inferior vena cava was removed). Identify the structures at the porta hepatis and find the continuous longitudinal fissure formed by the **round ligament of the liver** and the **ligamentum venosum.** Note that this fissure on the visceral surface marks the separation of the left lobe from the **caudate** and **quadrate lobes (ATLAS PLATE 217 #217.2).**

The round ligament of the liver is the fibrous remnant of the **left umbilical vein** that carried blood from the placenta to the **left vitelline vein** (left branch of the portal vein in the adult, **Figure 15-6**). The **ligamentum venosum** is the fibrous remnant of the fetal **ductus venosus,** which shunted blood from the left portal vein to the inferior vena cava. Oxygenated blood was routed from the umbilical vein to the left vitelline vein (left portal vein) and then short-circuited by the ductus venosus to the inferior vena cava and right atrium without coursing through liver tissue.

Identify the **quadrate lobe** of the liver as the quadrangular region on the visceral surface between the gall bladder and the fissure for the **round ligament.** Behind the quadrate lobe, identify the **caudate lobe** between the inferior vena cava and the fissure for the ligamentum venosum (**Figure 15-6**). Examine the posterior surface, and note that the **bare area of the liver** is bounded by the anterior and posterior leaves of the coronary ligament. Return to the visceral surface and see if you can identify impressions for the right kidney and suprarenal gland, duodenum, right colic flexure, and stomach (**Figure 15-6**). These may not be apparent because of the way organs hardened in position after fixation.

Examine the fundus of the gall bladder and note that the greenish color is formed by extravasated bile. Dissect the neck and cystic duct free of connective tissue and observe where the cystic duct joins the **common hepatic duct** to form the **common bile duct.** Follow the cystic artery to the neck and fundus of the gall bladder.

D. **Bile Passages, Duodenum, and Pancreas** (**Figure 15-8**). The bile passages, duodenum, and pancreas form an important functional group of structures that are best studied together. The duodenum receives bile from the liver along biliary ducts and exocrine secretions from the pancreas by the pancreatic ducts.

1. **Bile Passages.** Bile is formed by hepatic cells and secreted into small **canaliculi,** which form networks within the hepatic lobules. From canaliculi, **interlobular ductules** transport bile to

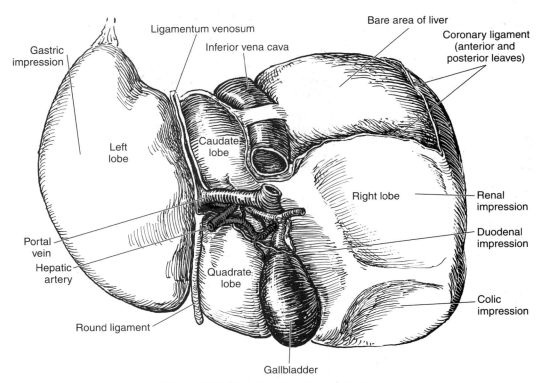

Figure 15-6. The visceral surface of the liver.

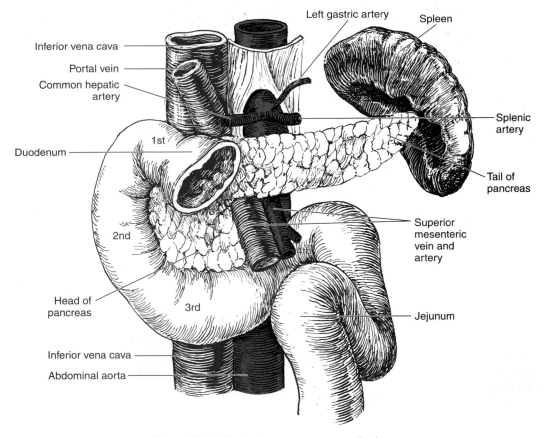

Figure 15-7. The duodenum, pancreas, and spleen.

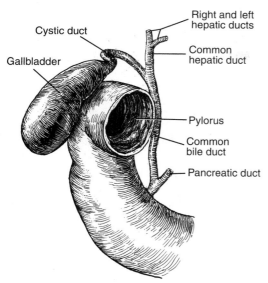

Cystic duct

Gallbladder

Right and left hepatic ducts

Common hepatic duct

Pylorus

Common bile duct

Pancreatic duct

Figure 15-8. The biliary duct system.

sequentially larger ducts until the **right** and **left hepatic ducts** emerge from their respective lobes at the hilum. These two hepatic ducts join to form the **common hepatic duct.** The **cystic duct** usually extends toward the left from the neck of the gall bladder to join the common hepatic duct, thereby forming the **common bile duct (ATLAS PLATES 221, 222).**

The common bile duct, which is approximately 8 cm in length and 6 mm in diameter, descends behind the first part of the duodenum (near the gastroduodenal artery) and then continues behind the head of the pancreas adjacent to the descending (second) part of the duodenum (**ATLAS PLATE 224 #224.2**). The common bile duct joins the **main pancreatic duct** midway down the duodenum and terminates in a dilatation called the **hepatopancreatic ampulla (ampulla of Vater).** Variations in this pattern are illustrated in **ATLAS PLATE 224.**

The ampulla communicates with the duodenum through an opening in the duodenal wall called the **major duodenal papilla,** which is approximately 9 to 10 cm below the pylorus. This is surrounded by a thickening of circular muscle called the **sphincter of Oddi.** The delicate **accessory pancreatic duct** empties into the duodenum 2 cm proximal to the major duodenal papilla.

2. **Duodenum.** The duodenum is the first and widest part of the small intestine (**Figure 15-7**). It measures approximately 25 cm (10 inches) in length or, as its name implies, the width of 12 fingers, and it is firmly fixed to the posterior abdominal wall being almost entirely retroperitoneal. The duodenum has four parts: first (superior), second

▶
Grant's 114, 126
Netter's 267, 270, 271
Rohen 311

▶
Grant's 126–129
Netter's 270, 271, 291, 292, 294
Rohen 311, 312, 316–318

◀
Grant's 143, 148, 149–151
Netter's 284–287
Rohen 296, 297, 299

▶
Grant's 126
Netter's 270, 271
Rohen 317

◀
Grant's 130, 131
Netter's 285, 287, 288
Rohen 296, 297, 316, 317

▶
Grant's 130
Netter's 270, 271
Rohen 317

◀
Grant's 126, 127, 130
Netter's 266, 270
Rohen 296, 317

(descending), third (horizontal), and fourth (ascending). It is C-shaped and, within the concavity of the C, is enclosed the head of the pancreas (**ATLAS PLATE 223 #223.2**).

a. **First (Superior Part).** The **first,** or **superior, part** of the duodenum is approximately 5 cm long. It begins at the pylorus, passes upward and to the right (**ATLAS PLATE 212 #212.1**), and is adjacent to the quadrate lobe of the liver and the gall bladder. Its anterior surface is often discolored (greenish) by bile that has seeped through the wall of the gall bladder. Posterior to the first part of the duodenum is found the **gastroduodenal artery,** the **common bile duct** and the **portal vein,** and inferiorly is the **head of the pancreas (ATLAS PLATES 223, 224).**

b. **Second (Descending Part).** The second, or descending, part is approximately 8 cm long and it courses downward from the 1st to the 3rd lumbar vertebra. It is crossed anteriorly by the transverse colon and the root of its mesocolon. Posteriorly, it is in contact with the hilum of the right kidney, the right renal vessels and the inferior vena cava. The medial surface of the descending part encloses the head of the pancreas and between these two organs are found the **superior** and **inferior pancreaticoduodenal vessels.** The **common bile duct** descends medial to the upper 5 cm of the second part before it opens (with the main pancreatic duct) into the duodenal wall (**ATLAS PLATE 224**).

c. **Third (Horizontal Part).** The third, or horizontal, part of the duodenum is approximately 10 cm long; it courses from right to left across the vertebral column at the 3rd lumbar vertebra. Over its anterior surface descend the superior mesenteric vessels and the root of the mesentery of the small intestine. Posteriorly are found the **abdominal aorta** and its **testicular** or **ovarian branches,** the **right ureter, right psoas major muscle,** and the **inferior vena cava.** Superiorly is located the **head of the pancreas (ATLAS PLATE 223 #223.2).**

d. **Fourth (Ascending Part).** The fourth, or ascending, part is only 3 cm in length. On the left side of the aorta at the L2 level, it bends forward at the **duodenojejunal flexure** to become continuous with the **jejunum (ATLAS PLATE 230, 232).** Superior to this part is the **body of the pancreas** and laterally the **left kidney** and **ureter.** Across its anterior surface passes the **transverse colon** and its **mesocolon.** Posteriorly, it rests on the **psoas major muscle** and the **left renal vessels.**

3. **Pancreas.** The pancreas is an elongated lobular gland (12 to 15 cm in length) situated posterior to the stomach. It extends across the posterior abdominal wall anterior to the L1 and L2 vertebrae and has a head, neck, body, and tail. The **head** of the pancreas is flat and is positioned within the curve of the duodenum (**ATLAS PLATES 223, 224**). The **common bile duct** passes behind the head of the pancreas or through its substance, and the **superior mesenteric vessels** descend through the gland. Posterior to these vessels is found the **uncinate process** of the head of the pancreas.

◄
Grant's 126, 127, 130, 131
Netter's 265, 266, 270, 288
Rohen 296, 297, 315, 317, 319

The **neck** and **body** of the pancreas pass anterior to the portal vein, aorta, and left suprarenal gland. Continuing to the left anterior to the middle part of the **left kidney,** the **tail** of the pancreas is directed to the hilum of the **spleen** (**ATLAS PLATE 223 #223.2**).

The pancreas secretes the hormone insulin directly into the blood stream, but its exocrine secretion (at least eight digestive enzymes) passes into small ducts in the lobules of the gland. These join the **main pancreatic duct** that courses along the length of the gland (**ATLAS PLATE 224 #224.1**). This duct unites with the common bile duct, and together, they pass through the wall of the descending part of the duodenum. The **accessory duct** originates in the neck of the pancreas and opens into the duodenum 2 cm above the main duct.

►
Grant's 126, 127, 131
Netter's 292, 295, 297, 300
Rohen 302, 309, 317

Dissect the biliary passages, duodenum, and head of the pancreas as an entire block of tissue. Make the stomach mobile by cutting across the greater omentum below the gastroepiploic vessels adjacent to the greater curvature. Elevate the stomach similar to that seen in **ATLAS PLATE 215 #215.1**, and expose the pancreas and duodenum by cutting through the peritoneum covering their anterior surfaces. Identify the gastroduodenal artery and find its **superior pancreaticoduodenal branches.**

◄
Grant's 126, 127, 129
Netter's 291, 292, 294
Rohen 316

►
Grant's 115, 123, 156
Netter's 264, 289
Rohen 296, 317

There are usually two superior pancreaticoduodenal branches, anterior and posterior; the posterior is sometimes called the **retroduodenal artery.** These branches descend on the anterior and posterior aspects of the head of the pancreas and supply both the pancreas and the duodenum (**Figure 15-4**). They anastomose with **anterior** and **posterior branches** of the **inferior pancreaticoduodenal artery** that ascends from the superior mesenteric artery. **Anterior** and **posterior arterial arcades** are formed by the anastomosis of these vessels (**Figure 15-4**).

Dissect the arterial arcades in the head of the pancreas and look for the **supraduodenal artery** that frequently descends to supply the anterior surface of the first part of the duodenum (**Figure 15-4**). Usually, this vessel arises from the gastroduodenal artery (approximately 60% of cases), and it is often the first artery beyond the pylorus to supply the duodenum.

Find the common bile duct and trace it inferiorly on the posterior aspect of the head of the pancreas. Dissect the **main pancreatic duct** by picking away small pieces of the pancreas along the longitudinal course of the duct. Commence near the middle of the body of the pancreas and use **ATLAS PLATE 224 #224.1** as a guide.

Open the first and second parts of the duodenum by cutting longitudinally along their anterior surface. Identify the **major duodenal papilla** approximately midway down the second part. Note this orifice internally opposite the site where the hepatic and pancreatic ducts join externally (**ATLAS PLATE 224**). Try to locate the opening of the **accessory duct** 2 cm proximal to the major papilla.

Find the **superior mesenteric artery** and **vein** as they cross anterior to the third (or horizontal) part of the duodenum. Find the origin of the **portal vein** by identifying the junction of the splenic and superior mesenteric veins (**ATLAS PLATE 223**). Find the splenic artery and identify one or more of its numerous pancreatic branches that descend into the gland. Follow the body of the pancreas to the left, and note the relationship of the tail of the pancreas to the middle part of the left kidney and the hilum of the spleen.

E. **Spleen** (**ATLAS PLATES 212, 213, 215**). The spleen is a soft, purplish organ located in the upper left quadrant of the abdomen, and its convex **diaphragmatic surface** lies deep to the 9th, 10th, and 11th ribs (**ATLAS PLATE 199 #199.2**). Its concave **visceral surface** is oriented toward other abdominal organs and presents **gastric, renal,** and **colic impressions,** as well as a small region of the splenic hilum where the **tail of the pancreas** contacts the spleen. The spleen is surrounded by peritoneum, the two folds of which are connected to the kidney (**lienorenal ligament**) and the stomach (**gastrosplenic ligament**).

Follow the **splenic artery** and **vein** across the abdomen toward the splenic hilum (**ATLAS PLATE 210**). Note whether **small accessory spleens** exist along their course (found in 25% of individuals).

Dissect the splenic branches at the hilum, and then find the **left gastroepiploic artery** branching from the splenic artery to the greater curvature. Find one or more **short gastric branches** of the splenic artery that supply the fundus of the stomach (**ATLAS PLATE 207**).

Elevate the stomach and palpate the visceral surface of the spleen. Pull the spleen forward from the diaphragm, and then remove it from the abdomen by severing its peritoneal ligaments and the splenic vessels at the hilum. Study its diaphragmatic and visceral surfaces (**ATLAS PLATES 212, 213**).

Make an incision through the spleen and examine its cut surfaces. Note its fibroelastic capsule, and note that connective tissue trabeculae pass inward from the capsule to form a branching reticular network, the interstices of which are filled with splenic pulp. In certain pathologic conditions, the spleen may enlarge enormously.

◀
Grant's 119, 122, 123, 127, 142, 144
Netter's 290–292
Rohen 315–317, 318

Clinical Relevance

Location of the liver. The liver lies directly below the diaphragm and deep to the anterior surfaces of the 7th to the 11th ribs on the right side. Its left lobe ascends deep to the sternum and the 5th rib on the left side. Its sharp inferior border is overlain by the costal margin of the thoracic cage and deep to this border is located the pylorus of the stomach and the proximal part of the gall bladder. If the liver can be palpated inferior to the costal margin, it may be enlarged.

Cirrhosis of the liver. This condition is marked by degeneration of the hepatic parenchyma, patches of which are then replaced by scar tissue. This condition frequently develops in chronic alcoholism and usually is caused by inadequate nutrition. This condition is also known as Laennec's cirrhosis. If portal hypertension develops from the impairment of venous blood return through the liver, enlargement of veins in the esophagus or rectum and around the umbilicus can occur. Of these varicosities, those on the inner aspect of the esophagus can be exceedingly dangerous and can lead to massive hemorrhage and death.

Gallstones. These concretions can develop but not cause pain, or they can obstruct the biliary tract and cause acute pain that is often referred to the right upper quadrant. Obstruction of the biliary tract by gallstones can cause an inflammatory reaction on the inner surface of the gall bladder because of its enlargement (cholecystitis). Excess bile in the biliary system can become absorbed in the bloodstream and cause a condition called jaundice.

The duodenum. The duodenum has four parts: superior, descending, transverse, and ascending. Its name implies that the length of the duodenum is equivalent to the breadth of 12 fingers. The horizontal 3rd part crosses the midline and is itself crossed anteriorly by the superior mesenteric vessels. If an individual quickly loses much weight, these vessels can constrict the duodenum and cause a blockage of the gastrointestinal tract.

Carcinoma of the pancreas. If this serious condition exists, it most often occurs in the head of the pancreas, and at this site it could obstruct the biliary system. A backup of bile absorbed by the vascular system causes the discoloration of the skin called jaundice. This condition is best observed by looking at the white sclera of the eyes, which appears yellowish.

Enlargement of the spleen. This organ of the reticuloendothelial system can become greatly enlarged from diseases that effect that system, such as lymphoma or leukemia. This enlargement is referred to as splenomegaly.

Abdominal aorta. The aorta enters the abdomen anterior to the body of the first lumbar vertebra (L1) or the disc between T12 and L1. This large vessel then descends retroperitoneally and to the right of the inferior vena cava to the level of the 4th lumbar vertebra where it divides into left and right common iliac arteries. The wall of the aorta (either above, below, or near the origin of the renal arteries) can weaken and bulge, forming an aortic aneurysm. These can be surgically repaired with a graft, but the most vulnerable are those that arise at or near the origin of the renal arteries.

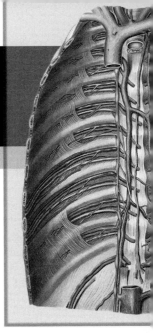

DISSECTION #16

Abdominal Cavity III: Intestinal Tract From Duodenojejunal Junction to Rectum

OBJECTIVES

1 Dissect the superior and inferior mesenteric vessels and their branches.

2 Dissect the small intestine within the abdomen; remove the jejunum and ileum and study their internal structure.

3 Dissect the cecum and appendix and the remainder of the large bowel as far as the rectum; remove the large intestine.

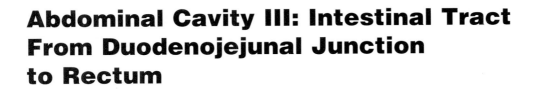
I. Superior and Inferior Mesenteric Vessels

The superior and inferior mesenteric arteries are unpaired branches from the abdominal aorta. The superior and inferior mesenteric veins drain the GI tract from the 2nd (descending) part of the duodenum to the mid-region of the rectum, and their blood flows into the portal vein.

A. Superior Mesenteric Artery and Vein. The superior mesenteric artery, which arises from the abdominal aorta 1 cm below the celiac trunk, is an unpaired vessel that supplies all of the small intestine except for the proximal 7 to 10 cm of duodenum (**ATLAS PLATES 230, 231**). It also supplies the cecum and appendix, the ascending colon, and most of the transverse colon. To the right of the artery courses the **superior mesenteric vein.** The superior mesenteric

◄
Grant's 126, 127, 152
Netter's 292, 295, 299, 300
Rohen 302, 309, 317
►
Grant's 126
Netter's 290–292, 297
Rohen 316

artery is crossed by the **splenic vein,** which joins the superior mesenteric vein to form the **portal vein** (**ATLAS PLATE 232**).

Surrounding the superior mesenteric artery at its source is the **superior mesenteric plexus,** containing both sympathetic and parasympathetic nerve fibers. Also found here are numerous lymphatic channels and nodes (**ATLAS PLATE 257**). Below the pancreas, the superior mesenteric vessels descend over the horizontal (3rd) part of the duodenum where they commence giving off branches (**ATLAS PLATES 223, 230, 231**). From the superior mesenteric artery arise 1) the **inferior pancreaticoduodenal artery,** 2) **intestinal arteries** (jejunal and ileal), 3) the **ileocolic artery,** 4) the **right colic artery,** and 5) the **middle colic artery.**

1. **Inferior pancreaticoduodenal artery.** Usually, this vessel is the first branch off of the superior mesenteric artery, and it arises near the upper border of the horizontal duodenum (**ATLAS PLATE 207**) (it may arise from the uppermost jejunal artery). It courses to the right, behind the superior mesenteric vein, and divides into anterior and posterior branches, which anastomose with the anterior and posterior superior pancreaticoduodenal vessels.

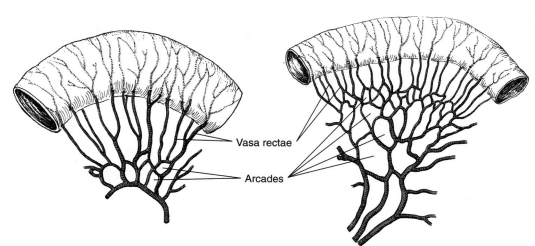

JEJUNUM   ILEUM

Figure 16-1. Comparison of the arterial arcades in the jejunum on the left and the ileum on the right.

Vasa rectae

Arcades

2. **Jejunal and ileal intestinal branches.** There are 12 to 16 jejunal and ileal intestinal branches that arise from the **left side** of the superior mesenteric artery and course between the two leaves of the mesentery (**ATLAS PLATES 230, 231**). Descending nearly parallel to each other, they divide to join neighboring branches and form a series of arches. These arches (or arcades) are initially simple in the jejunum but become more complex with three and sometimes four tiers of arches in the distal ilium (**Figure 16-1**). Straight branches, called **vasa rectae**, course to the intestinal wall from the outermost arch.

3. **The ileocolic artery.** The ileocolic artery arises midway down on the **right side** of the superior mesenteric artery, often the most inferior of the branches from this side of the main stem (**ATLAS PLATES 230, 231**). It courses toward the ileocecal junction, where its ascending branch anastomoses with the right colic artery to supply the ascending colon. Its descending branch anastomoses with the most distal ileal branch to supply the terminal ileum. The ileocolic artery gives rise to **anterior** and **posterior cecal arteries** and the important **appendicular artery**. This latter vessel passes behind the terminal ileum and supplies the **vermiform appendix** between the leaves of the **mesoappendix** (**Figure 16-2**).

4. **Right colic artery.** The right colic artery may arise from the superior mesenteric artery or from a common stem with the ileocolic. It courses behind the peritoneum to the right, anterior to the right ureter and gonadal vessels, to supply the ascending colon and the right colic (hepatic) flexure (**ATLAS PLATES 230, 231**). It anastomoses with the ileocolic and middle colic arteries.

◄
Grant's 127, 136, 137
Netter's 295, 296, 300
Rohen 302, 303, 309
►
Grant's 134, 135, 139, 140
Netter's 295, 296
Rohen 302, 303, 308
►
Grant's 138
Netter's 296, 313

◄
Grant's 135–137, 140, 141
Netter's 295, 296, 312
Rohen 302, 303, 309

►
Grant's 132, 140
Netter's 262, 270, 288
Rohen 296, 308, 311

◄
Grant's 126, 136, 137
Netter's 296, 312, 313
Rohen 302, 303, 309

5. **Middle colic artery.** The middle colic artery arises from the superior mesenteric artery just below the pancreas, and it divides into right and left branches to supply the transverse colon (**Figure 16-3**). It anastomoses with the right colic artery and with the left colic branch of the inferior mesenteric artery.

6. **Marginal artery.** Along the inner border of the large bowel, an anastomosis is formed that involves the ileocolic, right colic, and middle colic arteries, and branches from the inferior mesenteric artery. This anastomosis is called the **marginal artery** (of Drummond), and it circles the inner border of the large intestine, giving off straight branches (vasa rectae) to the bowel (**Figure 16-3**). At times, secondary arcades are formed by the anastomosing vessels so that the marginal artery may be found close to the border of the large colon or, because of an interposed arcade, at a short distance from it.

Reflect the stomach and the transverse colon upward, and push the coils of jejunum to the right. Locate the **duodenojejunal junction** 2 cm to the left of the midline just below the transverse mesocolon. Note if one or more duodenal fossae or recesses can be recognized at that junction (**ATLAS PLATE 228**).

In approximately 75% of cases, an **inferior duodenal recess** is located on the left side of the terminal part of the duodenum where the small intestine acquires its mesentery (**ATLAS PLATE 228**). This recess, located at the L3 vertebra, may be 2 cm deep, and its entrance allows the tips of one or more fingers.

Other fossae that may be present at this site include the **superior duodenal recess** (**ATLAS PLATE 228**),

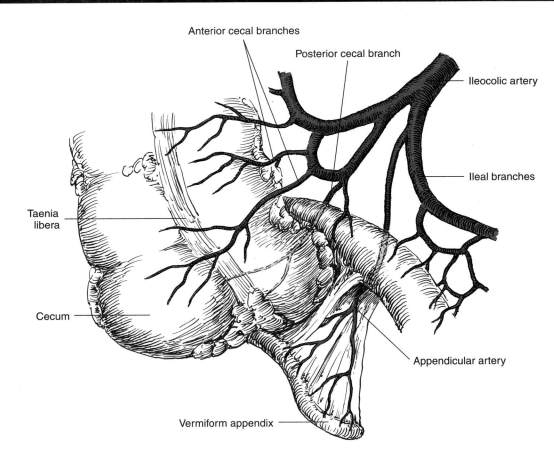

Anterior cecal branches

Posterior cecal branch

Ileocolic artery

Ileal branches

Taenia libera

Cecum

Appendicular artery

Vermiform appendix

Figure 16-2. The arterial supply to the ileocecal region and the vermiform appendix.

approximately 2 cm above the inferior duodenal recess; the important **paraduodenal recess,** which invaginates behind the inferior mesenteric vein (20% of subjects, most often in children); and the less frequent **retroduodenal recess,** located upward behind the fourth part of the duodenum. **These recesses are important because they are sites where herniation and possible strangulation of a loop of small intestine may occur.**

Dissect into the mesentery to the right of the duodenojejunal junction and expose the **superior mesenteric artery and vein** below the inferior border of the duodenum. Follow the artery superiorly to the interval between the neck of the pancreas and the upper border of the duodenum, and find the **inferior pancreaticoduodenal artery** and its branches. These vessels may be hidden by a dense network of nerve fibers called the **superior mesenteric plexus,** which surrounds the proximal part of the superior mesenteric artery (**ATLAS PLATE 242**). Carefully cut away the plexus from the vessels to visualize the anastomosis between the inferior and superior pancreaticoduodenal vessels.

◄
Netter's 262
Rohen 310, 318

►
Grant's 136, 137
Netter's 295
Rohen 302, 308

◄
Grant's 136, 137, 140, 141
Netter's 291–295, 299
Rohen 303, 309, 316, 317

Separate the descending part of the duodenum and the head of the pancreas from the right kidney, right ureter, and inferior vena cava. Reflect the right side of the duodenum and head of the pancreas to the left and see on their posterior surface the anastomosis of the vessels.

Push the coils of the jejunum and ileum across the midline to the left (**ATLAS PLATE 226**). Strip the peritoneum from one or two coils of upper jejunum to expose several **jejunal branches** of the superior mesenteric artery. Pick away the fat along these vessels and identify some of the numerous **mesenteric lymph nodes** and the complex web of **mesenteric nerve fibers** that accompany the vessels within the mesentery (**ATLAS PLATE 216**). Display the **vasa rectae** and the **single row of arterial arcades** that characterize the upper jejunum.

Similarly, dissect one or two loops of **ileum** 10 cm (4 inches) proximal to the **ileocecal junction.** Note that the arcades are more complex and that two or three rows of arcades often precede the shorter vasa rectae (**Figure 16-1**).

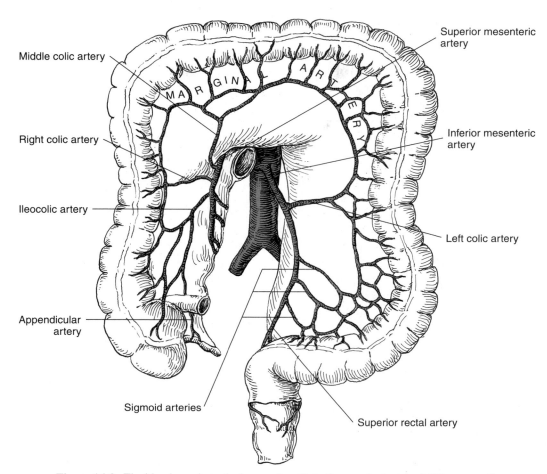

Figure 16-3. The blood supply to the large colon. Note the marginal artery (of Drummond).

By lifting a loop of small intestine in front of a bright light, a surgeon can recognize the degree of complexity of the vascular pattern and thereby know approximately which part of the small intestine is being manipulated.

Before dissecting the ileocolic artery, look for the **superior and inferior ileocecal recesses** and their associated peritoneal folds adjacent to the ileocecal junction (**ATLAS PLATE 226**). Also, determine the location of the **vermiform appendix** and its mesentery.

The superior and inferior ileocecal recesses are the most constant in the cecal region (**ATLAS PLATE 226**). The **superior ileocecal recess** is located above the ileocecal junction, and it is bounded anteriorly by the vascular peritoneal fold of the cecum that contains the anterior cecal artery and vein and posteriorly by the mesentery of the ileum. The **inferior ileocecal recess** is located below the ileocecal junction and it lies between the **inferior ileocecal fold** (the "bloodless fold of Treves") and the mesentery of the appendix (**ATLAS PLATE 237 237.2**). The ileocecal recesses are important as anatomic landmarks but not as sites for intestinal herniations.

◄
Grant's 132, 135, 136
Netter's 263, 273, 275
Rohen 307, 311, 318

◄
Grant's 135–137
Netter's 295, 296
Rohen 302. 303, 309

►
Grant's141, 152, 153
Netter's 299–304
Rohen 300–303, 309

Dissect the **ileocolic branch** of the superior mesenteric artery, often the lowest branch from the **right side** of the main stem (**ATLAS PLATES 230, 231, 234**). Find its branches to the **cecum** and identify the terminal ileum and ascending colon (**Figure 16-2**). Find the **appendicular branch** to the **vermiform appendix** that most often arises from the **posterior cecal artery** (**ATLAS PLATE 237 #237.2**).

Identify the **right colic** and **middle colic** branches, which arise superior to the ileocolic on the right side of the main stem (**ATLAS PLATES 230, 231, 234**). Trace these vessels to the ascending and transverse colons and observe their anastomosing branches (**Figure 16-3**).

Note that the tributaries of the **superior mesenteric vein** follow the arteries. Observe that this vein begins in the ileocolic region by the junction of the ileal and ileocolic veins (**ATLAS PLATE 230**). It enlarges as it ascends and behind the pancreas it joins the splenic vein to form the portal (**ATLAS PLATES 223 #223.2, 224 #224.2**).

B. Inferior Mesenteric Artery and Vein. The inferior mesenteric artery is smaller than the superior, and it supplies the left part of the transverse colon, the splenic flexure, and the descending and sigmoid colons. Its terminal branch is the **superior rectal artery,** which is distributed to the upper part of the rectum (**ATLAS PLATES 232, 233**). Arising from the abdominal aorta approximately 4 cm above the aortic bifurcation, the inferior mesenteric artery courses inferiorly and to the left behind the peritoneum and into the lesser pelvis between the two leaves of the sigmoid mesocolon.

The **inferior mesenteric vein** returns blood from the rectum and the sigmoid and descending colons. It courses superiorly behind the peritoneum anterior to the left psoas major muscle and flows into the splenic vein (**ATLAS PLATE 232**). It may terminate near the point of junction of the splenic vein with the superior mesenteric where the portal vein is formed.

The inferior mesenteric artery gives off the left colic branch, two to four sigmoid arteries, and the superior rectal artery.

1. **Left colic branch.** The **left colic branch** of the inferior mesenteric artery courses to the left and usually divides into ascending and descending branches. Its ascending branch supplies the left half of the transverse colon, the left colic (splenic) flexure, and the upper part of the descending colon. The descending branch supplies the lower part of the descending colon and anastomoses with the uppermost sigmoid artery (**ATLAS PLATES 232, 233**).

2. **Sigmoid arteries.** The sigmoid branches of the inferior mesenteric artery course inferolaterally to the left and supply the lower part of the descending colon. They anastomose with the left colic artery, enter the sigmoid mesocolon, and supply all of the sigmoid colon. Inferiorly, the sigmoid arteries anastomose with the superior rectal artery (**Figure 16-4**).

3. **Superior rectal artery.** The superior rectal artery is the continuation of the main stem of the inferior mesenteric artery beyond the sigmoid branches. It descends into the pelvis and divides into smaller branches. These anastomose on the rectum with the **middle rectal** branch of the internal iliac artery (**ATLAS PLATES 232, 310**).

Turn the coils of the small intestine to the right and identify the **inferior mesenteric artery** arising from the aorta approximately 4 cm above its bifurcation and at a site deep to the horizontal part of the duodenum (**ATLAS PLATES 232, 243**). Observe that the artery (with the **inferior mesenteric vein** to

◄
Grant's 138, 141
Netter's 296, 300, 302, 313
Rohen 301, 302, 308

◄
Grant's 138, 139, 141
Netter's 296, 313
Rohen 302, 308

◄
Grant's 138, 139
Netter's 296, 313
Rohen 302, 308

◄
Grant's 138, 139
Netter's 296, 313
Rohen 302, 308

►
Grant's 132, 133
Netter's 272

◄
Grant's 138, 139, 141
Netter's 296, 301, 302, 313
Rohen 302, 303, 308

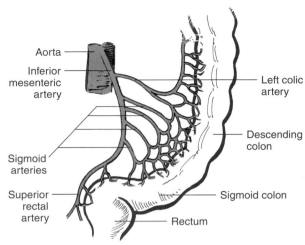

Figure 16-4. The branches of the inferior mesenteric artery to the descending and sigmoid colons and to the upper rectum.

its left) lies behind the peritoneum and that the **inferior mesenteric plexus** of autonomic nerves surrounds the vessel at its source. Dissect through the peritoneum, identify the **left colic artery,** and trace it to the descending colon where it divides into ascending and descending branches (**ATLAS PLATE 232**).

Find the **sigmoid branches** by dissecting into the layers of the sigmoid mesocolon (**ATLAS PLATE 232, Figure 16-4**). Trace the main stem of the inferior mesenteric artery inferiorly where its continuation becomes the **superior rectal artery.**

Follow the **inferior mesenteric vein** superiorly; observe that it lies to the left of the artery and medial to the left ureter (**ATLAS PLATES 232, 243**). Dissect it superiorly as it crosses the left gonadal vessels and ascends behind the duodenum and pancreas to enter the splenic vein.

II. Jejunum and Ileum

The **jejunum** and **ileum** are attached to the posterior abdominal wall by the mesentery of the small intestine and are arranged in coils that extend from the duodenum to the cecum (**ATLAS PLATES 226, 228**). The jejunum comprises the upper two-fifths of the small intestine beyond the duodenum, and the ileum comprises the distal three-fifths. The anatomy of the jejunum is different from that of the ileum but the change is gradual, and no specific line marks the boundary between these two parts of the small bowel. The jejunum has a thicker wall and a slightly larger diameter (4 cm) than the ileum (3.5 cm), is more vascular, and is redder in color in a living body. Solitary and aggregated lymphatic follicles (called **Peyer's patches**) are larger and more numerous in the ileum, especially in its most distal part. The inner surface of the jejunum is marked by many circular folds, called **plicae circulares.** These diminish in number in the upper ileum and are virtually absent in the lower ileum.

> Roll a coil of upper jejunum between your thumb and index finger and try to feel the folds of the mucous membrane on the internal surface of the jejunum. Compare it with the smoother distal ileum and note that the jejunum feels thicker.
>
> Remove the jejunum and ileum to study their internal surfaces. Tie two strings tightly (2 cm apart) around the jejunum 8 cm (3 inches) below the duodenojejunal junction. Similarly, tie a pair of strings around the ileum just above the cecum. Cut through the jejunum and ileum between the two ligatures of each pair. Remove the small intestine by severing the mesentery near its attachment to the small bowel (**ATLAS PLATE 235**).
>
> To study the inner surface of the jejunum, tie another pair of strings 15 cm (6 inches) below the upper end of the removed intestine and cut the jejunum between the new ligatures. Similarly, tie a pair of ligatures approximately 15 cm (6 inches) above the ileal end of the removed intestine and cut the ileum between these new ligatures.
>
> At a sink with running water remove the ligatures from the 6-inch pieces of jejunum and ileum. Cut open the two pieces of small intestine longitudinally. Note the circular folds on the inner mucosal surface of the jejunum and the smoothness of and lack of folds on the inner surface of the ileum. Spread the opened intestinal pieces on an absorbent surface (such as a paper towel) and allow to dry. Identify the lymphatic follicles, best seen by transillumination of the ileum. These are fewer, smaller, and difficult to see in the elderly.

III. Large Intestine

The large intestine extends from the ileocecal junction to the anus. It measures approximately 5 feet in length and varies in its diameter from 3 to 8 cm. The large intestine is arranged on the posterior abdominal wall in a horseshoe shape (**ATLAS PLATES 226, 228, 238, Figure 16-3**). Commencing at the **cecum,** the posterior abdominal wall parts include the **ascending colon, right colic flexure** (hepatic), **transverse colon, left colic flexure** (splenic), and **descending colon,** all of which surround the jejunum and ileum (**ATLAS PLATE 238**). On reaching the left iliac fossa, the descending colon turns medially as the **sigmoid colon,** which then bends acutely downward in the midline into the pelvis at the **rectum** (**ATLAS PLATES 228, 238, 239**).

▶
Grant's 132, 135, 136
Netter's 273, 276
Rohen 306, 310, 318

▶
Grant's 139
Netter's 273–276
Rohen 310

◀
Grant's 132
Netter's 261, 276, 296
Rohen 306–308

▶
Grant's 164
Netter's 255, 273
Rohen 307, 333

Except for the rectum and vermiform appendix, the external surface of the large intestine is marked by longitudinal muscle fibers arranged in three narrow bands called **taeniae coli.** On the cecum and ascending colon they are located anteriorly (**taenia libera),** posteromedially (**taenia mesocolica),** and posterolaterally (**taenia omentalis).** These longitudinal muscle bands alter the shape of the large bowel and transform its smooth external shape into a series of sacculations, called **haustrae coli,** which are readily visible through the peritoneum (**ATLAS PLATES 236, 238**). Also found on the surface of the large intestine (except the cecum, appendix, and rectum) are numerous small fat-filled projections called **appendices epiploicae.**

A. **Cecum and Vermiform Appendix (Figure 16-5).** The cecum is a blind pouch that projects into the right iliac fossa and is the first part of the large intestine. This large cul de sac (approximately 6 cm wide and 8 cm long) is interposed between the terminal ileum and the ascending colon (**ATLAS PLATE 236**). It is often mobile because it is enveloped by peritoneum, but at times its posterior surface is devoid of peritoneum, and it is then more fixed.

   On the inner surface of the cecum are situated the ileocecal orifice that is guarded by the **ileocecal valve,** and the small ostium into the vermiform appendix (**Figure 16-5, ATLAS PLATE 236**). The ileocecal valve is composed of superior and inferior flaps, which are folds of cecal wall, between which is the ileocecal orifice. At the margins of the valve, the flaps unite to form ridges called the **frenula of the valve (ATLAS PLATE 236 #236.1).**

   The **vermiform appendix** arises from the posteromedial wall of the cecum (**ATLAS PLATES 236, 237**). It may extend upward posterior to the cecum (retrocecal, 65%); inferiorly over the brim of the pelvis (descending or pelvic, 31%); inferiorly to the right and posterior to the cecum (subcecal, 2%); superior and anterior to the terminal ileum (1%); and superior and posterior to the terminal ileum (1%).

> Lift the cecum and note that it lies in the right iliac fossa over the peritoneum that covers the iliacus and psoas major muscles and the nerves of the lumbar plexus (**ATLAS PLATE 256**). Find the appendix and note that the three longitudinal muscle bands, or **taeniae,** converge at its origin on the cecum. Note that the ileocecal orifice projects onto the anterior abdominal wall at the point of intersection between the **intertubercular line** and the right lateral boundary of the rectus abdominis muscle. Observe that the root of the appendix lies approximately 1 inch inferior to the ileocecal junction (**ATLAS PLATE 236 #236.1**).

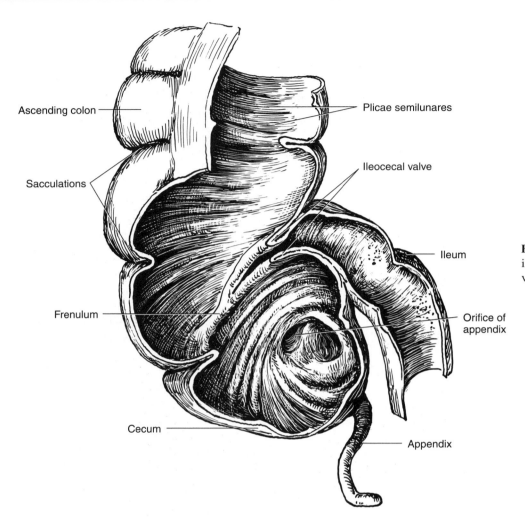

Ascending colon

Plicae semilunares

Sacculations

Ileocecal valve

Ileum

Frenulum

Orifice of appendix

Cecum

Appendix

Figure 16-5. An internal view of the ileocecal junction showing the ileocecal valve and the orifice of the appendix.

B. Ascending, Transverse, Descending, and Sigmoid Colons.

1. **Ascending colon.** The ascending colon passes superiorly above the iliac crest to the inferior border of the right lobe of the liver where it bends sharply forward and to the left forming the right colic (or hepatic) flexure (**ATLAS PLATES 235, 238**). It is 12 to 20 cm in length (5 to 8 inches), and it is covered ventrally and on its sides by peritoneum, but no peritoneum covers its posterior surface. It rests on fascia overlying the quadratus lumborum and iliacus muscles and the ilioinguinal and iliohypogastric nerves (compare **ATLAS PLATE 235 to PLATE 240**). The **right colic** (or **hepatic**) flexure lies anterior to the fat and fascia surrounding the right kidney. Anterior to the right colic flexure is the right lobe of the liver and the fundus of the gall bladder. Posterior to the right colic flexure courses the descending (2nd) part of the duodenum.

▶
Grant's 114, 132, 134, 140
Netter's 262, 263, 276
Rohen 292, 301, 306, 309

◀
Grant's 92, 132, 140, 152
Netter's 261, 263, 276
Rohen 307, 318

2. **Transverse colon.** The transverse colon measures 45 to 50 cm in length (18 to 20 inches), making it the longest part of the large intestine. It arches across the abdomen from the **right colic flexure** to the lower part of the spleen where it turns abruptly downward at the **left colic** (or **splenic**) **flexure** (**ATLAS PLATES 235, 238, 239**). The transverse colon is mobile because it is suspended from the posterior abdominal wall by the transverse mesocolon and its position therefore varies somewhat in different individuals. The root attachment of the transverse mesocolon from the posterior abdominal wall crosses the descending (2nd) part of the duodenum, the head of the pancreas, and the lower border of the body and tail of the pancreas (**ATLAS PLATE 240**). Between the leaves of the transverse mesocolon course the middle colic artery and vein along with lymphatics and visceral nerves that serve the transverse colon. The left colic flexure is located posterior to the greater curvature of the stomach and posterior to the left kid-

ney, splenic hilum, and tail of the pancreas. At this flexure, the transverse colon bends inferiorly to become the descending colon (compare **ATLAS PLATES 235, 240,** and **242**).

3. **Descending colon.** The descending colon is approximately 25 cm long (10 inches), and it courses from the left colic flexure to the brim of the pelvis, where it turns medially and posteriorly to become the sigmoid colon (**ATLAS PLATES 228, 232, 235**). Its diameter is less than that of either the ascending or transverse colons. It lies initially adjacent to the spleen and left kidney and then anterior to the quadratus lumborum, iliacus and psoas major muscles, and the nerves of the left lumbar plexus (compare **ATLAS PLATES 235, 240,** and **242**). Its anterior surface and sides are covered by peritoneum securing it to the posterior abdominal wall, but at times, its lower part has a short mesocolon, making it somewhat more mobile.

4. **Sigmoid colon.** The sigmoid colon, although variable, averages approximately 40 cm in length (16 inches), and it commences at the lower end of the descending colon in the lesser pelvis (**ATLAS PLATES 228, 232**). It is freely movable because it is surrounded by peritoneum that forms a mesentery called the **sigmoid mesocolon**. The attachment of the mesocolon is shaped as an inverted V, and it ends medially in front of the sacrum. At this site, the sigmoid colon bends inferiorly into the pelvis as the **rectum** (**ATLAS PLATES 228, 240**).

◄
Grant's 164
Netter's 255, 273, 276
Rohen 302, 308, 311

►
Grant's 132, 134, 138, 140
Netter's 263, 266, 276
Rohen 306–308, 310

◄
Grant's 134, 140, 141, 198
Netter's 263, 276
Rohen 308, 311, 318

Incise the peritoneum vertically along the right border of the **ascending colon.** Retract the colon medially and identify the lower pole of the right kidney, deep to which are located the longitudinal fascicles of the quadratus lumborum muscle. Below the iliac crest identify the iliacus muscle, and anterior and medial to the iliacus, observe the psoas major muscle (**ATLAS PLATE 250 #250.1**).

With the liver at its normal position in the right upper quadrant, observe the relationship of the right colic flexure to the right lobe of the liver and the gall bladder (**ATLAS PLATE 235**). Follow the transverse colon and its mesocolon across the abdomen to the left colic flexure. In doing so, manipulate the two layers of the mesocolon and note how they separate to enclose the transverse colon. Cut away the attachment of the transverse mesocolon from the anterior surfaces of the duodenum and pancreas. Just below the lower pole of the spleen, identify a double-fold of peritoneum called the **phrenicocolic ligament,** which attaches the abdominal surface of the diaphragm to the left colic flexure (**ATLAS PLATES 235, 240**).

◄
Grant's 115, 132, 133, 140
Netter's 319, 320
Rohen 318, 330, 331

◄
Grant's 115
Netter's 265, 266

Cut the peritoneum along the left border of the descending colon and reflect the colon medially. Verify by palpation the lower border of the left kidney and note the same muscles (quadratus lumborum, iliacus, and psoas muscles) seen on the right side. Follow the sigmoid colon medially toward the rectum and confirm that the attachment of the root of the **sigmoid mesocolon** outlines the shape of an inverted "V" (**ATLAS PLATE 240**).

Tie two ligatures (approximately 1/2 inch apart) 2 inches above the site where the sigmoid colon bends inferiorly to become the rectum. Cut across the sigmoid colon between the two ligatures. Then, remove the large intestine from the posterior abdominal wall by cutting away the peritoneal attachments of the ligated terminal ileum, cecum, and ascending colon. Cut the transverse mesocolon near its attachment to the transverse colon, detach the descending colon, and finally cut the sigmoid mesocolon along the border of the sigmoid colon. With the jejunum, ileum, and most of the large intestine removed, the posterior abdominal wall is exposed for further study (**ATLAS PLATE 240**).

Clinical Relevance

Lymphoid tissue in the small intestine. The collection of lymphoid nodules (called Peyer's patches) in the small intestine are most numerous in the lower ileum. These nodules are located on the antimesenteric border of the bowel and are not present in the upper part of the jejunum. More evident in younger persons, these nodules tend to involute and disappear as individuals grow older.

Meckel's diverticulum. This congenital condition, found in about 1 to 2% of the population, is a diverticulum of the small intestine located on the antimesenteric border of the ileum about 1.5 to 3 feet (average 2 feet) proximal to the ileocecal junction. Its length may vary from 0.5 to 4 inches, and it is the remnant of a narrow tube called the vitelline duct that normally is obliterated by the 7th prenatal week. If it persists in its entirety, it can lead to a fistula at the umbilicus, or if only the intestinal end of the duct remains open, it becomes a Meckel's diverticulum.

Cisterna chyli. A sac located to the right of the abdominal aorta anterior to the bodies of the L1 and L2 vertebrae the receives lymph from the gastrointestinal tract and the organs and the walls of the pelvic regions. After a fatty meal the lymph from the gastrointestinal tract is milky and is called chyle. The thoracic commences at the cisterna chyli and ascends in the posterior mediastinum to open into the left subclavian vein.

Duodenojejunal junction. This continuation of the duodenum, where it becomes jejunum, is located just below the transpyloric plane. Here the small intestine becomes intraperitoneal by becoming surrounded by two leaves of peritoneum from the mesentery that evaginate from the posterior abdominal wall.

Duodenal fossae. Several types of duodenal fossae can be found at the duodenojejunal junction. These are significant because hernias of the small bowel can occur into one or another of these fossae. These are surgically important because the herniated loop could become strangulated. When repaired, care must be taken not to injure the nearby inferior mesenteric vein.

Ligament of Treitz. This suspensory ligament of the small intestine at the duodenojejunal junction extends from the distal end of the duodenum or the proximal part of the jejunum superiorly to the right crus of the diaphragm. It passes superiorly posterior to the pancreas and anterior to the aorta.

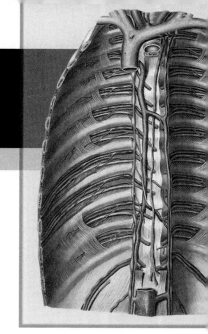

DISSECTION #17

Abdominal Cavity IV: Posterior Abdominal Wall

OBJECTIVES

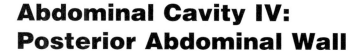

1 Dissect the gonadal vessels, kidneys, ureters, and suprarenal glands.

2 Dissect the muscles of the posterior abdominal wall and the nerves of the lumbar plexus.

3 Dissect the diaphragm from the abdominal aspect.

4 Dissect the abdominal aorta, inferior vena cava, and lumbar sympathetic chain.

Atlas Key:

Clemente Atlas, 5th Edition = Atlas Plate #

Grant's Atlas, 11th Edition = Grant's Page #

Netter's Atlas, 3rd Edition = Netter's Plate #

Rohen Atlas, 6th Edition = Rohen Page #

Cut through the esophagus just below the esophageal hiatus and sever the vascular attachments of the greater and lesser omenta, and the vessels along the lesser and greater curvatures of the stomach. Cut the splenic, hepatic, and superior mesenteric vessels and remove the stomach, duodenum, pancreas, and spleen.

After dissection of the gastrointestinal tract, there remains within the abdominal cavity the **kidneys, ureters, suprarenal glands,** the **abdominal aorta** and its paired branches, and the **inferior vena cava** and its tributaries. Behind these structures are located the muscles that comprise the posterior wall of the abdomen, the nerves of the **lumbar plexus,** and the **lumbar sympathetic chains.** Superior to these structures is found the **diaphragm** forming the muscular roof over the abdominal cavity.

The stomach, duodenum, pancreas, and spleen must still be removed (if not already done) before proceeding with a dissection of the posterior abdominal viscera and wall.

◄
Grant's 155
Netter's 319
Rohen 331

I. Gonadal Vessels, Kidneys, Ureters, and Suprarenal Glands

The testicular or ovarian vessels will be located first and then the kidneys, ureters, and suprarenal glands dissected free from the surrounding fat.

A. The Gonadal Vessels. The **testicular arteries** arise from the aorta anteriorly and diverge as they descend inferolaterally. The vessels cross the ureters, genitofemoral nerves, and the external iliac arteries on their way to the abdominal inguinal rings where they enter the inguinal canals (**ATLAS PLATE 243**). The **right testicular vein** accompanies the artery initially, but then ascends to enter the inferior vena cava. The

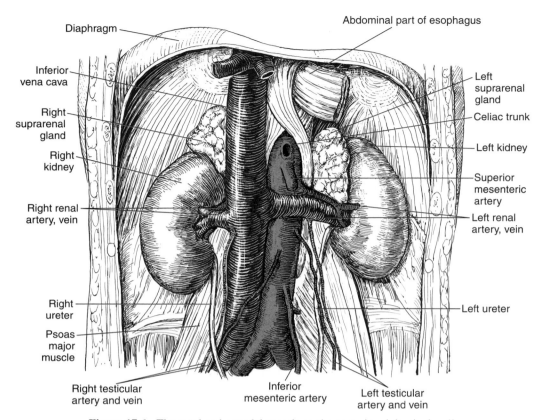

Diaphragm

Abdominal part of esophagus

Inferior vena cava

Right suprarenal gland

Right kidney

Right renal artery, vein

Right ureter

Psoas major muscle

Left suprarenal gland

Celiac trunk

Left kidney

Superior mesenteric artery

Left renal artery, vein

Left ureter

Right testicular artery and vein

Inferior mesenteric artery

Left testicular artery and vein

Figure 17-1. The renal and gonadal vessels on the posterior abdominal wall.

left testicular vein also ascends with its accompanying artery, but it drains into the left renal vein (**Figure 17-1, ATLAS PLATE 243**).

The two **ovarian arteries** also arise from the anterior aspect of the aorta. They descend over the brim of the pelvis and cross the external iliac arteries to enter the broad ligaments of the uterus within which they pass to the ovaries (**ATLAS PLATE 280**). The **right ovarian vein,** similar to the right testicular vein, enters the inferior vena cava, whereas the left ovarian vein flows into the left renal vein.

Remove the parietal peritoneum covering the posterior abdominal wall. Be cautious in dissecting the delicate testicular (**ATLAS PLATE 243**) or ovarian vessels that cross anterior to the ureters. Initially, look for the vessels through the peritoneal layer, and expose them inferiorly to the abdominal inguinal rings (testicular vessels) or the pelvic brim (ovarian vessels).

B. Kidneys, Ureters, and Suprarenal Glands. The **kidneys** are paired organs that excrete excess water and waste products resulting from metabolic functions. They are essential for maintaining electrolyte and water balance, and they help control the pH of

◄
Grant's 155, 167
Netter's 380, 381
Rohen 341, 360

►
Grant's 155, 157
Netter's 319, 321,
322, 328
Rohen 323–327,
331

►
Grant's 163
Netter's 332
Rohen 324,325

the blood and tissue fluids. This is done by the processes of **filtering** the blood plasma, **secreting** additional substances into the filtrate and then **reabsorbing** most of the filtrate and salt back into the blood. Approximately 1.3 liters of blood flows through the renal arteries per minute, resulting in nearly 180 liters of fluid that is filtered into the renal tubules every 24 hours. Reabsorption of most of the filtered water (approximately 99.5%) and NaCl allows the formation of approximately 1 liter of urine daily.

The kidneys are situated retroperitoneally on the posterior abdominal wall, one on each side of the vertebral column (**ATLAS PLATES 241–243**). They are reddish-brown and bean-shaped and measure 10 to 12 cm in length, 6 cm in width, and 3 cm in thickness. A concave region, the **renal hilum,** is located on the medial border of each kidney at the L1 vertebra, and through it the renal veins, arteries, and ureters traverse (**ATLAS PLATE 243**). The kidneys extend between the T12 and L3 vertebrae, but the right is slightly lower than the left because of the position of the liver.

The kidneys are embedded in considerable **perirenal fat (ATLAS PLATES 259, 260**), which extends superiorly over the suprarenal glands. A condensation of fascia, called the **renal fascia** (Gerota's fascia), surrounds

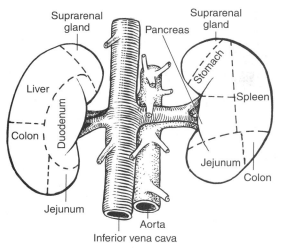

Figure 17-2. The anterior relationships of abdominal organs to the kidneys.

► Grant's 155, 157–160
Netter's 321, 323, 324
Rohen 326, 327, 331

► Grant's 93, 157–160, 239
Netter's 308, 319, 320
Rohen 330, 331

the kidney, its perirenal fat, and the suprarenal glands. Dorsal to the renal fascia is a large quantity of **para-renal fat.**

1. **Anterior relationships of the kidneys.** The relationship of the **anterior surface of the kidney** differs on the two sides **(Figure 17-2)**. Overlying the upper pole of the **right kidney** is the pyramidal-shaped **right suprarenal gland.** Below this, a large area of the anterior surface is in contact with the **right lobe of the liver.** Inferior to the hepatic impression is the **right colic flexure,** and, medially, the right renal hilum is covered by the descending part of the **duodenum (ATLAS PLATE 244 #244.1).**

   The upper pole of the **left kidney** is in contact medially with the **left suprarenal gland.** Inferior to the upper pole, the **stomach** and **spleen** lie anterior to the upper half of the left kidney. The left renal hilum lies posterior to the **pancreas (ATLAS PLATE 239)**, whereas the inferior third of the left kidney lies posterior to the **jejunum** and left colic flexure **(Figures 17-2, 17-3 and ATLAS PLATE 244 #244.1).**

2. **Posterior relationships of the kidneys.** The **posterior surface of the kidneys** is embedded in pararenal fat and overlies the 12th rib on the right side and the 11th and 12th ribs on the left (**ATLAS PLATE 246 #246.3**). The upper half of each kidney rests on the **diaphragm** and the **medial** and **lateral arcuate ligaments** (lumbocostal arches). Inferior to the diaphragm both kidneys lie on the **psoas major** and **quadratus lumborum muscles** and the tendons of the **transversus abdominis muscles (ATLAS PLATES 250–252).** Also coursing posterior to the kidneys are the

◄ Grant's 154
Netter's 319
Rohen 318

◄ Grant's 162, 163
Netter's 320
Rohen 324, 331, 335

subcostal vessels and **nerves (T12)** and the **ilio-hypogastric and ilioinguinal branches of the L1 nerves (ATLAS PLATE 241, 253).**

3. **Renal hilum.** Along the concave medial margin of the kidney is located the renal hilum, containing the **renal vein** and **artery** and the funnel-shaped upper end of the **ureter,** which is called the **renal pelvis (ATLAS PLATES 245, 246 #246.1).** Normally, the renal vein is anterior, the ureter posterior, and the renal artery in between; however, it is not unusual for secondary branches of the vessels to alter this pattern.

4. **Ureters.** The **ureters** are long narrow tubes that lead from the hilum of the kidney to the **urinary bladder.** They are approximately 25 cm (10 inches) in length, and their smooth muscular wall initiates peristaltic movements that convey urine

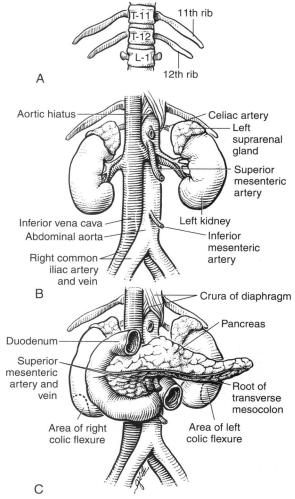

Figure 17-3. Organ relationships on the posterior abdominal wall at three levels. **A.** Vertebral level; **B.** Great vessels and kidneys; **C.** Duodenum and pancreas.

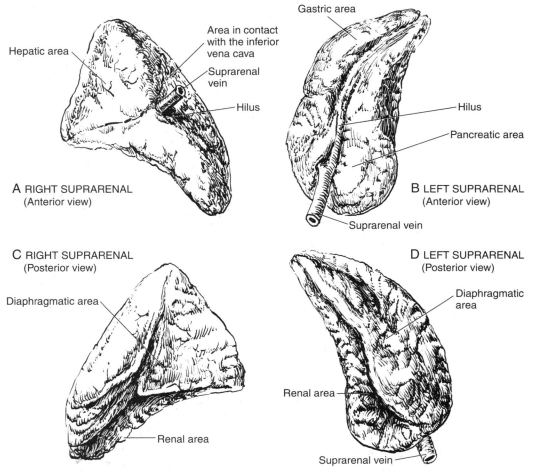

Figure 17-4. The suprarenal (adrenal) glands.

to the bladder. The ureters descend into the lesser pelvis by crossing the common iliac arteries near their bifurcation (**ATLAS PLATE 243**). Ureters receive their blood supply from several sources. The **upper third** gets small branches from the renal artery and from the gonadal arteries; the **middle third** is supplied by small vessels directly from the aorta and/or common iliac arteries; and the **lower third** is supplied by branches from the superior vesical arteries to the bladder, and in females from the uterine arteries as well.

5. **Suprarenal glands (Figure 17-4)**. The **suprarenal** (or adrenal) **glands** are endocrine organs situated between the vertebral column and the medial surface of the upper pole of each kidney. They secrete hormones that are essential to life. The right gland is pyramidal in shape, but the left is semilunar or crescent-shaped. Their combined weight is between 10 and 15 grams, but because they are surrounded by much fat, they appear to weigh more.

▶
Grant's 154, 155, 170, 171
Netter's 319, 322, 333, 334, 336
Rohen 326, 327, 331

▶
Grant's 123, 155, 156, 163, 171
Netter's 319, 322, 332–334
Rohen 324–327, 331

The suprarenal glands are highly vascular and receive blood from at least three sources: 1) directly from the abdominal aorta; 2) from the inferior phrenic arteries; and 3) from the renal arteries (**ATLAS PLATE 245**). The **suprarenal vein,** which emerges at the hilum of the gland, empties into the inferior vena cava on the right side and into the left renal vein on the left side (**ATLAS PLATE 243**).

Palpate both **kidneys** and feel for the suprarenal glands above and medial to their upper poles. Observe that the kidneys are embedded in perirenal fat and surrounded by the **renal fascia.** Note that the **suprarenal glands** are similarly surrounded by fat and renal fascia.

Make a longitudinal incision in the renal fascia of both kidneys and, using your fingers, free the organs from the surrounding perirenal fat. Clean each suprarenal gland being careful not to destroy its delicate arteries and the larger **suprarenal vein** at its hilum (**ATLAS PLATE 245**). Separate the suprarenal glands from the kidneys. Clean the structures at the **renal hilum** and turn each kidney over medially to expose their posterior surfaces.

Clean both ureters and the **renal pelvis** at the renal hilum. Note that the renal pelvis is the most posterior structure at the hilum although a branch of the artery or vein may lie behind the ureter. Follow the ureters to the pelvic brim and observe their relationship to the gonadal vessels and the common iliac vessels at their bifurcation. Clean the **renal artery** and note that most of its branches lie between the renal vein anteriorly and the ureter posteriorly (**ATLAS PLATES 245, 246 #246.1**).

◄
Grant's 157–160
Netter's 319–324
Rohen 326–331

Remove the **pararenal fat body** posterior to each kidney. Identify the crura of the diaphragm, the psoas major, and quadratus lumborum muscles. Envision how the 12th rib passes obliquely behind the kidney (**ATLAS PLATES 198, 198.2, 246 #246.2**) and that the uppermost part of the organ extends up to the 11th rib (somewhat higher on the left).

Return the kidneys to their normal position and dissect the two **renal veins.** Observe that the veins course anterior to the renal arteries (**ATLAS PLATE 243**) and that the left renal vein is three times the length of the right (7.5 cm to 2.5 cm). Follow the veins to their termination into the inferior vena cava. Identify the **left gonadal vein,** which flows into the left renal vein from below, and the **left suprarenal vein** and the **left inferior phrenic vein,** which drain into it from above. Sever the left renal vein and reflect it to the left to expose the left renal artery. Observe that the artery divides into two or more branches prior to entering the kidney (**ATLAS PLATES 245, 246**).

◄
Grant's 77, 155
Netter's 234, 257, 322
Rohen 326, 327, 330, 331

►
Grant's 141, 155
Netter's 319, 328
Rohen 330, 331

►
Grant's 171
Netter's 322
Rohen 329

Detach the left suprarenal gland from the upper pole of the left kidney. Without severing the renal vessels or ureter at the hilum, use a scalpel and split the kidney longitudinally into anterior and posterior halves (**Figure 17-5, ATLAS PLATE 247**). Do this by sectioning along the lateral convex border and cut medially toward the hilum. Open the halves and leave them still loosely attached at the renal pelvis of the ureter.

Note the thin **fibrous renal capsule,** which can easily be stripped from the underlying tissue. Observe that the kidney internally consists of an outer **renal cortex** and an inner **renal medulla.** Identify the **renal pyramids** that form the medulla and the **renal columns** (of Bertin), which consist of cortical tissue that separates the pyramids by extending inward as far as the renal pelvis (**ATLAS PLATE 247**

◄
Grant's 157, 158
Netter's 321, 323
Rohen 326, 327

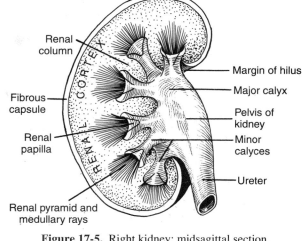

Figure 17-5. Right kidney: midsagittal section.

#247.2). At the renal pelvis, identify the **minor calyces.** Note that several of these join to form a **major calyx** and that three or more major calyces open into the renal pelvis (**Figure 17-5**).

Observe that the **ureters** are crossed from medial to lateral by the gonadal vessels. Look for small branches from the renal arteries that supply the upper parts of the ureters, and find other vessels from the aorta or the common iliac arteries that supply their middle parts. Realize that the lower part of the ureter in the pelvis gets blood from the superior vesical artery.

Look for small vessels descending to the suprarenal gland from the **inferior phrenic artery.** Note that others enter the medial surface of the gland from the **aorta,** and still other arteries ascend to the gland from the **renal artery** (**ATLAS PLATES 242, 243, 245**). Find the central **suprarenal vein** that emerges from the hilum of the gland and confirm that it drains into the inferior vena cava on the right side and into the left renal vein on the left (**ATLAS PLATE 243**). Remove one gland and cut across it with a scalpel. Identify the inner **adrenal medulla** and the surrounding shell of tissue that comprises the **adrenal cortex.**

II. Muscles of the Posterior Abdominal Wall and the Lumbar Plexus (Figure 17-6)

The muscles and fascia that form the posterior abdominal wall are located behind the kidney and below the diaphragm. In relationship to these muscles are the **subcostal (T12) nerves** as well as the **lumbar plexus** of nerves formed by the roots of the lumbar nerves.

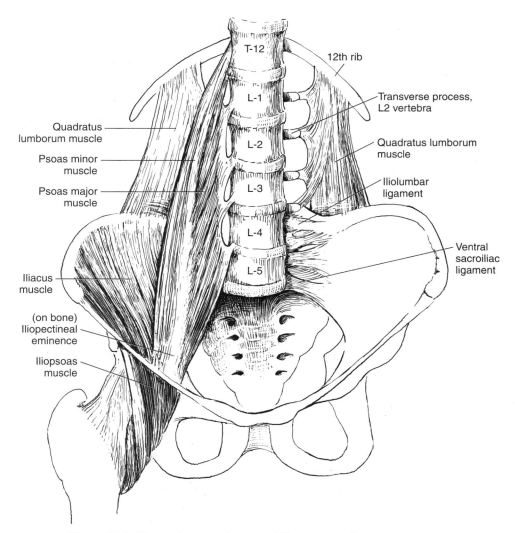

Quadratus lumborum muscle

Psoas minor muscle

Psoas major muscle

Iliacus muscle

(on bone) Iliopectineal eminence

Iliopsoas muscle

T-12

L-1

L-2

L-3

L-4

L-5

12th rib

Transverse process, L2 vertebra

Quadratus lumborum muscle

Iliolumbar ligament

Ventral sacroiliac ligament

Figure 17-6. The quadratus lumborum and iliopsoas muscles.

A. Muscles of the Posterior Abdominal Wall (Figure 17-6). The posterior abdominal muscles extend superiorly to the **diaphragm** and its **crura.** Coursing laterally at the level of the **12th ribs** are two fibrous arches (on each side), called the **medial** and **lateral arcuate ligaments** (**ATLAS PLATES 250–252**). The muscles include the origins and upper parts of the **psoas major** and **minor** and the entire **quadratus lumborum.** Inferior to the iliac crest is located the **iliacus muscle.**

1. **Psoas major and minor muscles.** The psoas major and minor function jointly with the iliacus and together are called the **iliopsoas muscle.** Acting from above, these muscles are the most powerful flexors of the thigh at the hip joint. When the muscles of both sides act from below, they flex the vertebral column such as in sitting up from a

◄
Grant's 164, 165
Netter's 255
Rohen 334, 335

◄
Grant's 264
Netter's 255
Rohen 330, 331, 439

►
Grant's 163, 164
Netter's 255–257
Rohen 331, 333, 335

supine position. The psoas major, located just lateral to the vertebral column, arises by muscular slips attached to each of the lumbar vertebrae and their intervertebral discs (**ATLAS PLATES 250–252**). It descends over the pelvic brim and continues into the thigh where it is joined by the iliacus muscle before inserting into the lesser trochanter of the femur (**ATLAS PLATE 371**). Along its anterior surface, when present (60% of cadavers), is located the small **psoas minor muscle** (**ATLAS PLATE 250 #250.1**). The psoas major is supplied by the upper three lumbar nerves, while the psoas minor receives a small branch from L1.

2. **Quadratus lumborum muscle.** The quadratus lumborum attaches below to the **iliac crest** and **iliolumbar ligament** and medially to the **transverse processes** of the upper four lumbar

vertebrae (**ATLAS PLATES 250 #250.1, 252**). It extends superiorly to the medial half of the 12th rib, and lies partially behind the psoas major. The quadratus is innervated by the upper 3 or 4 lumbar nerves, and acts as a lateral flexor of the vertebral column as well as an accessory muscle of respiration.

3. **Iliacus muscle.** The iliacus muscle lies inferior to the quadratus lumborum and its fibers arise from the iliac crest and the concave **iliac fossa** (**ATLAS PLATES 250 #250.1, 252**). The muscle descends deep into the inguinal ligament and its fibers attach to the lateral surface of the tendon of the psoas major muscle. It is innervated by the **femoral nerve.**

◄ Grant's 155, 164, 359
Netter's 255, 478, 480
Rohen 330, 331, 338

► Grant's 164, 165
Netter's 478–480
Rohen 471, 475

Reflect the kidneys medially and expose the muscles of the posterior abdominal wall by removing any remaining fat. Note that the fascia on the anterior surface of the quadratus lumborum is continuous with the **fascia transversalis,** the **psoas fascia** over the psoas muscles, and the **iliac** fascia covering the iliac muscles.

Find the **right** and **left crura of the diaphragm** over the bodies of the upper lumbar vertebrae (**ATLAS PLATES 250–252**). Identify the **inferior phrenic arteries,** which branch from the abdominal aorta and are directed laterally across the abdominal surface of the diaphragm (**ATLAS PLATE 253**).

◄ Grant's 155, 163
Netter's 255, 256, 332
Rohen 282, 331, 333

Immediately lateral to the vertebral column just below the diaphragm on the left, find two tendinous arches at the superior borders of the quadratus lumborum and psoas major muscles (**ATLAS PLATES 250 #250.1, 252**). These are the **lateral** and **medial arcuate ligaments.** Note that the **lateral arcuate ligament** (over the quadratus lumborum) is a thickened band attached medially to the transverse process of the L1 vertebra and laterally to the 1st rib. Verify that the adjacent **medial arcuate ligament** is a tendinous arch over the psoas major and that it attaches to the transverse process and body of the L1 vertebra. On the right side, the inferior vena cava must be pushed medially to see the medial arcuate ligament completely.

◄ Grant's 164
Netter's 255
Rohen 282

► Grant's 164, 165, 222, 352, 353
Netter's 259, 478–480
Rohen 330, 333, 475

Expose the posterior abdominal muscles by removing their fascial coverings. Be careful not to damage the **subcostal nerve** and the **genitofemoral** and other nerve trunks coursing through the psoas major muscle (**ATLAS PLATE 253**). Deep to the iliac fascia, identify the iliac branches of the iliolumbar vessels coursing laterally.

► Grant's 103–105, 353
Netter's 249, 259
Rohen 477, 479

◄ Grant's 164, 165
Netter's 259, 389, 478
Rohen 471, 475

B. Lumbar Plexus of Nerves (Figure 17-7). The **lumbar plexus** forms within the psoas major muscle

by the ventral primary rami of L1, L2, and L3 nerves and half of the L4 nerve (**ATLAS PLATE 254**). The other half of L4 joins the L5 nerve to form the **lumbosacral trunk** that contributes to the **sacral plexus.**

The 1st lumbar nerve divides to form the **iliohypogastric** and **ilioinguinal nerves** (**ATLAS PLATE 256**). Another branch from L1 joins a branch from L2 to form the **genitofemoral nerve** (**ATLAS PLATE 253**). The L2, L3, and L4 nerves divide to form **anterior** and **posterior divisions.** Parts of the posterior divisions of L2 and L3 form the **lateral femoral cutaneous nerve.** The other portions of the posterior divisions of the L2 and L3 nerves and all of the posterior division of L4 form the large **femoral nerve** (**ATLAS PLATE 256**). The anterior divisions of the L2, L3, and L4 nerves form the **obturator nerve.** When present, the **accessory obturator nerve** also arises from the anterior divisions of the L3 and L4 nerves. The remainder of L4 and all of L5 join to form the **lumbosacral trunk.** In summary:

- Iliohypogastric: L1
- Ilioinguinal: L1
- Genitofemoral: L1, L2
- Lateral femoral cutaneous: L2, L3
  (Dorsal divisions)
- Femoral (Dorsal divisions):   L2, L3, L4
- Obturator (Ventral divisions): L2, L3, L4
- Accessory obturator: L3, L4
  (Ventral divisions)
- Lumbosacral trunk: L4, L5

Identify the delicate **genitofemoral nerve** coursing along the anterior surface of the psoas major muscle. Observe that its roots course through the psoas muscle after branching from the L1 and L2 nerves. Preserve the genitofemoral nerve while dissecting the other lumbar nerves and note that it divides into **genital** and **femoral branches** (**ATLAS PLATES 253, 256**).

The **femoral branch** of the genitofemoral nerve supplies cutaneous innervation to the upper medial thigh. In both men and women, it enters the lower limb by passing deep to the inguinal ligament. The **genital branch** enters the inguinal canal through the deep inguinal ring and supplies the cremaster muscle in men and becomes sensory to the skin of the lateral scrotum. In women, the genital branch courses with the round ligament to the labium majus and mons pubis. The genitofemoral nerve contains the sensory (femoral branch) and motor fibers (genital branch) of the male cremasteric reflex, which, on stimulation, lifts the testes in the scrotum.

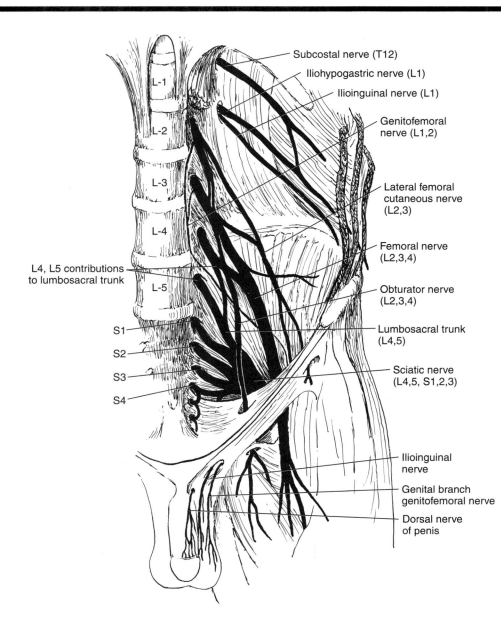

Subcostal nerve (T12)

Iliohypogastric nerve (L1)

Ilioinguinal nerve (L1)

Genitofemoral nerve (L1,2)

Lateral femoral cutaneous nerve (L2,3)

Femoral nerve (L2,3,4)

Obturator nerve (L2,3,4)

Lumbosacral trunk (L4,5)

Sciatic nerve (L4,5, S1,2,3)

L4, L5 contributions to lumbosacral trunk

Ilioinguinal nerve

Genital branch genitofemoral nerve

Dorsal nerve of penis

Figure 17-7. The lumbar plexus.

Palpate the 12th rib and identify the **subcostal nerve** (T12) and vessels that course along its lower border beneath the lateral arcuate ligament (**ATLAS PLATES 253, 256**). Remove fascicles of the psoas major muscle in a piecemeal manner by stripping them away longitudinally with "rat-toothed" forceps and scissors. **Carefully preserve the lumbar nerve roots and trunks as they course through the muscle (ATLAS PLATE 256).**

Below the subcostal nerve find the **iliohypogastric** and **ilioinguinal** branches of the L1 nerve. Note that the iliohypogastric nerve courses inferolaterally anterior to the quadratus lumborum muscle and pierces the transversus abdominis muscle near the iliac crest. Find the ilioinguinal nerve slightly below

▶

Grant's 164, 165, 352, 353
Netter's 259, 478–480
Rohen 331, 333, 415

◀

Grant's 164, 165
Netter's 259, 478–480
Rohen 333, 415

the iliohypogastric nerve and note that it also pierces the transversus abdominis.

Continue shredding the psoas major and find the **lateral femoral cutaneous nerve** coursing inferolaterally along the surface of the iliacus muscle. Observe that it descends into the lateral thigh 1 cm medial to the anterior superior iliac spine. Find the **femoral nerve** descending medial to the lateral femoral cutaneous nerve (**ATLAS PLATES 253, 256**). Note that it is the largest of the lumbar nerves arising from the posterior divisions of the anterior primary rami of the L2, L3, and L4 nerves. Trace the femoral nerve along the groove between the psoas and iliacus muscles, and observe that it enters the thigh 5 cm medial to the lateral femoral cutaneous nerve (**ATLAS PLATE 372**).

Shred away the lower **medial** part of the psoas major muscle from the L4 and L5 vertebrae to find the **obturator nerve** and, if present, the **accessory obturator nerve** as well as the **lumbosacral trunk** (**ATLAS PLATE 256**). Identify the obturator nerve emerging from the medial side of the psoas muscle. Follow it as far as the obturator foramen through which it enters the medial thigh (**ATLAS PLATES 256, 377**). Look for an **accessory obturator nerve** (in 10% of cadavers) descending between the obturator and femoral nerves.

Most medially and deep, along the lateral sides of the L4 and L5 vertebrae, find the **lumbosacral trunk** descending over the sacrum to join the upper three sacral nerves in the formation of the **sciatic nerve** (**ATLAS PLATE 255**).

III. The Diaphragm From the Abdominal Aspect (Figures 17-8, 17-9)

The diaphragm is a thin musculotendinous sheet that forms the partition between the thoracic and abdominal cavities. It is perforated by structures that descend into the abdomen from the thorax and others that ascend into the thorax. Its inner portion consists of a C-shaped **central tendon,** normally depressed by the heart, and the elevated lateral regions are muscular and called the **right** and **left domes** (**ATLAS PLATE 250**). The diaphragm arises by muscular fibers attached to structures around the border of the thoracic outlet (**ATLAS PLATES 251, 252**). The **sternal part** arises from the inner surface of the xiphoid process and the adjoining costal cartilages, the **costal part** from the inner surface of the lower 6 ribs, and the **lumbar part** by way of the

◄
Grant's 164, 165
Netter's 259,
478–480
Rohen 333, 470,
471, 475

◄
Grant's 164, 165
Netter's 189,
255–258
Rohen 282, 283,
327, 332

►
Grant's 164, 165,
168, 222
Netter's 259, 289,
479, 480
Rohen 334, 335

►
Grant's 155, 167,
171
Netter's 189, 233,
256, 322
Rohen 315, 329,
331, 333

right and **left crura** that attach to the bodies of the upper three lumbar vertebrae and from the **medial** and **lateral arcuate ligaments** (**ATLAS PLATE 250 #250.1**). From this circumferential origin, the muscle fibers insert in a radial manner into the central tendon.

The right crus is wider and longer than the left. It arises from the upper three lumbar vertebrae, wheras the left crus attaches only to L1 and L2 (**Figure 17-8**). An opening between the two crura, anterior to the T12 vertebra, is the **aortic hiatus,** and it transmits the **aorta** and **thoracic duct.** At the level of the T10 vertebra in the mid-line, the crural fibers form another opening, the **esophageal hiatus,** through which pass the **esophagus,** the two **vagus nerves,** and branches of the **left gastric vessels.**

The aperture for the **inferior vena cava** is located in the central tendon on the right side, 3 cm from the midline at the level of the T8 vertebra (**Figure 17-9**). The pericardium and the lower part of the right atrium attach to the thoracic surface of the diaphragm at this site (**ATLAS PLATE 134, 135**).

In the upper thorax, the **sympathetic trunks** lie lateral to the bodies of the thoracic vertebrae, but in the lower thorax, they shift more anteriorly to enter the abdomen behind the medial arcuate ligaments (**ATLAS PLATES 158, 255, 256**). The **splanchnic nerves** penetrate the crura to enter the abdomen (**ATLAS PLATE 158**). Behind the crura ascend the **lumbar veins** that become the **azygos** and **hemiazygos veins** in the posterior mediastinum (**ATLAS PLATE 159**).

Identify and preserve the **right** and **left inferior phrenic arteries** that supply the diaphragm as you remove the peritoneum from its abdominal surface. Find the left artery coursing on the diaphragm behind the esophagus and then to the left, and find the right

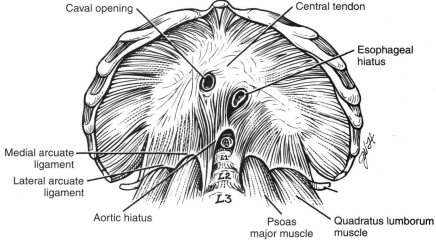

Figure 17-8. The diaphragm seen from below.

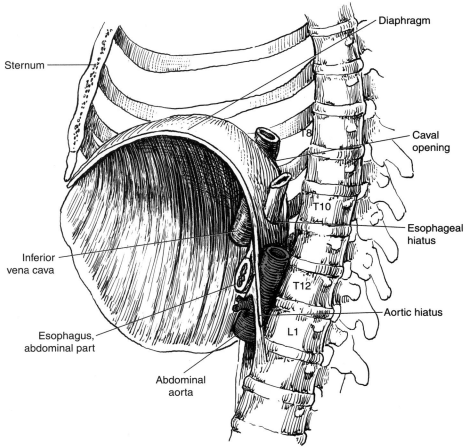

Sternum

Diaphragm

18

Caval opening

T10

Esophageal hiatus

Inferior vena cava

T12

Aortic hiatus

L1

Esophagus, abdominal part

Abdominal aorta

Figure 17-9. The diaphragm viewed from the left showing the vertebral levels of its openings (after Thorek).

artery behind the inferior vena cava and to the right (**ATLAS PLATE 253**). Determine whether the arteries are paired (69%) or arise by a single trunk (31%) and whether they arise directly from the aorta (45%) or from the celiac artery or some other vessel (more than 50%).

Commence on the thoracic side of the diaphragm and identify the following through to the abdominal side:

1) Sympathetic trunks on the upper lumbar vertebrae behind the medial arcuate ligaments,

2) Greater and lesser splanchnic nerves through the crura of the diaphragm (**ATLAS PLATE 158**),

3) Esophagus, vagus nerves, and **left gastric vessels** through the esophageal hiatus (**ATLAS PLATE 162**),

4) Aorta and **thoracic duct** through the aortic hiatus (**ATLAS PLATE 158**), and

◄
Grant's 72–75, 155, 168
Netter's 256–259, 290, 305, 309
Rohen 327, 331–335

►
Grant's 155
Netter's 257, 259
Rohen 333

5) Inferior vena cava through the caval opening (**ATLAS PLATE 243**).

Note that the muscle fibers of the diaphragm commence at their peripheral attachments and insert into the perimeter of the central tendon (**ATLAS PLATE 251**).

IV. Abdominal Aorta; Inferior Vena Cava; Lumbar Sympathetic Chain

The **abdominal aorta** courses along the posterior abdominal wall in the midline, the **inferior vena cava** ascends immediately to the right of the aorta, and the **sympathetic trunks** are located anterolaterally on the bodies of the lumbar vertebrae (**ATLAS PLATES 242, 243, 253**).

A. Abdominal Aorta. The **abdominal aorta** commences at the aortic hiatus of the diaphragm anterior to the body of the L12 vertebra and ends by dividing into the right and left common iliac arteries slightly to the left of the midline at the L4 vertebra (**ATLAS PLATE 243**). In a living person, the **level** of bifurcation can be determined by a line across the abdomen between the highest points of the iliac crest. The surface **site** of the bifurcation is approximately 1 inch below the umbilicus, slightly to the left of the linea alba.

Identify the cut stumps of the 3 unpaired branches that arise from the abdominal aorta, namely the **celiac trunk** immediately inferior to the aortic hiatus, the **superior mesenteric artery** 1 cm below the celiac trunk, and the **inferior mesenteric artery,** which arises 3 to 4 cm superior to the aortic bifurcation (**ATLAS PLATE 243**). Find the **celiac plexus,** which surrounds the celiac trunk and receives the **greater** and **lesser splanchnic nerves** of both sides (**ATLAS PLATE 242**). Separate the web of neural tissue on the surface of the vessels. Identify the autonomic fibers that constitute the **superior** and **inferior mesenteric plexuses** surrounding these aortic branches (**ATLAS PLATE 242**). Realize that, in addition to nerve fibers, these plexuses contain nerve cell bodies of postganglionic sympathetic neurons.

◄ Grant's 155, 167, 171
Netter's 256, 308
Rohen 331–335

Note that the aorta is crossed anteriorly by the **left renal vein** just below the origin of the inferior mesenteric artery (**ATLAS PLATE 243**). Review the origins of the **inferior phrenic, suprarenal,** and **renal arteries.** Dissect on the posterolateral aspect of the aorta to find pairs of **lumbar arteries** (**ATLAS PLATE 253**). Note that these arise opposite the bodies of the lumbar vertebrae and course posterior to the sympathetic trunks. On the right side, follow the lumbar arteries behind the inferior vena cava. Review the origin of the **gonadal arteries** and find the **median (middle) sacral artery** (**ATLAS PLATE 253**) that arises from the aorta near its bifurcation and descends anterior to the sacrum.

▶ Grant's 77, 171
Netter's 257, 322
Rohen 279

◄ Grant's 155, 171
Netter's 257, 322
Rohen 327, 329, 331

B. Inferior Vena Cava. The **inferior vena cava** is the largest vein in the body, and it carries blood back to the right atrium from the lower limbs, pelvis, and abdomen. It is formed by the junction of the **right** and **left common iliac veins** along the right side of the L5 vertebra (**ATLAS PLATE 243**). It ascends along the posterior abdominal wall to the right of the vertebral column and aorta. From the posterior surface of the liver, it traverses the diaphragm, penetrates the pericardium, and empties into the right atrium (**ATLAS PLATES 135, 137 #137.1**).

◄ Grant's 155, 171
Netter's 257
Rohen 331

Along this vein's ascent in the abdomen, it is crossed by the right gonadal vessels and the root of the mesentery of the small intestine. It also lies posterior to the transverse colon, duodenum, head of the pancreas, portal vein, and liver (**ATLAS PLATE, 241**). Adjacent to the hilum of the right kidney, the inferior vena cava lies anterior to the right renal artery. The right ureter descends along its right margin (**ATLAS PLATE 243**).

Confirm that the inferior vena cava forms by the junction of the **right and left common iliac veins,** 2 cm to the right of the midline and slightly below the intertubercular line (**ATLAS PLATE 243**). Identify the gonadal, renal, and suprarenal veins. Mobilize the posterior wall of the inferior vena cava and find several pairs of **lumbar veins** flowing into it posterior to the psoas muscles (**ATLAS PLATE 253**).

Note that the left lumbar veins are longer because they must cross the vertebral column to reach the inferior vena cava. Observe that the lumbar veins are interconnected longitudinally to form **ascending lumbar veins** and these flow superiorly to become the azygos and hemiazygos veins in the posterior thorax (**ATLAS PLATE 159**). Cut open the uppermost part of the inferior vena cava for a distance of approximately 5 cm below the diaphragm to see the openings of the **hepatic veins.**

C. Lumbar Part of the Sympathetic Trunks. The two sympathetic trunks extend below the diaphragm along the posterior abdominal wall anterior to the lumbar vertebrae. They continue into the pelvis anterior to the sacrum and reach the coccyx (**ATLAS PLATES 255, 256**). The lumbar sympathetic ganglia are variable in size and number, but most often, there are 3 to 5 on each side. The lumbar trunks receive **white rami communicantes only** from the L1, L2, and possibly L3 spinal nerves, but **gray rami** are distributed at all segmental levels.

In addition to the gray rami, which return to the segmental nerves, the lumbar sympathetic ganglia give off visceral branches, called the **lumbar splanchnic nerves.** These course from the ganglia to preaortic plexuses such as the intermesenteric, inferior mesenteric, hypogastric, and pelvic plexuses (**ATLAS PLATES 242, 255**). While the thoracic splanchnic nerves carry preganglionic sympathetic fibers, the lumbar splanchnic nerves contain both preganglionic and postganglionic fibers. The preganglionic fibers go through only the sympathetic chain and synapse with postganglionic neurons within the preaortic plexuses. The postganglionic fibers traverse only these plexuses on their way to the viscera.

Identify the sympathetic trunks in the upper abdomen by directing a probe from the thorax behind the diaphragm at their sites of penetration. Note that the trunks enter the abdomen deep to the medial arcuate ligament (**ATLAS PLATES 253, 255, 256**). Mobilize the aorta and inferior vena cava so that the **lumbar sympathetic chain** can be seen anterior to the lumbar vertebrae. Identify several of the **lumbar ganglia,** and note that the lumbar chain sends gray rami laterally to the lumbar nerves (**ATLAS PLATE 255**). Observe that other branches leave the sympathetic trunk, course medially, and join the sympathetic plexuses anterior to the aorta. Follow these inferiorly into the pelvis as the **superior hypogastric plexus (ATLAS PLATE 242**).

◄
Grant's 168, 170, 171
Netter's 308, 330, 389
Rohen 334, 335

Clinical Relevance

Nephrectomy. This operation is the surgical removal of a kidney, usually because of a malignancy or large stones.

Renal biopsy. Renal biopsies should be taken from the inferior pole of the kidney, if possible, because the superior pole is adjacent to the diaphragm, above which is the thoracic cavity. This step will avoid the possibility of penetrating the pleural cavity and causing a pneumothorax.

Congenital anomalies of the kidney. Some common anomalies include bifid renal pelvis and ureters, retrocaval ureter, pelvic kidney, horseshoe kidney, and accessory renal arteries and veins.

Cancer of the kidney. Most tumors of the kidney are renal cell carcinomas that develop in the proximal convoluted tubule. Early signs include blood in the urine (hematuria) and pain below the scapula in the lower back.

Peristaltic waves of the ureter. Often called ureteric or renal colic, this contraction of the muscular wall of the ureter frequently occurs when the ureter is attempting to pass a stone to the bladder. This painful condition is referred to the lower back on the side affected and to the upper thigh.

Suprarenal glands. These vital glands overlie the superior poles of the kidneys and lie adjacent to the vertebral column. During development the kidneys ascend to their normal location, but if they do not ascend, the suprarenal glands still develop in the upper medial aspect of the posterior abdominal wall near the vertebral column and lateral to the celiac axis where it branches from the aorta.

Aortic bruits. These are a variety of rhythmic sounds or murmurs audible upon auscultation of the abdomen. Among these is a blowing-type sound emanating from an aortic aneurysm or from a narrowed aorta.

Lumbar sympathectomy. This operation is often aimed at increasing the arterial blood supply to the lower limbs. It is done somewhat more easily on the left side because of the ascent of the inferior vena cava on the left. However, the abdominal aorta on the left side overlies part of the left lumbar trunk, so that surgeons must be careful not to injure these great vessels. Usually two or more ganglia are removed. The trunks are located in a sulcus medial to the psoas muscles and lateral to the bodies of the lumbar vertebrae.

Psoas sign. This swelling in the superior medial thigh is caused by a draining of blood and pus inferiorly within the psoas fascia at the site of insertion of the psoas major muscle onto the lesser trochanter of the femur. The source of the infection is often a diseased intervertebral disc (tuberculosis; salmonella discitis).

Diaphragmatic pain. The diaphragm is innervated by the C3, C4, and C5 segments by way of the phrenic nerves. Referred pain from the diaphragm is usually perceived in the lower neck and shoulder region where the sensory supraclavicular nerves, which are derived from the same segments, supply innervation to the skin.

Compression of the inferior vena cava. In the later stages of pregnancy, women often develop edema in the lower limbs or varicosities of the tributaries of the femoral vein. This is usually due to a compression of the inferior vena cava (IVC) by the enlarged uterus, which then impedes the return of venous blood from the lower limbs. More serious, however, is the compression of the IVC by a malignant posterior abdominal tumor. This syndrome is characterized by enlarged venous channels that normally drain into the IVC and anastomose with venous channels that drain into the superior vena cava, forming what is called a caval-caval shunt condition.

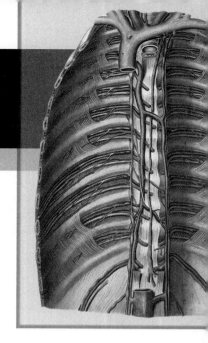

DISSECTION #18

The Pelvis: Male and Female

OBJECTIVES

1 **Both Male and Female Cadavers:** To learn features common to both the male and female pelvis and to examine the pelvic organs and peritoneal reflections *in situ.*

2 **Male Cadavers:** To dissect the male pelvic viscera: the urinary bladder, ureters, seminal vesicles, ductus deferens, prostate gland, prostatic urethra, and rectum.

3 **Female Cadavers:** To dissect the female pelvic viscera: the urinary bladder, ureters, urethra, ovaries, uterine tubes, uterus, uterine ligaments, vagina, and rectum.

4 **Both Male and Female Cadavers:** To dissect the lateral wall of the pelvis, the pelvic vessels, nerves, and muscles.

Atlas Key:

Clemente Atlas, 5th Edition = Atlas Plate #

Grant's Atlas, 11th Edition = Grant's Page #

Netter's Atlas, 3rd Edition = Netter's Plate #

Rohen Atlas, 6th Edition = Rohen Page #

BOTH MALE AND FEMALE CADAVERS

I. General Features Found in Both the Male and Female Pelvis

The pelvic cavity ("pelvis" means "basin") is the lower continuation of the abdominal cavity located inferior to the pelvic brim. The brim or **arcuate line** is formed by the crests of the pubic bones and the sharp pectineal lines (pecten pubis) which extend posteriorly to the promon-

▶
Grant's 190, 191
Netter's 340, 468
Rohen 435

▶
Grant's 187, 188,
242
Netter's 340, 341,
346, 367
Rohen 440
◀
Grant's 90, 191
Netter's 342
Rohen 435

tory of the sacrum (**ATLAS PLATES 265 #265.1**). This cavity is sometimes referred to as the **lesser, minor,** or **true pelvis** to differentiate it from the **greater** or **false pelvis,** located above the pelvic brim and simply that part of the lower abdomen between the flanged wings of the iliac bones (**ATLAS PLATES 270 #270.2, 271 #271.2**).

A. Walls and Floor of the Pelvis. The bony lateral and anterior walls of the true pelvis are formed by the two pubic bones and the lower internal surfaces of the ilium and ischium on both sides (**ATLAS PLATES 266, 267**). Posteriorly, the pelvic cavity is bounded by the sacrum and coccyx. Where walls of the bony pelvis are not complete they are covered by muscles, fascial membranes, and ligaments. Three deserve special mention: 1) anteroinferiorly, a triangular zone between the pubic rami contains the **urogenital diaphragm** or **perineal membrane** (**ATLAS PLATES 296 #296.2**); 2) anterolaterally, the obturator foramina are closed off by the **obturator membranes** and **obturator muscles** (**ATLAS PLATES 282, 287**); and 3) posteriorly, the space between the sacrum and ischium is transformed into the **greater** and **lesser sciatic foramina** by the **sacrospinous** and **sacrotuberous ligaments** (**ATLAS PLATES 271 #271.2, 272 #272.3**).

Two muscles on each side cover the inner surface of the bony pelvis. Posteriorly, the **piriformis muscle** overlies the sacrum and enters the gluteal region through the greater sciatic foramen. The **obturator internus muscle** arises from the inner surface of the anterolateral wall of the true pelvis (**Figure 18-1**). Its fibers course inferiorly and converge at the lesser sciatic foramen through which its tendon enters the gluteal region (**ATLAS PLATES 282, 314 #314.1**).

Nearly the entire floor of the pelvis is formed by the **levator ani muscles** and fascial layers that line them superiorly and inferiorly. This comprises the **pelvic diaphragm** (**ATLAS PLATES 287, 311 #311.2, 313 #313.2**). The levator ani muscle arises from the pubis anteriorly and the ischial spine posteriorly, and between these bones along a tendinous arch in the fascia covering the obturator internus muscle. The anterior part of the levator ani muscle is the **pubococcygeus,** while the part extending to the ischium is the **iliococcygeus** (**ATLAS PLATE 313 #313.2**).

The iliococcygeus inserts onto the coccyx and the midline **anococcygeal raphe,** which extends between

◄
Grant's 193–195, 372
Netter's 343, 345, 481
Rohen 343, 344, 470

◄
Grant's 193–195, 204
Netter's 343, 345
Rohen 342–344, 470

►
Grant's 186, 188, 190, 191
Netter's 240, 340, 341, 408
◄
Rohen 433, 438

◄
Grant's 193–195, 199, 259
Netter's 343–346, 361
Rohen 350, 351

the tip of the coccyx and the anus. Most of the pubococcygeus inserts on the coccyx and anococcygeal raphe, but its most anterior part swings around the rectum to form a U-shaped sling called the **puborectalis** (**ATLAS PLATE 289 #289.1**).

In continuity with the iliococcygeus posteriorly is the **coccygeus muscle.** It arises from the ischial spine and inserts posteriorly on the coccyx and sacrum (**ATLAS PLATE 313 #313.2**). At times, the coccygeus is called the **ischiococcygeus,** a term consistent with the two parts of the levator ani muscle, the pubococcygeus, and iliococcygeus.

Study the pelvis in an articulated skeleton. Refer to **Figures 18-2, 18-3,** and **ATLAS PLATES 265–273.**

1. Identify the **iliac crests** and the pelvic brim (or arcuate line). Realize that the cavity above the pelvic brim between the iliac crests constitutes the **greater** (false) **pelvis** and that the **lesser** (true) **pelvis** lies below the pelvic brim (**Figure 18-2**).

2. Identify the **iliopubic eminence, ischial tuberosities, ischial spines, sacrum,** and **coccyx.** Visualize the attachments of the **sacro-**

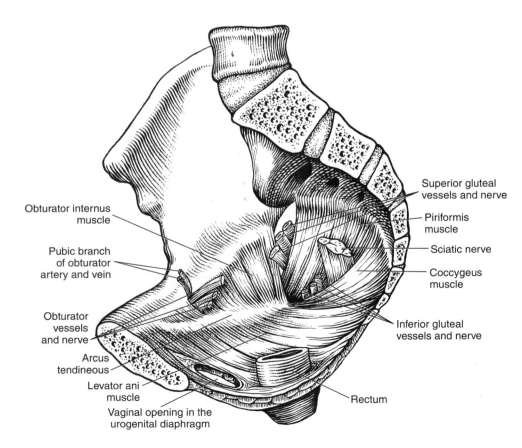

Obturator internus muscle

Pubic branch of obturator artery and vein

Obturator vessels and nerve

Arcus tendineous

Levator ani muscle

Vaginal opening in the urogenital diaphragm

Rectum

Inferior gluteal vessels and nerve

Coccygeus muscle

Sciatic nerve

Piriformis muscle

Superior gluteal vessels and nerve

Figure 18-1. Muscles that form the lateral wall of the pelvis.

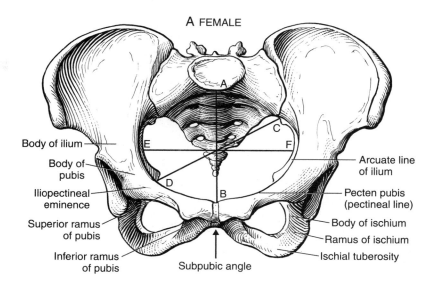

A FEMALE

Body of ilium

Body of pubis

Iliopectineal eminence

Superior ramus of pubis

Inferior ramus of pubis

Arcuate line of ilium

Pecten pubis (pectineal line)

Body of ischium

Ramus of ischium

Ischial tuberosity

Subpubic angle

Figure 18-2. The female pelvis (**A**) and the male pelvis (**B**).

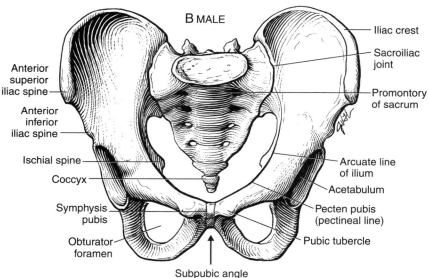

B MALE

Anterior superior iliac spine

Anterior inferior iliac spine

Ischial spine

Coccyx

Symphysis pubis

Obturator foramen

Iliac crest

Sacroiliac joint

Promontory of sacrum

Arcuate line of ilium

Acetabulum

Pecten pubis (pectineal line)

Pubic tubercle

Subpubic angle

tuberous and **sacrospinous ligaments** and define the **greater and lesser sciatic foramina** (**Figure 18-3, ATLAS PLATES 270–272**).

3. Look at **ATLAS PLATE 265** and identify the divisions of the hip bone into the **pubis, ischium,** and **ilium.** Identify the body and superior and inferior rami of the pubis and the body and ramus of the ischium (**Figure 18-2**).

4. Look for features that would help identify the gender of the pelvis being studied (**Figure 18-2**).
   (a) The female pelvis is more slender than the male.
   (b) Observe the **infrapubic angle** located below the symphysis pubis. The male angle is more acute and measures 50° to 60°, and

▶
Grant's 190, 191
Netter's 342
Rohen 434, 435

the female angle is wider, i.e., between 75° to 85°.

(c) Observe the shape of the pelvic inlet at the pelvic brim. The female superior aperture is more "transversely" oval, but the male pelvic inlet is more "heart-shaped." The greatest transverse diameter of the male pelvic inlet is located more posteriorly than in the female (compare **ATLAS PLATES 270 # 270.1, 271 #271.2**).

(d) The cavity of the lesser pelvis in the male is longer and more cone-shaped, but in the female, it is shallower and wider.

(e) Observe the greater sciatic notch. In the male, it is deep and narrow (approximately 50°); in the female, the notch is wider (approximately 75°) and less indented.

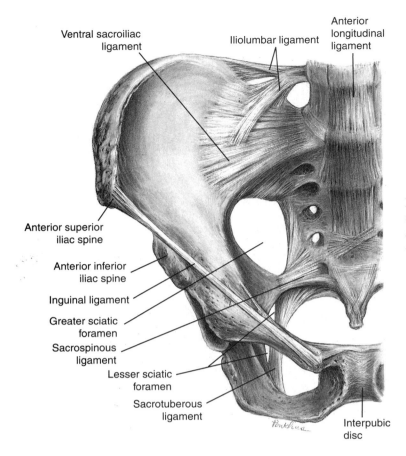

Ventral sacroiliac ligament

Iliolumbar ligament

Anterior longitudinal ligament

Anterior superior iliac spine

Anterior inferior iliac spine

Inguinal ligament

Greater sciatic foramen

Sacrospinous ligament

Lesser sciatic foramen

Sacrotuberous ligament

Interpubic disc

Figure 18-3. Ligaments of the pelvis. Note that the sacrospinous and sacrotuberous ligaments help define the greater and lesser sciatic foramina. (From Clemente CD. Gray's Anatomy. 30th U.S. Edition. Philadelphia: Lea and Febiger, 1985.)

OPTIONAL PROCEDURE

5. If time permits, measure three diameters of the pelvic inlet in both a male and female pelvis. Compare your measures with the following averages:
   (a) anteroposterior (**Figure 18-2, A and B**), or **true conjugate** (male 12.7 cm, female 13.3 cm), measured from the internal upper margin of the symphysis pubis to the sacral promontory.
   (b) oblique diameter (male 11.4 cm, female 12.1 cm) measured from the inner surface of the sacroiliac joint on one side to the iliopubic eminence on the other (**Figure 18-2, C and D**).
   (c) transverse diameter (male 12.7 cm, female 13.3 cm), which usually is the greatest width of the pelvic brim (**Figure 18-2, E and F**).

   Observe that each of these diameters is greater in the female pelvis.

B. Peritoneum Overlying the Pelvic Organs. In both males and females, the abdominal parietal peri-

▶
Grant's 197, 198, 224, 225
Netter's 347, 348, 350, 352
Rohen 336, 355

◀
Netter's 342
Rohen 434, 438

▶
Grant's 204, 205, 225
Netter's 245
Rohen 211, 293, 355

toneum is reflected over the pelvic organs. It covers the superior surface of the organs, descends between them, and produces certain fossae. The manner by which the peritoneum is arranged anteriorly over the bladder and posteriorly in front of the rectum is similar in both sexes. The peritoneal reflection between these two organs differs in males and females because of the interposition of the different pelvic genital organs (compare **ATLAS PLATES 277 #277.1** and **302 #302.1**).

MALE CADAVERS

Before dissection, visualize from above the male pelvic organs in place. Observe how the peritoneum is reflected over the pelvic viscera, thereby separating the pelvis from the abdomen (**ATLAS PLATE 302**).

Before dissecting the peritoneum below the pelvic brim in the true pelvis, identify the umbilicus on the inner surface of the anterior abdominal wall. Find the **urachus (median umbilical ligament),** covered by peritoneum, passing between the apex of the bladder in the midline to the umbilicus (**ATLAS PLATES**

204, 264). On both sides of the urachus, identify the **medial umbilical ligaments** ascending toward the umbilicus. Note that these fibrous cords, covered by peritoneum, are the continuations of the **superior vesical arteries** to the bladder and in fetal life were the **umbilical arteries.** More laterally, find the **inferior epigastric vessels** ascending to the umbilicus. Covered by peritoneum, these vessels form the **lateral umbilical ligaments.**

Identify the **ureters** descending over the pelvic brim at the bifurcation of the common iliac artery (**ATLAS PLATES 241, 243**). Note that they disappear beneath the peritoneum behind the **urinary bladder.** Find the **ductus deferens** by probing the peritoneum at both abdominal inguinal rings. Follow their course deep to the peritoneum across the external iliac vessels until they disappear behind the bladder (**ATLAS PLATE 303**).

See how the peritoneum reflects across the superior and lateral surfaces of the bladder from the anterior abdominal wall (**ATLAS PLATE 302**). Look for recesses called **paravesical fossae** between the bladder and the lateral pelvic wall. Palpate the posterior wall of the bladder and feel the rounded **seminal vesicles** beneath the peritoneum. Follow the peritoneum from the bladder to the anterior surface of the rectum across the **rectovesical fossa,** where it ascends into the greater pelvis (**ATLAS PLATE 302**). On both sides of the rectum look for the **pararectal fossae.**

Using forceps and fingers, remove the peritoneum from the surfaces of the male pelvic organs. Expose the **bladder, rectum, ureters, seminal vesicles,** and **prostate** and **ductus deferens.**

◄
Grant's 198, 204, 205, 208
Netter's 348, 350
Rohen 336, 337, 345, 354

►
Grant's 224, 225
Netter's 347, 352
Rohen 355, 356

◄
Grant's 198
Netter's 348, 350, 377
Rohen 336, 337, 344

FEMALE CADAVERS

The arrangement of peritoneum over the pelvic organs in the female is similar to that in the male except for the presence of the **uterus, ovaries, uterine tubes,** and the **broad ligaments** between the **rectum** and the **bladder** (**Figure 18-4**). The parietal peritoneum is reflected between the superior surface of the bladder and the anterior surface of the uterus as far as the vaginal fornix (**ATLAS PLATE 277**). It then continues between the uterus and the rectum, dipping downward to form a deep pouch called the **rectouterine pouch.** The peritoneum covers the rectum anteriorly and becomes continuous with the peritoneum covering the posterior abdominal wall (**Figure 18-5**). A shallow recess is formed between the anterior surface of the uterus and the posterior surface of the bladder called the **vesicouterine pouch,**

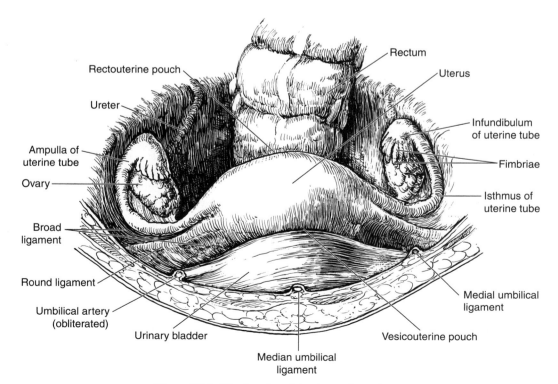

Figure 18-4. The female pelvic viscera from above.

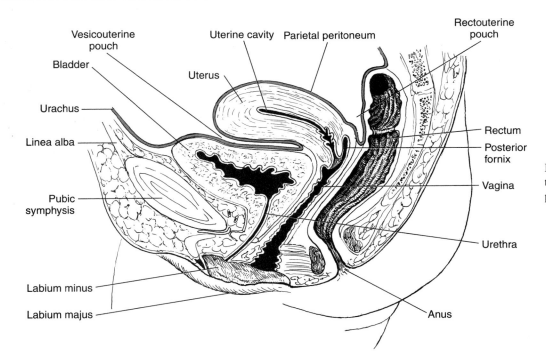

Vesicouterine pouch
Uterine cavity
Parietal peritoneum
Bladder
Uterus
Urachus
Linea alba
Pubic symphysis
Labium minus
Labium majus
Rectouterine pouch
Rectum
Posterior fornix
Vagina
Urethra
Anus

Figure 18-5. Midsagittal section of the female pelvis showing the peritoneal reflections.

somewhat emphasized by the anteverted uterus over the bladder. Realize two additional points:

1. The **posterior fornix** of the vagina comes into direct contact with the peritoneum in the depth of the rectouterine pouch (**Figure 18-5, ATLAS PLATE 274**). This "easy access" to the peritoneal cavity in women allows for the use of drains through the vagina for infections in the lower abdomen. However, vaginal injuries at the posterior fornix could lead to peritoneal infections.

2. The peritoneum covering the body and fundus of the uterus expands laterally as the **broad ligament (ATLAS PLATE 278 #278.1)**. Composed of two peritoneal layers, **anterior** and **posterior,** this ligament courses to the lateral walls of the pelvis. It divides the true pelvis into a posterior part containing the rectum and an anterior part containing the bladder. The broad ligament on each side encloses the **uterine tube** and the **ovary** and the **ovarian** and **uterine vessels.** The **mesosalpinx** and **mesovarium,** which, respectively, suspend the uterine tube and ovary, are separate parts of the broad ligament.

Follow the peritoneum from the anterior abdominal wall to the superior surface of the bladder. Identify the **median umbilical ligament** ascending to the umbilicus. Know that it contains the **urachus,** which in the fetus was a canal between the apex of the bladder and the allantois. Locate fibrous cords called the **medial umbilical ligaments,** which are

▶
Grant's 205, 209, 225
Netter's 245
Rohen 293

◀
Grant's 224
Netter's 347

◀
Grant's 224, 225, 233
Netter's 349, 356
Rohen 354, 358

▶
Grant's 224, 225
Netter's 347, 349, 351, 354
Rohen 354–357

▶
Grant's 224, 227, 228, 233
Netter's 347, 349, 354, 356
Rohen 355, 356, 359

◀
Grant's 205, 208, 225
Netter's 245
Rohen 293

covered by peritoneum, on both sides of the urachus. In fetal life, these were **umbilical arteries** and were extensions of the superior vesical arteries to the umbilicus (**ATLAS PLATES 204, 264**).

Palpate the superior surface of the bladder and, laterally, observe concave recesses called **paravesical fossae.** Elevate the uterus from its anteverted position and confirm the continuity of the peritoneum through the **vesicouterine pouch** and over the fundus of the uterus.

Palpate the depth of the **rectouterine pouch** and feel for the posterior fornix of the vagina on the anterior surface of the pouch (**Figures 18-4, 18-5, ATLAS PLATES 275, 277**). This is done by placing the index finger of your gloved left hand into the vagina as far as the posterior fornix and then palpating the deepest part of the rectouterine pouch within the pelvis with your gloved right hand. Follow the peritoneum covering the anterior surface of the rectum.

Turn your attention to the lateral margins of the uterus and to the broad ligaments. Follow their peritoneal layers to the lateral walls of the pelvis. Use **ATLAS PLATES 277, 278,** and **#279.3** for reference and do the following:

(a) Examine the upper free margin of one broad ligament and palpate the **uterine tube.**

(b) Identify the ovary attached to the **posterior layer** of the broad ligament.

(c) Trace the **mesosalpinx.** It is the broad ligament between the uterine tube and the ligament of the ovary and mesovarium (**ATLAS PLATE 279 #279.3**).

(d) Return to the ovary and feel the **ligament of the ovary,** a fibrous cord visible through the posterior layer of the broad ligament. It extends between the ovary and the upper lateral margin of the uterus just below the uterine tube (**ATLAS PLATE 278 #278.1**).

(e) Identify that part of the broad ligament from the upper lateral aspect of the ovary to the pelvic brim. This is the **suspensory ligament of the ovary** and between its peritoneal layers course the ovarian vessels (**ATLAS PLATES 277 #277.2, 278 #278.1**).

(f) Identify the **round ligament of the uterus.** This narrow flat band can be seen through the anterior peritoneal layer of the broad ligament. Note that it courses from the lateral angle of the uterus to the abdominal inguinal ring (**ATLAS PLATE 277 #277.2**).

(g) Palpate the two **rectouterine folds.** These pass from the uterine cervix posteriorly on both sides of the rectum to the posterior wall of the pelvis (**ATLAS PLATES 275 #275.1, 278 #278.1**). Forming the brim of the rectouterine pouch, they contain the fibrous **uterosacral ligaments** that attach the uterus to the sacrum.

MALE CADAVERS

II. Male Pelvic Organs: Urinary Bladder and Ureters; Seminal Vesicles and Ductus Deferens; Prostate Gland and Prostatic Urethra; Rectum (Figures 18-6, 18-7, 18-8)

The organs in the male pelvis **not found** in the female are the **seminal vesicles, ductus deferens,** and **prostate gland.** The seminal vesicles are situated on the posterior wall (base) of the bladder, and the two ductus deferens course to the posterior wall of the bladder from the abdominal inguinal rings (**ATLAS PLATE 304 #304.2**). The prostate gland surrounds the neck of the bladder and the prostatic urethra (**ATLAS PLATES 304, 305**). The rectum lies immediately posterior to the bladder, seminal vesicles, ampullae of the ductus deferens, and prostate gland, and it is separated from them

◄ Grant's 227, 233
Netter's 354, 356
Rohen 347

► Grant's 197, 204–208
Netter's 348, 350, 353, 367
Rohen 338, 339, 342

◄ Grant's 223, 227, 229
Netter's 347, 354
Rohen 355, 358, 359

► Grant's 155, 207, 208
Netter's 348, 367, 381
Rohen 326, 336, 342

◄ Grant's 225, 241
Netter's 347, 349, 351, 354
Rohen 356, 357

► Grant's 198, 215, 216
Netter's 381
Rohen 331

◄ Grant's 204, 205, 207, 208
Netter's 348, 367
Rohen 336, 337, 339, 342

► Grant's 198, 215, 216
Netter's 335, 338, 377

only by the **retrovesical pouch** (**ATLAS PLATES 302, 303**).

A. **Urinary Bladder and Ureters.** The **urinary bladder** is a hollow muscular organ that receives urine from the kidneys through the two ureters and disposes of urine through a single urethral orifice (**ATLAS PLATE 304**). Its shape and size vary with its degree of distention, but the average capacity is 500 to 550 cc (16 to 18 oz). Its triangular superior surface and two inferolateral surfaces converge anteriorly and superiorly at the **apex.** The **base** of the bladder, also triangular, is its posterior surface. The **neck** of the bladder is directed inferiorly and is fixed in males because its walls are surrounded by the prostate gland (**Figure 18-6, ATLAS PLATE 305**).

The **ureters** are narrow muscular tubes descending from the kidneys into the pelvis (**ATLAS PLATE 243**). They are 25 to 28 cm long; half of their course is abdominal and the other half pelvic. The pelvic part crosses the external iliac artery near the bifurcation of the common iliac (**ATLAS PLATE 303**). Remaining deep to the peritoneum, the ureter descends along the lateral wall of the pelvis and curves anteromedially to the base of the bladder. Near the posterior surface of the bladder, each ureter is crossed anteriorly from lateral to medial by the **ductus deferens** before it enters the bladder (**ATLAS PLATES 302 #302.1, 304 #304. 2**). The pelvic portion of the ureter receives small arteries from the internal or common iliac artery as it crosses the pelvic brim and from the inferior vesical artery near the bladder (**ATLAS PLATE 264**). The abdominal part is supplied by the renal artery.

Trace the ureters across the external iliac vessels and remove any peritoneum covering them. Expose the ductus deferens from the abdominal inguinal ring to the posterior surface of the bladder. Observe that the ureter is crossed by the ductus deferens and then trace it to its entrance into the bladder (**ATLAS PLATE 302 #302.1**). Separate the bladder from the inner surface of the anterior pelvic wall. Pass your fingers between the symphysis pubis and the bladder and remove any retropubic fat in this **retropubic space** (of Retzius).

Remove a wedge of bone **that includes the symphysis pubis** to expose better the bladder, prostate, and urethra. Initially, cut away the attachments of abdominal wall structures for 3 cm on both sides of the symphysis. Reflect the soft tissue structures from the perineal surface of the symphysis down to the inferior border of this joint. Be careful not to sever the dorsal vein of the penis. Push the penile structures downward and posteriorly and then

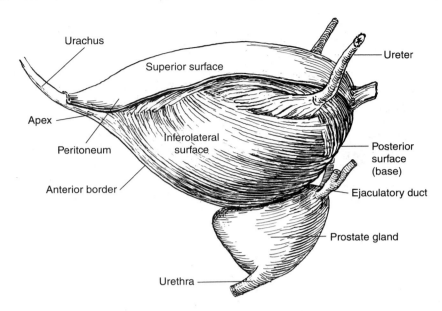

Figure 18-6. The urinary bladder and prostate gland (after Thorek).

insert a probe (just below the symphysis pubis) from outside into the pelvis. Extend the opening below the symphysis laterally. Using a handsaw, make vertical cuts on both sides through the anterior part of the bony pelvis 2 cm lateral to the symphysis pubis. As the saw approaches the subpubic region, be careful not to cut into the penis, prostate, or bladder.

With the wedge of bone removed, gently pull the lower limbs apart a few centimeters to expose the anterior pelvis more completely. Open the bladder by making a transverse cut with scissors across its superior surface 1 cm in front of the posterior wall. From each end of this transverse cut, make an additional incision downward (inferomedially) so that a triangular flap of the bladder can be pulled anteriorly. Identify the smoothened trigone on the interior of the bladder (**Figure 18-7, ATLAS PLATE 304 #304.1**). Find the orifices of the two ureters and the urethra that form the three points of the trigone. Dissect the obliterated **umbilical artery (medial umbilical ligament)** and follow it back to the **superior vesical** artery that supplies the upper part of the bladder. Also find the **inferior vesical artery** that supplies the base of the bladder and the prostate. It often arises in common with the middle rectal artery.

B. Seminal Vesicles and Ductus Deferens (Figure 18-8). The **seminal vesicles** are two sacculated tubes located on the base or posterior surface of the bladder (**ATLAS PLATES 302 #302.2, 304 #304.2**). Each coiled organ is 5 cm long and 2 cm wide, but when unfolded, measures 12 to 15 cm in length. The seminal vesicles produce an alkaline secretion that forms part of the seminal fluid; it

does not store the sperm. On each side, the ducts of the seminal vesicle and ductus deferens join to form an **ejaculatory duct,** which passes through the upper part of the prostate to open into the prostatic urethra (**Figure 18-8, ATLAS PLATES 306 #306.1, 307 #307.2**).

The thick-walled, muscular **ductus deferens** is the continuation of the epididymis (**ATLAS PLATE 194 #194.1**). It carries the sperm that mix with secretions of the seminal vesicles and prostate to form **semen.** From the scrotum, the duct enters the pelvis through the inguinal canal within the spermatic cord (**ATLAS PLATES 192, 307 #307.1**). From the abdominal inguinal ring, it crosses the inferior epigastric vessels and enters the true pelvis (**ATLAS PLATE 264**). The duct continues posteriorly and medially, crosses the

► Grant's 205–208
Netter's 367
Rohen 342

◄ Grant's 204–208
Netter's 348, 367
Rohen 336–339, 342

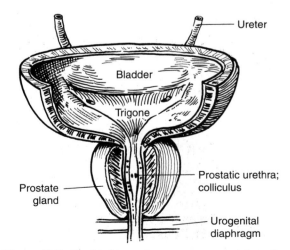

Figure 18-7. The bladder and prostate opened to show the trigone and the prostatic urethra.

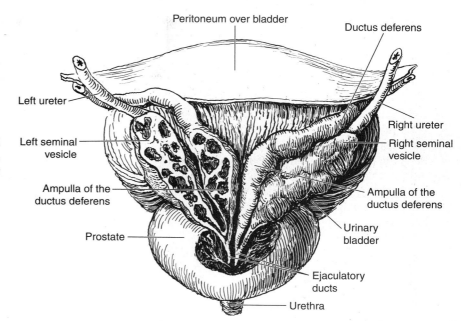

Figure 18-8. The ductus deferens and seminal vesicles on the posterior surface of the bladder. Note the formation of the ejaculatory ducts (after Grant).

obturator vessels and ureter to reach the posterior surface of the bladder (**ATLAS PLATE 303**). The ducts become dilated (ampullae), approximate each other, and each joins the duct of the seminal vesicle of that side to form an **ejaculatory duct.** In older men, the prostate often enlarges and this junction may be hidden by the prostate gland (**Figure 18-8**).

The seminal vesicle is supplied by the inferior vesicle and/or middle rectal arteries. The ductus deferens receives blood from the **deferential artery** and sometimes a branch from a vessel off the internal iliac artery (**ATLAS PLATE 303**).

◄
Grant's 215, 216
Netter's 370, 378, 381, 383
Rohen 341

◄
Grant's 205, 208, 215, 216
Netter's 348, 367
Rohen 336, 338, 339

> Clean the ductus deferens from the abdominal inguinal ring to the base of the bladder where it crosses the ureter. On the posterior bladder surface, observe the expansion of the deferens ducts to form ampullae adjacent to the seminal vesicles (**Figure 18-8**). Dissect the seminal vesicles and find their ducts inferiorly. To see the formation of the ejaculatory ducts, it may be necessary to dissect into the substance of the prostate gland.

C. Prostate Gland and Prostatic Urethra (Figures 18-6, 18-7). The **prostate gland** is an organ composed of glandular lobules encased by a fibrous and smooth-muscular stroma. It feels firm and dense when palpated and surrounds the proximal portion of the urethra (approximately 3 cm). The prostate gland consists of 15 to 20 alveolar segments each with a prostatic duct. The ducts open into the **prostatic sinus** alongside the urethral crest in the floor of the prostatic urethra (**ATLAS PLATE 306 #306.1**). The prostate is shaped like an inverted

◄
Grant's 197, 204–208, 210
Netter's 245, 253, 366–368
Rohen 336, 339, 342, 343

►
Grant's 197, 206–209
Netter's 353, 367, 368
Rohen 235–237, 343

cone with its base being the most proximal and widest part (approximately 4.5 cm) adjacent to the neck of the bladder (**Figure 18-6**). The apex of the prostate gland is its most inferior part and it lies on the superior fascia of the urogenital diaphragm (**ATLAS PLATE 305 #305.2**). The gland consists of a **median lobe** in direct contact with the trigone of the bladder, and **right** and **left lobes** interconnected by an isthmus. Its arterial supply comes from the inferior vesicle and middle rectal branches of the internal iliac artery. It is drained by a rich plexus of veins formed around the base and lateral surfaces of the gland that also receives the deep dorsal vein of the penis. The plexus flows into the internal iliac vein.

The prostatic secretion is forcefully delivered into the urethra during ejaculation by the smooth muscle of its stroma. It joins the combined secretions from the testis and seminal vesicles discharged through the ejaculatory ducts. After the age of 50 years the prostate commonly becomes enlarged (hypertrophied) and may project into the urethral end of the bladder, thereby partially blocking the flow of urine.

The prostatic urethra is oriented vertically and measures 3 cm in length (**Figure 18-7, ATLAS PLATE 306 #306.1**). Projecting from the posterior wall is a narrow ridge 3 mm high called the **urethral crest.** Along both sides of the crest are shallow longitudinal grooves called the **prostatic sinuses** that are perforated by the openings of the prostatic ducts. Midway along the urethral crest is a rounded enlargement, the **colliculus seminalis,** and on its summit is found a small (5 mm) blind pouch or cul-de-sac called the **prostatic utricle.** On both sides of the utricle are the openings of the ejaculatory ducts. The physician palpates the prostate gland and seminal vesicle by performing a digital rectal examination. These organs, anterior to the finger, are felt as firm masses 6 cm deep to the anal opening.

Note how the bladder and prostate gland in the pelvis are firmly attached to the pelvic floor (**ATLAS PLATE 305**). Clean the fascia around the prostate and seminal vesicles and expose the **lateral** and **medial puboprostatic ligaments.** Follow these bands of thickened endopelvic fascia as one extends anteriorly and the other laterally from the neck of the bladder to the posterior pubis (**ATLAS PLATE 302 #302.1**). The medial puboprostatic ligaments can be seen only if the wedge of bone was **not** removed. Palpate the **pubococcygeus part** of the **levator ani muscles** located lateral and posterior to the prostate, and note that the gland lies directly superior to the urogenital diaphragm (**ATLAS PLATE 305 #305.2**).

Cut longitudinally through the prostate gland along the midline to the **prostatic urethra.** Open the prostatic urethra and examine its posterior wall (**ATLAS PLATE 306 #306.1**). Identify the **urethral crest, colliculus, prostatic utricle,** and lateral to the crest, the **prostatic sinuses.** Probe the blind pouch of the utricle and find the **openings of the ejaculatory ducts** on each side of the utricle. Observe the minute **openings of the prostatic ducts** in the floor of the prostatic sinuses.

D. Rectum (From Within the Pelvis). The rectum is the continuation of the sigmoid colon; it begins anterior to the sacrum. It is approximately 12 cm (5 inches) long and, regardless of its name, the rectum does not follow a straight course but, more or less, an S-shaped curve (**ATLAS PLATE 239, 305 #305.2**). The upper two-thirds of the rectum is covered laterally and anteriorly by peritoneum. In males, the rectum and bladder come into contact when either organ is full, thus reducing the size of the rectovesical pouch. The pelvic rectum is supplied by the middle rectal branch of the inferior vesical or internal iliac artery (**ATLAS PLATE 310**). The superior rectal vein drains into the inferior mesenteric vein and the portal circulation, and the middle rectal vein drains into the caval circulation through the internal iliac vein (**ATLAS PLATE 311 #311.1**).

Trace the course of the inferior mesenteric artery and confirm that the continuation of the main vessel itself becomes the **superior rectal artery** (**Figure 18-9, ATLAS PLATES 243, 310**). Remove the peritoneum from the rectum, but do not destroy the middle rectal arteries, which may arise from the

◄ Grant's 197, 206, 249
Netter's 353
Rohen 342

◄ Grant's 209
Netter's 353, 367
Rohen 338

◄ Grant's 196–199, 201, 202, 206, 207, 210
Netter's 374, 375, 377–379
Rohen 343, 345

► Grant's 224, 225, 232
Netter's 247, 249, 354
Rohen 355, 357

◄ Grant's 138, 201, 203
Netter's 296, 301, 378, 379
Rohen 302, 308

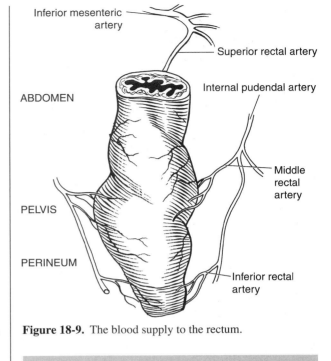

Figure 18-9. The blood supply to the rectum.

internal iliac, inferior vesical, or internal pudendal artery.

OPTIONAL PROCEDURE

Perform a digital examination of the rectum. Place a gloved index finger of one hand into the anal canal and simultaneously with the other hand feel the prostate gland and seminal vesicles inside the pelvis.

FEMALE CADAVERS

III. Female Pelvic Organs: Urinary Bladder, Ureters, and Urethra; Ovaries and Uterine Tubes; Uterus and Vagina; Rectum

Between the urinary bladder and rectum in the female pelvis are located the ovaries, uterine tubes, uterus, and vagina, and their peritoneal and fibrous ligaments (**ATLAS PLATES 274, 276–278**). Similar to males, in females the ureters course from the posterior abdominal wall to the bladder. Before entering the bladder, however, **the female ureter is crossed by the uterine artery, whereas the male ureter is crossed by the ductus deferens.**

A. Urinary Bladder, Ureters, and Urethra. The female **urinary bladder** is a hollow muscular organ and its shape, position, and size are similar to that seen in the male. The attachments at its neck and base, however, and its relationships to organs posteriorly are not the same. In the male the neck of the bladder is fixed by lateral ligaments attached to a rather immobile prostate. The neck of the female bladder is more loosely attached to the cervix of the uterus and the anterior fornix of the vagina, and is more mobile. The base of the female bladder is directed posteriorly, adjacent to the anterior vaginal wall (**ATLAS PLATE 274**), whereas it lies adjacent to the rectum in the male. The internal anatomy of the female bladder is similar to that in the male, the smooth trigone being bounded by the urethral and two ureteric openings.

The abdominal course of the ureters is similar in both sexes, but the relationship of the ureters along their pelvic course is different. On crossing the internal iliac artery and vein deep to the peritoneum, the ureter in the female lies initially behind the ovary. As it passes forward and medially toward the bladder, **it courses deep to the broad ligament and the uterine artery crosses it. Thus, as the ureter approaches the bladder, it passes below or inferior to the uterine artery** (**ATLAS PLATES 274, 275, 281**).

The female urethra measures slightly less than 4 cm in length and 6 mm in diameter and commences at the internal urethral opening of the bladder. It courses inferiorly along the anterior wall of the vagina (**ATLAS PLATE 274**) and then through the urogenital diaphragm just inferior to the symphysis pubis. The urethra opens anterior to the vagina, 2.5 cm posterior to the glans clitoris (**ATLAS PLATES 290, 291**). The anterior and posterior walls of the urethra are in apposition except during urination. When the **detrusor muscle** of the bladder wall contracts, the **sphincter urethrae** relaxes, resulting in the passing of urine.

Remove the peritoneum from the pelvic wall to expose the bladder and rectum. Identify and trace the ureters over the pelvic brim (**ATLAS PLATES 281, 285 #285.1**). Follow their course behind the ovary, to the pelvic floor and then anteromedially below the broad ligament. At this site the ureters lie adjacent to the lateral fornices of the vagina. Note that before entering the bladder, **the ureters are crossed superiorly from lateral to medial by the uterine arteries.**

Remove the peritoneum from the urinary bladder and separate the organ from the symphysis pubis. Identify the **urachus,** a fibrous cord that extends from the apex of the bladder to the umbilicus deep to the peritoneum. This is the postnatal remnant of the allantoic duct. Manually explore the fascial plane between the symphysis pubis and bladder, which is called the **retropubic space.**

◄
Grant's 224, 228, 241
Netter's 347, 349, 352, 353
Rohen 354, 357

◄
Grant's 232, 241
Netter's 354, 380, 382, 384
Rohen 356

►
Grant's 228
Netter's 352, 353
Rohen 354

◄
Grant's 224
Netter's 347, 351
Rohen 354, 355, 357

◄
Grant's 225, 228
Netter's 354, 380, 382, 384
Rohen 356

►
Grant's 225, 227, 233
Netter's 354, 356
Rohen 355, 358, 359

◄
Grant's 225
Netter's 245, 349

To expose the bladder, urethra, and urogenital diaphragm, remove a wedge of bone containing the symphysis pubis as described in the section on the male. Clean the soft tissues from the symphysis pubis by severing the attachments of abdominal wall muscles for 3 cm lateral to the symphysis. Carefully reflect the tissues on the anterior aspect of the symphysis down to the inferior margin of the joint. **Do not damage the clitoris or its dorsal vein.** Push the genitalia downward and insert a probe below the symphysis pubis into the pelvis from outside. Extend this opening laterally on both sides below the symphysis. Using a handsaw, make two cuts vertically through the anterior part of the pelvic wall 2 cm on each side of the symphysis pubis. As the saw approaches the subpubic region, be careful not to cut the clitoris externally or the bladder internally. Remove the wedge of bone containing the symphysis and pull the lower limbs apart gently to open the pelvis further.

Open the bladder by making a transverse cut across its superior surface. From the ends of this transverse cut make two additional cuts downward (inferomedially) so that a triangular flap of the bladder wall can be pulled forward. Within the bladder identify a smoothened triangular area, the **trigone,** located above and posterior to the urethral orifice. Find the openings of the two ureters that complete the three points of the trigone.

Open the urethra distally by cutting its anterior wall longitudinally from the urethral opening at the bladder. Note that its walls are distensible and that the posterior urethral wall blends with the anterior wall of the vagina.

B. Ovaries and Uterine Tubes. The ovaries are located one on each side of the female pelvis lateral to the uterus (**ATLAS PLATES 277 #277.2, 278**). They are flattened organs (2.5 cm long) attached to the posterior aspect of the broad ligament by a short fold of peritoneum, the **mesovarium.** The rounded medial surface of the ovary is adjacent to the fimbriated end of the uterine tube. Its upper or **tubal pole** is attached to the pelvic brim by the **suspensory ligament of the ovary,** which contains the **ovarian artery and vein.** Its lower or **uterine pole** is attached to the uterus by a fibrous cord called the **ligament of the ovary (ATLAS PLATES 275 #275.1, 277–279).**

The **uterine tubes** transmit ova from the ovaries to the internal wall of the uterus. Each tube is 10 cm long and their medial ends are attached to the superior angles of the uterus. Passing horizontally across the pelvis along the superior border of the broad ligament, the fimbriated end of the uterine tube, called **the infundibulum,** communicates with the abdominal cavity (**ATLAS PLATES 277, 278**). Normally, however, the fimbria are closely applied to the ovary in order to catch each ovum as it ruptures from the Graafian follicle.

> Identify the ovaries and confirm their attachment to the posterior surface of the broad ligament. Find the ovarian vessels, follow them to the pelvic brim, and note that they are surrounded by a fold of peritoneum which forms the **suspensory ligament of the ovary** (**ATLAS PLATES 277 #277.2, 278 #278.1**). Expose the ovarian vessels and trace them to the ovary and the upper part of the uterine tube (**ATLAS PLATE 280**). Do not sever the ureters that cross the pelvic brim adjacent to these vessels.
>
> Expose the **ligament of the ovary** (ovarian ligament), which is a fibrous cord between the two layers of the broad ligament. Note that it courses from the inferomedial aspect of the ovary to the wall of the uterus (**ATLAS PLATE 277 #277.2**).
>
> Clean the **uterine tube** along the upper free margin of the broad ligament and note that its fimbriated end, the **infundibulum,** is funnel-shaped and located near the ovary. With a fine pair of scissors open one uterine tube from its fimbriated end to its uterine attachment and note its mucosal folds (**ATLAS PLATE 279 #279.3**).

C. Uterus, Uterine Ligaments, and Vagina. The **uterus** is a thick-walled muscular organ interposed between the bladder and rectum in the female pelvis (**ATLAS PLATE 277 #277.2**). Its muscular wall is continuous below with the **vagina,** and the uterine tubes open into its upper lateral angles (**ATLAS PLATE 279 #279.1**). The nonpregnant uterus is pear-shaped and is 8 cm long, 5 cm wide, and 2.5 cm thick. The rounded part of the uterus is called the **fundus.** Below this is the **body of the uterus,** which tapers downward to the **cervix** (**ATLAS PLATE 279**). Projecting into the vagina, the cervix is surrounded by the innermost part of the vagina to form the vaginal fornix (**ATLAS PLATES 274, 279 #279.1**).

The upper part of the uterus is attached to the lateral pelvic walls by the broad ligaments (**ATLAS PLATE 277 #277.2**), while the cervix is held firm posteriorly by the **uterosacral ligaments** (**ATLAS PLATE 289 #289.2**) and laterally by the **transverse cervical ligaments** (cardinal ligaments of **Mackenrodt**). Additionally, the **round ligaments** are narrow, flat bands that attach to the uterus just below the uterine tubes and course laterally and anteriorly to enter the inguinal canal at the deep inguinal ring (**ATLAS PLATE 277 #277.2**).

► Grant's 227, 230, 233
Netter's 347, 352, 355
Rohen 355, 357–359

◄ Grant's 225, 227, 229, 233
Netter's 349, 354, 356, 380
Rohen 358, 359

► Grant's 228, 229, 232, 233
Netter's 351, 354, 358, 380
Rohen 356, 360, 361

► Grant's 224, 225, 228, 232, 233
Netter's 347, 352, 354
Rohen 354–360

◄ Grant's 224, 225
Netter's 347, 349
Rohen 354–357

► Grant's 227, 233
Netter's 356
Rohen 358–360

◄ Grant's 241
Netter's 351, 354, 356, 357

► Grant's 224
Netter's 347, 352, 373
Rohen 355, 357

The **vagina** is a fibromuscular organ that extends upward and backward from its opening between the labia minora to the cervix of the uterus, which it surrounds to form a groove, the **vaginal fornix** (**ATLAS PLATE 274**). The vagina measures 7.5 cm in length but is highly distensible. The vaginal wall contains smooth muscle, connective tissue, and many elastic fibers and normally its anterior and posterior surfaces are in contact. The anterior vaginal wall is adjacent to the posterior surface of the bladder, whereas the posterior vaginal wall is separated from the rectum by the rectouterine pouch superiorly and by fascia inferiorly (**ATLAS PLATE 274**).

The uterus is supplied by the two uterine arteries from the internal iliac arteries. Each uterine artery passes along the pelvic wall to the lateral side of the cervix (**Figure 18-10**) where it crosses (from lateral to medial) superior to the ureter to enter the uterus. The uterine arteries anastomose with the ovarian arteries superiorly and the vaginal arteries inferiorly (**ATLAS PLATE 280**).

> Place the index finger of your gloved hand into the vagina and palpate within the pelvis with your other hand. Feel the bladder anterior to the vagina. Palpate the cervix of the uterus and, within the pelvis, the body of the uterus. Dissect the uterine arteries at the lateral border of the cervix by probing through the posterior layer of the broad ligament (**ATLAS PLATES 280, 281**). Note the relationship of the vessels to the ureters and trace the arteries along the lateral uterine borders toward the ovary and the vagina (**Figure 18-10**).
>
> Identify the **round ligaments** and follow them to the deep inguinal ring. Cut the attachments of the broad ligaments along the lateral surfaces of the uterus, but do not sever the uterine arteries, ureters, ovarian vessels, or round ligaments.
>
> Open the cavity of the uterus by cutting across the top of the uterus through the wall of the fundus between the attachments of the two uterine tubes (**Figure 18-11**). Continue this incision downward along the two lateral borders of the uterus (anterior to the uterine arteries) through the cervix and into the vagina. This will divide the uterus into anterior and posterior parts.
>
> Probe the uterine cavity and identify the **external ostium** of the cervix into the vagina; the **cervical canal; isthmus; cavity of the uterine body;** and **openings of the uterine tubes** (**ATLAS PLATE 279 #279.3**).

D. Female Rectum. The female rectum is similar to the male rectum. The principal difference is that the anterior rectal wall in females is directly posterior to

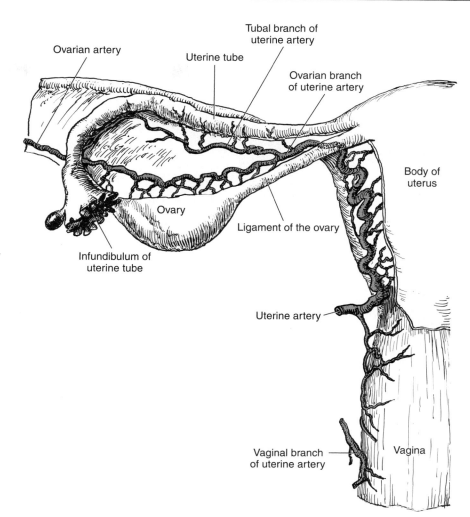

Figure 18-10. The uterine artery and its anastomoses above with the ovarian artery and below with the vaginal artery.

the vaginal fornix, cervix, and vagina, whereas in the male it lies behind the bladder, seminal vesicles, and prostate gland (**ATLAS PLATE 274**).

Read the section on the rectum in the male pelvis. Trace the inferior mesenteric artery over the pelvic brim where it becomes the **superior rectal artery** (**Figure 18-9, ATLAS PLATES 281, 310**). Strip the peritoneum from the rectum, being careful to preserve the delicate middle rectal arteries which arise from the internal iliac or one of its branches (**ATLAS PLATES 281, 285 #285.1**).

◄
Grant's 199, 201
Netter's 296, 327,
375, 380
Rohen 361, 410

OPTIONAL PROCEDURE

Perform a rectal examination of the female pelvic organs. Place the gloved index finger of one hand through the anus and feel the muscular external anal sphincter upon penetrating the anus (**ATLAS PLATE 308**). Palpate anteriorly the posterior wall of the vagina and the cervix of the uterus (**ATLAS**

PLATE 274). Place your other hand in the rectouterine pouch within the pelvis. Realize how closely approximated are the anterior wall of the rectum, the peritoneal cavity, and the posterior fornix of the vagina (**ATLAS PLATE 274**).

BOTH MALE AND FEMALE CADAVERS

IV. Lateral Pelvic Wall and Floor: Vessels, Nerves, and Muscles

Overlying the muscular floor and lateral pelvic wall are the **internal iliac vessels** and their branches. Located posterolaterally are the anterior primary rami of the five sacral nerves forming the **sacral plexus,** the **lumbosacral trunk** superiorly and the **coccygeal nerve** inferiorly.

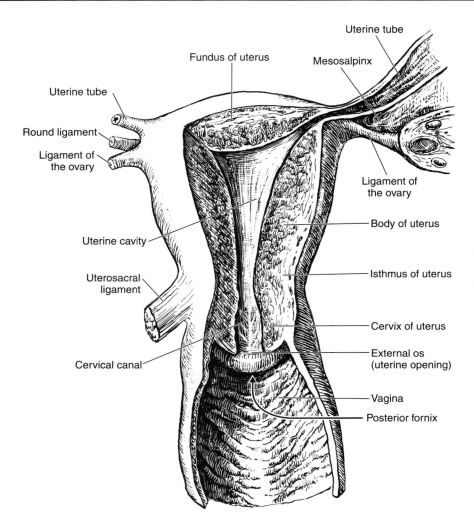

Uterine tube

Fundus of uterus   Mesosalpinx

Uterine tube

Round ligament

Ligament of
the ovary

Ligament of
the ovary

Body of uterus

Uterine cavity

Isthmus of uterus

Uterosacral
ligament

Cervix of uterus

External os
(uterine opening)

Cervical canal

Vagina

Posterior fornix

Figure 18-11. The uterus and vagina
opened to show the uterine cavity and its
tubal and vaginal orifices.

A. Pelvic Vessels. The internal iliac artery arises at the bifurcation of the common iliac and descends into the pelvis to supply its walls and viscera (**ATLAS PLATE 282**). Three other arteries branch directly from the aorta. These are the **superior rectal artery,** which is the continuation of the inferior mesenteric to the upper rectum; the **ovarian artery;** and the **median sacral artery,** which descends in the midline, anterior to the sacrum (**ATLAS PLATE 282**).

The internal iliac artery courses inferiorly for approximately 4 cm where it usually divides into a **posterior trunk** and an **anterior trunk** (**ATLAS PLATES 282, 283**). The **posterior trunk of the internal iliac artery** gives rise to parietal branches that supply the pelvic walls:

1. **Iliolumbar artery,** which courses laterally to the iliac fossa and superiorly, posterior to the psoas major (**ATLAS PLATES 253, 283**).
2. Two **lateral sacral arteries** that descend on the sacrum, sending branches into sacral foramina (**ATLAS PLATE 282**).

◄
Grant's 201, 202,
215, 216, 234
Netter's 378, 380,
382, 383
Rohen 344–346,
360

3. **Superior gluteal artery** that courses through the greater sciatic foramen above the piriformis muscle (**Figure 18-12, ATLAS PLATES 282, 283**).

The **anterior trunk of the internal iliac artery** gives rise to three parietal branches that leave the pelvis and at least four (and sometimes five) visceral branches (**Figure 18-12**).

The **parietal branches** from the anterior trunk are as follows:

1. **Inferior gluteal artery,** which leaves the pelvis through the greater sciatic foramen below the piriformis muscle (**ATLAS PLATES 282, 283**).
2. **Obturator artery** that courses with the obturator nerve along the lateral pelvic wall to the obturator foramen and enters the adductor compartment of the thigh (**ATLAS PLATE 285 #285.1**). In 25% of cases, the obturator artery arises from the inferior epigastric artery and passes around the femoral ring to reach the obturator foramen (**ATLAS PLATE 283 #283.2**).

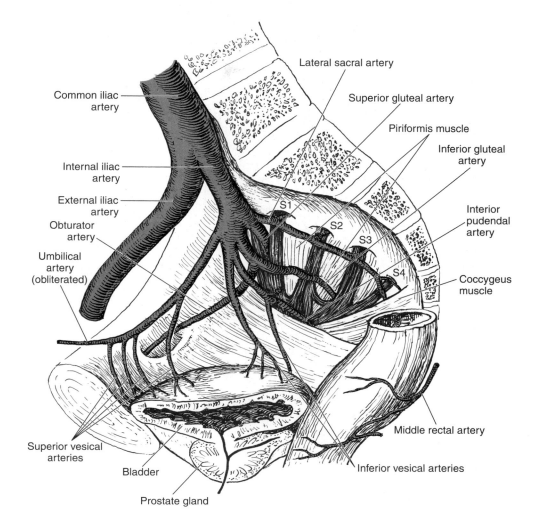

Figure 18-12. The branches of the internal iliac artery and the sacral nerves on the lateral surface of the pelvis.

Surgeons must be aware of this variation during repairs of hernias.

3. **Internal pudendal artery,** which often is one of the terminal branches of the anterior trunk. It leaves the pelvis through the greater sciatic foramen below the piriformis (**ATLAS PLATES 282, 283**).

The **visceral branches** from the anterior trunk are directed medially and supply the pelvic organs (**Figure 18-12**). These include the following:

4. **Superior vesical artery,** which sends branches to the bladder, ductus deferens, and ureters (**ATLAS PLATE 283**).

5. **Inferior vesical artery,** which often arises with the middle rectal artery. It supplies the inferior part of the bladder, the prostate, and seminal vesicles.

6. **Middle rectal artery,** which may arise directly from the anterior trunk. More frequently, it arises from the inferior vesical or internal pudendal artery and helps supply the lower rectum.

◄
Grant's 201, 215, 216, 234
Netter's 378–380, 382–384
Rohen 344, 345, 360

7. **Uterine artery,** which descends from the internal iliac and courses medially, crossing the ureter 1 cm lateral to the uterine cervix (**ATLAS PLATE 281**).

8. **Vaginal artery,** which may arise directly from the anterior trunk, but more frequently is a branch of the uterine artery (**Figure 18-10, ATLAS PLATE 280 #280.1**).

Pull the bladder, rectum, and uterus away from the lateral pelvic wall and follow the **common iliac artery** to its bifurcation into **external** and **internal iliac arteries.** Cut away the internal iliac vein and its tributaries to expose the arteries better. Observe the division of the internal iliac artery into posterior and anterior trunks in your cadaver and expect variation from textbook descriptions. Use **Figure 18-12** and **ATLAS PLATES 282 and 283** as guides to identify branches of the internal iliac artery.

Find the **iliolumbar artery** arising from the posterior side of the internal iliac. It is the only artery that ascends out of the true pelvis and sends branches to the iliac fossa (**ATLAS PLATES 282, 283**). Find the **lateral sacral arteries** (often two) descending medially anterior to the sacrum.

The **superior gluteal, inferior gluteal,** and **internal pudendal arteries** can be identified because they arise from above-downward in that order and all leave the pelvis through the greater sciatic foramen. To identify them find the piriformis muscle and follow the superior gluteal through the foramen above the muscle, while the inferior gluteal and internal pudendal arteries leave the pelvis inferior to the muscle.

Find the **obturator artery** accompanied by the **obturator nerve** passing forward to the obturator foramen along the lateral wall of the pelvis. Look for its anastomosis with the pubic branch of the inferior epigastric artery (**ATLAS PLATES 279, 282**).

Identify the **medial umbilical ligaments** on the inner surface of the anterior abdominal wall ascending to the umbilicus lateral to the urachus. These are the fibrosed remnants of the **umbilical arteries** in the fetus (**ATLAS PLATE 264**). Note that at the level of the bladder this vessel gives rise to two or more small **superior vesical arteries.**

In **male cadavers,** locate the **inferior vesical** and **middle rectal arteries.** These may arise from a common stem and course medially in the fatty tissue just above the pelvic floor (**ATLAS PLATE 283**).

In **female cadavers,** identify the **uterine arteries** and find their **vaginal branch.** Find the **middle rectal artery** in the female pelvis, and note that the vaginal vessels may help supply the rectum.

B. Pelvic Nerves. The nerves found in the true pelvis are derived from the lumbosacral trunk (L4, L5 nerves), the five sacral nerves, and one coccygeal nerve (**ATLAS PLATE 255**). Additionally, the obturator nerve descends to the obturator foramen. The upper four sacral nerves emerge from the spinal column by way of the pelvic sacral foramina (**Figure 18-12**). The small fifth sacral perforates the coccygeus muscle between the sacrum and coccyx and the coccygeal nerve emerges inferior to the transverse process of the coccyx.

The nerve cords of the **sacral plexus** converge over the surface of the piriformis muscle (**Figure 18-12**) near the greater sciatic foramen in the form of two flattened bands. The larger upper band continues through the greater sciatic foramen as the **sciatic nerve** and the lower band leaves the pelvis through the same foramen as the **pudendal nerve.** The sciatic nerve is formed by

the lumbosacral trunk (L4, L5) plus S1, S2, and most of the S3 nerve, whereas the pudendal nerve gets a small part of S2, and larger contributions from S3 and S4 (**Figure 18-13**). The sacral plexus also gives rise to nerves that will be studied when the gluteal and posterior thigh regions are dissected.

The **sacrococcygeal plexus** consists of nerve loops derived from a branch of S4, all of S5 and the coccygeal nerve. From this plexus come nerves that supply the levator ani, coccygeus, and the external anal sphincter muscles.

The sympathetic nerves in the pelvis consist of extensions of the ganglionated sympathetic trunks located anterior to the sacrum and medial to the anterior sacral foramina (**ATLAS PLATE 255**). Four sacral ganglia usually give gray rami to the sacral nerves. Also, the **superior hypogastric plexus** of autonomic fibers (**ATLAS PLATE 242**), located anterior to the bifurcation of the abdominal aorta, descends into the pelvis and divides into right and left **inferior hypogastric plexuses.** These plexuses contain sympathetic fibers and ganglion cells and parasympathetic fibers from the **pelvic splanchnic nerves** (S2, S3, and S4) to innervate the lower gastrointestinal tract. From the inferior hypogastric plexus, collections of autonomic fibers form plexuses to supply the pelvic viscera.

Identify the piriformis muscle on the ventral surface of the sacrum and remove the fascia and fat from the anterior sacral region. Find the **lumbosacral trunk** as it crosses the pelvic brim to join the upper three sacral roots to form the **sciatic nerve** anterior to the piriformis muscle (**ATLAS PLATES 255, 282**).

Note that the superior gluteal artery courses posteriorly to the greater sciatic foramen between the lumbosacral trunk and the 1st sacral root (**Figure 18-12, ATLAS PLATE 282**) or between the 1st and 2nd sacral roots. Observe that the inferior gluteal artery courses through the same foramen between sacral roots one segment below those separated by the superior gluteal artery.

Find the **pudendal nerve** and note its origin from the ventral rami of S2, S3, and S4. Follow this nerve to the greater sciatic foramen through which it also leaves the pelvis (**ATLAS PLATE 282**).

Identify the **obturator nerve** coursing anteriorly and inferiorly along the obturator internus muscle with the obturator vessels. Note that it leaves the pelvis through the obturator foramen to enter the adductor compartment of the thigh (**ATLAS PLATE 377**).

Find the pelvic extensions of the **sympathetic trunks** adjacent to the anterior sacral foramina

◄
Grant's 215, 216, 234
Netter's 382, 383
Rohen 345

►
Grant's 168, 201, 219, 221
Netter's 330, 389, 390, 392, 394–397
Rohen 334, 335, 365

◄
Grant's 212
Netter's 382, 383
Rohen 345, 356

►
Grant's 164, 165, 168, 220
Netter's 479, 481
Rohen 470, 472

►
Grant's 192, 220, 222
Netter's 479–481, 484, 485
Rohen 470, 472

►
Grant's 192, 221, 222
Netter's 380, 390, 479–481, 521
Rohen 466, 472

◄
Grant's 220, 222
Netter's 479, 481
Rohen 470, 472

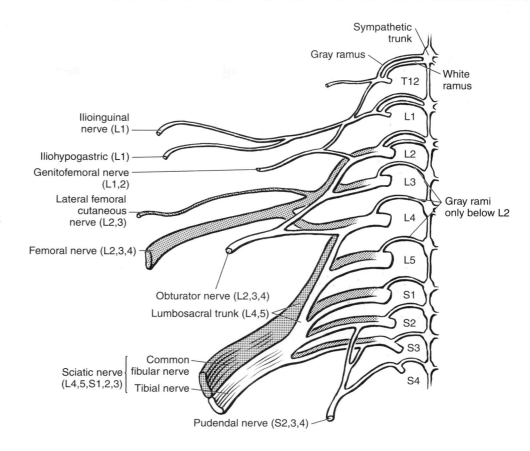

Figure 18-13. The lumbar and sacral plexuses.

(ATLAS PLATES 255, 256). Identify the autonomic nerves that comprise the **superior hypogastric plexus** anterior to the aortic bifurcation (**ATLAS PLATE 242**). Follow this plexus into the pelvis where it divides to form right and left **inferior hypogastric plexuses** that innervate the pelvic organs (**ATLAS PLATE 313, #313.1**).

◄
Grant's 168, 201, 202, 236, 239
Netter's 330, 389, 390, 392
Rohen 334, 335, 345

C. **Muscles of the Walls of the Pelvic Cavity.** The muscles that form the floor and walls of the pelvis include the piriformis, obturator internus, levator ani, and coccygeus muscles. These were all described in Section IA of this dissection.

To study the floor and walls of the pelvis, remove the pelvic viscera as follows:

1. Free the rectum of its peritoneal attachments and separate it from the anterior sacrum. In **males** separate the rectum from the bladder, seminal vesicles, and prostate, and in **females** from the vagina. Tie two ligatures tightly (3 cm apart) around the most distal part of the rectum (just above the pelvic floor). Sever the organ between the two ligatures.

►
Grant's 192, 194, 195, 220
Netter's 344–346
Rohen 342, 343, 345, 470

2. **IN MALE CADAVERS,** remove the bladder and prostate by cutting through the urethra distal to the prostate.

3. **IN FEMALE CADAVERS,** cut through the neck of the bladder, urethra, and vagina just superior to the urogenital diaphragm and remove these organs. Also remove the uterus, uterine tubes, and ovaries.

Define the **piriformis muscle** stretching from the anterior aspect of the sacrum to the greater sciatic foramen (**ATLAS PLATES 282, 283**). Find the **coccygeus muscle** located anterior to the piriformis.

Remove the fascia overlying the **levator ani muscle** and note that it consists of two parts, the **iliococcygeus** posteriorly and the **pubococcygeus** anteriorly. Observe how their fibers arise from the ischial spine and the pubis, and between these two bony sites along a **tendinous arch** in the fascia over the obturator internus (**ATLAS PLATE 289 #289.1**). Follow the muscle to its insertion on the coccyx and into the midline anococcygeal raphé. Note that the most anterior part of the pubococcygeus forms a U-shaped sling around the posterior surface of the rectum called the **puborectalis muscle.**

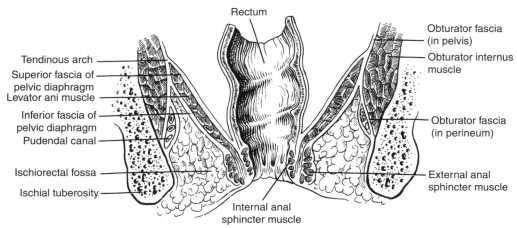

Figure 18-14. Frontal section through the pelvis and perineum.

Realize that the levator ani muscle separates the pelvis from the perineum. Note also that the upper part of the obturator internus is in the pelvis and the lower part in the perineum (**Figure 18-14, ATLAS PLATE 313 #313.1**).

Clinical Relevance (Both male and female)

Bony pelvis. The bony pelvis is shaped similar to a basin with walls and a floor. It is lined on its inner surface by muscles, and its floor is formed by the levator ani muscles. Openings in the posterior wall of the pelvis are bound by ligaments, and these openings transmit important structures to and from the gluteal region. One opening, the greater sciatic foramen, transmits the sciatic nerve that descends to the lower limb, the pudendal vessels and nerves, and the gluteal vessels and nerves to the buttocks. The lesser sciatic foramen then transmits the pudendal vessels and nerves to the perineum.

Fractures of the pelvis. There are several types of pelvic fractures. One can result from a heavy fall on the upper lateral hip region where the head of the femur can fracture the bones of the acetabulum. Fractures of the rami of the pubis can occur from a crush accident or when a heavy object falls on a person who is reclined. Fractures of the inferior bony ring (pubic rami, ischium, acetabulum, ilium, or sacrum) often involve more than one break or are combined with joint dislocation. At times fractures of the pubis also involve injury to the urinary bladder or urethra.

Fractures of the sacrum or coccyx. After fractures of the sacrum, fibrosis can occur around the sacral nerve roots, resulting in persistent pain. These fractures often require bed rest followed by the use of crutches.

Constriction of the ureter. The lumen of the ureter has three sites where it may be constricted: a) where the renal pelvis joins the ureter; b) where the ureter crosses the pelvic brim; and c) where the ureter courses through the bladder wall to gain access to the interior of the bladder. Kidney stones may cause obstruction at any of these sites.

Cancer of the colon or rectum. This is a common and often fatal disease. Tumors of the colon generally develop from nonmalignant polyps that then change and become malignant. Important features with respect to prognosis relate to the severity of the disruption of the wall of the colon, the degree of penetration of the tumor, and the possible metastases that may have spread by way of the lymphatics.

Rupture of the bladder. Because the bladder extends superiorly into the lower abdomen, it is subject to injury as a result of an automobile accident that causes fractures of the pelvis. When the bladder is ruptured anteriorly, urine can pass into the peritoneal cavity. If the bladder is ruptured posteriorly, urine passes into the pelvis and perineum.

Sigmoidoscopy. Examination of the sigmoid colon is achieved by this procedure using a sigmoidoscope that is placed through the anus and elevated to the sigmoid colon. The instrument is a flexible tube that is fitted with illumination and lenses. It can also be used to obtain a biopsy of the mucosal wall.

Bladder cancer. Cancer of the bladder is usually found in older patients. It can be small and superficial and be readily treated, or it can be more advanced and have spread outside the bladder saved. More advanced cancers might have invaded the ureter, resulting in the obstruction and consequent retrograde urination retention damage to the kidneys.

Male Pelvis
Clinical Relevance

Pelvic fractures in males. These fractures can result in injury to other pelvic organs such as the urethra as it traverses the urogenital diaphragm. The bladder, located retropubically, can be punctured by bone fragments. Additionally, blood vessels such as tributaries to the internal iliac vein, or pelvic nerves such as the pelvic splanchnic nerves, can be injured by pelvic fractures. These nerves carry important preganglionic parasympathetic nerve fibers that will synapse and then supply male pelvic organs.

Cancer of the prostate. This condition can be suspected after a routine anal digital examination in which the posterior surface of the prostate feels uneven or irregular and the organ has hardened to the touch. During defecation or during sneezing or coughing, increased pelvic pressure releases metastatic cells to other organs such as the vertebral column and the spinal cord and brain.

Transurethral resection of the prostate. This operation is performed by passing an endoscope through the penile urethra to the prostatic urethra, where a portion of the prostate or the entire prostate is resected.

Benign prostate enlargement. Hypertrophy of the prostate often is benign and common in men over 50 years of age. Its principal symptoms are difficulty in the commencement of urination and an increased frequency of urination during the night. Difficulty in commencement of urination is caused by the compression of the enlarged prostate on the urogenital urethra, and frequency in the urge to urinate usually results in only a few milliliters of urine expressed.

Female Pelvis
Clinical Relevance

Pelvic measurements. Measurements of the true or lesser pelvis are especially important in obstetrics when a transvaginal birth is being considered. These measurements include the true or obstetric conjugate (distal tip of the sacral promontory to the inferior margin on the posterior surface of the symphysis pubis), the diagonal conjugate (the distance from the posterior surface of the symphysis pubis to the sacral promontory), and the interspinous distance (the distance between the two ischial spines), which must be wide enough for passage of the baby's head.

Caudal anesthesia. In this technique the anesthetic agent is introduced into the sacral canal from below. This anesthetizes the 2nd to the 5th sacral nerves. Used in obstetrics, this technique blocks pain in the pelvis and perineum.

Prolapse of the uterus. This is a displacement of the uterine cervix into the vaginal canal. Support for the uterus within the pelvis is maintained by the levator ani muscles along with the ligaments attaching the cervix to the pubis (pubocervical ligaments), the sacrum (uterosacral ligaments), and the lateral pelvic wall (transverse cervical ligaments). Loss in the support of these structures during childbirth is often the cause of prolapse of the uterus.

Cystitis. This inflammatory condition in the urinary bladder results in painful urination. It is more common in women because bacteria can more easily access the bladder through the short urethra.

Tubal ligation. Ligation of the uterine tube is a method of achieving birth control. After ligation, discharged ovarian follicles degenerate in the uterine tube and never reach the uterus. This procedure is done laporoscopically through the abdomen.

Ectopic pregnancy. This is the implantation of a blastocyst into the wall of the uterine tube most commonly into the ampulla. If this type of pregnancy is not diagnosed early, the uterine tube may rupture and cause hemorrhage into the abdominal cavity. At times if the tube ruptures on the right, it can be misdiagnosed as appendicitis.

Hysterectomy. Surgical removal of the uterus is a common operation, and it can be done either through the abdomen or transvaginally. Especially important is the ligation of the uterine vessels and their proximity to the ureters. This can be a potential danger if the ureters are not identified.

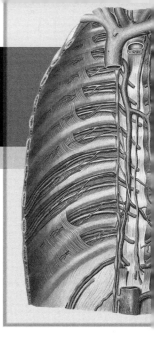

DISSECTION #19

The Perineum: Male and Female

OBJECTIVES

1 **Both Male and Female Cadavers:** To study the surface anatomy of the perineum.

2 **Both Male and Female Cadavers:** To dissect the **anal triangle,** including its vessels and nerves and the muscles and fascia that bind the **ischiorectal fossa.**

3 **Male Cadavers:** To dissect and study the **male urogenital triangle.** This region includes the penis and the muscles, vessels, and nerves in the superficial and deep perineal compartments.

4 **Female Cadavers:** To dissect and study the **female urogenital triangle.** This region includes the female genitalia and the associated muscles, vessels, and glands in the superficial and deep perineal compartments.

I. General Information and Surface Anatomy (Figures 19-1, 19-2)

► Grant's 242, 243, 245, 257, 260
Netter's 359, 361
Rohen 345, 351, 364, 365

The **perineum** is a diamond-shaped region located between the upper thighs and between the lower parts of the buttocks. It consists of structures that constitute the region below the pelvic floor. These surround the urethral, anal, and vaginal orifices. The perineum is bounded by the **symphysis pubis** anteriorly, the **coccyx** posteriorly, and the two **ischial tuberosities** laterally. Between the symphysis pubis and ischial tuberosities are the **rami of the pubic bones** and the **rami of the ischia.** Extending from the ischial tuberosities to the coccyx (and sacrum) are the **sacrotuberous ligaments,** over

which are spread the gluteus maximus muscles (**ATLAS PLATES 294, 318 #318.2**).

If a transverse line is drawn across the perineum anterior to the anus between the ischial tuberosities, the diamond-shaped perineum is divided into two triangular areas, the posterior **anal triangle** and the anterior **urogenital triangle** (**Figures 19-1, 19-2**). The anatomy of the anal region is not especially complex, and it is similar in the two sexes. In contrast, the urogenital regions are quite different and more complex, and they contain: (a) the **external genitalia** and other structures within a **superficial perineal compartment;** and (b) the fascia-covered muscular urogenital diaphragm between the pubic rami that constitutes the **deep perineal compartment.**

BOTH MALE AND FEMALE CADAVERS

Place the cadaver in a lithotomy position. This is done with the cadaver lying on its back and a wooden block placed under the gluteal region to elevate the

192

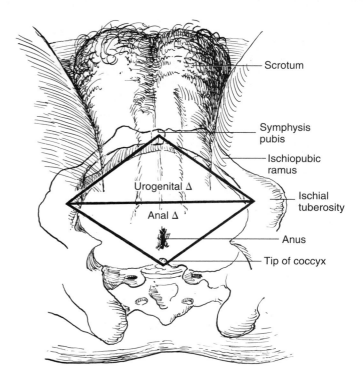

Figure 19-1. The male perineum, showing the urogenital and anal triangles.

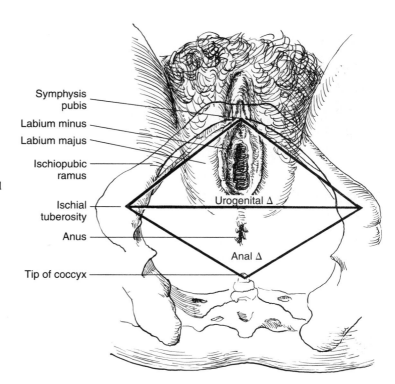

Figure 19-2. The female perineum, showing the urogenital and anal triangles.

perineum. Spread the lower limbs as far as possible without injuring the hip joints. Tie the spread limbs to stable structures with rope or gauze strips.

Study the regional anatomy of the perineum by using an articulated pelvis. Compare the locations of the bony landmarks that define the inferior pelvic outlet with the surface anatomy of the perineum on the cadaver (**ATLAS PLATES 256, 290, 318**).

1. Identify the **ischial tuberosities**, the **coccyx,** and the **symphysis pubis** on the articulated pelvis (**ATLAS PLATE 291 #291.1**). Try to palpate these important bony landmarks on the cadaver. (The symphysis pubis may have been removed during dissection of the pelvis.)

2. Observe that the **anal orifice** on the cadaver is located in the midline, about 4 cm anterior to the coccyx. Palpate the **central tendinous point (perineal body) of the perineum** just anterior to the anus (**ATLAS PLATE 290**).

MALE CADAVERS

3. Observe that the **body of the penis** is attached to the anterior aspect of the symphysis pubis. Note that the anterior surface of the flaccid penis is called the **dorsum** of the penis, and the opposite surface, oriented toward the scrotum is the **urethral** (or **scrotal**) **surface.** Identify the **glans penis,** the **external opening** of the **urethra,** and the **prepuce** (or **foreskin**), if present, attached to the glans penis by a midline fold called the **frenulum** (**ATLAS PLATE 323 #323.4**).

4. Note the median raphe of the **scrotal sac** that was dissected with the anterior abdominal wall. The raphe is the line of fusion of the two scrotal halves.

FEMALE CADAVERS

5. Identify the female external genital organs. Note that the **labia majora** are thickened, fat-filled cutaneous folds. These extend from a rounded mound called the **mons pubis** into the perineum to a site 2.5 cm anterior to the anus (**ATLAS PLATES 290, 291**).

6. Identify the **labia minora.** These small cutaneous folds are located between the labia majora. Note that the two folds approach each other anteriorly, and at the **clitoris** each labium

◄
Grant's 186–189
Netter's 342
Rohen 436, 437

►
Grant's 258, 259, 261
Netter's 361, 365
Rohen 350, 362

◄
Grant's's 243, 250, 251
Netter's's 363–365
Rohen 348–350

►
Grant's 245, 261
Netter's 384, 385, 391, 393
Rohen 352, 363

►
Grant's 245
Netter's 376
Rohen 350

◄
Grant's 243, 257, 259, 260
Netter's 359
Rohen 362, 364

divides into two parts. The upper parts from each side unite over the **glans** to form the **prepuce of the clitoris,** while the two lower parts pass below the clitoris to form its **frenulum** (**ATLAS PLATES 290, 291, 294**).

7. Realize that the clitoris is an erectile structure about 2.5 cm in length embedded in the tissues of the labia minora. The small, free extremity, called the **glans,** can be seen only if the prepuce covering it is retracted (**ATLAS PLATE 291 #291.1**).

8. Probe the **vestibule,** enclosed by the labia minora, and note the **urethral orifice** anteriorly and the opening of the **vagina** posteriorly (**ATLAS PLATE 290**).

II. Anal Triangle and Region

Posterior to a line across the perineum that passes anterior to the anus and interconnects the two ischial tuberosities is the **anal triangle.** Its three points are the two ischial tuberosities laterally and the tip of the coccyx posteriorly (**Figures 20-1, 20-2**). Most of the region deep to the surface consists of fat-filled spaces, one on each side of the midline, called the **ischiorectal fossae** (**ATLAS PLATES 291, 318**). The base of each fossa is directed toward the surface of the anal triangle and the apex oriented deeply (superiorly). In the midline of the anal triangle is located the anal orifice surrounded by the **external anal sphincter** (**ATLAS PLATES 291, 309, 318**). Each ischiorectal fossa is bounded by muscular walls and fascia and is crossed from lateral to medial by the **inferior rectal branches** of the **pudendal nerve** and **internal pudendal vessels** (**ATLAS PLATES 295, 319**).

A. Ischiorectal Fossa

1. **Boundaries and recesses.** Each ischiorectal fossa occupies a space 5 cm long, 2.5 cm wide, and 5 cm deep. It is filled with fat and fibrous connective tissue. The two fossae communicate posterior to the anal canal. The **lateral wall** of each ischiorectal fossa is formed by the fascia covering the surface of the **obturator internus muscle** and is almost vertical in orientation (**ATLAS PLATES 291, 311 #311.2, 318 #318.2**). The **medial wall** of each fossa is formed by the inferior fascia of the pelvic diaphragm that covers the perineal surface of the **levator ani muscle** and, superficially, by the fibers of the **external anal sphincter muscle.** Posterior to the anus, the two levator ani muscles insert into the midline **anococcygeal raphe** (**ATLAS PLATES 291,**

318 #318.2, 319). The **anterior boundary** of the fossa is the **urogenital diaphragm,** and **posteriorly** the fossa is limited by the **gluteus maximus muscle**.

The **anterior recess** of the ischiorectal fossa extends forward superior to the urogenital diaphragm. The **posterior recess** is located between the coccygeus muscle deeply and the more superficial gluteus maximus. The ischiorectal fossae, which are filled with loose, soft, fatty tissue, are located adjacent to the anal canal, allowing it to expand easily when necessary during defecation.

2. **Central tendinous point.** The **central tendinous point of the perineum** or the **perineal body** is located in the midline 1 cm anterior to the anus, behind the bulb of the penis in males and behind the posterior commissure of the labia majora in females (**ATLAS PLATES 290, 291, 318 #318.2**). It consists of fibrous tissue that receives the insertions of the external anal sphincters, the anterior fibers of the levator ani muscles, the bulbospongiosus muscles, and the superficial and

▶
Grant's 245
Netter's 384, 385,
391, 393
Rohen 339, 340,
343

◀
Grant's 259
Netter's 359–361,
365
Rohen 234, 235,
248, 249

deep transverse perineal muscles. The anal canal is supported by its attachment into the posterior part of the central tendinous point, as is the vagina by its attachment into the anterior part of this point. Obstetricians refer to the central tendinous point as **"the perineum"** in women.

3. **Inferior rectal vessels and nerves.** The vessels and nerves in the ischiorectal fossa are branches of the **internal pudendal vessels** and the **pudendal nerve (Figure 19-3).** They leave the pelvis through the greater sciatic foramen below the piriformis muscle, curve over the sacrospinous ligament, enter the lesser sciatic foramen, and course to the perineum within the **pudendal canal** (Alcock's canal) (**ATLAS PLATE 282**). This canal is a tunnel formed by a sheath of fascia fused with the fascia covering the obturator internus muscle (**ATLAS PLATE 311 #311.2**). Within the canal, the pudendal vessels and nerve give off the **inferior rectal vessels** and the **inferior rectal nerve** (**ATLAS PLATE 319**).

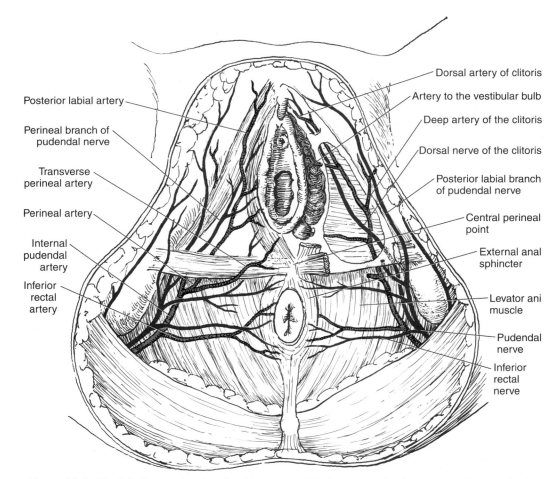

Figure 19-3. The inferior rectal and perineal branches of the internal pudendal vessels and nerves in the female perineum.

The internal pudendal vessels and the pudendal nerve continue forward in the perineum to supply urogenital structures. Their inferior rectal branches, however, cross the ischiorectal fossa from lateral to medial to supply the external anal sphincter and levator ani muscles around the anus (**ATLAS PLATES 295, 319**). The inferior rectal veins may become varicose, resulting in **hemorrhoids** or piles (**ATLAS PLATE 309.1**). Most frequently these varicosities are located in the submucosa of the anal canal and lower rectum. They may develop during pregnancy or as a result of portal vein obstruction, because these veins do not contain valves and are surrounded by loose connective tissue within the wall of the bowel.

4. **Internal and external anal sphincters.** The lower end of the smooth circular muscle in the wall of the rectum and anal canal is thickened and constitutes the **internal anal sphincter** (**ATLAS PLATE 309 #309.1**). Sympathetic fibers contract the muscle and parasympathetic fibers relax it.

◄
Grant's 245
Netter's 373–375
Rohen 343

The **external anal sphincter** is a tubular muscle that surrounds the most inferior part (2.5 cm) of the anal canal (**ATLAS PLATES 309 #309.1 and 309.2**). It is striated and consists of three parts: subcutaneous, superficial, and deep. The **subcutaneous part** is a cylindrical band of fibers that lies just deep to the skin at the anal opening. The **superficial part** lies deep to the subcutaneous part and is elliptical. Its anterior fibers insert into the central tendinous point, and its posterior fibers attach to the tip of the coccyx. The **deep part** also is an annular band of striated muscle. It surrounds the upper part of the internal

◄
Grant's 245, 248, 255, 259
Netter's 364, 365, 373–376
Rohen 343, 350–353, 364, 365

sphincter near the anorectal junction and is deep (i.e., more superior) to the superficial part (**ATLAS PLATE 309 #309.3**).

BOTH MALE AND FEMALE CADAVERS

Begin dissection of the anal triangle by making a transverse incision through the skin between the two ischial tuberosities in front of the anus (**Figures 19-4, A–B, 19-5, A–B**).

MALE CADAVERS

Make a second skin incision in the midline, at right angles to the first, which extends from the root of the glans penis to the tip of the coccyx, encircling the anus (**Figure 19-4, C–E**).

FEMALE CADAVERS

Make a second incision from the symphysis pubis anteriorly around the lateral borders of both labia majora to the anus in the midline. Continue this incision posteriorly, encircling the anal orifice, to the coccyx in the midline (**Figure 19-5, C–E**).

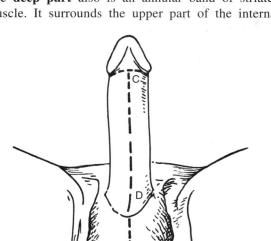

Figure 19-4. Skin incisions in the male perineum.

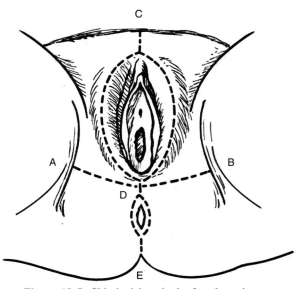

Figure 19-5. Skin incisions in the female perineum.

BOTH MALE AND FEMALE CADAVERS

Reflect the four triangular skin flaps: the two urogenital flaps anterolaterally and the two anal flaps posterolaterally. Take care around the anus because the external anal sphincter lies immediately under the skin.

Grant's 245
Netter's 365, 375, 376, 396

Make a transverse incision 1.5 cm deep across the ischiorectal fossa penetrating into the fatty tissue. Probe the fossa with your gloved index finger and loosen the fatty tissue. With forceps and probe, pick away the fat, being careful to identify and retain the **inferior rectal vessels and nerve.** These cross the fossa from **lateral to medial** at a depth of about 3 to 4 cm (**ATLAS PLATES 295, 319, Figure 19-3**).

Grant's 245
Netter's 384, 385, 391, 393
Rohen 353, 354, 365

Remove the fascia from around the anal orifice and uncover the **external anal sphincter (ATLAS PLATES 291, 318 #318.2, 319)**. Trace the elliptical fibers of the superficial part of this muscle from the central point of the perineum to the coccyx.

Grant's 245, 248
Netter's 364, 365, 373–377
Rohen 364, 365

Expose the walls of the ischiorectal fossa and note that the **lateral wall** is lined by the fascia over the **obturator internus muscle.** Observe that the **medial wall** is the fascia on the inferior surface of the **levator ani** and **coccygeus muscles (ATLAS PLATES 311 #311.2, 318 #318.2)**. Expose the border of the **gluteus maximus muscle** that forms the **posterior boundary** of the fossa. You may encounter the **inferior clunial** branches of the **posterior femoral cutaneous nerve.** These are sensory to some of the skin overlying the fossa (**ATLAS PLATES 295, 319**).

Grant's 107, 111
Netter's 335, 348, 370
Rohen 218, 219

Grant's 245
Netter's 361, 376
Rohen 350

III. Male Urogenital Triangle and Region

The three bony points of the **urogenital triangle** are the **symphysis pubis** anteriorly and the two **ischial tuberosities** laterally. The male urogenital region contains the bulb and crura of the penis, the superficial perineal muscles, and the perineal branches of the internal pudendal vessels and nerves, all of which are said to lie within the **superficial perineal compartment,** or **pouch.** This compartment is to be differentiated from the **deep perineal compartment,** also called the **urogenital diaphragm.** The deep perineal compartment contains the deep transverse perineal muscles, the external urethral sphincter, the membranous part of the urethra, and the bulbourethral glands. Through it course the deep and dorsal arteries of the penis (from the internal pudendal) and the dorsal nerve of the penis. The deep compartment lies beneath the deep fascia (perineal membrane) of the perineum. To visualize the boundaries of the superficial

Grant's 243, 245
Netter's 361, 364–366
Rohen 351, 352

and deep perineal compartments and their contents, one must understand the reflections of fascia in this region.

A. **Fascial Reflections in the Male Urogenital Region.** The **superficial fascia** of the urogenital region is an extension of the superficial fascia over the lower anterior abdominal wall. It consists of an outer fatty layer, similar to Camper's fascia, and an inner (deeper) membranous layer, continuous with Scarpa's fascia (**Figure 19-6**). In the perineum the deeper layer of superficial fascia is called **Colles' fascia.**

The superficial fatty layer descends from the lower anterior abdominal wall and is continuous with the fatty superficial fascia of the thigh and of the perineum in both the urogenital and anal regions. In contrast, as the membranous layer passes down from the abdominal wall, it courses over the inguinal ligament and attaches firmly to the deep fascia of the thigh. Thus, the potential space between Scarpa's fascia and the deep fascia over the anterior abdominal wall is closed off from the comparable fascial plane in the thigh. No such arrangement is found medially. The membranous layer passes into the urogenital region (Colles' fascia) and forms a tubelike fascial sleeve for the penis, which becomes continuous with the **fascia penis** (Buck's fascia) and with the **dartos layer** in the scrotal sac (**Figure 19-6**). Colles' fascia attaches securely to the pubic and ischial rami and spreads posteriorly across the urogenital triangle to the urogenital diaphragm and central point of the perineum, where it terminates.

MALE CADAVERS

Study **Figures 19-6** and **19-7** and understand why the attachments of Colles' fascia are important. If there is a rupture of the penile part of the urethra just distal to the urogenital diaphragm, the attachments determine the path that extravasated urine would spread (**Figure 19-7A**). Escaping urine deep to Colles' fascia would spread posteriorly only as far as the urogenital diaphragm and laterally to the ischial and pubic rami because of these attachments. It would spread deep to the fascia penis (Buck's fascia), around the scrotum, and then ascend over the anterior abdominal wall deep to Scarpa's fascia (**Figure 19-7B**). **This is because the dartos, the fascia penis, and Scarpa's fascia are all coextensive with Colles' fascia.** From the anterior abdominal wall, urine would not extend inferiorly over the inguinal ligaments into the thigh, because Scarpa's fascia attaches tightly to the deep fascia of the thigh (fascia lata), 2 cm below and parallel to the inguinal ligament (**Figure 19-6**).

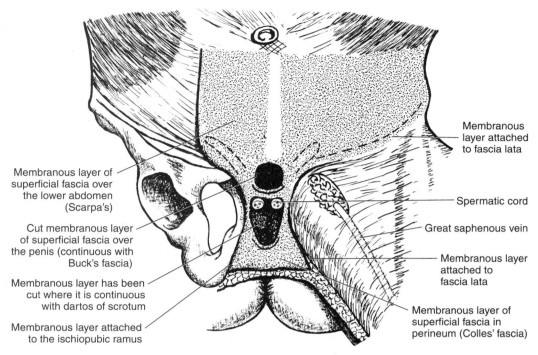

Membranous
layer attached
to fascia lata

Spermatic cord

Great saphenous vein

Membranous layer
attached to
fascia lata

Membranous layer of
superficial fascia in
perineum (Colles' fascia)

Membranous layer of
superficial fascia over
the lower abdomen
(Scarpa's)

Cut membranous layer
of superficial fascia over
the penis (continuous with
Buck's fascia)

Membranous layer has been
cut where it is continuous
with dartos of scrotum

Membranous layer attached
to the ischiopubic ramus

Figure 19-6. Diagrammatic figure showing the continuation of the membranous layer of superficial fascia of the abdomen (Scarpa's) into the perineum (Colles') in the male (after Cunningham).

Deep to the skin, fatty layer, and Colles' fascia in the urogenital region is located the superficial perineal compartment containing the **ischiocavernosus, bulbocavernosus,** and **superficial transverse perineal muscles.** Deep to these muscles is found the **inferior fascia** of the urogenital diaphragm (often called the **perineal membrane**). This fascia forms the innermost boundary of the superficial compartment (**ATLAS PLATE 318 #318.2**). Thus, the superficial perineal compartment lies between Colles' fascia superficially and the inferior fascia of the urogenital diaphragm deeply. Also found in the superficial compartment are the **posterior scrotal branches of the perineal vessels and nerves** and the **perineal branch** of the **posterior femoral cutaneous nerve** (**ATLAS PLATE 319**).

◄
Grant's 245
Netter's 344, 385, 391
Rohen 350-353

►
Grant's 245
Netter's 364, 377
Rohen 352

With the skin removed from the urogenital triangle, dissect the fatty superficial and membranous layers of the superficial fascia. These are to be reflected posteriorly from the scrotal raphe to the anal triangle and removed. Upon severing the attachments of Colles' fascia the superficial perineal compartment is opened. Probe the connective tissue deep to Colles' fascia and identify the **posterior scrotal branches of the perineal vessels** and the **posterior scrotal nerve** (**ATLAS PLATE 319**).

◄
Grant's 345
Netter's 385, 391
Rohen 353-355

►
Grant's 245
Netter's 364, 377
Rohen 352

B. Muscles in the Male Superficial Perineal Compartment (Figures 19-8, 19-14). There are three pairs of muscles in the superficial perineal compartment. These are the superficial transverse perineal muscles posteriorly and the bulbospongiosus and ischiocavernosus muscles that overlie the bulb and the crura of the penis (**ATLAS PLATE 318 #318.2**).

The **superficial transverse perineal muscles** are narrow muscular slips oriented transversely in front of the anus. They extend from the anterior part of the ischial tuberosities to the central point of the perineum (**ATLAS PLATE 318 #318.2**).

The **bulbospongiosus muscles** are located in the midline of the urogenital region anterior to the anus. The two muscles are joined by a longitudinal raphe (**Figure 19-14**). Their fibers arise from both the central tendinous point and the raphe, diverge around the bulb of the penis, and end in an aponeurosis over the corpus spongiosum penis (**ATLAS PLATES 318 #318.2, 319**). The posterior fibers expel the last drops of urine from the penile urethra, while the intermediate and anterior fibers help to maintain penile erection by tightening the aponeurosis covering the deep dorsal vein.

The two **ischiocavernosus muscles (Figure 19-14)** each overlie one crus of the penis. The muscle fibers arise on the ischial tuberosities and rami and course anteriorly and insert over the crura (**ATLAS PLATE 318**

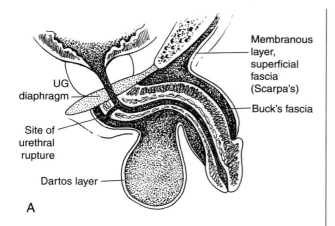

A

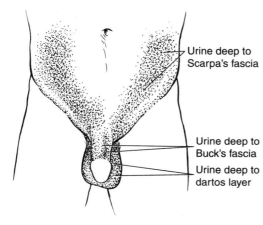

B

Figure 19-7. Extravasation of urine following rupture of the penile urethra. **A.** Urine is seen to spread deep to the dartos layer and Buck's fascia which are coextensive with Colles' fascia and with Scarpa's fascia. **B.** Urine is seen to spread over the anterior abdominal wall deep to Scarpa's fascia.

#318.2). The ischiocavernosus muscles compress the crura and may assist in maintaining erection.

> Within the superficial perineal compartment, identify the branches of the perineal vessels and nerves, and look for the fibers of the **superficial transverse perineal muscles.** These course transversely from the ischial tuberosities to the central point of the perineum anterior to the anus but may be difficult to demonstrate (**ATLAS PLATE 319**). Note that the bulbospongiosus and ischiocavernosus muscles are embedded in thin fascia that becomes somewhat thicker over the penile shaft. This is the **fascia penis (Buck's fascia),** and it should be incised and removed from the bulb and crura of the penis to expose the muscles fully.

▶ Grant's 252, 254
Netter's 365
Rohen 339, 340

▶ Grant's 250–252, 254
Netter's 364, 365
Rohen 338-340

▶ Grant's 252, 254
Netter's 348, 368
Rohen 337, 339

▶ Grant's 251
Netter's 364, 365
Rohen 336, 337

◀ Grant's 245
Netter's 385, 391
Rohen 353, 354

◀ Grant's 251
Netter's 363–365
Rohen 348

> Cut the fibers of the **bulbospongiosus muscle** in the midline to expose the bulb, and separate the fibers of the **ischiocavernosus muscle** on one side to expose one crus of the penis (**ATLAS PLATE 321**). Note the small, triangular region between the bulb and the crus on each side. If you probe the depth of these small triangles, you will touch the inferior fascia of the urogenital diaphragm (**ATLAS PLATE 318 #318.2**).

C. The Penis (Figures 19-9, 19-10, 19-11). The **penis** is composed of (a) the **root** (consisting of the bulb and two crura), which is attached to the urogenital diaphragm and pubic arch; (b) the **body (or shaft)** formed by three cylindrical masses of erectile tissue: two **corpora cavernosa penis** and the **corpus spongiosum penis;** and (c) a terminal enlargement, the **glans penis,** which is a conical expansion of the corpus spongiosum over the ends of the corpora cavernosa (**ATLAS PLATE 321**).

From their attachments on the ischium and pubis the two crura converge anteriorly as the corpora cavernosa penis and are joined by the corpus spongiosum (**Figure 19-9**). At their junction, the two corpora cavernosa form the dorsal part of the penile shaft. The corpus spongiosum unites with the corpora cavernosa along a median groove on their ventral surface (**Figure 19-10**). The tight fascial layer that binds the three corpora together makes up the fascia penis or Buck's fascia (**Figure 19-11**).

Through the entire length of the corpus spongiosum penis to the external urethral orifice courses the **penile part of the urethra** (**ATLAS PLATE 305 #305.2**). The surface of the penis along the corpus spongiosum is the **urethral surface,** while the surface dorsal to the corpora cavernosa is the **dorsum of the penis.**

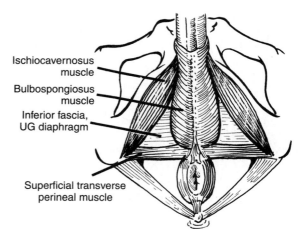

Figure 19-8. The muscles of the male urogenital triangle and the inferior fascia of the urogenital diaphragm (perineal membrane).

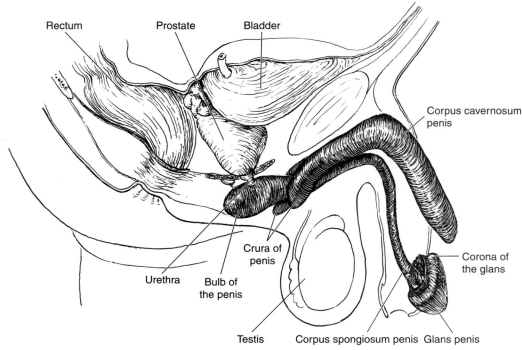

Figure 19-9. The erectile bodies of the penis distal to the urogenital diaphragm.

The arteries supplying the penis on each side are the **artery to the bulb of the penis,** the **deep artery of the penis,** and the **dorsal artery of the penis** (**ATLAS PLATES 320 #320.2, 323, Figure 19-11**). These are all terminal branches of the internal pudendal artery that course through the urogenital diaphragm to reach the penis.

The **artery to the bulb of the penis** is a short vessel that enters the bulb of the penis and supplies the erectile tissue of the proximal part of the corpus spongiosum.

◄
Grant's 250-252, 254
Netter's 385, 389
Rohen 348, 349, 353

►
Grant's 274, 275
Netter's 364, 383, 385
Rohen 348, 349

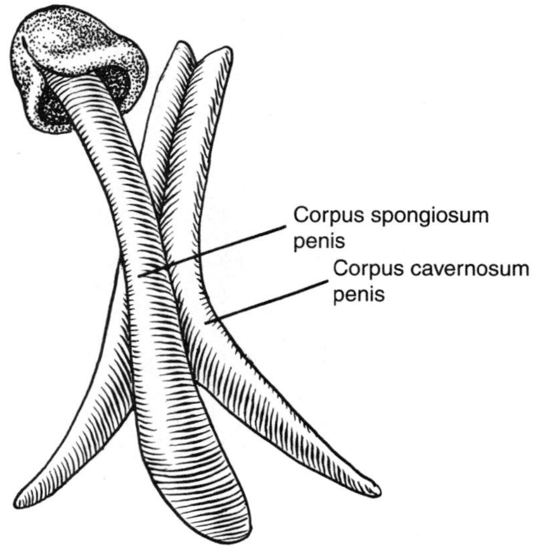

The **deep artery of the penis** enters the crus of the penis on each side, courses through the interior of the corpus cavernosum, and supplies blood to the erectile tissue (**ATLAS PLATE 322 #322.2**).

On each side the **dorsal artery of the penis** ascends between the crus and the pubic arch to reach the dorsum of the penis. The two arteries course distally as far as the glans and are accompanied on their lateral sides by the **dorsal nerves of the penis.** The **deep dorsal vein** courses between the two arteries (**ATLAS PLATES 320 #320.2, 323 #323.1**).

The **deep dorsal vein** drains posteriorly in the median plane and divides into right and left branches that

Figure 19-10. The corpora cavernosum penis and spongiosum penis.

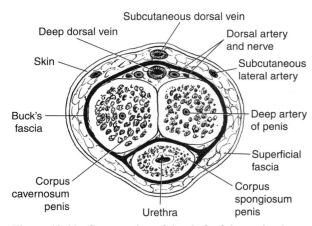

Figure 19-11. Cross section of the shaft of the penis, showing its arteries and veins.

flow into the prostatic plexus. The dorsal vein, two dorsal arteries, and two dorsal nerves are all encased tightly with the three corpora by the fascia penis.

The penis is supported on its dorsal surface by the **fundiform** and **suspensory ligaments.** The fundiform ligament (**ATLAS PLATES 176, 178**) is continuous downward over the symphysis pubis from the linea alba. It divides into right and left bands that diverge on the sides of the penis and attach on the urethral surface to the septum of the scrotum. The suspensory ligament (**ATLAS PLATES 181, 192, 320 #320.2**) is deep to the fundiform. It attaches above to the symphysis pubis and below to the fascia penis on the dorsolateral aspect of the organ.

Superficial to the three corpora and the dorsal vessels and nerves is the loose superficial fascia that attaches the shaft to the overlying skin (**Figure 19-11**). The skin is thin, loose, and freely movable, and on the urethral surface it forms a raphe that is continuous with the median raphe of the scrotum. Distally the skin attaches around the circumference of the **corona of the glans** and then overlaps it as the **prepuce** (**ATLAS PLATE 323 #323.4**).

Superficial arteries in the skin along the dorsum of the penis external to the fascia penis are branches of the **superficial external pudendal arteries** from the femoral artery. Between the superficial arteries is the **superficial dorsal vein** that drains into the external pudendal vein and then into the great saphenous vein (**Figure 19-11**).

> If the median wedge of bone that included the symphysis pubis was not removed, identify the **fundiform** and **suspensory ligaments** that attach the dorsum of the penis to the symphysis pubis (**ATLAS PLATES 176, 181**). Cut these ligaments and sever the skin of the penis in the midline along the urethral surface as far as the glans (**Figure 19-4**). Cut the **prepuce** from the margin of the glans penis and reflect

▶
Grant's 250, 254
Netter's 364, 381, 383
Rohen 217, 219, 349
◀
Grant's 101, 107, 250
Netter's 241, 242, 335, 348
Rohen 211, 212

▶
Grant's 252
Netter's 365
Rohen 340

▶
Grant's 254
Netter's 365
Rohen 339
◀
Grant's 97
Netter's 241, 247
Rohen 478

▶
Grant's 197, 206, 242
Netter's 366
◀ Rohen 350–353
Grant's 251
Netter's 364, 383
Rohen 349

the skin. Along its inner surface identify the **superficial dorsal vein** and the **superficial external pudendal arteries** coursing longitudinally.

Identify the **(deep) dorsal vein,** the **dorsal arteries,** and the **dorsal nerves** deep to the fascia penis (**ATLAS PLATES 320 #320.2, 322 #322.2**). Clean and separate these vessels and nerves along the dorsum as far as the glans.

With forceps and scalpel, separate the corpora cavernosa from the corpus spongiosum by cutting longitudinally through the tightly investing fascia (**ATLAS PLATE 321, Figure 19-10**). Note that the glans is the expanded terminal part of the corpus spongiosum. Dissect a corpus cavernosum penis back to its crus. Remove the ischiocavernous muscle over one crus and identify the tough tunica albuginea surrounding the crus. Transect one crus proximal to its junction with the crus from the opposite side. Study the cross section of the crus and look for the deep artery of the penis within the substance of the corpus cavernosum (**ATLAS PLATES 322 #322.2, 323**).

Cut along the midline raphe of the bulbospongiosus muscle and expose the enlarged bulb of the penis (**ATLAS PLATE 321**). When exposed, transect the corpus spongiosum just distal to the perineal membrane and probe the spongy tissue for the urethral channel.

D. Male Urogenital (UG) Diaphragm. The urogenital diaphragm and deep perineal compartment are two terms for the same region. The **UG diaphragm** is a fibromuscular structure that consists of two layers of fascia between which are located the deep transverse perineal muscle and other structures (**ATLAS PLATES 308 #308.1, 318 #318.2, Figure 19-12**).

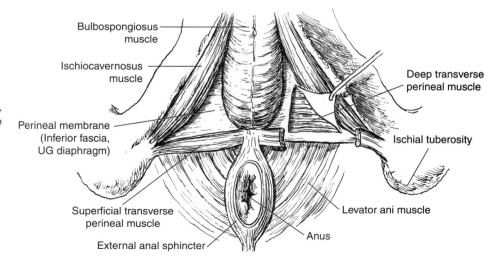

Figure 19-12. The urogenital diaphragm, showing its inferior fascia and the deep transverse perineal muscle.

Bulbospongiosus muscle

Ischiocavernosus muscle

Perineal membrane (Inferior fascia, UG diaphragm)

Superficial transverse perineal muscle

External anal sphincter

Deep transverse perineal muscle

Ischial tuberosity

Levator ani muscle

Anus

The two fascial layers are the inferior fascia of the UG diaphragm or perineal membrane **(Figure 19-12)** and a similar layer, the superior fascia of the UG diaphragm. These fascial sheets stretch horizontally across the pubic arch, one below and the other above the deep transverse perineal muscle. Thus, the UG diaphragm (or deep compartment) is bounded laterally by the ischiopubic rami and lies below the symphysis pubis (**ATLAS PLATE 308 #308.1**). The deep transverse perineal muscle occupies most of the space in the deep compartment, but the circular **urethral sphincter** is an important voluntary muscle around the membranous urethra. Injury to it results in urinary incontinence.

The perineal branches of the internal pudendal vessels and pudendal nerve (described above) course through the deep compartment, penetrate the inferior fascia of the UG diaphragm, and enter the superficial compartment to supply the scrotum, the bulb of the penis, and the muscles in the superficial compartment (**ATLAS PLATES 319**).

The two small (5 to 6 mm in diameter) **bulbourethral glands (of Cowper)** are located on the lateral sides of the membranous urethra, within the UG diaphragm (**ATLAS PLATE 308 #308.1**). Their ducts (4 cm long) pass distally through the inferior fascia of the UG diaphragm and open into the proximal part of the penile urethra.

◄
Grant's 242, 243, 245
Netter's 348, 366–368
Rohen 338

►
Grant's 242, 254
Netter's 366
Rohen 348–353

►
Grant's 242
Netter's 366
Rohen 350–353

◄
Grant's 204, 206, 255
Netter's 348, 353
Rohen 336, 339, 342

Upon erotic stimulation the glands secrete a mucoid secretion that precedes ejaculation.

Palpate the UG diaphragm. Insert your index finger into the anterior recess of the ischiorectal fossa. Press down with your thumb and feel the UG diaphragm between your thumb and index finger.

Remove the bulbocavernosus and ischiocavernosus muscles. Detach the crura of the penis from the pubic rami and section the bulb of the penis along the plane of its attachment to the UG diaphragm. Reflect the bulb forward and expose the inferior fascia of the UG diaphragm and the severed urethra at its entrance into the bulb.

Identify the **inferior fascia** of the UG diaphragm stretching between the pubic arches. Remove this fascia and expose the contents of the deep perineal compartment (**ATLAS PLATES 308 #308.1**). Observe the fibers of the deep transverse perineal muscle (**Figure 19-12**). Look for the circular sphincter around the urethra and the bulbourethral glands. These may be difficult to identify grossly. Note the vessels and nerves of the penis that penetrate the UG diaphragm.

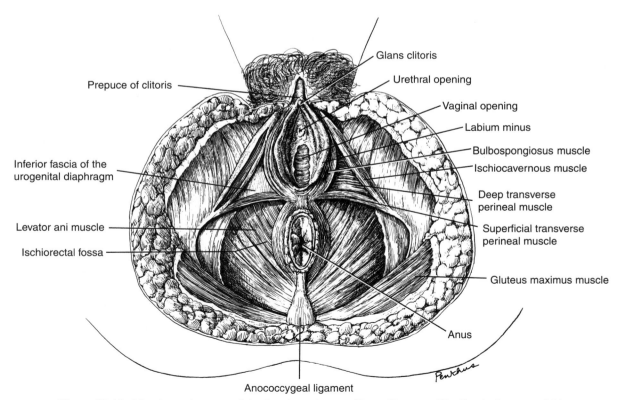

Figure 19-13. Muscles and organs of the female perineum. (From Clemente CD. Gray's Anatomy. 30th U.S. Edition. Philadelphia: Lea & Febiger, 1985.)

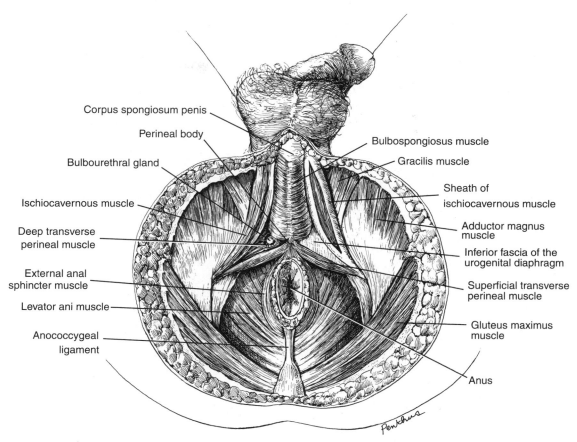

Corpus spongiosum penis

Perineal body

Bulbourethral gland

Ischiocavernous muscle

Deep transverse
perineal muscle

External anal
sphincter muscle

Levator ani muscle

Anococcygeal
ligament

Bulbospongiosus muscle

Gracilis muscle

Sheath of
ischiocavernous muscle

Adductor magnus
muscle

Inferior fascia of the
urogenital diaphragm

Superficial transverse
perineal muscle

Gluteus maximus
muscle

Anus

Figure 19-14. The male perineum. (From Clemente CD. Gray's Anatomy. 30th U.S. Edition. Philadelphia: Lea & Febiger, 1985.)

IV. Female Urogenital Triangle and Region

As in the male, the three landmarks that define the female urogenital triangle are the **symphysis pubis** anteriorly and the two **ischial tuberosities** laterally. The urogenital region deep to the surface contains the **mons pubis, the labia majora, the labia minora, the bulbs of the vestibule, the greater vestibular glands,** and the **crura, body,** and **glans of the clitoris.** These are all positioned around the **vestibule,** which is the cleft between the labia minora, containing the **urethral** and **vaginal orifices** (**ATLAS PLATES 290, 291**). Additionally, the female urogenital region contains three pairs of muscles homologous to those in the male (**ATLAS PLATE 294, Figure 19-15**), perineal vessels and nerves (**ATLAS PLATE 295**), as well as the deep and dorsal vessels and nerves of the clitoris. All of these structures are contained in the **superficial perineal compartment.**

Deep to the superficial compartment is located the **deep perineal compartment** containing the structures of the UG diaphragm. These structures located be-

◀
Grant's 242–244,
256
Netter's 359, 361,
384, 393
Rohen 350–354

▶
Grant's 256–258
Netter's 360

◀
Grant's 242, 243,
256, 258
Netter's 361
Rohen 363, 365,
366

tween two layers of fascia include the deep transverse perineal and sphincter urethrae muscles, as well as the vessels and nerves that traverse this space to supply the genital organs in the superficial compartment (**ATLAS PLATE 296**). The fascial layers in the female urogenital region are comparable to those in the male. Compare the following paragraphs to the section on fascial reflections in the male urogenital region.

A. Fascial Reflections in the Female Urogenital Region. The superficial fascia in the female urogenital region, as in males, is continuous with that over the anterior abdominal wall. It consists of an outer fatty layer that extends downward from Camper's fascia and an inner membranous layer continuous with Scarpa's fascia. This fatty layer is a thick stratum that contributes to the contours of the mons pubis and labia majora. It continues posteriorly to the anal triangle, where it is coextensive with the fat in the ischiorectal fossa and below the inguinal ligament with the superficial fascia in the thigh.

The deeper membranous layer of superficial fascia (Scarpa's) descends from the anterior abdominal wall

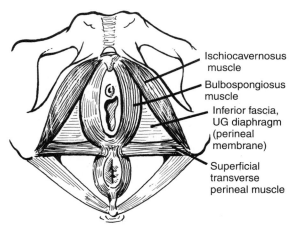

Figure 19-15. The muscles of the urogenital region in the female. UG, urogenital.

▶
Grant's 256–258
Netter's 359
Rohen 350

over the inguinal ligaments and attaches securely to the deep fascia of the thigh. Medially, it descends into the perineum as the membranous layer of superficial fascia. On each side this membranous layer attaches to the pubic and ischial rami and spreads posteriorly around the superficial transverse perineal muscle to join the posterior margin of the UG diaphragm and central point of the perineum. This membranous layer lies superficial to the vestibular bulbs and glands, the other external genital organs, and the superficial perineal muscles, vessels, and nerves. These are all located in the **superficial perineal compartment.**

◀
Grant's 105, 258, 260
Netter's 360, 361, 393
Rohen 365, 366

Deep to the superficial perineal compartment is the inferior layer of the UG diaphragm (perineal membrane) **(ATLAS PLATE 291 #291.1, Figure 19-16)**. As in males, the superficial perineal compartment is the space bounded superficially by the membranous layer of superficial fascia (Colles') and deeply by the inferior fascia of the UG diaphragm.

FEMALE CADAVERS

With the skin removed from the female urogenital region, reflect the fatty layer of superficial fascia from the mons pubis anteriorly down to the labia majora. Carefully cut away the skin of the labia majora by making a shallow incision along the medial border of each labium in the cleft that separates it from the labium minor. Leave the labia minora completely intact. Most of the labia majora consists of subcutaneous fat to be cut away with the superficial fatty layer, **but be careful not to destroy the crura and body of the clitoris** embedded in the tissues anterior to the labia minora (see **ATLAS PLATES 290, 291, 294**). Complete the reflection of the superficial fascia posteriorly to the anal triangle.

Dissect through the membranous layer of superficial fascia to enter the superficial perineal compartment and identify the female urogenital muscles and the perineal vessels and nerves (**ATLAS PLATES 294, 295**).

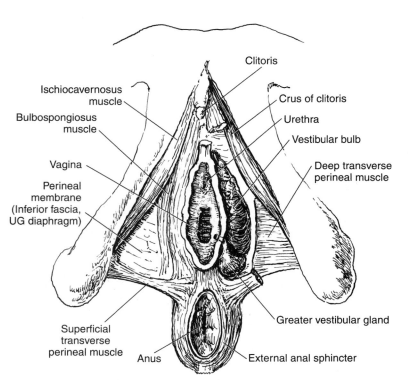

Figure 19-16. The vestibular bulb and greater vestibular gland following removal (on the reader's right) of the bulbospongiosus muscle in the female urogenital triangle.

B. Muscles in the Female Superficial Perineal Compartment. Deep to the fatty and membranous layers of superficial fascia are located the **ischiocavernosus, bulbocavernosus,** and **superficial transverse perineal muscles.** The female urogenital muscles correspond to similarly named muscles in the male, but they are smaller and less distinct (**Figures 19-13, 19-14, 19-16**).

The **superficial transverse perineal muscles** are narrow bands that course transversely across the perineum just anterior to the anus (**ATLAS PLATES 294, 295**). They arise from the anterior aspect of the ischial tuberosities and insert into the central point of the perineum.

The **bulbospongiosus muscles** course forward around both sides of the vagina from their origin posteriorly at the central tendinous point. Their fibers surround the labia minora and vestibule and overlie the vestibular bulbs (**ATLAS PLATES 294, 295**). These thin muscular layers on each side attach to the corpora cavernosa clitoridis and are capable of compressing the vaginal orifice. A small fascicle on each side also attaches onto the fibrous tissue dorsal to the clitoris. These may contribute to erection of the clitoris by compressing the deep dorsal vein.

The **ischiocavernosus muscles** are considerably smaller than the comparable muscles in males (**Figure 19-13**). They arise from the inner surface of the ischial rami and tuberosities and overlie the crura of the clitoris (**ATLAS PLATES 294, 295**). They attach onto the inferior surfaces of the corpora cavernosa clitoridis before the latter join to form the body of the clitoris. These muscles may compress the crura of the clitoris and assist in maintaining its erection.

Open the superficial perineal compartment and find the perineal branches of the internal pudendal artery coursing forward just medial to the ischiopubic ramus (**ATLAS PLATE 295**). Realize that the **posterior labial branches** to the labia majora were cut when the labia were removed. Identify the **artery to the vestibular bulb,** which supplies its erectile tissue and also the greater vestibular gland (of Bartholin). Continuing anteriorly, try to find the **deep artery of the clitoris,** which enters the corpus cavernosum, and the **dorsal artery of the clitoris,** which supplies the dorsum and glans of the clitoris.

Identify the **perineal branch of the pudendal nerve,** which gives off **posterior labial branches** and **motor branches to the urogenital muscles** (**ATLAS PLATE 295**). Try to find the small **dorsal nerve to the clitoris** (on each side), which supplies sensory innervation to its body and glans.

Clean the connective tissue from the surface of the **superficial transverse perineal muscles.** These are

◄
Grant's 256
Netter's 361, 393
Rohen 364–366

►
Grant's 260
Netter's 361, 376, 384
Rohen 364–366

►
Grant's 258
Netter's 361, 384
Rohen 363–366

►
Grant's 258, 261
Netter's 361, 384
Rohen 362–364
◄
Grant's 258, 261
Netter's 384
Rohen 365, 366

◄
Grant's 256, 257, 261
Netter's 393
Rohen 365, 366

often poorly developed and may be only a few muscle strands coursing transversely anterior to the anus. Clean the **bulbospongiosus muscles,** which are formed from fibers that course anteriorly from the central point of the perineum and curve around the vagina over the surface of the vestibular bulbs and greater vestibular glands (**ATLAS PLATES 291, #291.1, 294, 295**). Observe that their fibers converge to insert onto the clitoris. More laterally, identify the **ischiocavernosus muscles** coursing anteromedially as they cover the surfaces of the crura of the clitoris (**ATLAS PLATES 291, #291.1, 294**).

C. Vestibular Bulbs and Greater Vestibular Glands. Immediately deep to the bulbospongiosus muscles on both sides are located the **vestibular bulbs.** The two bulbs together are the homologue of the single penile bulb in the male. The female urethra does not course through the vestibular bulb, but it is positioned in the midline between the two bulbs. The vestibular bulbs are elongated masses of highly vascularized connective tissue that lie on each side of the vestibule and functionally serve as erectile tissue (**ATLAS PLATE 291 #291.1**). Their anterior ends are prolonged past the urethral orifice and unite to form a commissure along the ventral surface of the body of the clitoris to join the glans clitoridis (**Figure 19-17**). The vestibular bulbs are supplied by a branch of the perineal artery (**artery of the bulb**) that crosses the urogenital region to reach the bulb.

The **greater vestibular glands (of Bartholin)** are two oval bodies (5 to 6 mm in diameter) located on each side of the vestibule, adjacent to the posterior ends of the vestibular bulbs (**ATLAS PLATE 291 #291.1, Figure 19-16**). Homologues of the male bulbourethral glands, each gland has a duct 2 cm long that opens into the vestibule just lateral to the vaginal orifice.

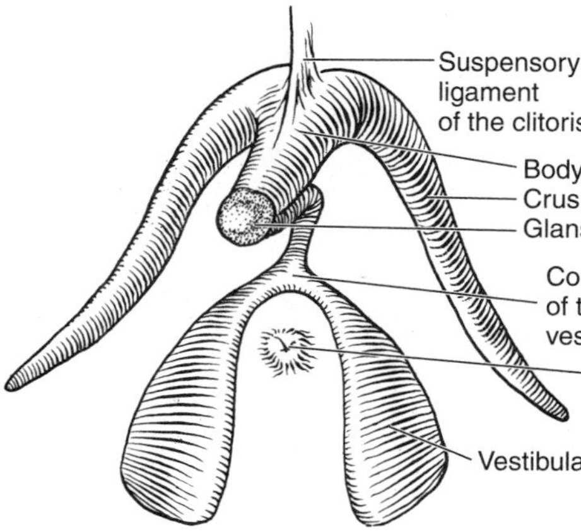

Figure 19-17. The body, crura, and glans of the clitoris. Note also the vestibular bulbs and their commissure.

On one side, cut the fibers of the bulbospongiosus muscle posteriorly at the central point of the perineum. Separate the muscle from the surface of the vestibular bulb (**ATLAS PLATE 291 #291.1**). Observe that the bulb is oblong, is formed by erectile tissue, and rests on the inferior fascia of the urogenital diaphragm.

Look for the greater vestibular gland in the tissue posterior and deep to the vestibular bulb (**ATLAS PLATE 291 #291.1**). These glands are often quite difficult to find because they assume the color of the surrounding tissue and because they become atrophied in older women. If identified, the gland will appear as a small round body underlying the posterior end of the vestibular bulb on each side of the vagina.

D. Labia Minora and Clitoris.

The **labia minora** are two thin folds of skin that surround a cleft called the **vestibule**, into which open the urethra and the vagina (**ATLAS PLATES 290, 294, 295**). Each labium minor blends with the labium majus posteriorly, but a fold of skin (the **frenulum of the labia minora**) may join the two labia minora across the midline adjacent to the central point of the perineum. Anteriorly, each labium minor divides to form two folds that join similar folds from the other side. One pair of folds unites on the dorsum of the clitoris to form the **prepuce**, and the other forms the **frenulum clitoridis** that attaches to the urethral surface of the clitoris (**ATLAS PLATES 290, 291, 291.1**).

The **clitoris** is an erectile organ homologous to the penis, and it is embedded in surrounding tissues. It consists of two **crura**, a **body**, and the **glans** (**ATLAS PLATE 291, Figure 19-17**). Each crus measures about 3 cm, attaches to the ischiopubic rami, and is covered by the ischiocavernosus muscle. The two crura join the body of the clitoris, which is also about 3 cm long. The body is cylindrical and is formed by the union of two corpora cavernosa surrounded by connective tissue. A small suspensory ligament attaches the body of the clitoris to the pubic symphysis. At the rounded distal end of the corpora cavernosa is a small mass of erectile tissue called the glans clitoris.

The labia minora are supplied by medial branches of the perineal arteries derived from the internal pudendal. The clitoris receives the **dorsal artery of the clitoris** on each side, and the erectile tissue of the crura is supplied by the **deep artery of the clitoris** (**ATLAS PLATES 188, 295**). The **small dorsal nerve of the clitoris** is a branch of the pudendal nerve. A small **dorsal vein of the clitoris** courses in

▶
Grant's 258, 260
Netter's 361, 384, 393
Rohen 362, 363, 366

◀
Grant's 258, 261
Netter's 361, 384
Rohen 363–366

▶
Grant's 242, 258, 261
Netter's 361
Rohen 364–366

◀
Grant's 259
Netter's 359
Rohen 362, 365, 366

◀
Grant's 258–262
Netter's 359, 361, 384
Rohen 362, 366

▶
Grant's 242, 258, 261
Netter's 361
Rohen 364, 365

◀
Grant's 258
Netter's 384, 393
Rohen 365, 366

the midline and is flanked on each side by the dorsal arteries and dorsal nerves (**ATLAS PLATE 188**).

Identify the glans clitoris and its prepuce and feel for the body of the clitoris deep to the subcutaneous tissue. Remove the ischiocavernosus muscles from the crura of the clitoris. Trace the crura forward to their union in the formation of the body of the clitoris. Look for the vessels and nerves on the dorsum of the clitoris (**ATLAS PLATE 188**).

E. Female Urogenital Diaphragm (Deep Perineal Compartment).

The UG diaphragm in women is comparable to that found in men, but it differs in two respects. In women, it is traversed by the vagina and does not contain bulbourethral glands. Similar to that in males, the female UG diaphragm is formed by the **deep transverse perineal muscle** with layers of fascia superior and inferior to the muscle. The **inferior fascia of the UG diaphragm** (perineal membrane) is not as tough as in males, but the breadth of the diaphragm is greater because of the wider subpubic angle in women.

The urethra courses through the UG diaphragm, and surrounding it are the circular fibers of the voluntary **sphincter urethrae muscle.** The vagina occupies a significant portion of the central region of the UG diaphragm, and some deep transverse perineal muscle fibers blend into the vaginal wall (**ATLAS PLATE 296**). Also found coursing through the deep perineal compartment are the perineal vessels and nerves directed toward the superficial perineal compartment to supply the external genitalia.

To palpate the female UG diaphragm, place your index finger into the anterior recess of the ischiorectal fossa, then press down with your thumb. Between your thumb and finger is located the deep perineal compartment. **To dissect the female UG diaphragm,** reflect forward the crura of the clitoris and the vestibular bulbs and expose the underlying triangular inferior fascia of the UG diaphragm or perineal membrane (**Figure 19-18**). Open the deep perineal compartment by reflecting the fascia. Identify the transversely coursing fibers of the deep transverse perineal muscle and try to locate the circular fibers of the sphincter urethrae around the urethra (**ATLAS PLATES 291, #291.1, 296**).

Clinical Relevance (Both Male and Female)

Perineal body. This central point of the perineum consists of fibromuscular tissue and is the site of attachment of the levator ani and superficial and deep

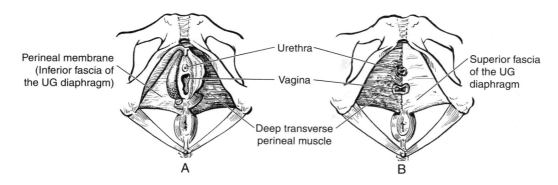

Figure 19-18. The urogenital diaphragm in the female seen from below. **A.** The inferior fascia *(left)* and the deep transverse perineal muscle *(right)* after removal of the inferior fascia. **B.** The external genitalia are removed to show the urethra and vagina penetrating the diaphragm. On *right,* the deep transverse perineal muscle is removed showing the superior fascia of the UG diaphragm. UG, urogenital.

transverse perineal muscles. It is located in the midline, just anterior to the anus, and obstetricians call this point the perineum.

Deep perineal pouch. The deep perineal pouch (or compartment) is located between the superior and inferior fascias of the urogenital diaphragm. In the male it contains the membranous part of the urethra, the external urethral sphincter, the bulbourethral glands (of Cowper), and branches of the internal pudendal vessels and the pudendal nerve. The sphincter surrounds the urethra and is under voluntary control. It is important during resection of the prostate to avoid injury to the circular sphincter. In the female the urogenital diaphragm contains the muscles and nerves described above, and through the diaphragm course not only the female urethra but also the vagina.

Hemorrhoids. The rectum is supplied by the superior, middle, and inferior rectal arteries and is drained by the same named veins. These vessels anastomose along the length of the rectum and when a problem occurs with venous return through the liver or some obstruction in the inferior vena cava, the backup of blood results in the engorgement of the inferior rectal veins (among other veins) both internally in the rectum (internal hemorrhoids) and in the region of the anus (external hemorrhoids).

Prolapse of the rectum. Partial prolapse of the rectum outside of the anus can occur in older men and women whose muscles, such as the levator ani, have lost their tone. This condition can also occur in younger women who have had difficulty at childbirth.

Abscesses in the ischiorectal fossa. Hard feces can injure the mucosa of the anus, and an infection can develop in the ischiorectal fossa. Any surgical intervention in the fossa must be transverse incisions because vertical incisions will sever the inferior pudendal vessels and nerves. These have emerged

from the pudendal canal laterally and course medially across the fossa to the levator ani and external sphincter muscles.

Male Perineum

Superficial perineal pouch. The superficial perineal pouch (or compartment) in the male contains the superficial transverse perineal, ischiocavernosus and bulbospongiosus muscles, and the bulb and crura of the penis. When the urethra is injured in the perineum (e.g., from a straddle injury), urine extravasates into the superficial perineal compartment, around the penis and deep to the membranous layer of superficial fascia on the anterior abdominal wall.

Pelvic splanchnic nerves. Injury to these nerves in the male can result in the loss of bladder control and the inability to develop an erection. These sacral nerves, derived from the S2–S4 spinal segments, are known as pelvic splanchnic nerves and they contain somatic afferent, somatic efferent, visceral afferent, and visceral efferent (parasympathetic) nerve fibers. These nerves are important for male perineal sensory and motor functions.

Vasectomy. This procedure, which in males causes sterilization, ligates the ductus deferens as it emerges from the superior part of the scrotal sac. After the operation the male ejaculate still contains the prostatic and seminal secretions, but it no longer contains sperm from the testis. These degenerate in the epididymis.

Sensory innervation of the scrotum. The scrotum is supplied anteriorly by the ilioinguinal nerve (L1) and the genital branch of the genitofemoral nerve (L1, L2). The perineal branches of the pudendal nerve and the posterior femoral cutaneous nerve supply the posterior surface of the scrotum.

Male ejaculation. This is the reflexive propulsion of semen through the urethra and involves a closure of the neck of the bladder so that semen courses forward in the urethra and not back into the bladder. It also involves the stimulation and contraction of the urethral muscular wall along with a contraction of the bulbospongiosus muscle. Sympathetic fibers from the L1 and L2 segments along with parasympathetic fibers from the S2 to S4 segments play an important part of this phenomenon. Visceral and somatic afferent fibers transmit the sensory impulses from the penis and perineal muscles that are characteristic of male ejaculation and orgasm.

Hypospadias. This developmental defect in the penis has the external orifice not opening at the tip of the glans, but instead along the ventral surface of the penis.

Female Perineum

Incontinence of urine. During labor and during a difficult delivery, the muscles in the floor of the pelvis become stretched. At times this results in a loss of some strength in the deep transverse perineal muscle and especially the fibers of the external sphincter of the urethra. This loss of strength causes a partial incontinence for urine when these women are acutely stressed or when they increase intraabdominal pressure when they sneeze or cough.

Fistulae involving the vagina. Vaginal fistulae can occur between the vagina and some of the pelvic organs adjacent to it. Vesicovaginal, urethrovaginal, and rectovaginal fistulae at times may result in the discharge of urine or feces from the vagina.

Pap smear test. This test is performed by inserting a narrow spatula through a distended vagina and scraping the uterine cervix and its opening. A small brush capable of retrieving cells is then used to gather the cervical cells, and these cells are placed on slides, then stained and examined under the microscope.

Episiotomy. This procedure is a conventional surgical incision of the posterior (inferior) wall of the vagina to enlarge the vaginal orifice, thereby allowing delivery of the baby during childbirth. It cuts into the peroneal body and then, upon repair, the scar blends with the connective tissue of this central tendinous point.

Greater vestibular glands. These glands (of Bartholin) can become infected when their ducts are obstructed, resulting in their enlargement so that they can be palpated. Usually the blockage is caused by an accumulation of a mucous secretion that leads to a pathogenic inflammation and pain.

Female urethra. This organ is about $1^1/_2$ inches long and it passes from the neck of the bladder through the urogenital diaphragm (surrounded by its external sphincter). It opens at the urethral orifice inferior to the clitoris and superior to the vagina. It is easier to catheterize than in the male patient.

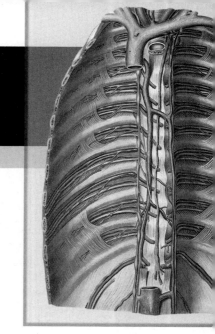

The Gluteal Region, Posterior Thigh, and Popliteal Fossa

OBJECTIVES

1 Study the surface anatomy of the buttocks and posterior thigh and learn their cutaneous innervation.

2 Dissect the gluteal muscles and learn their actions at the hip joint, and identify the gluteal vessels and nerves, including the sciatic nerve.

3 Dissect the muscles of the posterior thigh, learn their actions, and follow the course of the sciatic nerve.

4 Dissect the popliteal fossa and learn the relationships of the popliteal vessels and nerve.

Atlas Key:

Clemente Atlas, 5th Edition = Atlas Plate #

Grant's Atlas, 11th Edition = Grant's Page #

Netter's Atlas, 3rd Edition = Netter's Plate #

Rohen Atlas, 6th Edition = Rohen Page #

The gluteal region and posterior thigh contain muscles that act at the hip and knee joints. Also found in the gluteal region are the **gluteal vessels and nerves.** The **pudendal vessels and nerve** pass from the pelvis into the gluteal region and then into the perineum. The large **sciatic nerve** and **posterior femoral cutaneous nerve** also emerge from the pelvis and descend through the gluteal region and thigh. The sciatic nerve divides into **tibial** and **common fibular** branches, and they supply motor innervation to all the muscles of the leg and foot.

►
Grant's 365, 366
Netter's 476, 477, 527
Rohen 226, 454, 455

I. Surface Anatomy; Skin Incisions; Cutaneous Innervation

A. Surface Anatomy. The gluteal region contains the soft tissues of the buttocks and extends from the crest of the ilium superiorly to the gluteal sulcus (or crease) inferiorly (**ATLAS PLATES 365, 366 #366.2**). Laterally, the bony landmarks of the gluteal region are the anterior superior iliac spine superiorly and the greater trochanter of the femur inferiorly. The gluteal region is bounded medially by a deep groove, the natal cleft, oriented longitudinally between the two buttocks. In the depth of the cleft is found the posterior surface of the sacrum, while inferiorly is the coccyx, and beyond this the perineum.

Below the gluteal sulcus extends the posterior thigh. More inferiorly is the space behind the knee joint, called the **popliteal fossa (ATLAS PLATES**

365, 394). The posterior thigh region contains the hamstring muscles and the large sciatic nerve.

With the body in the prone position (face down), elevate the buttocks and place a wooden block under the anterior surface of the pelvis. Study the posterior surface of the pelvis and the femur in an articulated skeleton and palpate or trace the following structures:

1. The **crest of the ilium,** which forms the upper border of the gluteal region (**ATLAS PLATES 267, 386**). Note that a line drawn between the highest points on the two iliac crests (**intertubercular line**) crosses the 4th lumbar vertebra (**ATLAS PLATE 267**).

2. The **anterior superior iliac spine,** by tracing the iliac crest forward to its anterior extremity (**ATLAS PLATES 267, 364 #364.1**).

3. The **posterior superior iliac spine** (**ATLAS PLATES 272 #272.1, 328**). This is located posteriorly, deep to a dimple in the skin 5 cm from the midline.

4. The **gluteus maximus muscle** and its overlying fat that form the contour of the gluteal region. Note that the curved **gluteal sulcus** separates the gluteal region from the posterior thigh inferiorly (**ATLAS PLATES 365 #365.1, 366 #366.2**).

5. The **ischial tuberosity,** a large, rounded bony prominence located on the inferior aspect of the pelvis. It can be felt on the cadaver by pressing your thumb upward just above the medial end of the gluteal crease (**ATLAS PLATES 265 #265.1, 267**). Because we sit on our ischial tuberosities, these bony structures can be palpated easily on ourselves.

6. The **greater trochanter** of the femur. This can be felt on the lower lateral aspect of the hip region as a rounded bony prominence 10 cm below the iliac crest (**ATLAS PLATES 273 #273.1, 432**). Knowledge of its location is important in the recognition of fractures of the hip or upper femur.

It is clinically significant to be able to visualize the course of the sciatic nerve so that it is not injured by intramuscular injections in the gluteal region or by longitudinal incisions along the posterior thigh (**Figure 20-1**).

On the cadaver visualize the gluteal region divided into four quadrants. Realize that only the upper lateral quadrant should be used for intramuscular injections.

◄
Grant's 363, 366
Netter's 468, 469
Rohen 435–438

◄
Grant's 365, 366
Netter's 476, 477
Rohen 454, 455

►
Grant's 372
Netter's 484
Rohen 485

◄
Grant's 362, 363
Netter's 468–471
Rohen 438, 439

◄
Grant's 366, 367, 372
Netter's 484, 527
Rohen 480, 483, 485

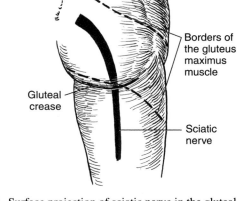

Figure 20-l. Surface projection of sciatic nerve in the gluteal region and upper thigh, posterior view.

This avoids injury to the sciatic nerve in the lower quadrants and the gluteal vessels and nerves in the upper medial quadrant (**ATLAS PLATE 389**).

At the gluteal crease palpate the ischial tuberosity with one hand and the greater trochanter with the other. Realize that the sciatic nerve enters the posterior thigh midway between these two bony structures. At this site it is covered only by skin and superficial fascia (**ATLAS PLATE 386**). The course of the sciatic nerve can now be imagined by tracing your finger down the middle of the posterior thigh to a point 10 cm superior to the knee joint, where the nerve often divides into two large branches (**ATLAS PLATE 387**). Along the upper half of the posterior thigh all branches from the sciatic nerve are directed medially. This makes the upper lateral quadrant of the posterior thigh relatively safe for longitudinal incisions.

B. **Skin Incisions** (**Figure 20-2**). The skin of the gluteal region is thick, is securely attached to superficial fascia, and often contains much fat. The superficial fascia contains the cutaneous nerves (see below), and it covers the **gluteus maximus muscle** that overlies most of the other gluteal structures (**ATLAS PLATE 382**). The skin and superficial fascia of the posterior thigh are continuous with those of the gluteal region and cover a thick strong aponeurosis over the hamstring muscles, called the **fascia lata.**

Make four incisions through the skin only. The cutaneous nerves will be dissected before the superficial fascia is reflected.

1. Make a curved incision from medial to lateral along the iliac crest (**Figure 20-2, A–B**). Start at

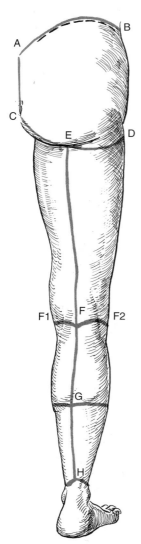

Figure 20-2. Incision lines: gluteal region and posterior thigh and leg.

the posterior superior iliac spine (L5) and course around to the anterior superior iliac spine.

2. Make a vertical incision in the midline of the lower back from the medial end of the first incision over the sacrum to the coccyx (**Figure 20-2, A–C**).

3. Make an oblique inferolateral incision from the tip of the coccyx, over the ischial tuberosity to the lateral part of the thigh, 10 cm below the greater trochanter (**Figure 20-2, C–D**). **Do not cut too deeply** because the **posterior femoral cutaneous nerve** descends just deep to the fascia below the border of the gluteus maximus muscle in the middle of the posterior thigh (**ATLAS PLATE 382**).

4. Make a vertical cut down the posterior thigh 3 cm medial to the midline of the thigh to avoid the posterior femoral cutaneous nerve (**Figure 20-2, E–F**). Carry the incision medially and laterally around the knee joint (**Figure 20-2, F1–F2**).

Reflect the skin from the gluteal and posterior thigh regions and dissect the cutaneous nerves.

C. **Cutaneous Nerves of the Gluteal Region.** Cutaneous nerves approach the gluteal region superiorly, medially, laterally, and inferiorly.

1. **Superiorly:** (a) lateral cutaneous branches of the subcostal (T12) and iliohypogastric (L1) nerves and (b) posterior primary rami of L1, -2, and -3 descend over the iliac crest. The subcostal and iliohypogastric branches descend laterally, and the posterior primary rami of L1, -2, and -3, medially. The latter three nerves are the **superior cluneal nerves (ATLAS PLATES 367 #367.2, 382).**

2. **Medially:** small posterior primary rami of the S1, -2, and -3 nerves supply the skin over the sacrum and medial part of the gluteus maximus muscle. These nerves are the **medial cluneal nerves (ATLAS PLATES 367 #367.2, 382).**

3. **Laterally:** lateral femoral cutaneous nerve branches supply the skin over the greater trochanter and posterolateral thigh (**ATLAS PLATES 367 #367.2, 382**).

4. **Inferiorly:** branches of the posterior femoral cutaneous nerve ascend to the gluteal region over the lower border of the gluteus maximus muscle. These are the **inferior cluneal nerves (ATLAS PLATES 367 #367.2, 382).**

D. **Cutaneous Nerves of the Posterior Thigh.** Branches of the posterior femoral cutaneous nerve (S1, -2, -3) are found in the superficial fascia of the posterior thigh. These supply skin down to the middle of the calf. In the thigh they are overlapped medially by cutaneous branches of the femoral nerve and laterally by branches from the lateral femoral cutaneous nerve (**ATLAS PLATE 367 #367.2**).

Thus, skin in the middle area of the posterior thigh is supplied by upper sacral segments, while both laterally and medially, the 2nd and 3rd lumbar segments innervate the skin. This break in sequential segmental innervation is important clinically to the neurologist trying to localize spinal lesion levels because two spinal cord

▶
Grant's 340
Netter's 527
Rohen 226, 229, 480

▶
Grant's 340
Netter's 527
Rohen 484

◀
Grant's 371
Netter's 485, 527
Rohen 483–485

segments (L4 and -5) are not represented between the field of the posterior femoral cutaneous nerve (S1, -2, -3) and the medial (L2, -3) and lateral (L2, -3) cutaneous fields of the overlapping nerves.

Make a transverse incision 15 cm long (6 inches) through the superficial fascia midway between the iliac crest and the gluteal crease. Cut only as deep as the obliquely coursing fibers of the gluteus maximus muscle. Before removing the upper part of this fascia, identify some of the five cutaneous nerve branches that descend over the iliac crest. The two most lateral are branches of the subcostal (T12) and iliohypogastric (L1) nerves. The three medial branches are posterior primary rami of S1, S2, and S3, called the **superior cluneal nerves (ATLAS PLATES 367 #367.2, 382)**. Reflect and remove the upper half of the superficial fascia over the gluteus maximus.

Before removing the lower half of the superficial fascia over the gluteus maximus find the **posterior femoral cutaneous nerve.** Probe through the fascia midway between the ischial tuberosity and the greater trochanter at the level of the gluteal crease. Note that the nerve descends deep to the lower border of the gluteus maximus into the thigh (**ATLAS PLATE 382**). Find branches of this nerve that ascend over the lower margin of the gluteus maximus (**inferior cluneal nerves**) and, more medially, the **perineal branch.** Reflect the lower fascia over the gluteus maximus, but preserve the posterior femoral cutaneous nerve.

Remove the superficial fascia over the posterior thigh by making an initial longitudinal incision 3 cm lateral to the midline of the thigh, but only as deep as the deep fascia. Extend the cut down to the lower end of the popliteal fossa, preserving the posterior femoral cutaneous nerve.

II. Gluteal Region

The muscles of the gluteal region serve as extensors, medial and lateral rotators, and abductors of the femur at the hip joint. Deep to the gluteus maximus are found the gluteus **medius** and **minimus** and five other muscles. Two take origin within the pelvis (the **piriformis** and **obturator internus**), then leave the pelvis and insert on the femur. The three others (**gemellus superior** and **inferior** and **quadratus femoris**) are small lateral rotators of the femur that arise on the spine and posterior surface of the ischium and insert laterally on the femur (**Figure 20-3**). All arteries and the nerves that supply these muscles enter the gluteal

▶
Grant's 186, 188, 294, 298, 299
Netter's 340, 341
Rohen 444, 445

◀
Grant's 340, 371
Netter's 527
Rohen 226, 480, 484

▶
Grant's 294, 298, 299
Netter's 340, 341
Rohen 438, 444

▶
Grant's 366–371
Netter's 476, 477, 484, 485
Rohen 454, 455
◀
Grant's 366–373
Netter's 477
Rohen 454, 456

region from the pelvis, and the veins drain into the pelvis along the same routes.

A. **Sacrotuberous and Sacrospinous Ligaments.** Deep to the gluteus maximus, the lower posterior surface of the pelvis is marked by a pointed bony process called the ischial spine, below which is located the ischial tuberosity (**ATLAS PLATE 272 #272.2**). The powerful **sacrotuberous** and **sacrospinous ligaments** attach the sacrum to these ischial bony processes and transform the notches above and below the ischial spine into the **greater** and **lesser sciatic foramina (ATLAS PLATES 271 #271.2, 272 #272.2).** Traversing these foramina are the muscles, nerves, and vessels that pass between the pelvis and the gluteal region.

The sacrotuberous ligament is a strong band that attaches the ischial tuberosity to the sides of the sacrum. It is directed vertically and medially. Its main function is to retain the inferior part of the sacrum in position and counteract the weight of the trunk at the lumbosacral and sacroiliac joints, because the trunk would tend to push the superior part of the sacrum forward and its inferior part backward. The sacrospinous ligament is triangular and is located anterior to the sacrotuberous ligament. It interconnects the spine of the ischium to the lower sacrum and coccyx and separates the greater and lesser sciatic foramina.

Look at the posterior surface of an articulated pelvis and identify the ischial spine. Envision the **sacrospinous ligament** attaching to the spine and crossing over to the lower segments of the sacrum and the coccyx (**ATLAS PLATES 270–273**). Note that the greater sciatic foramen is formed from the greater sciatic notch and is located above the ischial spine. Visualize the **sacrotuberous ligament** extending from the ischial tuberosity to the sacrum; it creates the lesser sciatic foramen (below the ischial spine) from the lesser sciatic notch.

B. **Gluteus Maximus Muscle.** The gluteus maximus muscle is broad and thick and is the largest muscle by weight in the body. It forms the contour and prominence of the buttocks (**ATLAS PLATES 383, 384, 385 #385.1**). It arises from the posterior surfaces of the ilium, sacrum, coccyx, and sacrotuberous ligament. Its fibers pass inferolaterally, become aponeurotic, and insert onto the iliotibial band. A bursa separates its insertion from the greater trochanter (**ATLAS PLATE 391**). Deeper fibers of the lower part of the muscle insert on the gluteal tuberosity of the femur.

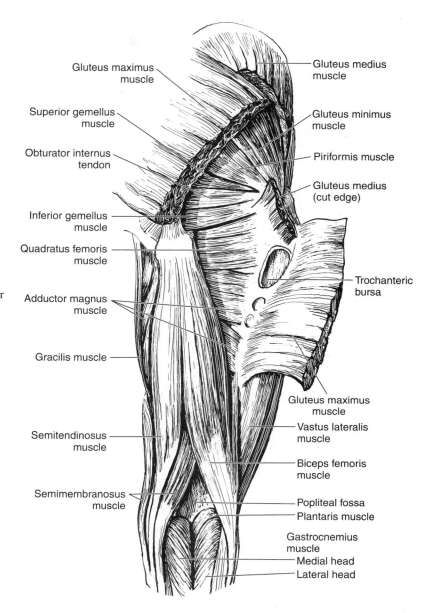

Figure 20-3. Muscles of the gluteal region and posterior thigh with gluteus maximus cut.

The gluteus maximus is a powerful extensor, adductor, and lateral rotator of the femur at the hip joint. When acting from below with the thigh fixed, it serves as an extensor of the flexed trunk. It is used more powerfully in running than in walking and, with the thigh fixed, in lifting heavy objects from the floor. Its insertion on the iliotibial tract helps balance the trunk by stabilizing the pelvis. The muscle is innervated by the inferior gluteal nerve (L5, S1, S2) but receives blood from both the inferior and superior gluteal arteries (**ATLAS PLATE 393**).

Remove the fascia from the surface of the gluteus maximus muscle. Define its superior border, and use your fingers and sharp dissection to separate the deep surface of the upper part of the muscle from underlying

◄
Grant's 366, 367
Netter's 477
Rohen 454

structures. Continue separating the lateral half of the muscle along this deep plane. **Cut the entire muscle vertically about 3 cm medial to its femoral insertion.**

Reflect the lateral part of the muscle and find the **trochanteric bursa** over the greater trochanter. Lift the medial part of the muscle, and separate its deep surface from the posterior femoral cutaneous and sciatic nerves (**ATLAS PLATE 393**). Identify and cut the inferior gluteal vessels and nerves entering the deep surface of its lower part and the superior gluteal vessels entering its upper part. Reflect the muscle mass medially over the ischial tuberosity and sacrotuberous ligament. Do not remove the muscle completely, but leave it attached along its most medial border.

C. Piriformis Muscle, Gluteal Vessels and Nerves, Sciatic Nerve. The triangular piriformis muscle enters the gluteal region from the pelvis through the greater sciatic foramen **(Figure 20-6)**. In the gluteal region, it crosses laterally to insert onto the greater trochanter of the femur **(ATLAS PLATES 287, 386)**. The piriformis muscle serves as the key to locating other structures in the gluteal region. Above its upper border emerging from the pelvis are the superior gluteal vessels and nerves, while below its lower border are the inferior gluteal vessels and nerves, the large sciatic nerve, the nerve to the quadratus femoris, the posterior femoral cutaneous nerve, and most medially, the internal pudendal vessels and pudendal nerve **(ATLAS PLATES 386, 387, 393)**.

◄
Grant's 367, 371
Netter's 484, 485
Rohen 481, 482

Define the superior border of the piriformis muscle. Identify the **superior gluteal** artery, vein, and nerve. Remove the vein and its branches to expose the artery and nerve. Below the inferior border of the piriformis remove the branches of the **inferior gluteal** vein and find the inferior gluteal artery and nerve. Note that the superior gluteal nerve and the superior and inferior gluteal vessels sent branches (now cut) into the gluteus maximus. Clean the large **sciatic nerve** and, more medially, the **posterior femoral cutaneous nerve.** Both of these emerge from the pelvis through the greater sciatic foramen below the piriformis muscle **(ATLAS PLATES 386, 393)**.

◄
Grant's 370, 371
Netter's 484
Rohen 483

The sciatic nerve is the largest nerve in the body (L4, -5; S1, -2, -3) and it consists of a **tibial** and a **common fibular** trunk **(Figure 20-6)**. Usually the two emerge as a single large nerve, but occasionally the fibular division pierces the piriformis muscle and joins the tibial portion below the muscle. Most often the sciatic nerve **does not** supply branches to the gluteal muscles. It **does** supply all of the muscles in the posterior compartment of the thigh, all of the muscles of the leg and foot, and the skin of the foot and much of the leg.

►
Grant's 367–371
Netter's 484
Rohen 481

Follow the trunk of the sciatic nerve into the thigh where it disappears deep to the long head of the biceps femoris muscle **(ATLAS PLATE 386)**.

D. Gluteus Medius and Gluteus Minimus Muscles. The **gluteus medius** is a broad, powerful muscle located above the piriformis muscle **(ATLAS PLATE 386)**. It arises from the posterior surface of the ilium and inserts on the lateral surface of the greater trochanter. Its inferior part is covered by the gluteus maximus. It is an abductor and medial rotator of the thigh when the pelvis is fixed and the

limb free to move. When acting from below, as in walking, the gluteus medius tilts its side of the pelvis laterally and downward, enough to raise the opposite hip joint and opposite foot off the ground.

The **gluteus minimus (Figure 20-4)** lies deep to the gluteus medius, and it arises from the posterior surface of the pelvis anterior to the gluteus medius **(ATLAS PLATES 391, 392)**. Its tendon inserts onto the greater trochanter, and its actions are similar to those of the gluteus medius. Both the gluteus medius and minimus are supplied by the superior gluteal nerve and artery **(ATLAS PLATE 387)**. The artery splits into a superficial branch that supplies the gluteus maximus muscle and a deep branch (joined by the superior gluteal nerve) that **courses forward in the plane between the gluteus medius and minimus.** This deep division of the artery and the nerve serves as a convenient guide to determine the plane of separation between the gluteus medius and minimus.

Identify the gluteus medius and remove the fascia from its outer surface. Separate its border from the piriformis muscle. With your fingers, follow the plane of the deep branches of the superior gluteal artery and nerve between the gluteus medius and minimus muscles. Upon separating the gluteus medius from the gluteus minimus, cut across the gluteus medius, using a curved incision about 5 cm above the greater trochanter **(ATLAS PLATE 391)**. Reflect the two parts of the muscle and expose the gluteus minimus.

►
Grant's 370, 371, 374
Netter's 479, 481
Rohen 471, 485

E. External Rotators, Pudendal Nerve, and Internal Pudendal Vessels. Below the piriformis muscle are five muscles, all of which serve as lateral rotators of the thigh **(ATLAS PLATE 391)**. These are, from above downward, the **superior gemellus,** the tendon of the **obturator internus,** the **inferior gemellus,** the **quadratus femoris,** and, deep (anterior) to the quadratus femoris, the **obturator externus (ATLAS PLATE 386)**.

►
Grant's 367, 371, 373
Netter's 477
Rohen 454, 456

◄
Grant's 367–371
Netter's 477, 485
Rohen 454, 456, 481

The **obturator internus muscle** arises within the pelvis from most of the inner surface of the obturator membrane **(ATLAS PLATE 282)**. Its tendon enters the gluteal region through the lesser sciatic foramen and courses laterally to the greater trochanter of the femur **(ATLAS PLATES 386, 387)**. Just superior to this tendon is located the **superior gemellus** and just inferior to it, the **inferior gemellus**. These two small muscles cross the gluteal region to insert on the greater trochanter **(ATLAS PLATES 391, 392)**. The four-sided **quadratus femoris** arises from the ischial tuberosity. Its fibers

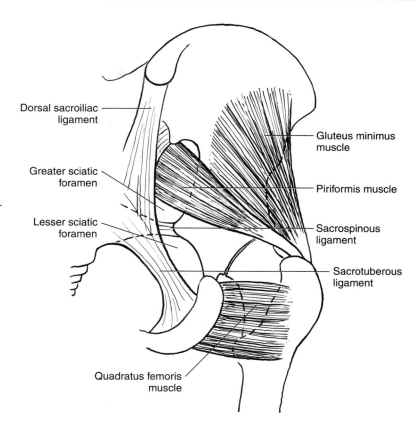

Figure 20-4. The gluteus minimus, piriformis, and quadratus femoris muscles.

extend horizontally to insert on the intertrochanteric crest of the femur below the greater trochanter (**ATLAS PLATES 391, 393, 431**).

The **obturator externus** arises from the anterior (external) surface of the fibrous membrane covering the obturator foramen. It is a fan-shaped muscle and its fibers course laterally deep (anterior) to the quadratus femoris across the neck of the femur to insert in the trochanteric fossa (**ATLAS PLATE 392**).

The **internal pudendal artery** accompanied by its vein, the **pudendal nerve,** and the nerve to the **obturator internus** muscle enter the most inferior part of the greater sciatic foramen (**Figure 20-5**). The pudendal vessels and nerve immediately cross the sacrospinous ligament and pass through the lesser sciatic foramen. Under cover of the obturator internus fascia (within the **pudendal canal**) they course to the perineal region (**Figure 20-6**). The nerve to the obturator internus sends an additional branch to the superior gemellus muscle. Another small nerve in this region is the **nerve to the quadratus femoris** and **inferior gemellus muscle.** It leaves the pelvis through the greater sciatic foramen ventral (deep) to the sciatic nerve.

Identify the **tendon of the obturator internus muscle** inferior to the piriformis muscle. Note that attached to its upper border is the small **superior**

◀ Grant's 228, 373, 376
Netter's 475, 521
Rohen 343, 453

◀ Grant's 215, 221, 370, 371
Netter's 373, 374, 484, 485
Rohen 481

▶ Grant's 330, 332–334
Netter's 484, 485
Rohen 492

◀ Grant's 367, 371, 373
Netter's 477, 485
Rohen 454, 456

gemellus muscle, and along its lower border, the **inferior gemellus muscle** (**ATLAS PLATES 386, 391**). Separate the three structures and note that the obturator internus tendon emerges from the pelvis and takes a right angle turn through the lesser sciatic foramen to enter the gluteal region. Trace the obturator tendon with the gemelli to their insertion on the greater trochanter. Cut the tendon and the gemelli at their insertion and retract them to the lesser sciatic foramen where a bursa lies adjacent to the bone (**ATLAS PLATE 392**).

Find the **internal pudendal vessels and nerve** emerging from the most medial part of the greater sciatic foramen. Follow these structures across the sacrospinous ligament as they enter the lesser sciatic foramen toward the perineum (**Figures 20-5 and 20-8**). Note that the pudendal nerve courses on the medial side of the artery, while lateral to the artery and adjacent to the bone is the small **nerve to the obturator internus.**

Identify and clean the **quadratus femoris muscle** below the inferior gemellus (**ATLAS PLATE 391**). Note that the sciatic nerve descends across its posterior surface. Separate the upper border of the quadratus from the inferior gemellus to expose the tendon of

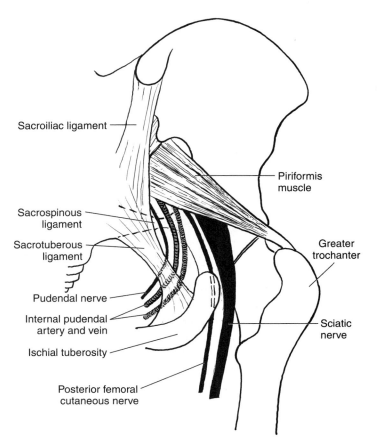

Figure 20-5. The sciatic and posterior femoral cutaneous nerves and the pudendal vessels and nerve emerging below the piriformis muscle.

Labels on figure: Sacroiliac ligament; Piriformis muscle; Sacrospinous ligament; Sacrotuberous ligament; Greater trochanter; Pudendal nerve; Internal pudendal artery and vein; Ischial tuberosity; Sciatic nerve; Posterior femoral cutaneous nerve

the **obturator externus muscle** more deeply between them (**ATLAS PLATE 392**). Expose the obturator externus more clearly by cutting the quadratus femoris near its insertion on the femur.

III. Posterior Compartment of the Thigh (Figures 20-6, 20-7)

The region between the hip joint and the knee joint is the **thigh,** and the part of the lower limb between the knee and ankle joints is called the **leg.** The posterior compartment, or back of the thigh, contains muscles that flex the leg at the knee joint and, upon continued action, extend the thigh at the hip joint (**Figure 20-9**). The **sciatic nerve** descends through the posterior thigh and it has already divided into tibial and common fibular nerves before reaching the back of the knee (**ATLAS PLATE 393**).

A. Posterior Thigh Muscles. Three muscles compose the posterior compartment of the thigh: the **biceps femoris,** the **semitendinosus,** and the **semimembranosus** (**ATLAS PLATES 384, 391, 392**). They are frequently referred to as the hamstring muscles. To be a hamstring, the muscle must (a) arise from

◄
Grant's 333–335, 367, 372
Netter's 477, 484, 485, 521
Rohen 453, 454, 456

◄
Grant's 366
Netter's 484, 522
Rohen 484, 485

►
Grant's 360, 369
Netter's 475, 521
Rohen 453

►
Grant's 366, 367, 372
Netter's 477
Rohen 455, 456

◄
Grant's 366, 367, 372
Netter's 477
Rohen 455, 456

the ischial tuberosity, (b) cross both the hip and knee joints, and (c) be innervated by the medial or tibial division of the sciatic nerve. Both the semitendinosus and semimembranosus as well as the long head of the biceps femoris fulfill these conditions, but the short head of the biceps does not, because it arises from the femur and is supplied by the lateral or fibular division of the sciatic nerve (**ATLAS PLATE 393**).

The most medial part of the **adductor magnus muscle** is also considered a hamstring. It arises from the ischial tuberosity and is supplied by the tibial division of the sciatic nerve. Its insertion, however, into the adductor tubercle on the medial condyle of the femur does not cross two joints. Its tendon is continuous and in direct line with the **tibial collateral ligament.** During development these were a single structure that did cross the knee joint to attach to the tibia (**ATLAS PLATE 437 #437.2**).

The **biceps femoris muscle** consists of long and short heads. The long head arises from the ischial tuberosity and passes obliquely downward to the lateral side of the posterior thigh. It crosses the sciatic nerve and joins the short head, which arises from the linea aspera of the femur (**ATLAS PLATES 392, 393**). The

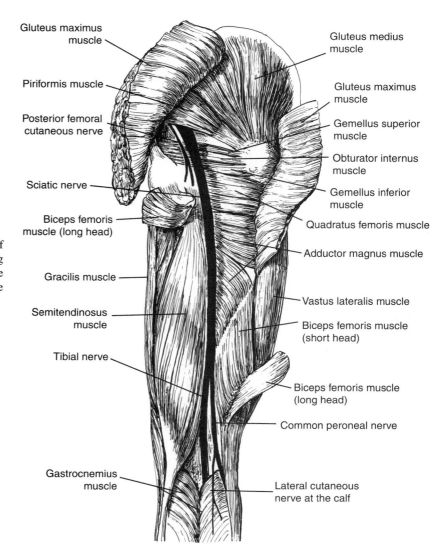

Figure 20-6. The posterior thigh. Note the course of the sciatic nerve with the gluteus maximus and long head of the biceps femoris cut. Observe that the nerve divides into common peroneal and tibial nerves above the popliteal fossa.

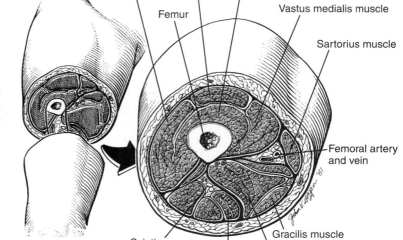

Figure 20-7. Cross section though the middle third of the thigh. Note the quadriceps muscles in the anterior (extensor) compartment, the hamstrings posteriorly, and the adductor magnus, gracilis, and the neurovascular structures medially.

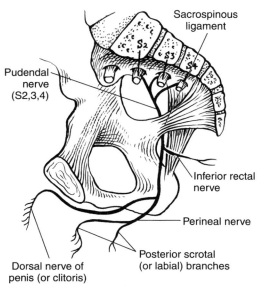

Figure 20-8. The course of the pudendal nerve from pelvis to perineum.

common tendon of insertion attaches to the lateral surface of the head of the fibula (**ATLAS PLATE 404**).

The **semitendinosus muscle** arises from the ischial tuberosity. Its muscle fibers end just below the middle of the thigh to form a long cylindrical tendon that descends on the surface of the semimembranosus muscle (**ATLAS PLATES 384, 391**). Its insertion on the medial surface of the tibia is located behind the tendons of the gracilis and sartorius muscles. The webbed expansion of these three tendons is called the **pes anserina** (goose's foot) and is frequently used surgically to strengthen the medial aspect of the knee joint (**ATLAS PLATE 414**).

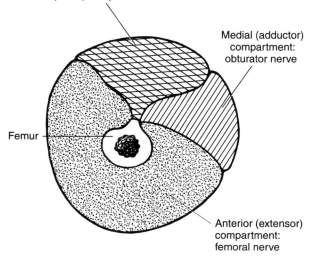

Figure 20-9. Cross section of thigh, showing its three compartments.

The **semimembranosus muscle** descends as a broad aponeurosis from the ischial tuberosity deep to the upper parts of the biceps and semitendinosus (**ATLAS PLATE 392**). Muscle fibers arise from this aponeurosis midway down the thigh and continue below the knee, where the semimembranous inserts on the medial condyle of the tibia (**ATLAS PLATE 414**). From this site expansions of the insertion course upward and laterally to form the **oblique popliteal ligament** that reinforces the posterior part of the joint capsule. Another expansion continues downward to form the fascia over the popliteus muscle (**ATLAS PLATE 418**).

> Remove the superficial fascia over the posterior thigh and sever the deep fascia vertically. Avoid cutting the posterior femoral cutaneous nerve (**ATLAS PLATE 382**). Open the posterior compartment and trace the sciatic nerve inferiorly from the gluteal region deep to the long head of the biceps femoris muscle. Pull the muscle to one side and find the **tibial** and **common fibular divisions** of the nerve below the middle of the thigh (**ATLAS PLATES 386, 393**).

▶
Grant's 367, 370,
371, 375
Netter's 584
Rohen 481, 485

B. Sciatic Nerve and Perforating Arteries in Posterior Thigh

1. **Sciatic nerve in the thigh.** In its descent in the thigh, the **sciatic nerve** lies along the posterior surface of the adductor magnus muscle (**ATLAS PLATE 393**). The nerve may divide into its tibial and common fibular divisions as high as the gluteal region, but usually this occurs in the middle of the thigh. It gives off branches to the three hamstring muscles and the medial (hamstring) portion of the adductor magnus. The branches that supply the hamstring muscles course medially from the tibial division of the sciatic nerve, whereas the branch to the short head of the biceps is directed laterally from the common fibular division (**Figure 20-10**).

The tibial division (L4, -5; S1, -2, -3) of the sciatic nerve is the larger of the two divisions. Beyond the split it descends through the middle of the posterior thigh and popliteal fossa (**ATLAS PLATE 393**). The common fibular division (L4, -5; S1, -2) courses obliquely laterally in the posterior thigh to the upper lateral side of the popliteal fossa. The sciatic nerve receives arterial branches from the inferior gluteal artery and from the perforating arteries (**ATLAS PLATE 393**).

▶
Grant's 346, 360
Netter's 484, 494
Rohen 467, 481

2. **Perforating arteries.** The posterior thigh does not have a large through-going artery descend-

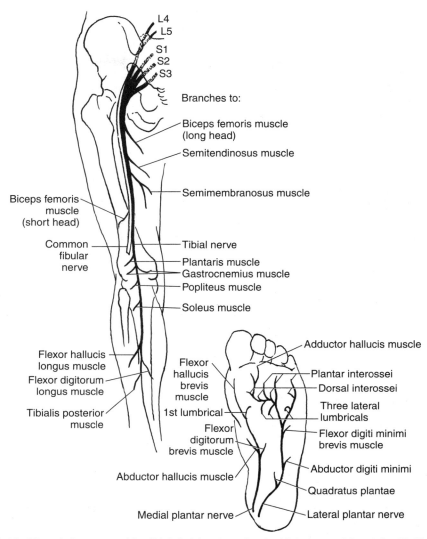

Figure 20-10. The sciatic nerve and its tibial division: branches in thigh, leg, and foot (after Hollinshead).

ing with the hamstring muscles. Instead, a series of vessels derived from the profunda femoral branch of the femoral artery on the anterior aspect of the thigh perforate the adductor magnus muscle to reach the posterior thigh. There are usually four **perforating arteries,** and they pass through the substance of the muscle close to the linea aspera of the femur (**ATLAS PLATES 377, 393**).

The perforating arteries anastomose with each other and with branches of the popliteal artery inferiorly. The first perforating artery also anastomoses superiorly with the inferior gluteal artery and the medial and lateral circumflex branches of the profunda femoral artery to form the **cruciate anastomosis.** This anastomosis supplies blood to the hip joint.

▶
Grant's 366, 367, 384, 385
Netter's 477, 484
Rohen 456, 485

Lift the long head of the biceps femoris and cut it away from the ischial tuberosity. Reflect the muscle to its junction with the short head that arises from the femur. Find the branch from the tibial nerve that supplies the long head and the branch from the common fibular division that supplies the short head (**ATLAS PLATE 393**).

Separate the semitendinosus from the underlying semimembranosus. Note that the long tendon of the semitendinosus overlies the lower muscular portion of the semimembranosus. Pick up the upper muscular part of the semitendinosus and examine the broad membranous tendon of the semimembranosus deep to it (**ATLAS PLATE 392**). Identify the nerve branches from the tibial division that supply these two muscles.

Detach both muscles from the ischial tuberosity to expose the adductor magnus. Find the branch from the sciatic nerve that supplies the medial part of the adductor magnus. It often comes from the branch that supplies the semimembranosus. See the broad insertion of the adductor magnus on the femur, and identify the perforating arteries that penetrate it to reach the posterior compartment (**ATLAS PLATE 363**).

Follow the insertion of the biceps femoris onto the bicipital tuberosity on the head of the fibula (**ATLAS PLATE 404**). Another small slip inserts on the lateral condyle of the tibia. Trace the insertion of the semitendinosus to the medial aspect of the tibia (**ATLAS PLATE 414**) and the insertion of the semimembranosus to the posterior surface of the medial tibial condyle. Observe that the latter insertion extends upward and laterally to form the **oblique popliteal ligament** and downward over the popliteus muscle (**ATLAS PLATE 418**).

IV. Popliteal Fossa (Figure 20-11)

A. Location and Boundaries. The popliteal fossa is a fat-filled, diamond-shaped space that lies behind

▶
Grant's 384, 385
Netter's 477, 484,
494, 522
Rohen 456, 485,
487, 488

◀
Grant's 361, 390,
391, 396, 397
Netter's 477, 488,
486, 493
Rohen 456–458,
478

▶
Grant's 386, 398,
399
Netter's 477, 494,
500
Rohen 466, 467,
487, 488

the knee joint. It extends superiorly behind the lower one-third of the femur and inferiorly behind the upper part of the tibia. Through the fossa course the popliteal vessels and the tibial and common fibular divisions of the sciatic nerve (often called **medial** and **lateral popliteal nerves** in this region). **Superiorly,** the popliteal fossa is bounded by the biceps femoris muscle laterally and by the semitendinosus and semimembranosus muscles medially. **Inferiorly** the two bellies of the gastrocnemius muscle and the small plantaris muscle form the medial and lateral borders of the fossa (**ATLAS PLATE 395 #395.2**).

B. Popliteal Vessels. The **popliteal artery** is the continuation of the femoral artery. It enters the popliteal fossa through the hiatus in the adductor magnus muscle at the superior apex of the diamond-shaped space (**ATLAS PLATES 395 #395.2, 396**). The vessel descends through the popliteal fossa and, at the lower border of the popliteus muscle, bifurcates into the anterior and posterior tibial arteries (**ATLAS PLATES 396, 419**).

The popliteal artery supplies branches to the muscles that bound the popliteal fossa, and it gives rise to

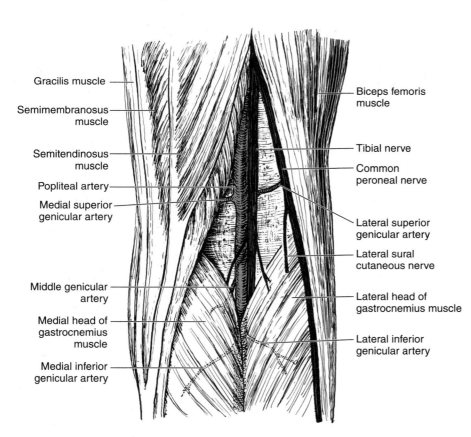

Figure 20-11. The popliteal fossa.

genicular branches that supply the knee joint (**ATLAS PLATES 396, 397**). There are usually five of these: two **superior genicular** (medial and lateral), a **middle genicular,** and two **inferior genicular** (medial and lateral) branches. An anastomosis around the knee joint includes these vessels, the **descending genicular artery** from the femoral artery (**ATLAS PLATES 363, 377, 379**), and the **anterior** and **posterior tibial recurrent branches** that ascend from the **anterior and posterior tibial arteries** in the upper leg (**ATLAS PLATE 363**).

The **popliteal vein** lies superficial to the artery in the popliteal fossa, and it is closely bound to it by connective tissue. It forms near the lower border of the popliteus muscle at the junction of the **anterior and posterior tibial veins.** Ascending through the popliteal fossa, it enters the adductor canal to become the femoral vein. The popliteal vein receives the **small saphenous vein** (**ATLAS PLATE 412**) and the **genicular veins** that accompany the genicular arteries.

C. Common Fibular and Tibial Nerves (Lateral and Medial Popliteal).

Deep to the biceps femoris muscle, about midway down the thigh, the sciatic nerve divides into the common fibular and tibial nerves.

The **common fibular nerve** courses obliquely along the lateral side of the popliteal fossa, crosses the lateral head of the gastrocnemius muscle, and leaves the fossa by winding around the neck of the fibula (**ATLAS PLATES 393, 402**). It passes deep to the fibularis longus muscle, where it divides into the superficial and deep fibular nerves (**ATLAS PLATE 402**). The common fibular nerve gives rise to **articular branches** and to two cutaneous branches. These are the **lateral sural cutaneous nerve,** which supplies the posterolateral aspect of the leg, and a **communicating branch** that joins the **medial sural cutaneous nerve** (from the tibial nerve) to form the **sural nerve** (**ATLAS PLATE 412**). The latter nerve accompanies the small saphenous vein along the calf.

The **tibial nerve** descends into the popliteal fossa and continues inferiorly along the same line as the sciatic nerve (**ATLAS PLATE 393**). It lies posterior to the popliteal vein and is the most superficial of the large popliteal neurovascular structures (**ATLAS PLATE 394**). As it enters the fossa, it lies lateral to the vessels, but in its descent, it crosses the posterior surface of the vessels from lateral to medial. The tibial nerve sends motor branches to both bellies of the **gastrocnemius muscle** and to the small **plantaris muscle.** In the lower part of the popliteal fossa it also supplies the **popliteus** and **soleus muscles** (**ATLAS PLATES 416, 417**).

▶
Grant's 340, 342, 343, 384
Netter's 522, 527
Rohen 469, 487

◀
Grant's 342–344, 354
Netter's 477, 498, 499
Rohen 467, 485, 487, 490

▶
Grant's 306, 361, 366, 416
Netter's 488, 489, 498
Rohen 457, 458

◀
Grant's 384–386
Netter's 484, 498, 522, 523
Rohen 467, 485, 487

▶
Grant's 348, 384, 385
Netter's 522, 527
Rohen 469, 489

▶
Grant's 385, 418, 419
Netter's 522, 523
Rohen 467, 485, 487

◀
Grant's 385, 417, 419
Netter's 522, 523
Rohen 487, 490, 491

▶
Grant's 384, 386
Netter's 477, 484, 494, 500
Rohen 485, 487, 488

The tibial nerve gives three articular branches (sensory) to the knee joint, which course with the middle and medial genicular arteries, and it contributes to cutaneous innervation in the leg by giving off the **medial sural cutaneous nerve** which helps form the **sural nerve** (**ATLAS PLATE 412**).

Incise the skin down the middle of the popliteal region and posterior leg to the ankle (**Figure 20-2, F–H**). Make lateral and medial skin incisions at both the midcalf and ankle levels (**Figure 20-2, G and H**) and reflect the skin flaps laterally and medially. Be careful not to sever the **small saphenous vein,** which is accompanied by the **sural nerve** along the lower third of the calf (**ATLAS PLATE 412**).

Follow the small saphenous vein to its entrance into the **popliteal vein** and remove fat from the fossa with probe and forceps in a piecemeal manner.

Define the tendons of the hamstring muscles to their insertions. Expose the medial and lateral heads of the gastrocnemius muscle inferiorly as well as the belly of the small plantaris muscle located above and medial to the lateral head of the gastrocnemius (**ATLAS PLATE 395 #395.2**). Identify two tendons that insert onto the tibia anterior to the insertion of the **semitendinosus.** These are the **gracilis** and the **sartorius muscles** (**ATLAS PLATE 414**).

Identify and free the **common fibular nerve** that courses obliquely in the popliteal space (**ATLAS PLATE 394 #394.2**). Identify its communicating branch to the **sural nerve** and the lateral sural cutaneous nerves that branch from the main trunk. Follow the common fibular nerve as it winds around the head of the fibula deep to the fibularis longus muscle. Note that it is vulnerable to injury at this site because it lies immediately under the skin and adjacent to bone (**ATLAS PLATE 404**).

Follow the **tibial nerve** down the middle of the popliteal fossa and find motor branches from it that descend to the two heads of the gastrocnemius muscle and to the plantaris muscle. Slightly lower, find a branch to the soleus muscle (**ATLAS PLATE 416**). Additionally, find the cutaneous branch that helps form the **sural nerve** within the sulcus between the two heads of the gastrocnemius muscle (**ATLAS PLATE 412**).

Deep (i.e., anterior) to the tibial nerve find the **popliteal vein and artery.** Separate these two vessels by opening the connective tissue vascular sheath that surrounds them. Then identify the **genicular branches** (2 superior, 1 middle, and 2 inferior) of the popliteal artery (**ATLAS PLATE 396 #396.1**). Cut away the tributaries of the popliteal vein to make this easier.

The following will help you identify the genicular arteries (**see ATLAS PLATE 396 #396.1**).

The **superior medial genicular** arises from the popliteal artery above the medial condyle of the femur. It courses medially around to the anterior aspect of the knee superior to the gastrocnemius and deep to the semimembranosus.

The **superior lateral genicular** arises superior to the lateral condyle of the femur. It courses laterally above the gastrocnemius and passes beneath the biceps femoris and ascends to the lower thigh.

The **middle genicular** is a short vessel that arises from the deep surface of the popliteal artery in the midregion of the popliteal fossa. It courses anteriorly and pierces the oblique popliteal ligament and articular capsule to enter the joint cavity.

The **inferior medial genicular** courses obliquely inferiorly and medially deep to the gastrocnemius muscle, along the upper margin of the popliteus muscle to reach the front of the leg (**ATLAS PLATE 417**).

The **inferior lateral genicular** courses deep to the lateral head of the gastrocnemius over the surface of the popliteus muscle. It reaches the front of the leg by coursing deep to the fibular collateral ligament superior to the head of the fibula.

◄
Grant's 386, 398, 399
Netter's 494, 500
Rohen 487, 488

Study the floor of the popliteal fossa. Observe that the upper one-third is bony and formed by the popliteal surface of the femur and that the middle one-third is formed by the posterior surface of the capsule of the knee joint.

Clean the fascia away from the surface of the flat **popliteus muscle** and note

1. That it forms the floor of the inferior third of the popliteal fossa (**ATLAS PLATES 418, 421**)

2. That the nerve to the popliteus muscle (from the tibial) descends over the muscle and then turns around its distal border to enter its anterior surface.

3. That the popliteus arises from the lateral condyle of the femur, the lateral part of the joint capsule, and the lateral meniscus (**ATLAS PLATES 418, 438 #438.1, 440**). Its fibers cross the floor of the popliteal fossa to insert on the posteromedial surface of the tibia above the soleus (**ATLAS PLATE 418**).

◄
Grant's 367, 375, 386, 397, 414
Netter's 499, 500, 523
Rohen 457, 460

Clinical Relevance

Superior gluteal nerve injury. This injury causes a weakening in abduction of the thigh by diminishing the function of the gluteus medius and minimus muscles. The result is a characteristic gluteus medius limp in which the person compensates by bending the trunk to the affected weakened side. When the person walks, the pelvis on the side with the defect is unsupported and it descends because the gluteal muscle is denervated. A waddling gait is described and is referred to as a positive Trendelenburg gait.

Intramuscular injections. The gluteal region is a common site for the intramuscular injection of drugs because the gluteus maximus is a thick muscle. The upper lateral quadrant is the safest site for these injections. Injections in the inferior medial or lateral quadrants can endanger the gluteal vessels and nerves.

Trochanteric bursitis. The bursa overlying the greater trochanter can become inflamed, resulting in a painful bursitis. This condition can occur from overuse or excessive straining of the gluteus maximus muscle. Acts such as lifting oneself repeatedly, as in climbing stairs or walking on a steep treadmill for a long time, can result in inflammation of the trochanteric bursa.

Compression of the sciatic nerve. The sciatic nerve enters the gluteal region through the greater sciatic foramen immediately inferior to the piriformis muscle. At this site the muscle can put pressure on the nerve in persons that use the gluteal muscle excessively, such as professional sports figures.

Hamstring injury. A pulled hamstring is a common sports injury. These often result from straining or tears of the tendinous origin of the muscle from the ischial tuberosity. Another hamstring injury is the extravasation of blood into a hamstring muscle, resulting in painful flexion of the leg at the knee joint. This is commonly referred to as a "charley horse."

Baker's cyst. This is a swelling in the popliteal fossa caused by the extravasation of synovial fluid from the synovial cavity of the knee joint.

Popliteal aneurysm. Aneurysm of the popliteal artery is thought to result from the constant flexion of the leg at the knee joint and the stretching and weakening of the arterial wall. This may enlarge significantly and, perhaps, be misdiagnosed as a Baker's cyst.

Popliteal abscesses. These infections within the popliteal fossa are painful because the tough popliteal fascia contains many pain nerve endings. The abscesses tend to spread superiorly into the inferior part of the posterior thigh or inferiorly into the posterior compartment of the leg.

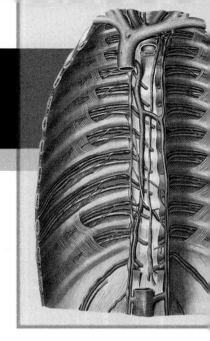

DISSECTION #21

Anterior and Medial Compartments of the Thigh

OBJECTIVES

1 Study the surface anatomy and dissect the superficial vessels and nerves of the anterior and medial thigh, the fascia lata, and its tensor.

2 Dissect the femoral triangle and its contents; trace the femoral and deep femoral vessels; open the adductor canal and identify its contents.

3 Dissect the quadriceps femoris muscle in the anterior compartment and identify the motor branches from the femoral nerve that supply its four heads.

4 Dissect the muscles and nerves of the medial or adductor region of the thigh.

Atlas Key:

Clemente Atlas, 5th Edition = Atlas Plate #

Grant's Atlas, 11th Edition = Grant's Page #

Netter's Atlas, 3rd Edition = Netter's Plate #

Rohen Atlas, 6th Edition = Rohen Page #

The anterior and medial compartments of the thigh contain muscles that act on the hip and/or knee joints. Of the **anterior compartment muscles** (**ATLAS PLATE 371**), the **sartorius, rectus femoris,** part of the **quadriceps femoris,** and **tensor fasciae latae** act across both joints. The **vastus lateralis, vastus medialis,** and **vastus intermedius** portions of the quadriceps femoris act only at the knee joint. The **iliopsoas** arises in the pelvis, inserts on the femur, and acts only across the hip joint (**ATLAS PLATE 374**). Coursing through the anterior compartment are the **femoral artery** and **vein** and the **femoral nerve** (**ATLAS PLATE 372**).

The **medial compartment** contains muscles that adduct the thigh at the hip joint (**adductors longus, brevis,** and **magnus**). The **gracilis muscle** also crosses the knee joint and adducts the thigh and flexes and medially rotates the leg (**ATLAS PLATES 374, 375,**

◄
Grant's 354, 355, 357, 360
Netter's 474, 482
Rohen 452, 480

►
Grant's 350, 353, 354
Netter's 241
Rohen 474

378). The medial compartment also contains the short **pectineus muscle**, the obturator artery, and nerves that supply this region (**ATLAS PLATE 379**).

I. Surface Anatomy; Superficial Vessels and Nerves

Before dissecting the anterior and medial thigh, examine its surface anatomy.

A. Surface Anatomy. Using **ATLAS PLATES 366 #366.1, 368–372** as guides, identify or outline the surface projections of the following:

> **1.** The **fold of the groin** and the **inguinal ligament.** The oblique fold of the groin is a flexion crease of skin and fascia, and it should not be mistaken for the inguinal ligament. Note that the ligament is the inferior border of the aponeurosis of the external oblique muscle folded internally on itself. Palpate the attachments of the ligament: **anterior superior iliac spine** laterally and **pubic tubercle** medially (**ATLAS PLATES 178, 179**). Note that the fold of the groin is somewhat more

transverse and lies 5 cm below the anterior superior iliac spine but only 2.5 cm below the pubic tubercle.

2. **Surface Projection of the Femoral Vessels and Nerve.** Identify the midinguinal point (midway between the anterior superior iliac spine and the pubic tubercle). Visualize the **femoral artery** descending from the pelvis just medial to this point. Note that medial to the artery courses the **femoral vein** (**ATLAS PLATES 372, 377**) and immediately lateral to the artery descends the large **femoral nerve** (**ATLAS PLATE 372**).

3. Compare the anterior femoral region on your cadaver with **ATLAS PLATES 364 #364.1, 370, and 372**. Outline the surface projection of the femoral triangle: **superiorly,** the inguinal ligament; **medially,** the adductor longus muscle; **laterally,** the sartorius muscle. On **ATLAS PLATE 371** note that the iliopsoas, pectineus, and adductor longus muscles form the floor of the triangle and that the femoral neurovascular structures traverse it (**ATLAS PLATE 372**).

B. Superficial Vessels and Nerves: The superficial fascia of the upper anterior thigh contains numerous superficial veins, inguinal lymph nodes, and cutaneous nerves. Make the following incisions and reflect the skin.

Incise the skin from the anterior superior iliac spine along a line parallel but slightly below the inguinal ligament (**Figure 21-1, A–B**). Then make a vertical cut along the middle of the anterior thigh that extends down to a site 5 cm below the patella (**Figure 21-1, C–D**). From this lower point, cut laterally and medially around the leg to calf (**Figure 21-1, D–E and D–F**). Reflect the skin flaps and expose the superficial fascia.

1. **Superficial Fascia and the Great Saphenous Vein.** The outer fatty layer of superficial fascia is continuous with Camper's fascia on the anterior abdominal wall. In contrast, the deeper membranous layer of superficial fascia of the anterior abdominal wall (Scarpa's fascia) fuses with the fascia lata of the thigh along a line below the inguinal ligament. If urine is extravasated from a ruptured urethra in the perineum, it can spread over the anterior abdominal wall deep to Scarpa's fascia. It is, however, prevented from passing into the anterior thigh because Scarpa's fascia fuses to the fascia lata.

◄ Grant's 342, 352–354
Netter's 482, 483
Rohen 466, 474

◄ Grant's 354, 355
Netter's 474
Rohen 452

► Grant's 342, 350
Netter's 526, 528
Rohen 478, 479

◄ Grant's 340, 342, 350, 351
Netter's 520, 526, 528
Rohen 468, 476, 479

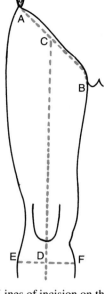

Figure 21-1. Lines of incision on the anterior thigh.

The **great saphenous vein** arises from a venous plexus on the medial surface of the foot (**ATLAS PLATE 398**). It ascends 2 cm anterior to the medial malleolus to the medial side of the knee and enters the thigh. It inclines laterally on the thigh and passes through the saphenous opening of the fascia lata to enter the femoral vein (**ATLAS PLATE 368**). In the upper medial thigh the great saphenous vein receives three small tributaries: the **superficial epigastric** and **superficial iliac circumflex,** which drain the lower anterior abdominal wall, and the **superficial external pudendal,** which drains the scrotum and skin of the penis (**Figure 21-2**). Small arteries with the same names accompany these veins (**ATLAS PLATES 9, 368**). These superficial veins anastomose with the **thoracoepigastric vein** to establish an important venous connection between the femoral and axillary veins (**ATLAS PLATES 9, 20**). This communication between veins that drain into the inferior vena cava and the superior vena cava allows passage of venous blood from one drainage system into the other in the event that either vena cava becomes blocked.

The great saphenous vein contains between 10 and 20 valves along its course. These valves and others between the superficial and deep veins of the lower limb may become incompetent and cause engorgement of the great saphenous vein. This venous stasis may result in ulceration and the painful condition of **varicose veins.**

Dissect the great saphenous vein along the medial thigh and note that several accessory veins drain into it as it ascends to the groin (**Figure 21-2**). Find the

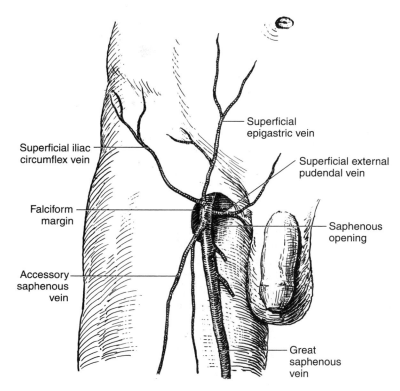

Figure 21-2. The superficial veins in the groin.

Superficial iliac circumflex vein

Falciform margin

Accessory saphenous vein

Superficial epigastric vein

Superficial external pudendal vein

Saphenous opening

Great saphenous vein

following three smaller veins in the upper thigh that drain into the great saphenous vein (**ATLAS PLATES 368, 370**): (a) the **superficial circumflex iliac** (coursing medially and inferiorly from the anterior superior iliac spine), (b) the **superficial epigastric** (descending over the inguinal region), and (c) the **superficial external pudendal** (draining the upper medial thigh and scrotum or labium majus).

About 4 cm inferior to the pubic tubercle, identify the saphenous opening and the saphenous vein passing through it to join the femoral vein (**ATLAS PLATE 369 #369.2**). Clean the sharp lateral border of the saphenous opening (called the **falciform margin**) anterior to the femoral sheath. Note the loose connective tissue (called the **cribriform fascia**) overlying the opening.

Open a segment of the saphenous vein with scissors to visualize one or more of its bicuspid venous valves (see **ATLAS PLATE 16 #16.1**).

The saphenous opening is important because an enlarging femoral hernia can penetrate through the loose fascia and become subcutaneous at this site.

2. **Superficial nerves of the anterior thigh.** The cutaneous nerves that supply most of the anterior thigh (**ATLAS PLATE 367 #367.1**) are the **lateral femoral cutaneous nerve** (L2, -3) and the **anterior cutaneous branches of the femoral**

◄ Grant's 342, 350–353 Netter's 526, 528 Rohen 466, 479

► Grant's 340 Netter's 526 Rohen 478, 479

► Grant's 340, 344 Netter's 528 Rohen 479

◄ Grant's 340 Netter's 526 Rohen 478, 479

nerve (L2, -3, -4). Smaller areas of the uppermost thigh (**ATLAS PLATE 367 #367.1**) are supplied, from lateral to medial, by the **iliohypogastric nerve** (L1), the **femoral branch of the genitofemoral nerve** (L1, -2), the **ilioinguinal nerve** (L1), and, most medially, the **cutaneous branch of the obturator nerve** (L2, -3, -4).

Guided by **ATLAS PLATE 368** probe the fascia longitudinally adjacent to the great saphenous vein and find the **anterior cutaneous branches of the femoral nerve** piercing the fascia lata. More medial branches perforate the deep fascia inferiorly. Free the nerves from the fascia and **cut them distally.**

Find the **lateral femoral cutaneous nerve** by probing the superficial fascia 7–10 cm below and medial to the anterior superior iliac spine (**ATLAS PLATE 367 #367.1**). Cut it distally also.

Look for some of the superficial inguinal lymph nodes within the superficial fascia (**ATLAS PLATE 369**). These are more readily seen in younger subjects. Although variable in number, they may be found below the inguinal ligament adjacent to the saphenous opening.

Reflect the superficial fascia from the anterior and medial thigh to expose the deep fascia, or **fascia lata** (**ATLAS PLATE 370**).

3. **Fascia lata, tensor fasciae latae, femoral sheath.** The broad deep fascia of the thigh (**fascia lata**) is a strong fibrous layer that invests all of the thigh muscles. It varies in thickness in different regions. Over the adductor muscles medially and over the hamstrings posteriorly it is relatively thin, but laterally it is remarkably thick and strong, forming the **iliotibial tract** that descends to the knee (**ATLAS PLATE 370**). Superiorly, the iliotibial tract encases the tensor fasciae latae muscle, and most of the gluteus maximus muscle inserts into it. Inferiorly, the iliotibial tract attaches to the patella, lateral condyle of the tibia, and head of the fibula.

The **tensor fasciae latae** is a thick, short muscle in the upper lateral aspect of the thigh (**ATLAS PLATE 371**). Its longitudinal fibers arise from the iliac crest and the anterior superior iliac spine and insert into the iliotibial tract 5 cm inferior to the greater trochanter. It is supplied by a branch of the superior gluteal nerve, and its pulling action on the iliotibial tract helps maintain extension of the leg at the knee joint.

The **femoral sheath** is an inferior prolongation of the **fascia transversalis** anterior to the femoral vessels. The **iliopsoas fascia** descends behind the vessels. These fascial layers form a funnel-shaped sheath around the femoral vessels for a distance of 4 to 5 cm below the inguinal ligament (**Figure 21-3**), but it does not surround the femoral nerve.

The femoral sheath allows the vessels to glide freely deep to the inguinal ligament during movement of the thigh at the hip joint. The most medial compartment of the femoral sheath, called the **femoral canal,** contains some extraperitoneal fat and a deep inguinal lymph node. The canal may be the site of herniation of a loop of bowel

◄
Grant's 350, 352, 353, 365
Netter's 241–243, 510
Rohen 452, 455, 480

►
Grant's 101, 350, 352–354
Netter's 241, 252, 482, 526, 528
Rohen 217, 218, 479

◄
Grant's 355, 357–359
Netter's 474, 476, 482, 483
Rohen 452, 455, 481

◄
Grant's 350, 352, 353
Netter's 242, 243, 252, 482, 528
Rohen 215, 218, 219

into the thigh, resulting in a **femoral hernia,** which occurs most often during childbearing. Superiorly, the upper entrance into the femoral canal (femoral ring) is larger in women than in men, and this type of hernia is three times more frequent in females than in males.

Cut the margins of the saphenous opening and follow the **great saphenous vein** to its entrance into the **femoral vein** by opening the femoral sheath (**ATLAS PLATE 369 #369.2**). Laterally expose the **femoral artery** and visualize the femoral canal medially. Observe that septa of the sheath form separate compartments for the femoral artery, femoral vein, and femoral canal. Insert a probe upward in the femoral canal and note that the inguinal ligament lies anterior to the probe, the pectineus fascia lies posterior, the femoral vein lateral, and the lacunar ligament medial (**ATLAS PLATE 369 #369.2**). To feel the sharp edge of the lacunar ligament insert a finger in the femoral canal and press medially.

Dissect the fascia in the floor of the femoral triangle and expose the vessels and muscles more completely. Uncover the sartorius muscle by cutting open the fascia overlying it (**ATLAS PLATES 370, 371**).

II. Femoral Triangle; Femoral Vessels and Their Branches; Adductor Canal; Femoral Nerve

The femoral nerve, artery, and vein course through the femoral triangle. Inferiorly, the vessels traverse the **adductor canal** accompanied by two branches of the femoral nerve: the **saphenous nerve** and the **nerve to the vastus medialis** (**ATLAS PLATES 372, 377**).

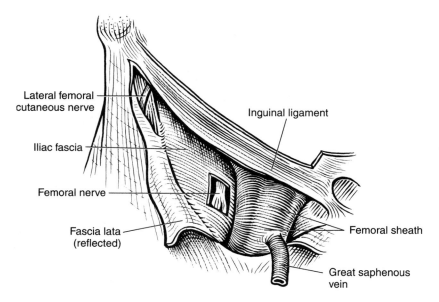

Figure 21-3. The femoral sheath surrounding the femoral vessels.

Lateral femoral cutaneous nerve

Iliac fascia

Femoral nerve

Fascia lata (reflected)

Inguinal ligament

Femoral sheath

Great saphenous vein

Because of their superficial location, these neuro-vascular structures, covered only by soft tissues, are especially vulnerable to injury.

A. Femoral Triangle. The femoral triangle is an area bounded **superiorly** by the **inguinal ligament, laterally** by the medial border of the **sartorius muscle,** and **medially** by the medial border of the **adductor longus muscle (ATLAS PLATE 372).** The apex of the triangle is directed downward and leads to a fascial tunnel called the **adductor** (or subsartorial) **canal (ATLAS PLATE 377).**

> Remove the fascia from the sartorius and adductor longus muscles. Note that with the inguinal ligament they bound the **femoral triangle (ATLAS PLATE 372).** Clean and separate the femoral vessels. Behind them identify from lateral to medial the **iliacus, psoas major** (iliopsoas), and **pectineus muscles.** These form the floor of the triangle and the adductor longus its medial border (**ATLAS PLATE 374**).

B. Femoral Vessels and Their Branches. The **femoral artery** is the continuation of the external iliac artery below the inguinal ligament. It courses down two-thirds of the thigh and then pierces the adductor magnus muscle to reach the popliteal fossa behind the knee (**ATLAS PLATE 363**). In its descent the vessel lies on the psoas major, the pectineus, and, more inferiorly, the adductor longus (**ATLAS PLATES 372, 377**). Just below the inguinal ligament, the artery usually gives off four small superficial branches: the **superficial iliac circumflex,** the **superficial epigastric,** and the **superficial** and **deep external pudendal (ATLAS PLATES 9, 368).**

The large **profunda femoris artery** arises from the posterolateral aspect of the femoral artery 3 to 4 cm below the inguinal ligament (**ATLAS PLATES 377, 379**). Two vessels, the **lateral** and **medial femoral circumflex arteries** frequently (55% of cadavers) branch from the profunda femoris (**ATLAS PLATE 379**). If the profunda femoris arises somewhat lower in the femoral triangle, the lateral femoral circumflex branches directly from the femoral (14% of cadavers). In other cadavers the medial femoral circumflex arises directly from the femoral artery (22% of specimens).

The profunda femoris descends posterior to the adductor longus muscle. From it are derived muscular branches, among which are four **perforating arteries.** These perforate the adductor magnus to enter the posterior thigh and supply the hamstring muscles (**ATLAS PLATE 363**).

The **femoral vein** is the superior continuation of the popliteal vein. In the adductor canal it lies behind and slightly lateral to the artery. As it ascends, the vein

◄
Grant's 354, 355, 357
Netter's 474
Rohen 452, 479, 480

►
Grant's 346, 354, 360, 364
Netter's 482, 483, 494
Rohen 466, 480, 481

◄
Grant's 354, 355, 357
Netter's 474
Rohen 452, 480

◄
Grant's 346, 354, 382
Netter's 482, 494
Rohen 466

►
Grant's 382, 383
Netter's 486

◄
Grant's 352–354
Netter's 482, 526
Rohen 466, 468

crosses behind the artery to its medial location in the upper part of the femoral triangle (**ATLAS PLATE 377**). The femoral vein receives the profunda femoral vein and the great saphenous vein. The medial and lateral femoral circumflex veins may drain into either the femoral or the profunda femoral vein (**ATLAS PLATE 379**).

> Place a wooden block behind the knee to reduce tension in the upper thigh. Separate the femoral vein from the femoral artery in the femoral triangle. Identify the **profunda femoris artery** and **vein** located behind the main trunk of the femoral artery and posterior to the adductor longus muscle. Retain the femoral and great saphenous veins, but cut away their tributaries to follow the arteries better. Identify the **medial** and **lateral femoral circumflex arteries** (**ATLAS PLATE 379**), but remove their accompanying veins. Determine the source and pattern of the femoral circumflex arteries in your cadaver.

1. **The cruciate anastomosis.** The **cruciate anastomosis** is formed by branches from the internal iliac artery and others from the femoral artery around the hip region. It involves descending branches from the **superior** and **inferior gluteal arteries,** the **ascending branch of the first perforating artery,** and transverse branches from both the **medial** and **lateral femoral circumflex arteries.** If the external iliac or femoral artery proximal to the profunda femoris branch is blocked or needs to be ligated, blood can still reach the lower limb from the internal iliac artery into the gluteal arteries and then, through the cruciate anastomosis, to vessels below the femoral artery. The pathway between the gluteal vessels and the femoral artery is through the ascending branch of the first perforating artery and then the transverse branches of the femoral circumflex arteries.

2. **The trochanteric anastomosis.** The important **trochanteric anastomosis** provides most of the blood to the head of the femur. In this formation descending branches from the superior and inferior gluteal arteries join with ascending branches from the medial and lateral femoral circumflex arteries on the greater trochanter and trochanteric fossa of the femur. Longitudinal branches ascend along the femoral neck and course beneath the retinacular capsule of the hip joint to supply the head of the femur. A small branch from the obturator artery accompanies the ligament of the head of the femur to help supply the femoral head in young people, but in the aged this vessel is rarely functional, and the trochanteric anastomosis becomes the essential source of blood for the head of the femur.

C. Adductor Canal. The **adductor canal** (or **sub-sartorial canal**) is a narrow muscular tunnel in the lower medial thigh behind the fascia of the sartorius muscle (**ATLAS PLATES 374, 377**). The canal extends from the apex of the femoral triangle down to an opening in the adductor magnus muscle, the **adductor hiatus.** The canal communicates with the popliteal fossa and through it course the femoral vessels. Also found within the canal are the **saphenous nerve** and the **nerve to the vastus medialis,** both branches of the femoral nerve (**ATLAS PLATE 377**).

> Lift the sartorius muscle from its fascial sheath. Divide the fascia on the deep surface of the muscle longitudinally, and note that it forms the roof of the adductor canal. Within the canal identify the **femoral vessels,** the **saphenous nerve** (sensory), and the **nerve to the vastus medialis** (motor), both branches of the femoral nerve (**ATLAS PLATE 377**).

D. Femoral Nerve and Its Branches. The **femoral nerve** supplies muscles in the extensor compartment of the thigh (**Figure 21-4**). It passes behind the inguinal ligament deep to the iliac fascia and enters the femoral triangle of the thigh lateral to the femoral artery (**ATLAS PLATE 372**). It then divides into anterior superficial branches and posterior deep branches.

Anterior branches of the femoral nerve include motor nerves to the pectineus (**ATLAS PLATE 372**) and

◀ Grant's 355, 364, 375
Netter's 382, 383, 387
Rohen 452, 453, 468

▶ Grant's 354, 364
Netter's 482, 483, 520
Rohen 478–481

▶ Grant's 364
Netter's 520

◀ Grant's 355, 364
Netter's 482, 483
Rohen 480, 481

sartorius muscles (**ATLAS PLATE 377**) and anterior cutaneous branches, called intermediate and medial femoral cutaneous nerves (**ATLAS PLATE 368**).

Posterior branches of the femoral nerve include the **saphenous nerve,** a long sensory nerve to the medial knee, the medial leg, and the medial malleolar surface of the foot (**ATLAS PLATE 379**), and **motor branches** to the four heads of the quadriceps femoris muscles (**ATLAS PLATES 377, 379**).

> To find the femoral nerve, probe longitudinally through the iliac fascia 1 cm lateral to the femoral artery, below the inguinal ligament. Note that the nerve divides into numerous branches. Find the **nerve to the pectineus muscle** by pushing the femoral vessels medially and probing behind them for a slender branch that arises from the medial side of the femoral nerve trunk near the inguinal ligament (**ATLAS PLATE 372**). Next, find the **nerve to the sartorius muscle,** which enters the medial border of the muscle. This often arises from the main trunk with the intermediate branch of the anterior cutaneous nerve of the thigh. Now turn your attention to the quadriceps femoris muscle and the posterior branches of the femoral nerve.

III. Quadriceps Femoris Muscle and Its Motor Nerves

Most of the mass of the anterior compartment of the thigh consists of the four bellies of the **quadriceps femoris muscle** (**ATLAS PLATE 371**). It is the powerful extensor of the leg at the knee joint and completely covers the anterior surface of the femur. The most superficial of the four bellies has a straight course downward from its origin on the ilium and is called the **rectus femoris.** The other three all take origin from the shaft of the femur and are called the **vastus lateralis, vastus medialis,** and, between these two, the **vastus intermedius.**

A. The Four Parts of Quadriceps Femoris (Figure 21-5)

1. The **rectus femoris** arises by two tendons, one from the anterior superior iliac spine and the other from the upper surface of the acetabulum and joint capsule (**ATLAS PLATE 375**). The two tendons join, and the muscle belly descends to terminate in an aponeurosis, which becomes a tendon that attaches to the anterior surface of the patella (**ATLAS PLATE 374**). Thus, the rectus femoris crosses two joints, but is not attached to the femur.

2. The **vastus lateralis** is the largest of the four bellies, and it arises from the upper half of the lateral lip of the linea aspera on the femoral shaft.

▶ Grant's 357–359
Netter's 474
Rohen 452, 453

▶ Grant's 357, 358, 362–364
Netter's 472–474
Rohen 452

▶ Grant's 355, 357–359, 364
Netter's 474, 482, 483, 520
Rohen 442, 443, 480, 481

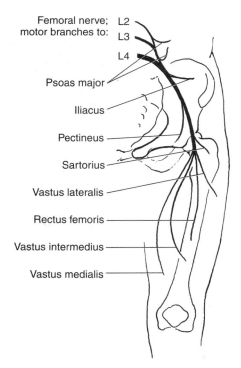

Femoral nerve;
motor branches to: L2
                     L3
                     L4

Psoas major
Iliacus
Pectineus
Sartorius
Vastus lateralis
Rectus femoris
Vastus intermedius
Vastus medialis

Figure 21-4. The femoral nerve and its motor branches.

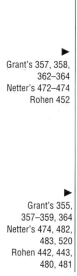

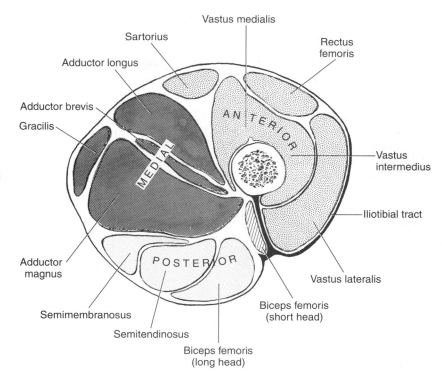

Figure 21-5. Cross section of thigh, showing its anterior, posterior, and medial compartments.

Its fibers descend and terminate in a flat tendon that inserts on the lateral aspect of the patella (**ATLAS PLATE 375**).

3. The **vastus medialis** arises along most of the medial lip of the linea aspera. Its fibers pass downward and forward to become tendinous and insert onto the medial surface of the patella (**ATLAS PLATE 374**).

4. The **vastus intermedius** lies deep to the rectus femoris and is interposed between the vastus lateralis and medialis. It arises from the anterior and lateral surfaces of the femur, and its fibers end in an aponeurosis that forms the deep part of the patellar tendon (**ATLAS PLATE 375**).

B. The Patellar Ligament. The four tendons of the quadriceps femoris converge inferiorly and form a common tendon that encases the **patella,** a sesamoid bone. This common quadriceps tendon becomes the **patellar ligament,** and it descends to insert on the **tuberosity of the tibia,** located on the upper anterior surface of that bone (**ATLAS PLATES 399 #399.2**).

C. Action, Innervation, and Blood Supply of the Quadriceps Femoris. The three vasti muscles act only across the knee joint, and they extend the leg. The rectus femoris, arising from the ilium, not only extends the leg but also assists in flexing the thigh at the hip joint. If the lower limb is fixed, it acts as a flexor of the trunk at the hip.

▶
Grant's 364
Netter's 482, 483
Rohen 481

▶
Grant's 346, 354
Netter's 483, 494
Rohen 481

◀
Grant's 356–359, 388, 393
Netter's 474, 475, 483, 489
Rohen 448, 449, 452, 479

The quadriceps femoris muscle is supplied by motor branches from the posterior division of the femoral nerve. The **nerve to the rectus femoris** divides into several branches that penetrate the deep surface of the muscle (**ATLAS PLATE 377**). The **nerve to the vastus lateralis** courses down with the descending branch of the lateral femoral circumflex artery to the deep surface of the muscle (**ATLAS PLATE 379**). The **nerve to the vastus medialis** descends in the adductor canal with the femoral vessels and saphenous nerve and enters the medial surface of the muscle (**ATLAS PLATE 377**). The **nerve to the vastus intermedius** consists of two or three branches that descend to enter the anterior surface of the muscle (**ATLAS PLATE 379**).

The arterial supply to the quadriceps femoris muscle is derived principally from the **profunda femoris artery** and its **lateral femoral circumflex branch** (**ATLAS PLATES 377, 379**). Along its descent in the adductor canal, the femoral artery sends some muscular branches to the vastus medialis.

Leave a strip (about 4 cm wide) of iliotibial band below the tensor fasciae latae muscle as far as the knee. Remove the remaining deep fascia from the anterior thigh to expose the underlying parts of the quadriceps femoris.

Free the sartorius muscle within its fascial sheath. Cut the muscle near its middle, and reflect its two parts. Separate the underlying rectus femoris from the rest of the quadriceps and find the motor nerve that enters its deep surface (**ATLAS PLATE 377**).

Cut the rectus femoris transversely below the site of entrance of its nerve, and reflect its two heads of origin proximally. Pull the lower part down to the quadriceps tendon proximal to the patella.

Separate the vastus lateralis from the vastus intermedius. Find its motor nerve and determine if it is coursing with the descending branch of the lateral femoral circumflex artery (**ATLAS PLATE 377**). Follow the muscle inferiorly to its tendon, which joins that of the rectus femoris near the lateral surface of the patella.

Note that the vastus medialis joins the vastus intermedius. They may be separated by cutting upward from the tendon of insertion below. Observe that the muscle fibers of the vastus medialis extend 5 cm or more below those of the vastus lateralis, forming a slight bulge medial to the patella.

When the quadriceps femoris is relaxed, the patella can be moved slightly from side to side. Lateral movement is limited, however, by the lateral condyle of the femur. This bony structure and the medial pull on the patella by the vastus medialis during extension of the leg keep the patella in its groove on the femur and prevents lateral dislocation.

Trace the vastus intermedius to its tendinous insertion and see how the tendons of the rectus femoris and the three vasti join with the patella to form the **patellar ligament.** Identify the motor branches to the vastus medialis and intermedius as they enter the muscles (**ATLAS PLATE 379**). Lift the patellar ligament, separate it from any attached tissues, and trace it to its insertion on the tibial tuberosity.

IV. The Medial (Adductor) Region of the Thigh (Figure 21-6)

The medial region of the thigh contains the gracilis and the adductors longus, brevis, and magnus. Also the pectineus muscle is located lateral to the adductor longus muscle (**ATLAS PLATES 372, 374**). The principal nerve of this region is the **obturator nerve** (**ATLAS PLATE 379**) and, in 10% of cadavers, the **accessory obturator nerve.** The medial femoral circumflex and the perforating branches of the profunda femoris artery supply blood to this region (**ATLAS PLATE 379**).

A. **Muscles of the Medial Thigh.** Five muscles are found in the medial region of the thigh: the **pectineus, adductor longus, adductor brevis, adductor magnus,** and the **gracilis.**

◄
Grant's 359, 364
Netter's 483, 520
Rohen 452, 453, 480

◄
Grant's 359, 364
Netter's 474, 482, 483, 520
Rohen 452, 453, 481

◄
Grant's 359, 360
Netter's 474, 489
Rohen 448, 452

►
Grant's 356, 357, 359, 360
Netter's 474
Rohen 452, 453

◄
Grant's 356, 357, 359, 360, 364
Netter's 474, 475, 483, 521
Rohen 452, 453, 481

◄
Grant's 356, 357, 359, 360
Netter's 474, 475
Rohen 452, 453

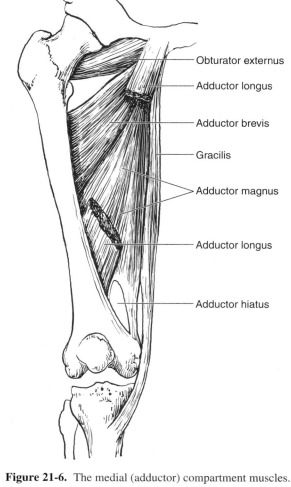

Figure 21-6. The medial (adductor) compartment muscles.

Labels on figure:
Obturator externus
Adductor longus
Adductor brevis
Gracilis
Adductor magnus
Adductor longus
Adductor hiatus

1. The **pectineus muscle** is a flat four-sided muscle extending from the pectineal line of the pubis to the posterior shaft of the femur (**ATLAS PLATES 372, 374**). It helps form the floor of the femoral triangle, and it lies behind the femoral vein and the femoral canal. The pectineus is supplied by a branch of the femoral nerve and (at times) by a twig from the obturator nerve. It flexes, adducts, and medially rotates the thigh at the hip joint.

2. The **adductor longus** lies medial to the pectineus and in the same plane (**ATLAS PLATES 372, 374**). It arises from the anterior aspect of the pubis and also inserts on the posterior shaft of the femur. It is supplied by the obturator nerve and is a strong adductor and flexor of the thigh at the hip joint.

3. The **adductor brevis** is located deep to the pectineus and adductor longus (**ATLAS PLATE 375**). It is shorter but thicker than the adductor longus. It arises along the inferior ramus of the pubis and descends to insert along the linea aspera lateral to the insertions of the pectineus and adductor longus. It is supplied by the obturator nerve and serves as an adductor and flexor of the thigh.

4. The **adductor magnus** is a massive, triangular muscle (**ATLAS PLATE 378, Figure 21-6**). It arises from the inferior ramus of the pubis, the ramus of the ischium, and the ischial tuberosity. The uppermost part is sometimes called the **adductor minimus**. Most of the muscle fans out inferiorly and laterally to insert along the linea aspera and medial supracondylar line of the femur (**ATLAS PLATE 378**). The most medial part of the muscle descends vertically to the adductor tubercle on the inferior medial aspect of the femur and is considered a "hamstring." Most of the muscle is supplied by the obturator nerve; however, the "hamstring" portion receives innervation from the tibial division of the sciatic nerve, similar to the other "hamstrings."

5. The **gracilis muscle** is long, narrow, and flat and is the superficial muscle of the medial compartment (**ATLAS PLATES 374, 378**). It arises from the inferior rami of the pubis and ischium, and its tendon inserts on the upper medial surface of the tibia between the insertions of the sartorius and semitendinosus muscles (**ATLAS PLATE 414**). The gracilis is supplied by the obturator nerve and serves as a flexor and medial rotator of the leg and an adductor of the thigh.

B. **Obturator Nerve** (**Figure 21-7**). The obturator nerve is derived from the L2, L3, and L4 spinal segments. It enters the thigh through the obturator canal deep to the pectineus muscle (**ATLAS PLATE 379**) and divides into anterior and posterior branches.

The **anterior branch** descends in the medial thigh and sends a sensory branch to the hip joint and muscular branches to the gracilis, adductors longus and brevis, and occasionally the pectineus. The terminal branch becomes cutaneous to supply the skin of the middle third of the medial thigh (**ATLAS PLATE 367 #367.2**) but may descend to the middle of the calf.

The **posterior branch** of the obturator nerve descends along the anterior surface of the adductor magnus (**ATLAS PLATES 256, 379**). It gives motor branches to both the adductor brevis and magnus. Superiorly, the posterior branch supplies the obturator externus muscle, and, inferiorly, it gives an articular branch to the knee joint.

◄
Grant's 364
Netter's 474, 475
Rohen 452, 453

◄
Grant's 359, 361, 364
Netter's 474
Rohen 452, 453

►
Grant's 346, 360
Netter's 483, 489
Rohen 466

►
Grant's 346, 364, 382
Netter's 483, 494
Rohen 466, 481

◄
Grant's 359–361, 364
Netter's 483, 521
Rohen 481

►
Grant's 355, 357, 364
Netter's 474
Rohen 452

►
Grant's 359
Netter's 483
Rohen 452, 453

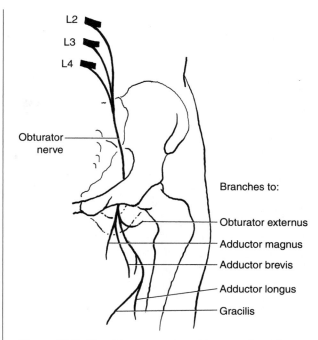

Figure 21-7. The obturator nerve and its motor branches.

C. **Blood Supply to Medial Compartment Structures.** The **deep femoral artery** and its **perforating branches** and, to a lesser extent, the **medial femoral circumflex branch** supply the large muscle mass of the medial compartment (**ATLAS PLATE 379**). The deep femoral artery descends anterior to the iliopsoas, pectineus, and adductor brevis muscles and continues along the surface of the adductor magnus adjacent to the shaft of the femur. Muscular branches supply the medial compartment, and **perforating branches** pierce the adductors brevis and magnus to supply the posterior thigh (**Figure 21-8**).

The **medial femoral circumflex artery** sends muscular branches to the adductor brevis and longus muscles (**ATLAS PLATE 379**). Then it winds around the medial aspect of the femur to the gluteal region, where it participates in the trochanteric and cruciate anastomoses.

Define the borders of the **adductor longus** muscle and expose the **gracilis muscle** along the medial aspect of the thigh (**ATLAS PLATE 374**). Dissect the gracilis to its insertion on the medial surface of the tibia. Define the borders of the **pectineus muscle** lateral to the adductor longus (**ATLAS PLATE 374**).

Cut the adductor longus 3 cm below its origin. Reflect the distal part and find its motor nerve entering its deep surface (**ATLAS PLATE 377**). Deep to the adductor longus, identify the **adductor**

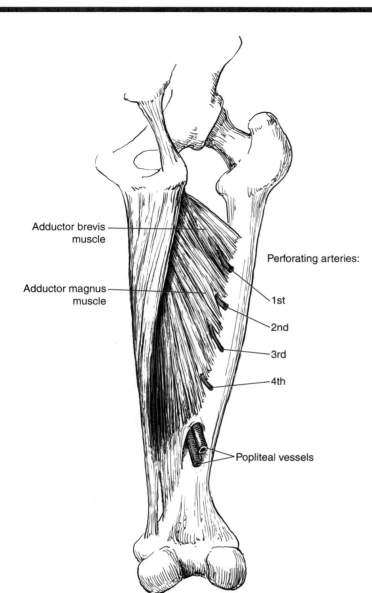

Adductor brevis muscle

Adductor magnus muscle

Perforating arteries:

1st

2nd

3rd

4th

Popliteal vessels

Figure 21-8. The perforating branches from the deep femoral artery (posterior view).

brevis and the insertions of the **iliopsoas** and pectineus muscles. Trace branches of the obturator nerve to the gracilis and adductor brevis muscles (**ATLAS PLATE 377**).

Dissect the **profunda femoris artery** and remove its accompanying veins. Identify one or more of its **perforating branches** that perforate the adductor brevis and magnus adjacent to the femoral shaft (**ATLAS PLATES 374, 393**). Cut the pectineus muscle along its origin. Reflect it laterally, and note that a branch from the femoral nerve supplies it.

◄
Grant's 346, 360, 364
Netter's 483, 494
Rohen 466, 481

►
Grant's 360, 361, 364
Netter's 475
Rohen 453

►
Grant's 373, 376
Netter's 475, 521
Rohen 453

Sever the origin of the adductor brevis muscle, reflect it downward, and expose the **adductor magnus** (**ATLAS PLATE 378**) and the posterior branch of the obturator nerve. Note that this sends motor branches to both the adductor brevis and magnus.

Identify the **obturator externus muscle** on the outer surface of the obturator membrane (**ATLAS PLATE 378**). Note that the posterior branch of the obturator nerve passes through the obturator externus muscle, while the anterior branch passes anterior to the muscle. Follow the tendon of the obturator externus laterally posterior to the neck of the femur.

Clinical Relevance

Varicose veins. Superficial veins in the lower limb drain to deeper veins by way of perforating vessels. The deep veins ascend to the femoral vein, which then drains into the iliac veins of the pelvis. Valves in the veins are important to prevent back flow and to retain a continuous ascent of the blood. If the superficial veins (especially the great saphenous vein and its tributaries) become dilated and tortuous they are called "varicose veins." The reason this occurs is because the intravenous valves become stretched by the dilatation of the veins and then they become incompetent. They do not close completely and leak blood back downward in the vessels.

Deep vein thrombosis. The formation of clots (thrombi) in the deep veins of the lower limb occur when a venous stasis or injury (e.g., in a fracture) occurs and there is an increased coagulation factor in the blood. This process can begin in the muscular region of the posterior compartment of the leg. The clot then ascends in the inferior vena cava through the right ventricle and occludes the pulmonary artery of one of its important branches.

Fracture of the femur. Fractures of the femur are common. The neck of the femur id fractures more commonly in older persons, especially in women who have weakened bones because of osteoporosis. Fractures occur not only in the femoral neck but also between the two trochanters and across the femoral shaft. Fractures of the femoral neck also interrupt the blood supply to the femoral head. Fractures of the shaft or the greater trochanter are usually caused by direct trauma.

Transplantation of the gracilis muscle. The function of the gracilis muscle is the least important of the muscles that adduct the thigh. This long and relatively narrow muscle, therefore, has been used surgically as a source of transplanted muscle with its vessels and nerve still attached distally to the muscle. It has been used in other regions of the limbs elsewhere in the body.

Groin injury. This injury usually involves the straining of a muscle in the anterior or medial aspects of the thigh. The adductors longus and magnus medially along with flexor muscles at the hip joint (iliopsoas, pectineus, rectus femoris, or sartorius) can be strained in sports events such as track where athletes sprint (100 meter dash) or in basketball, football, and baseball where speed is essential to the sport.

Femoral hernia. This hernia occurs through the femoral ring and protrudes into the femoral canal. Significantly more frequent in women, this injury often happens as a result of a difficult birth. The danger is the possible strangulation of the loop of bowel by the inguinal ligament and other connective tissue in the region.

Paralysis of the quadriceps. Paralysis of the quadriceps muscle can occur as a result of stab wounds that partially or completely sever the sciatic nerve. A person with such an injury cannot extend the leg at the knee joint against resistance. Often the syndrome requires a person to press the distal end of the thigh (femur) during walking to prevent inadvertent flexion at the knee joint.

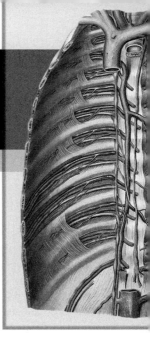

DISSECTION #22

Anterior and Lateral Compartments of the Leg and Dorsum of the Foot

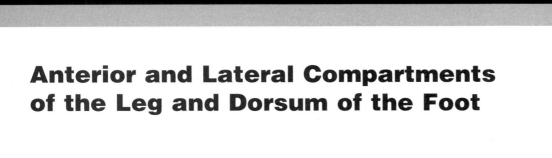

OBJECTIVES

1 Study the surface anatomy of the anterior and lateral compartments of the leg, ankle region, and dorsum of the foot; dissect the superficial vessels and nerves and the fasciae of these regions.

2 Study the features of the tibia and fibula, and learn the names and positions of the bones of the foot.

3 Dissect the muscles, vessels, and nerves in the anterior compartment of the leg, and visualize the extensor retinacula at the ankle.

4 Dissect the muscles and nerves of the lateral compartment of the leg and visualize the fibular retinacula.

5 Learn the relationship of the tendons, vessels, and nerves at the ankle.

6 Dissect the structures on the dorsum of the foot.

Atlas Key:

Clemente Atlas, 5th Edition = Atlas Plate #

Grant's Atlas, 11th Edition = Grant's Page #

Netter's Atlas, 3rd Edition = Netter's Plate #

Rohen Atlas, 6th Edition = Rohen Page #

The **tibia** and **fibula** are the long bones of the leg, and these articulate inferiorly with the **talus (Figure 22-1).** The talus is sustained by the **calcaneus,** which is the bone that forms the heel (**ATLAS PLATES 450, 451**). Tarsal bones distal to the talus are the **navicular, cuboid,** and the **three cuneiform bones.** Beyond these are 5 **metatarsals** and 14 **phalanges (ATLAS PLATE 450).**

▶

Grant's 405–407
Netter's 478, 501, 502, 524
Rohen 459, 462, 494

◀

Grant's 362, 363, 426, 427
Netter's 495, 497, 505, 506
Rohen 440–443

The tibia is located medial to the fibula, and its anterior border forms a sharp crest commonly known as the "shin bone" (**ATLAS PLATE 394, Figure 22-1**). Distally the tibia curves inward toward the **medial malleolus.** Proximally, its upper end is enlarged to form the **medial and lateral condyles,** and inferior to these is located the **tibial tuberosity** onto which inserts the patellar tendon (**ATLAS PLATE 446**).

The **anterior compartment** of the leg contains the muscles that dorsiflex and invert the foot and the extensors of the great toe and lesser toes. The **lateral compartment** muscles also aid in dorsiflexion but serve importantly as the everters of the foot. The principal artery of the anterior compartment is the **anterior tibial artery.** The **fibular artery,** which branches from the posterior tibial, sends perforating branches into the lateral compartment (**ATLAS PLATE 363**). The **common fibular nerve** winds around the neck of

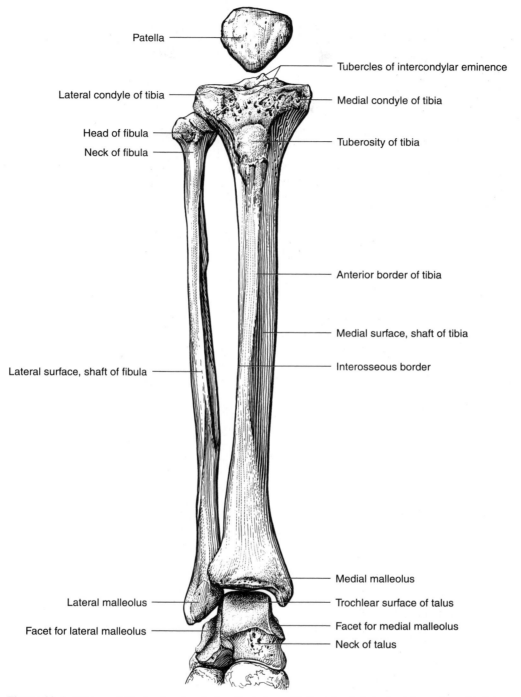

Patella

Tubercles of intercondylar eminence

Lateral condyle of tibia

Medial condyle of tibia

Head of fibula

Neck of fibula

Tuberosity of tibia

Anterior border of tibia

Medial surface, shaft of tibia

Lateral surface, shaft of fibula

Interosseous border

Medial malleolus

Lateral malleolus

Trochlear surface of talus

Facet for lateral malleolus

Facet for medial malleolus

Neck of talus

Figure 22-1. Tibia and fibula, showing their articulation with the talus inferiorly to form the ankle joint.

the fibula and divides into superficial and deep fibular branches. The **deep fibular nerve** is the nerve of the anterior compartment, and the **superficial fibular nerve** innervates the lateral compartment muscles (**ATLAS PLATE 402**).

I. Surface Anatomy; Superficial Vessels and Nerves; Anterior Leg, Ankle, and Dorsum of the Foot (Figures 22-2, 22-3)

The leg is the region between the knee joint and the ankle joint. Several bony structures of the leg are immediately under the skin and easy to palpate.

A. Surface Anatomy. The soft tissues of the leg occupy compartments **lateral** to the anterior border of the tibia (anterior and lateral compartments) and **medial** to that border extending behind the tibia and fibula (posterior compartment). The latter comprises the calf of the leg and is studied in the

▶
Grant's 460, 490, 522, 524
Netter's 495, 496
Rohen 440, 462, 492

◀
Grant's 408, 410, 412
Netter's 526, 527
Rohen 489, 492, 493

▶
Grant's 403, 405, 407
Netter's 488, 489, 491, 495
Rohen 440, 441, 492

next dissection. Before dissection, palpate on yourselves or the cadaver the following structures:

1. **Patella (ATLAS PLATE 364 #364.1).** With the quadriceps muscle relaxed, observe that the patella may be moved slightly from side to side. Movement laterally is limited by the lateral condyle of the femur and by the vastus medialis. These prevent lateral dislocation of the patella when the leg is flexed. The **prepatellar bursa** is located in front of the patella. Bursitis at this site is called "housemaid's knee."

2. **Tibial tuberosity (ATLAS PLATE 446, Figure 22-2).** Palpate this structure 4 cm below the lower end of the patella on the anterior tibia. The tuberosity can be felt by moving the loose skin over its surface. The **infrapatellar bursa** is located between the tuberosity and the skin (**ATLAS PLATE 399 #399.1**).

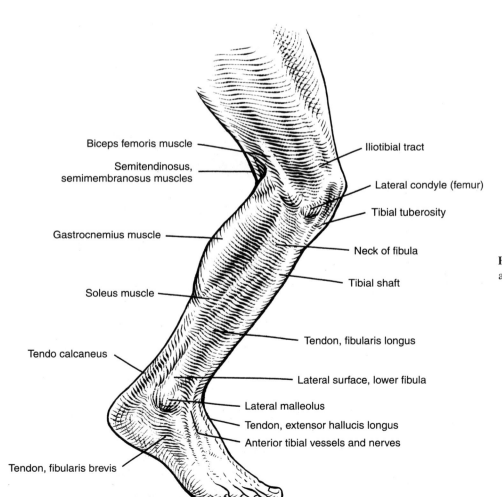

Biceps femoris muscle
Semitendinosus, semimembranosus muscles
Gastrocnemius muscle
Soleus muscle
Tendo calcaneus
Tendon, fibularis brevis

Iliotibial tract
Lateral condyle (femur)
Tibial tuberosity
Neck of fibula
Tibial shaft
Tendon, fibularis longus
Lateral surface, lower fibula
Lateral malleolus
Tendon, extensor hallucis longus
Anterior tibial vessels and nerves

Figure 22-2. Surface anatomy of the leg and foot dorsum, lateral view.

3. **Condyles of the tibia (ATLAS PLATE 435 #435.2).** Feel for the patellar ligament above the tibial tuberosity, and note slight depressions on both sides of the ligament. Palpate laterally and medially from these depressions, and feel the rounded upper borders of the lateral and medial condyles of the tibia.

4. **Anterior border of the tibial shaft (ATLAS PLATE 446).** Feel this sharp surface deep to the skin, down the leg from the tibial tuberosity to the medial ankle region, the **medial malleolus (ATLAS PLATE 399)**. Palpate the tendons across the front of the ankle joint to the **lateral malleolus (Figure 22-2).**

5. **Fibula.** The lateral malleolus is the enlarged lower end of the fibula, and it can easily be felt subcutaneously as the lateral ankle bone (**Figure 22-2**). From the lateral malleolus upward, note that most of the shaft of the fibula lies deep to muscle, but its upper end again becomes subcutaneous. Feel the head of the fibula at its articulation on the posterior surface of the lateral tibial condyle (**ATLAS PLATE 404**).

6. **Common fibular nerve.** About 2 cm down from the head of the fibula palpate the **common fibular nerve** by rolling the skin over the nerve and bone with your fingers (**ATLAS PLATE 402**).

7. **Tendons of hamstring muscles.** Palpate the tendon of the biceps femoris muscle above the head of the fibula on the lateral aspect of the knee (**Figure 22-2**). Feel the **tendon of the semitendinosus muscle** behind the knee on the medial side and the adjacent tendon of the **semimembranosus muscle (ATLAS PLATE 414).**

While sitting with your right foot crossed over your left knee, palpate anterior to the ankle joint for the **tendon of the tibialis anterior,** located just lateral to the medial malleolus. Lateral to this tendon feel the tendon of the **extensor hallucis longus muscle,** and find it again along the dorsum of the 1st metatarsal by flexing the big toe (**ATLAS PLATES 399 #399.2, 407**).

8. **Sustentaculum tali.** On the medial side of the ankle joint, palpate the sustentaculum tali of the calcaneus by pressing 2.5 cm directly below the medial malleolus (**ATLAS PLATES 451 #451.2, 453 #453.2**). Feel the large tuberosity of the calcaneus, which forms the bony infrastructure of the heel posterior and inferior to the malleoli (**ATLAS PLATES 452, 453**).

◄ Grant's 405, 415, 417
Netter's 491, 495
Rohen 440, 441, 446

► Grant's 421, 426, 427
Netter's 505, 506, 510
Rohen 442

◄ Grant's 405, 407, 411
Netter's 495, 496
Rohen 440, 462, 492

◄ Grant's 405, 407, 415
Netter's 495, 496
Rohen 440, 492, 494

► Grant's 340, 342, 346
Netter's 520, 524, 526
Rohen 468, 469, 478, 489, 492, 493

◄ Grant's 405, 410, 416, 417
Netter's 502, 524
Rohen 485, 487, 494

◄ Grant's 410, 484, 485
Netter's 477, 498
Rohen 455, 456, 488

◄ Grant's 406, 408, 421
Netter's 511–513
Rohen 462, 492, 493

◄ Grant's 426, 427, 435, 436
Netter's 506–510
Rohen 449, 450

9. **Tuberosity of the navicular.** To feel the tuberosity of the navicular bone, palpate the dorsomedial surface of the foot 6 to 7 cm distal to the medial malleolus.

10. **Tuberosity of the base of the 5th metatarsal.** Palpate the lateral border of the foot. Midway between the back of the heel and the distal end of the small toe feel the tuberosity of the base of the 5th metatarsal protruding laterally (**ATLAS PLATE 450 #450.2**).

B. **Superficial Vessels and Nerves.** The superficial veins on the dorsal foot drain medially into the **great saphenous vein (ATLAS PLATE 398)** and laterally into the **small saphenous vein (ATLAS PLATE 412).** The great saphenous vein ascends on the leg from 2 cm anterior to the medial malleolus. Medially, at the knee, the vein is joined by the **saphenous nerve,** a sensory branch of the femoral nerve that supplies cutaneous innervation to the medial side of the leg down to the malleolus (**ATLAS PLATE 398, Figure 22-3**).

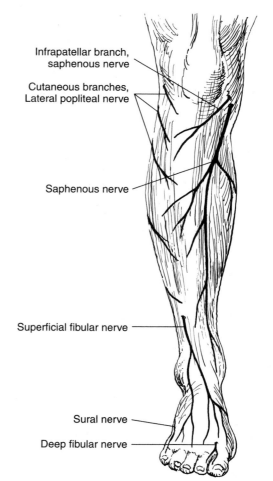

Infrapatellar branch, saphenous nerve

Cutaneous branches, Lateral popliteal nerve

Saphenous nerve

Superficial fibular nerve

Sural nerve

Deep fibular nerve

Figure 22-3. The cutaneous nerves of the leg and foot dorsum.

Laterally, the dorsal venous arch of the foot drains into the small saphenous vein behind the lateral malleolus (**ATLAS PLATE 412**). The vein ascends along the middle of the calf and is accompanied by the **sural nerve,** a cutaneous nerve formed by branches from both tibial and common fibular nerves. The small saphenous vein penetrates the deep fascia between the two heads of the gastrocnemius and opens into the popliteal vein (**ATLAS PLATE 413 #413.1**).

In addition to the saphenous and sural nerves, other cutaneous nerves that branch on the anterior and lateral leg and the dorsum of the foot include the **superficial fibular, deep fibular,** and **lateral sural nerves** (**ATLAS PLATE 406**).

The **superficial fibular nerve** pierces the deep fascia of the lateral compartment about 13 cm above the lateral malleolus (**ATLAS PLATE 406**). It then divides into **dorsal medial** and **intermediate branches** that descend anterior to the ankle joint to supply the skin over the dorsal foot and toes.

The **deep fibular nerve** descends in the anterior compartment, accompanied by the anterior tibial artery (**ATLAS PLATE 402**). On the dorsum of the foot, the nerve divides into a **tarsal branch** that crosses the foot to supply the tarsal and metatarsophalangeal joints of the 2nd, 3rd, and 4th toes and a **cutaneous branch** that supplies the skin on the adjacent surfaces of the large and 2nd toes (**ATLAS PLATES 406, 411**).

The **lateral sural cutaneous nerve of the calf** is a branch of the common fibular nerve. It supplies cutaneous twigs not only to the skin of the lateral calf but also to the lateral surface of the foot (**ATLAS PLATES 367 #367.2, 412**).

◄
Grant's 340–343, 406, 407
Netter's 502, 513, 524, 526
Rohen 471, 478, 492, 494

◄
Grant's 340, 346, 384, 385
Netter's 484, 503, 522, 526, 527
Rohen 478, 488, 489

Figure 22-4. Skin incisions on the anterior leg and foot dorsum.

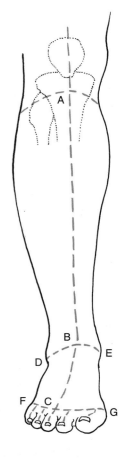

Locate the **superficial fibular nerve** by probing the fascia on the anterior leg, lateral to the anterior border of the tibia, about 12 to 13 cm (5 inches) above the lateral malleolus. Trace its **medial** and **intermediate branches** over the ankle joint onto the dorsum of the foot (**ATLAS PLATE 406**).

Find the **sural nerve** in the fascia behind the lateral malleolus (**ATLAS PLATE 406**). Follow the nerve forward along the lateral margin of the foot, where it is called the **lateral dorsal cutaneous nerve** (**ATLAS PLATE 406**).

Find the cutaneous branch of the **deep fibular nerve** by dissecting the space between the metatarsal bones of the large and 2nd toes (**ATLAS PLATES 406, 411**). Dissect it distally, and note that it supplies the adjacent sides of these two toes.

Skin incisions. Make skin incisions similar to those shown in **Figure 22-4.** Cut through the skin from the patella down the middle of the anterior leg and along the dorsum of the foot to the site of attachment of the middle toe (**Figure 22-4, A–B–C**). Make cuts laterally and medially at the ankle (**Figure 22-4, B–D and B–E**) and at the proximal ends of the toes (**Figure 22-4, C–F and C–G**). Incise the skin along the dorsum of the toes and remove the skin from the anterior leg and dorsum of the foot and toes.

Superficial veins. Identify the venous network on the **medial side** of the foot that forms the **great saphenous vein.** Dissect the **small saphenous vein** laterally, and trace it behind the lateral malleolus to the posterior leg (**ATLAS PLATES 398, 412**).

Cutaneous nerves. Find the **saphenous nerve** in the fascia anterior to the great saphenous vein on the medial surface of the leg. Dissect it free to the lower leg near the medial malleolus (**ATLAS PLATE 398**).

◄
Grant's 342, 343
Netter's 526, 527
Rohen 468, 469, 489

◄
Grant's 342, 346
Netter's 503, 520, 521, 524, 526
Rohen 478, 492–494

C. Deep Fascia of the Anterior Leg, Extensor, and Fibular Retinacula. The muscles of the leg are invested by deep fascia, called **crural fascia,** that is continuous with the fascia lata of the thigh (**ATLAS PLATE 399 #399.1**). Intermuscular septa from the deep fascia pass deeply to the bone and enclose the anterior and lateral compartments.

At the ankle, the deep fascia thickens to form strong restraining bands called **retinacula** that bind the tendons close to the bones. **Extensor** and **fibular retinacula** are formed on the anterior and lateral aspects of the leg. Each consists of superior and inferior thickened bands (**ATLAS PLATES 399, 401, 404, 408**).

The **superior extensor retinaculum** (**ATLAS PLATE 399 #399.1**) is located just above the ankle joint on the anterior leg. Its transverse fibers attach to the lower end of the fibula laterally and the anterior border of the tibia medially. It binds down the tendons of the anterior compartment muscles, and the anterior tibial vessels and deep fibular nerve course deep to it.

The **inferior extensor retinaculum** is a Y-shaped band located anterior to the ankle joint, about 4 cm below the superior retinaculum (**ATLAS PLATES 399, 407**). The stem of the Y extends below the lateral malleolus and attaches to the upper surface of the calcaneus. Medially, the upper arm of the Y attaches to the medial malleolus, and the lower arm extends downward to blend with fascia on the medial foot.

Two fibular retinacula (**ATLAS PLATE 408, #408.1**) bind the tendons of the fibularis longus and brevis as they descend from the leg into the lateral foot. The **superior fibular retinaculum** extends from the lateral malleolus downward and posteriorly to the calcaneus. The **inferior fibular retinaculum** is located more distally along the lateral side of the foot. Its fibers extend downward from the inferior extensor retinaculum and bind the fibular tendons to the lateral surface of the calcaneus.

Remove the superficial fascia from the anterior leg and dorsum of the foot to expose the deep **crural fascia.** Define the thickened bands of deep fascia called the **superior and inferior extensor retinacula** above and below the ankle joint. Retain both the transverse superior extensor retinaculum (above the ankle) and the Y-shaped inferior retinaculum (over the foot dorsum).

Remove the deep fascia surrounding the muscles of the anterior and lateral compartments. To do this, cut the deep fascia longitudinally from just below the knee to the superior extensor retinaculum. Cut through the deep fascia 2 cm below the tibial tuberosity laterally to the neck of the fibula. **Be careful not to cut the common fibular nerve as it comes around the fibula.** Cut the deep fascia laterally above the transverse fibers of the superior extensor retinaculum, and expose the muscles, vessels, and nerves of the anterior and lateral compartments.

◄ Grant's 408, 410, 412
Netter's 501, 503, 504, 511, 512, 526
Rohen 493, 494, 496, 497

► Grant's 406, 407, 410
Netter's 501, 502, 504, 524
Rohen 459, 462, 494

► Grant's 405, 406, 410
Netter's 501, 502, 504
Rohen 459, 462, 494

◄ Grant's 412, 413
Netter's 509, 511

◄ Grant's 408–410
Netter's 498, 503, 511, 512
Rohen 459, 462, 494

► Grant's 405, 406, 410
Netter's 501, 503
Rohen 462, 494, 495

◄ Grant's 407, 410, 411
Netter's 502, 524
Rohen 459, 494

II. Anterior Compartment of the Leg (Figures 22-5, 22-6)

The anterior compartment of the leg contains the muscles that **dorsiflex** the foot at the ankle joint, **invert** the foot, and **extend** the toes. All of the muscles are supplied by the **deep fibular nerve** and the **anterior tibial artery** (**ATLAS PLATES 401, 402, Figure 22-7**).

A. Anterior Compartment Muscles. The anterior muscles of the leg include the tibialis anterior, extensor hallucis longus, extensor digitorum longus, and the fibularis tertius.

The **tibialis anterior muscle** (**Figure 22-6**) arises from the lateral condyle and shaft of the tibia and from the interosseous membrane. At the ankle, its flattened tendon passes beneath the superior extensor retinaculum and both arms of the inferior extensor retinaculum. It descends just lateral to the medial malleolus to the medial margin of the foot and inserts on the medial cuneiform bone and base of the 1st metatarsal bone. The tibialis anterior dorsiflexes and inverts the foot.

The **extensor hallucis longus** (**ATLAS PLATES 399 #399.2, 403, 410, Figure 22-6**) arises from the anterior surface of the fibula and the interosseous membrane between the tibialis anterior and extensor digitorum longus. The deep fibular nerve and anterior tibial vessels are located medial to the extensor hallucis longus tendon as it passes beneath the extensor retinaculum (**ATLAS PLATE 402**). The tendon crosses medially over the vessels and nerves, descends on their medial side, and inserts on the base of the distal phalanx of the large toe (**ATLAS PLATES 410, 411**). The extensor hallucis longus extends the large toe and dorsiflexes the foot.

The **extensor digitorum longus** (**ATLAS PLATES 399 #399.2, 407, 409, Figure 22-6**) arises from the upper medial surface of the fibula and from the lateral condyle of the tibia. It descends lateral to the extensor hallucis longus, and its tendon passes beneath the retinacula before dividing into four slender tendons. These insert onto the dorsal digital expansions of the four lateral toes (**ATLAS PLATES 407, 409**). The extensor digitorum longus extends the toes and dorsiflexes the foot.

The **fibularis tertius** is often described as a part of the extensor digitorum longus. It arises from the medial side of the lower fibula and accompanies the extensor digitorum longus beneath the extensor retinacula. It inserts on the dorsal surface of the base of the 5th metatarsal bone (**ATLAS PLATES 399 #399.2, 402, 404**). The fibularis tertius helps to dorsiflex and evert the foot.

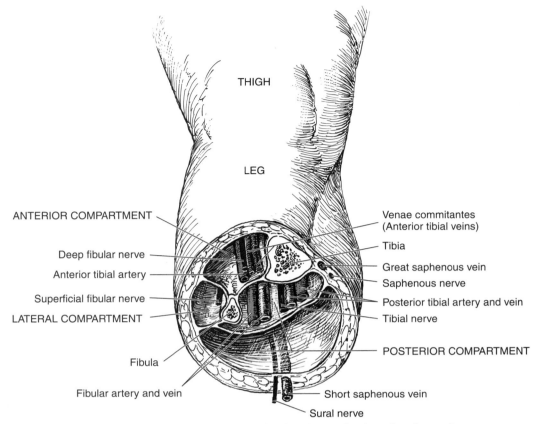

THIGH

LEG

ANTERIOR COMPARTMENT

Deep fibular nerve

Anterior tibial artery

Superficial fibular nerve

LATERAL COMPARTMENT

Fibula

Fibular artery and vein

Venae commitantes
(Anterior tibial veins)

Tibia

Great saphenous vein

Saphenous nerve

Posterior tibial artery and vein

Tibial nerve

POSTERIOR COMPARTMENT

Short saphenous vein

Sural nerve

Figure 22-5. Cross section of the leg (from below), showing the anterior, lateral, and posterior compartments.

B. Nerves and Vessels of the Anterior Compartment.

The anterior tibial vessels and the deep fibular nerve descend anterior to the interosseous membrane (**ATLAS PLATE 402, Figures 22-5, 22-7**).

The **anterior tibial artery** arises from the popliteal artery and passes forward to the anterior compartment by piercing the upper part of the interosseous membrane (**ATLAS PLATE 419**). As the artery descends, it gradually approaches the tibia so that anterior to the ankle joint it enters the dorsum of the foot as the **dorsalis pedis artery** midway between the two malleoli (**ATLAS PLATE 411**). Superiorly the anterior tibial artery gives off the **anterior tibial recurrent branch** that ascends to anastomose with the inferior genicular vessels off the popliteal artery (**ATLAS PLATE 402**). Inferiorly, **medial and lateral malleolar branches** arise from the anterior tibial about 5 cm above the ankle joint and participate in the anastomosis around the ankle (**ATLAS PLATE 411**).

The **deep fibular nerve** branches from the common fibular nerve between the fibularis longus muscle and the neck of the fibula (**ATLAS PLATE 402**). Passing into the anterior compartment in front of the interosseous membrane, the nerve descends adjacent to the anterior tibial artery as far as the ankle joint.

▶
Grant's 406, 410
Netter's 501, 502,
504
Rohen's 459, 462,
494

◀
Grant's 406, 407,
410
Netter's 502, 504
Rohen 494

▶
Grant's 346, 406,
407
Netter's 494, 502

◀
Grant's 406, 407,
411
Netter's 502, 504,
524
Rohen 494

It supplies all four muscles of the anterior compartment, and it sends a sensory branch to the ankle joint.

Identify the tendon of the **tibialis anterior muscle** lying immediately lateral to the medial malleolus. Lateral to this tendon identify the **deep fibular nerve** and dissect the **anterior tibial artery** by removing the accompanying veins (**ATLAS PLATE 401**). Lateral to the artery find the tendons of the **extensor hallucis longus, extensor digitorum longus,** and **fibularis tertius** in that order (**ATLAS PLATE 399 #399.2**). Free the tendons of all these muscles by cutting through the retinacula.

Separate the bellies of the anterior compartment muscles, and expose the proximal half of the anterior tibial artery and deep fibular nerve. Follow these neurovascular structures superiorly along the interosseous membrane to their entrance into the anterior compartment, cutting muscle fibers if necessary (**ATLAS PLATE 402**). Find the **anterior tibial recurrent branch** from the anterior tibial artery, which ascends to the knee in front of the interosseous membrane.

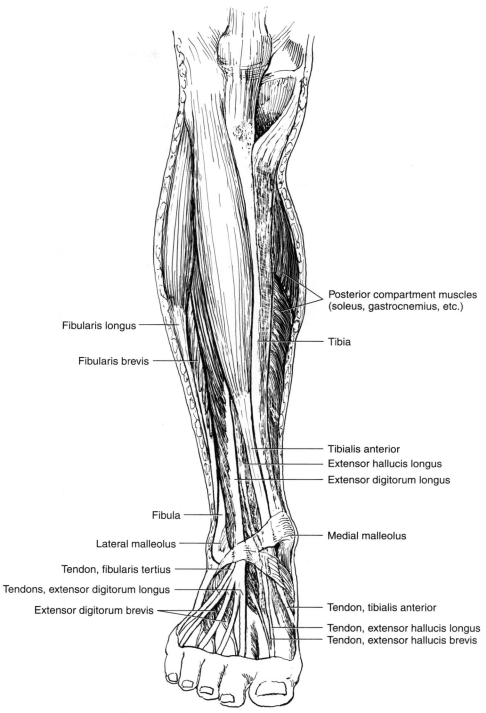

Figure 22-6. The muscles of the anterior and lateral compartments.

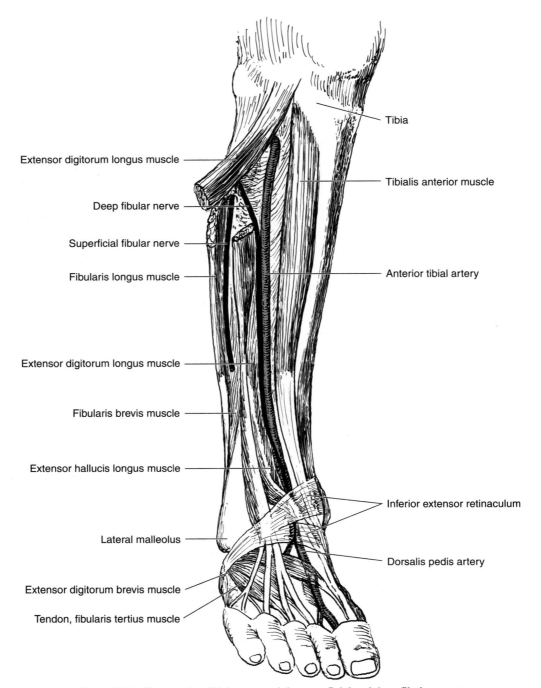

Figure 22-7. The anterior tibial artery and the superficial and deep fibular nerves.

> Learn the sequence of structure from medial to lateral anterior to the ankle joint: tibialis anterior, anterior tibial artery and deep fibular nerve, extensor hallucis longus, extensor digitorum longus, and fibularis tertius.

III. Lateral Compartment of the Leg (Figures 22-5 to 22-7)

The lateral compartment of the leg contains muscles that evert and weakly plantarflex the foot and the **superficial fibular nerve** that supplies them. The muscles descend lateral to the fibula, and the compartment is bounded by deep fascia, the anterior and posterior intermuscular septa.

A. Lateral Compartment Muscles. The lateral compartment contains the fibularis longus and brevis muscles (**ATLAS PLATE 404**). The **fibularis longus muscle** is the most superficial muscle in the lateral leg. It arises from the lateral surface of the upper fibula and the intermuscular septum. Its tendon descends to the foot, deep to the superior fibular retinaculum and behind the lateral malleolus and tendon of the fibularis brevis. The tendon courses to the cuboid bone, where it turns medially within a sulcus on the plantar surface of that bone (**ATLAS PLATE 427**). The sulcus becomes converted into a canal by the attachments of the long plantar ligament (**ATLAS PLATE 455 #455.1**). The tendon inserts medially on the plantar surface of the medial cuneiform bone and on the base of the 1st metatarsal bone. The fibularis longus is an everter of the foot, and, importantly, its tendon helps to maintain the lateral longitudinal and transverse arches of the foot.

The **fibularis brevis muscle** arises from the lateral surface of the lower fibula, anterior to the fibularis longus. Its tendon descends deep to the fibularis longus, behind the lateral malleolus, to insert on the tuberosity of the 5th metatarsal bone (**ATLAS PLATES 404, 408 #408.1**). The fibularis brevis helps to evert the foot.

B. Nerves and Vessels in the Lateral Compartment. The **superficial fibular nerve** supplies both the fibularis longus and brevis muscles. It descends in the lateral compartment between these muscles and the extensor digitorum longus (**ATLAS PLATE 402**). About two-thirds down the leg, it pierces the deep fascia, becomes superficial, and divides into medial and intermediate branches that supply cutaneous innervation to most of the dorsal foot (**ATLAS PLATE 406**).

► Grant's 419
Netter's 500
Rohen 490, 491

► Grant's 407, 410, 413
Netter's 501, 503, 504
Rohen 459, 460, 462

◄ Grant's 406, 407, 410, 411, 413
Netter's 501–504, 524
Rohen 459, 462, 494

► Grant's 340, 348, 407
Netter's 502, 524
Rohen 492–494

◄ Grant's 406, 410, 413
Netter's 501, 503, 504
Rohen 459, 462

► Grant's 362, 405, 409, 422, 436
Netter's 505–507
Rohen 440, 443

◄ Grant's 406, 407, 410, 413
Netter's 501, 504
Rohen 459, 460

◄ Grant's 406, 407, 410, 411
Netter's 502, 524
Rohen 494

► Grant's 413, 444, 445
Netter's 418, 419,
Rohen 450, 451, 495

Blood reaches the lateral compartment by vessels that branch from the **fibular artery** in the posterior compartment (**ATLAS PLATE 419**). These are perforating branches that pierce the posterior intermuscular septum to enter the lateral compartment, since there is no through-going vessel in the lateral compartment.

> Make a longitudinal incision in the deep fascia covering the lateral compartment of the leg. Also make transverse cuts in the fascia superiorly and inferiorly and expose the **fibularis longus** and **brevis muscles** (**ATLAS PLATE 404**). Note that the two muscles are only clearly separated inferiorly after they have formed tendons. Push a scalpel handle upward between the two tendons to separate the muscles as far as their fleshy bellies will allow. Cut the superior fibular retinaculum and separate the two tendons behind the lateral malleolus (**ATLAS PLATE 408 #408.1**).
>
> Identify the **superficial fibular nerve** where it leaves the muscles to become cutaneous in the lower leg. Follow it superiorly between the fibularis brevis and extensor digitorum longus muscles to the common fibular nerve near the neck of the fibula.
>
> **Taking care not to cut either the common or superficial fibular nerves,** carefully sever the bellies of the fibularis longus and extensor digitorum longus muscles as shown in **ATLAS PLATE 402**. Observe the branching of the common fibular nerve into the superficial and deep fibular nerves.

IV. Ankle Region and Dorsum of the Foot

A. Bones of the Foot. Study the skeleton of the foot (**Figure 22-8**) and the articulations at the ankle joint (**Figure 22-1**). Note that the lower ends of the tibia and fibula form prominences at the ankle region, called the **malleoli**. The inner surfaces of the two malleoli and the inferior surface of the tibia form a clasp, like an inverted U, that fits over the trochlea of the talus (**Figure 22-1**). These form the bony parts of the saddle-shaped **ankle joint** (**ATLAS PLATE 448**).

The talus overlies the posterior facet on the superior surface of the calcaneus to form the **subtalar joint** (**ATLAS PLATES 453, #453.1, 458**). The plantar surface of the head of the talus articulates with the anterior and middle articular facets on the calcaneus. The distal surface of the head of the talus articulates with the navicular bone to form the important

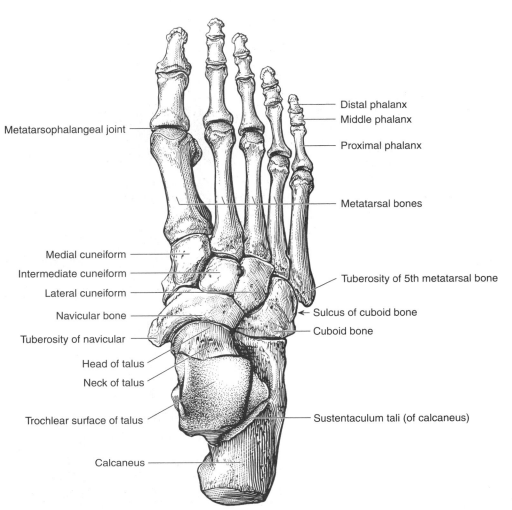

Metatarsophalangeal joint

Distal phalanx
Middle phalanx
Proximal phalanx

Metatarsal bones

Medial cuneiform
Intermediate cuneiform
Lateral cuneiform
Navicular bone
Tuberosity of navicular
Head of talus
Neck of talus
Trochlear surface of talus
Calcaneus

Tuberosity of 5th metatarsal bone
Sulcus of cuboid bone
Cuboid bone
Sustentaculum tali (of calcaneus)

Figure 22-8. Bones of the foot, dorsal view.

talocalcaneonavicular joint (ATLAS PLATE 454, Figure 22-8).

Anterior to the calcaneus laterally is found the **cuboid bone,** while in front of the navicular are located the medial, intermediate, and lateral **cuneiform bones.** Distal to these bones are the five metatarsal bones; distal to these are the phalanges (**ATLAS PLATES 450, 451**).

On an articulated skeleton:

1. Observe the trochlea of the talus gripped between the tibia and fibula of the leg and how it is interposed between these bones and the calcaneus and navicular bones (**Figure 22-1**). Note that the talus carries the body weight while standing.

2. Observe that the foot bones may be divided into medial and lateral groups. Anterior to the calcaneus, talus, and navicular are the three cuneiform bones and distal to these,

◄
Grant's 440, 441, 445
Rohen 434, 443,

►
Grant's 409, 426, 427, 441
Netter's 505, 506–510
Rohen 442, 443, 449, 450

◄
Grant's 432, 433, 436
Netter's 505, 506
Rohen 442, 443, 449, 450

►
Grant's 439, 440, 441
Netter's 505, 506
Rohen 442, 443

◄
Grant's 405, 409, 426, 427
Netter's 505, 506
Rohen 442, 443

the three medial metatarsals and the phalanges of these toes. Note that these bones form the elevated **medial longitudinal arch of the foot (ATLAS PLATE 459, Figure 22-9A).**

3. Study the **sustentaculum tali** of the calcaneus. Anterior to the calcaneus laterally identify the cuboid bone and its sulcus, which transmits the tendon of the fibularis longus. Distal to the cuboid identify the metatarsals and phalanges of the 4th and 5th digits. Note that the calcaneus, cuboid, and metatarsals and phalanges of the lateral two toes form the flat **lateral longitudinal arch of the foot** (**Figure 22-9B**).

4. From the dorsum of the foot, identify the trochlea, body and head of the talus, the tuberosities of the navicular, and the 5th metatarsal bones (**ATLAS PLATES 450, 451**).

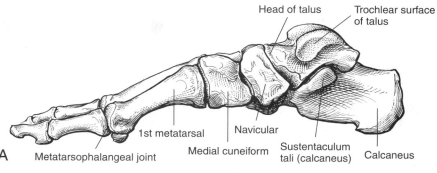

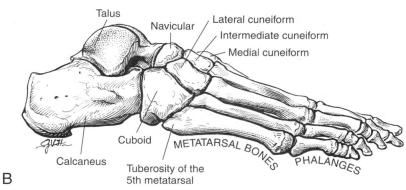

Figure 22-9. Bones of the foot, showing the medial arch (**A**) and the lateral arch (**B**).

B. Dorsum of the Foot: Nerves, Vessels, Tendons, and Muscle. A regional dissection of the dorsum of the foot should start with identification of the cutaneous branches of the superficial and deep fibular nerves (**ATLAS PLATE 406**). Simultaneously, the continuation of the anterior tibial artery is to be dissected distal to the ankle joint to the toes and then along the dorsum of one or more of the toes (**ATLAS PLATE 411**). The tendons of the six muscles occupying the anterior and lateral compartments of the leg are to be followed to their insertions. Finally, a single muscle on the dorsum of the foot, the **extensor digitorum brevis,** is to be cleaned and its tendons dissected distally (**ATLAS PLATE 410**).

Remove the skin from the dorsum of the foot, and dissect the superficial fascia for the cutaneous branches of the superficial and deep fibular nerves.

1. **Nerves on the dorsum of the foot.** Find the main trunk of the **superficial fibular nerve** as it emerges from the deep fascia midway down the leg. Trace its **dorsal medial branch,** which supplies the medial side of the large toe, and a second branch, which supplies the adjacent sides of the 2nd and 3rd toes. Trace the **dorsal intermediate branch** as its two digital nerves supply the skin along the adjacent sides of the 3rd and 4th toes and

◄
Grant's 307, 309, 340, 346, 367
Netter's 501–503, 511–513, 524
Rohen 459, 460, 492, 493, 496, 498

►
Grant's 408–410, 412, 413
Netter's 501, 502, 512, 513
Rohen 459, 462, 494

►
Grant's 348, 406, 407
Netter's 502, 512, 513, 524
Rohen 495

◄
Grant's 340
Netter's 524, 526
Rohen 492, 493, 496

►
Grant's 346, 407, 409
Netter's 502, 512, 513
Rohen 494, 495

the skin along the adjacent sides of the 4th and 5th toes (**ATLAS PLATE 406**).

Along the lateral border of the foot find the **lateral dorsal cutaneous nerve.** It is the continuation of the **sural nerve** and is the cutaneous innervation to the lateral surface of the foot and little toe (**ATLAS PLATE 406**).

Cut the **inferior extensor retinaculum** and free the tendons of the **tibialis anterior** and the **extensors digitorum longus** and **hallucis longus.** Find the **deep fibular nerve** and **anterior tibial artery** adjacent to the tendon of the extensor hallucis longus anterior to the ankle joint (**ATLAS PLATE 411**).

Trace the deep fibular nerve to its division into lateral and medial terminal branches. Follow the **lateral branch** across the dorsum to the **extensor digitorum brevis muscle,** which it supplies along with branches to the tarsal and metatarsophalangeal joints. Follow the **medial branch** distally, adjacent to the dorsalis pedis artery, to its division into dorsal digital nerves that supply the adjacent surfaces of the large and 2nd toes (**ATLAS PLATE 411**).

2. **Anterior tibial–dorsalis pedis artery.** Trace the **anterior tibial artery** in the anterior compartment, and find the **anterior medial malleolar branch** about 5 cm above the ankle joint. Note that it passes medially around the

tibia behind the tendons of the extensor hallucis and tibialis anterior to supply the ankle joint. Identify the **anterior lateral malleolar branch** coursing around the tibia and fibula behind the extensor digitorum longus to supply the lateral ankle region (**ATLAS PLATE 411**).

Follow the **dorsalis pedis artery** into the foot, and dissect it to the first intermetatarsal space where it pierces the 1st dorsal interosseous muscle to achieve the plantar surface of the foot (**ATLAS PLATE 411**). About an inch below the ankle joint (over the navicular bone) look for **lateral** and smaller **medial tarsal branches.**

Find the **arcuate branch,** which arches laterally over the metatarsal bones from the site where the dorsalis pedis artery pierces the 1st dorsal interosseous muscle. Dissect the 2nd, 3rd, and 4th **dorsal metatarsal** arteries, which descend from the arch in the intermetatarsal spaces (**ATLAS PLATE 411**). Find the 1st dorsal metatarsal artery arising directly from the dorsalis pedis artery before that vessel passes from the dorsum as the **deep plantar artery** to the sole of the foot.

3. **Muscles and tendons.** Follow the tendon of the tibialis anterior to its insertion on the medial cuneiform bone and the 1st metatarsal bone (**ATLAS PLATE 408 #408.2**).

Dissect the **tendon of the extensor hallucis longus** along the medial side of the foot to its insertion on the dorsal surface of the distal phalanx of the large toe. Dissect the four individual **tendons of the extensor digitorum longus muscle** to the distal phalanges of the lateral four toes (**ATLAS PLATE 409**).

Dissect the belly of the **extensor digitorum brevis,** and follow its tendons to the dorsal expansions over the phalanges of the 2nd, 3rd, and 4th toes. Another tendon, sometimes called the **extensor hallucis brevis,** inserts onto the large toe (**ATLAS PLATE 410**).

Sever the peroneal retinacula, and dissect the **tendon of the fibularis brevis** to the tuberosity of the 5th metatarsal bone and the tendon of the **fibularis longus** to the sulcus on the plantar surface of the cuboid bone (**ATLAS PLATES 404, 408 #408.1**).

◄
Grant's 346, 407, 408
Netter's 502, 512, 513
Rohen 456, 496, 497

◄
Grant's 406, 410, 412, 413
Netter's 501, 503, 511–513, 524
Rohen 459, 462, 494, 495

Clinical Relevance

Fibular fractures. These fractures most often occur in the inferior part of the bone and at times involve ankle bone dislocation or tibial fractures. Fractures happen when there is a strong inversion turning of the foot, breaking the lateral malleolus away from the lower part of the fibular shaft. Basketball, football, and soccer players are often subject to these painful fibular fractures. If the neck of the fibula is fractured just below the knee joint, the common fibular nerve is endangered.

Tibial fractures. These fractures are frequently compound fractures and often result from direct compression injury of the tibia, such as being hit by a blunt object in the shin bone or from falls from a considerable height. The inferior half of the bone is most vulnerable, and injury to its blood supply may delay healing of a tibial fracture. Fractures of the tibial plateau, on which rests the femur, are also common after forced flexion, hyperextension, or rotational injuries, and they are usually combined with damage to the collateral ligaments. Tibial fractures often occur in persons engaged in sports activities (e.g., skiing, football, and rock climbing) or in long forced marches in the military before the person is well conditioned and not "in shape."

Fracture of the patella. Fractures of the patella usually result from direct anterior trauma to the knee. A transverse fracture of the patella, however, can occur because of a quick and powerful contracture of the quadriceps muscle, which creates an excessive strain on the quadriceps tendon and patellar ligament that encase the bone.

Deep fibular nerve entrapment. When the anterior muscles of the leg are excessively used in sports activities, muscle injuries and extravasation of blood can cause edema in the anterior compartment of the leg, resulting in compression of the deep fibular nerve. Not infrequently compression of this nerve can occur when a skier wears tight-fitting ski boots—at times the condition is referred to as the "ski boot entrapment syndrome."

Fracture of the 5th metatarsal. This common fracture of the lateral tuberosity on the 5th metatarsal is usually caused by the pull of the fibularis brevis muscle that inserts on it. Usually the tuberosity is avulsed by an intense inversion of the foot.

Common fibular nerve injury. This injury results in the condition called "foot drop." The common fibular nerve is the most frequently injured nerve in the body because the nerve courses around the neck of the fibula where it is just deep to the skin and hard pressed against bone. At this site it is subject to direct trauma or is injured when the fibula is fractured. Injuries to the nerve or its severance result in paralysis of the anterior and lateral compartment muscles that dorsiflex and evert the foot. Foot drop occurs during the swing phase of walking when the toes drop to the ground in an uncontrolled manner before the heel strikes. Afflicted persons often lift the advancing knee and foot high in a steppage gait so that the toes clear the ground.

Anterior compartment syndrome. Anterior compartment muscles of the leg are tightly bound by fibrous connective tissue. Increase in intracompartmental pressure can occur because of edema caused by the extravasation of tissue fluids into the compartment. This often happens when the muscles are injured accompanying a fracture of the bone or bones Dorsiflexion of the foot at the ankle joint results in severe pain. The return of venous blood can also be impeded, adding to the increased pressure in the compartment. Surgeons can make longitudinal incisions through the deep fascia, thereby relieving the pressure in the compartment.

The value of the great saphenous vein. Segments of the great saphenous vein that ascends in the leg are frequently used as grafts to bypass occluded coronary arteries in patients who have coronary artery disease. The venous segments, however, must be placed so that the intravenous valves do not impede the flow of arterial blood flow. Segments of this vein can also be used to bypass problems in other large arteries when necessary.

Hammer toe. This deformity is characterized by the permanent dorsiflexion of a toe at the metatarsophalangeal joint. The distal phalanx might also be hyperextended, where the middle phalanx is plantarflexed at the proximal interphalangeal joint.

Fracture of the neck of the talus. This fracture can occur when a strong dorsiflexion at the ankle joint occurs. The usual example of this type of trauma is pushing on a pedal with the ball of the foot in an automobile at the time of a head-on collision.

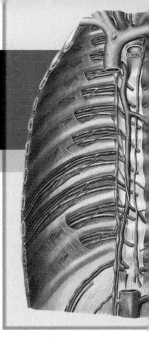

The Posterior Leg and Sole of the Foot

OBJECTIVES

1 Learn the muscles (and their actions), vessels, and nerves in the posterior compartment of the leg.

2 See the structures that course behind the medial malleolus as they enter the sole of the foot.

3 Visualize the muscle layers on the plantar foot and dissect the nerves and vessels that supply them.

Atlas Key:

Clemente Atlas, 5th Edition = Atlas Plate #

Grant's Atlas, 11th Edition = Grant's Page #

Netter's Atlas, 3rd Edition = Netter's Plate #

Rohen Atlas, 6th Edition = Rohen Page #

The posterior leg region contains muscles that **plantarflex the foot** at the ankle joint and **flex the toes** at the metacarpophalangeal and interphalangeal joints. Two muscles, the gastrocnemius and popliteus, can also act at the knee joint. The posterior leg muscles are arranged into superficial and deep groups. Through this region course the nerves and vessels that supply these muscles and the muscles in the sole of the foot.

► Grant's 405–407, 416
Netter's 495–500
Rohen 440, 457, 458

► Grant's 416, 417, 421
Netter's 498, 499, 503
Rohen 457, 458

◄ Grant's 414, 416–419
Netter's 498–500
Rohen 461, 467, 490, 491

► Grant's 410, 413
Netter's 498
Rohen 457

I. Surface Anatomy

Before dissecting the calf and sole of the foot, observe several surface anatomic features.

While sitting, flex your right leg and rest your right foot and its lateral malleolus on your left knee.

1. Palpate the right tibial shaft down to the medial malleolus and manipulate the fleshy mass of the calf. This mass contains the muscles and neurovascular structures of the posterior compartment of the leg (**ATLAS PLATE 365 #365.1**).

2. Grasp the **calcaneus tendon** (or Achilles tendon) located in the fossa behind the two malleoli. Trace this tendon of the gastrocnemius and soleus muscles to its attachment on the posterior surface of the calcaneus, the bone of the heel (**ATLAS PLATE 413**).

3. Ask your laboratory partner to stand on his or her toes. Note the two heads of the gastrocnemius muscle that accentuate the upper calf, and the calcaneous tendon that is prominently exposed.

4. Sit again with your right foot resting on your left knee. Palpate the sole of the foot and note

its flat lateral border and its arched medial border.

5. Tense the plantar surface of the foot by dorsiflexing the toes. Feel the tough **plantar aponeurosis** palpable in the central part of the sole (**ATLAS PLATE 422**).

6. Palpate the **tuberosity of the navicular bone** by passing a finger along the upper medial border of the foot, 4 cm distal to the medial malleolus. Continuing forward another 10 cm, feel the prominent **head of the 1st metatarsal bone** behind the metatarsophalangeal joint of the large toe (**ATLAS PLATE 450 #450.2**).

7. Examine the sole of the foot and feel the **tubercles of the calcaneus** proximally and the **heads of the metatarsal bones** distally (**ATLAS PLATE 458**). Often called the **ball of the heel** and the **ball of the toes,** these structures and the lateral border of the sole are in contact with the ground when we stand. At a convenient time when the plantar surface of the foot is wet, observe the imprint made on the floor by the sole of the foot. Note the arch (or degree of flatness) formed by the medial border of the foot during normal standing.

◄
Grant's 424
Netter's 514
Rohen 463, 500

◄
Grant's 426, 427
Netter's 505, 506
Rohen 442, 443

◄
Grant's 424, 429, 431
Netter's 505
Rohen 442, 443

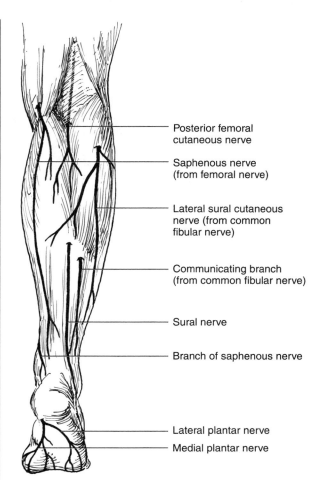

- Posterior femoral cutaneous nerve
- Saphenous nerve (from femoral nerve)
- Lateral sural cutaneous nerve (from common fibular nerve)
- Communicating branch (from common fibular nerve)
- Sural nerve
- Branch of saphenous nerve
- Lateral plantar nerve
- Medial plantar nerve

Figure 23-1. Superficial nerves of the right posterior leg.

II. Incisions and Superficial Dissection of the Posterior Leg

The superficial structures of the posterior leg that are to be dissected during the removal of the skin and superficial fascia are the **small saphenous vein** and the **sural nerve** (**ATLAS PLATE 412**).

The **small saphenous vein** commences on the lateral side of the dorsum of the foot, behind the lateral malleolus and lateral to the calcaneal tendon. It ascends in the fascia near the midline on the back of the leg. Behind the knee the small saphenous vein passes between the two heads of the gastrocnemius and opens into the popliteal vein (**ATLAS PLATES 412, 413 #413.1**).

Along the lower half of the posterior leg, the small saphenous vein is accompanied by the **sural nerve.** It is the main sensory nerve of the calf and lateral border of the foot (**ATLAS PLATE 412**). It is most often formed by branches coming from both the tibial and common fibular nerves, but at times the branch from the common fibular descends as a separate branch as far as the heel (**Figure 23-1**). The continuation of the sural nerve in the foot is the **lateral dorsal cutaneous branch** to the lateral foot and little toe.

◄
Grant's 340, 342
Netter's 527
Rohen's 468, 469, 489

►
Grant's 340, 342, 385
Netter's 527
Rohen 468, 469, 489, 493

◄
Grant's 340, 384, 385
Netter's 527
Rohen's 489, 493

Make a vertical incision down the middle of the posterior leg, being careful not to cut the **small saphenous vein** and **sural nerve** (**ATLAS PLATE 412**). Make lateral and medial incisions at the ankle and remove the skin entirely. Dissect the small saphenous vein to its junction with the popliteal vein and follow the sural nerve superiorly to its component branches from the tibial and common fibular nerves. Trace the sural nerve inferiorly behind the lateral malleolus to its entrance into the foot.

Remove the superficial fascia and sever the deep fascia overlying the bellies of the gastrocnemius muscle. Expose this muscle and its tendon completely by removing the deep fascia (**ATLAS PLATE 413**).

III. Posterior Compartment: Muscles, Vessels, and Nerves

The posterior compartment consists of superficial and deep muscles that are separated by a deep transverse

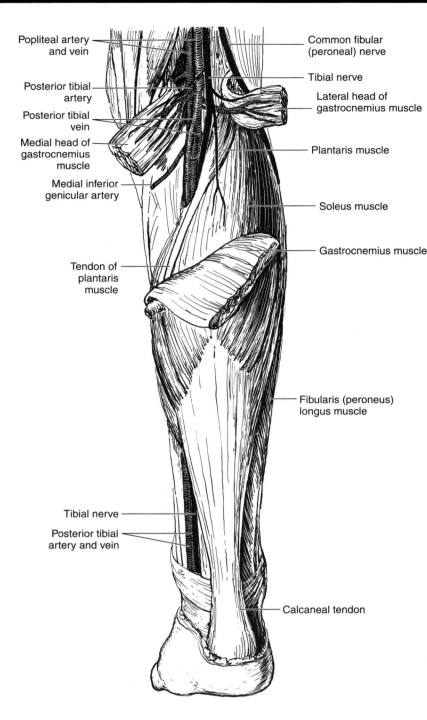

Popliteal artery
and vein

Posterior tibial
artery

Posterior tibial
vein

Medial head of
gastrocnemius
muscle

Medial inferior
genicular artery

Tendon of
plantaris
muscle

Tibial nerve

Posterior tibial
artery and vein

Common fibular
(peroneal) nerve

Tibial nerve

Lateral head of
gastrocnemius muscle

Plantaris muscle

Soleus muscle

Gastrocnemius muscle

Fibularis (peroneus)
longus muscle

Calcaneal tendon

Figure 23-2. The superficial compartment of the posterior leg.

fascial plane. The **posterior tibial vessels** supply the region, and the muscles are innervated by the **tibial nerve**.

A. Superficial Compartment Muscles. There are three muscles in the superficial compartment. Two are large, the **gastrocnemius** and the **soleus,** whereas the third is the small **plantaris muscle** that lies between the other two (**Figure 23-2**).

   1. The **gastrocnemius muscle** is the most superficial of the posterior leg muscles, and it forms the principal mass of the calf (**ATLAS PLATE 413**). It arises

▶
Grant's 416
Netter's 498
Rohen 457

◀
Grant's 416, 417, 453, 455
Netter's 498, 499, 504
Rohen 457, 458

by two heads from the posterior surface of the femoral condyles. Its tendon of insertion begins midway down the leg as a wide aponeurosis that becomes a thick, rounded tendon that joins the tendon of the underlying soleus muscle to form the **tendo calcaneus** (or **Achilles tendon**). It is the strongest and thickest tendon in the body, and it attaches onto the posterior surface of the calcaneus (**Figure 23-2**).

   2. The **soleus muscle,** deep to the gastrocnemius, is a broad, flat muscle that arises from the posterior surface of the upper fibula and the soleal line of the tibia (**ATLAS PLATES 415, 416**). Its fibers descend, become tendinous, and merge with the gastrocnemius to form the tendo calcaneus.

3. The **plantaris muscle** is a small muscle with an elongated, thin tendon. From its fleshy belly (7 to 9 cm long) descends a long, slender tendon (20 to 25 cm long) between the soleus and gastrocnemius muscles (**ATLAS PLATE 415**). The tendon is inserted into the calcaneus with the tendo calcaneus.

Clean the surface of the gastrocnemius, gently pull apart its two heads, and find their motor nerves, which enter at their deep (anterior) surface (**ATLAS PLATE 416**). Note that these nerves are branches from the tibial nerve. Cut across the bellies of the gastrocnemius 5 to 7 cm below their origin (or below the entrance of their nerves) and reflect the upper parts proximally (**ATLAS PLATE 416**). Turn the lower end of the muscle distally to its junction with the tendon of the underlying soleus muscle. Locate the slender tendon of the plantaris along the **medial border of the tendo calcaneus.** Follow the plantaris tendon proximally, and note that its muscle belly lies deep to the **lateral head** of the gastrocnemius muscle (**ATLAS PLATE 415**).

Cut the tendon of the plantaris and the tendo calcaneus about 2 cm below the level where the tendons of the gastrocnemius and soleus meet. Dissect the tendo calcaneus distally to the calcaneus, and identify the bursa between the tendon and the bone.

Lift the proximal end of the tendo calcaneus, and with your hand behind the soleus, separate it from the underlying deep posterior leg muscles. Sever the origin of the soleus muscle along its tibial attachment, leaving the fibular origin of the soleus intact. Turn the gastrocnemius and soleus muscle mass laterally (**ATLAS PLATE 417**).

With the superficial muscles reflected laterally, identify the **popliteus muscle** covered with fascia (**ATLAS PLATE 418**) and the posterior tibial vessels and tibial nerve (**ATLAS PLATES 418, 419**).

B. Popliteus Muscle, Posterior Tibial Vessels, and Tibial Nerve. The floor of the lower one-third of the popliteal fossa is formed by the popliteus muscle. Along its posterior surface descend the posterior tibial vessels and the tibial nerve.

1. The **popliteus** is an important muscle. It must "unlock" the fully extended knee joint when a person is standing erect before any flexion of the leg can be initiated, as in taking a step forward. It is a triangular, flat muscle attached inferiorly along the **soleal line** of the tibia. Its fibers course superiorly

◄
Grant's 417, 418
Netter's 499
Rohen 457, 490

◄
Grant's 416, 417, 419
Netter's 499, 522, 523
Rohen 457, 458

►
Grant's 418–420, 422
Netter's 500, 504, 511
Rohen 460, 461, 490, 491

►
Grant's 346, 419
Netter's 494, 500
Rohen 488, 491
◄
Grant's 437
Netter's 503, 511

►
Grant's 346
Netter's 500
Rohen 467, 491

◄
Grant's 397, 414, 419
Netter's 499, 500
Rohen 457, 460

►
Grant's 418, 419
Netter's 500, 523
Rohen 460, 461, 490, 491

◄
Grant's 414, 418, 419, 422
Netter's 499, 500, 523
Rohen 457, 460

and laterally and end in a rounded tendon that splits. Half of the tendon attaches to the lateral condyle of the femur, while the other half attaches to the lateral meniscus of the knee joint (**ATLAS PLATE 440**). **The popliteus rotates the femur laterally to unlock the knee joint and, simultaneously, retracts the lateral meniscus posteriorly so that it does not become crushed between the lateral condyles of the femur and tibia.**

2. **Posterior Tibial Vessels and Tibial Nerve.** The **posterior tibial artery** is one of the two terminal branches of the popliteal artery, and it commences at the lower border of the popliteus muscle (**ATLAS PLATE 419**). The anterior tibial artery also arises from the popliteal at this site and courses through the interosseous membrane to get to the anterior leg. Descending to the medial ankle region, the posterior tibial vessels and nerve course behind the medial malleolus to enter the plantar aspect of the foot (**ATLAS PLATE 419**). The **posterior tibial veins** receive the **medial and lateral plantar veins** from the foot and the **deep plantar venous arch.**

Dissect the popliteal artery to the lower border of the popliteus muscle and identify its terminal branches, the **anterior and posterior tibial arteries.** Confirm that the anterior tibial branch is the vessel you dissected in the anterior compartment. Follow the posterior tibial artery and its veins and the tibial nerve to the medial ankle region (**Figure 23-3**).

About 2.5 cm inferior to the popliteus muscle, find the **fibular artery** branching from the posterior tibial. Its origin may be as high as the popliteal fossa or as low as midcalf. Follow it toward the fibula and then deep (anterior) to the flexor hallucis longus muscle (**ATLAS PLATE 419**). Note that along its course the fibular artery gives off one or more **perforating branches** to supply the lateral compartment.

C. Deep Posterior Compartment of the Leg (Figure 23-3). In addition to the **popliteus muscle,** there are three other posterior compartment muscles in the leg: the **flexor digitorum longus,** the **flexor hallucis longus,** and the **tibialis posterior** (**ATLAS PLATE 418**). These latter three muscles act across the ankle joint and across other joints in the foot. Their tendons along with the posterior tibial vessels and the tibial nerve enter the foot by coursing behind the medial malleolus.

1. The **flexor digitorum longus** arises medially from the posterior surface of the tibia and the fascia covering the tibialis posterior muscle. Its

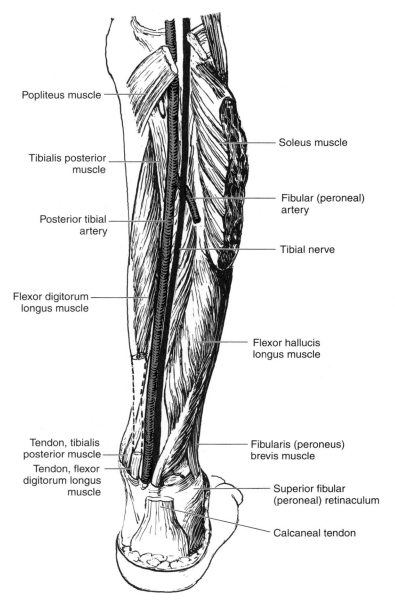

Popliteus muscle

Tibialis posterior muscle

Posterior tibial artery

Flexor digitorum longus muscle

Tendon, tibialis posterior muscle

Tendon, flexor digitorum longus muscle

Soleus muscle

Fibular (peroneal) artery

Tibial nerve

Flexor hallucis longus muscle

Fibularis (peroneus) brevis muscle

Superior fibular (peroneal) retinaculum

Calcaneal tendon

Figure 23-3. The posterior tibial artery and tibial nerve.

fibers end in a tendon that crosses to the lateral side of the tibialis posterior and passes into the plantar surface of the foot behind the medial malleolus. In the foot the tendon divides into four smaller tendons that insert onto the distal phalanges of the four lateral toes (**ATLAS PLATE 424**). It flexes these toes and helps to plantarflex the foot at the ankle joint when the foot is firmly on the ground (e.g., during the takeoff phase of walking).

2. The **flexor hallucis longus** arises from the posterior surface of the lower fibula and the interosseous membrane (**ATLAS PLATE 421**). Its fibers form a tendon that grooves the posterior

◄
Grant's 418–421
Netter's 500, 504, 511
Rohen 460, 461, 490, 491

►
Grant's 414, 418–420, 438
Netter's 500, 504, 511, 523
Rohen 460, 461, 490, 491

surface of the tibia, the talus, and the lower surface of the **sustentaculum tali** of the calcaneus. Behind the medial malleolus the tendon lies lateral to the posterior tibial vessels and nerve (**ATLAS PLATE 419**). It courses along the medial border of the plantar foot and inserts onto the distal phalanx of the large toe, which it strongly flexes (**ATLAS PLATE 424**).

3. The **tibialis posterior** lies between the previous two muscles and is more deeply placed in the posterior compartment. It arises from the interosseous membrane and from the surfaces of the fibula and tibia adjacent to that membrane. Its tendon enters the foot by passing immediately be-

hind the medial malleolus (**ATLAS PLATE 421**). Coursing forward in the foot, the tendon inserts onto the tuberosity of the navicular and several surrounding bones (**ATLAS PLATE 455 #455.2**). The tibialis posterior inverts the foot at the intertarsal joints and helps to plantarflex the foot at the ankle joint.

◄ Grant's 414, 418–421, 438 Netter's 500, 504, 511, 523 Rohen 460, 461, 491

Expose and separate the deep compartment muscles by dissecting the fascial layer deep to the soleus (**ATLAS PLATE 418**). Identify the **flexor hallucis longus** found on the fibular side of the deep compartment and then the **flexor digitorum longus** on the tibial side of the leg. Dissect the **tibialis posterior** that lies between these two muscles.

◄ Grant's 414, 418, 419 Netter's 500, 523 Rohen 460, 461, 490, 491

Follow the tendons and the posterior tibial vessels and nerve deep to the flexor retinaculum behind the medial malleolus (**ATLAS PLATE 414**). Expose the flexor retinaculum, and observe that it extends from the medial malleolus posteriorly and inferiorly to the medial surface of the calcaneus (**ATLAS PLATES 408 #408.2, 414**).

Cut through the flexor retinaculum and identify the order of structures behind the medial malleolus. Confirm the following:

1. Tendon of tibialis posterior
2. Tendon of flexor digitorum longus
3. Posterior tibial artery and veins
4. Tibial nerve
5. Tendon of flexor hallucis longus

◄ Grant's 420, 421 Netter's 500, 511 Rohen's 460, 461, 490, 491

IV. Plantar Aspect of the Foot

A. **Superficial Structures.** The skin on the sole of the foot is thick and cornified and adheres closely to a dense layer of superficial fascia. Deep to the superficial fascia is the exceedingly strong **plantar aponeurosis** (**ATLAS PLATE 422**). Its longitudinally oriented, glistening aponeurotic fibers spread forward from the calcaneus to the plantar surface of each digit and the borders of the plantar surface. The sole is innervated by the **medial and lateral plantar branches of the tibial nerve,** which perforate the plantar aponeurosis to reach the skin. The nerves are accompanied by branches of the medial and lateral plantar vessels (**ATLAS PLATE 422**).

◄ Grant's 470, 491, 531, 532 Netter's 514–517, 523 Rohen 463, 500–502

With the cadaver lying face downward, place a wooden block under the ankle region so that the plantar surface is elevated.

◄ Grant's 414, 418–421, 438 Netter's 500, 504, 511, 523 Rohen 460, 461, 491

Make a longitudinal incision in the midline of the plantar foot from the calcaneus to the base of the 2nd toe (**Figure 23-4, A–B**). Make transverse incisions to the lateral and medial borders of the foot at the base of the toes (**Figure 23-4, B–C and B–D**). Cut the skin in the midline along the plantar surface of the digits to the tip of each toe.

Reflect the skin and superficial fascia together, beginning at the heel. The depth of dissection should be along the plane just superficial to the glistening layer of the **plantar aponeurosis** (**Figure 23-5**). Also remove the skin from the toes. Using a scalpel, scrape along the surface of the plantar aponeurosis to expose its fascicles to the base of the toes. Find the **plantar metatarsal vessels** and the **common plantar digital nerves** that extend distally between the fascicles (**ATLAS PLATE 422 #422.2**). These are branches of the medial and lateral plantar vessels and nerves.

► Grant's 424, 428 Netter's 514, 515 Rohen 463, 500

Separate the central part of the plantar aponeurosis from the underlying muscles with a probe to determine its depth. Cut across the aponeurosis in the heel region and reflect it forward to the base of the toes as a sheet.

B. **First Layer of Plantar Muscles.** The first layer of muscles in the foot includes two abductors and a flexor: the **abductor hallucis,** the **abductor**

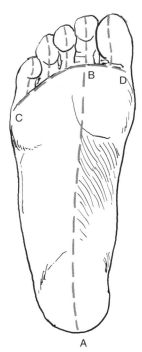

Figure 23-4. Incision lines on the plantar surface of the foot.

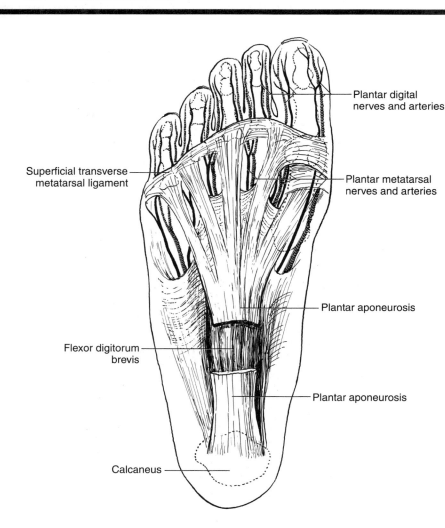

Plantar digital nerves and arteries

Superficial transverse metatarsal ligament

Plantar metatarsal nerves and arteries

Figure 23-5. The plantar aponeurosis and superficial plantar vessels and nerves to the toes.

Plantar aponeurosis

Flexor digitorum brevis

Plantar aponeurosis

Calcaneus

---

digiti minimi, and the **flexor digitorum brevis (Figure 23-6).**

1. The **abductor hallucis** forms the medial contour of the foot, and it overlies the plantar vessels and nerves as they enter the foot (**ATLAS PLATES 423–425**). It arises from the flexor retinaculum and the medial aspect of the calcaneus and inserts on the proximal phalanx of the large toe (**ATLAS PLATE 424**). It abducts and flexes the large toe at the metatarsophalangeal joint and is supplied by the medial plantar nerve.

2. The **abductor digiti minimi** is located along the lateral border of the foot. It also arises from the calcaneus and plantar aponeurosis, and its tendon inserts on the proximal phalanx of the 5th digit. It abducts and flexes the little toe and is supplied by the lateral plantar nerve (**ATLAS PLATES 423, 424**).

3. The **flexor digitorum brevis** is located in the middle of the plantar surface between the two

▶
Grant's 428
Netter's 515
Rohen 463, 500

◀
Grant's 428, 430, 431
Netter's 515–517
Rohen 463, 464

◀
Grant's 428, 430, 431
Netter's 515, 516, 523
Rohen 463, 464, 500, 501

▶
Grant's 428, 430,
Netter's 515, 516
Rohen 500, 501

abductors and is exposed as the plantar aponeurosis is removed (**ATLAS PLATE 423**). It arises from the calcaneus and the plantar aponeurosis and divides into tendons that insert onto the middle phalanx of the lateral four toes. At the level of the proximal phalanges, each tendon splits at the base of the toe to allow the respective tendon of the flexor digitorum longus to pass through on its way to the distal phalanx. The flexor digitorum brevis flexes the middle and proximal phalanges of the lateral four toes and is innervated by the medial plantar nerve.

Separate the **abductor hallucis** from deeper structures along the medial border of the foot. Follow its tendon to the base of the proximal phalanx of the large toe. At its insertion do not be confused by the tendon of the medial head of the **flexor hallucis brevis,** which inserts just deep to the abductor (**ATLAS PLATE 427**). Dissect the **abductor digiti minimi** along the lateral border of the foot. Trace

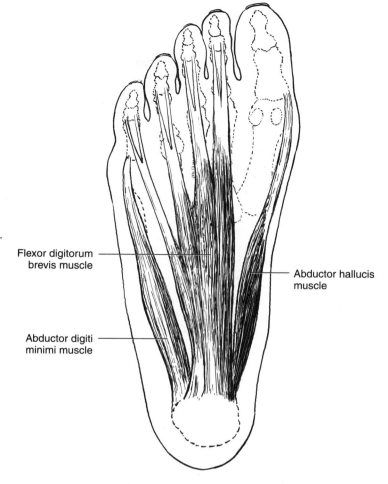

Figure 23-6. The first layer of plantar muscles.

Flexor digitorum brevis muscle

Abductor hallucis muscle

Abductor digiti minimi muscle

its tendon distally to the proximal phalanx of the little toe, where it inserts near the tendon of the underlying **flexor digiti minimi brevis (ATLAS PLATE 423)**.

Dissect the **flexor digitorum brevis** along the middle of the plantar surface and trace its four tendons to the lateral four toes. Dissect the tendon to the 2nd toe by severing longitudinally the digital fibrous sheath (**ATLAS PLATE 423**). Observe how the tendon of the flexor brevis splits, inserts on the middle phalanx, and allows the tendon of the flexor longus to pass to the distal phalanx.

Identify the **medial plantar nerve and vessels** between the abductor hallucis and the flexor digitorum brevis (**ATLAS PLATE 425**). Find the **lateral plantar nerve and vessels** between the flexor digitorum brevis and the abductor digiti minimi. **Being careful not to sever the neurovascular structures,** cut across the abductor hallucis near its middle and reflect the two ends. Sever the flexor digitorum brevis near

◄
Grant's 428
Netter's 497
Rohen 463, 500

►
Grant's 421
Netter's 516
Rohen 464, 501

◄
Grant's 428
Netter's 515, 516
Rohen 500, 501

its origin and turn the muscle forward to the bases of the toes. This requires severing the nerve that supplies it. Transect the abductor digiti minimi near its middle and reflect both ends.

C. Second Layer of Plantar Muscles, Medial and Lateral Plantar Nerves, and Vessels. Deep to the first layer of muscles are found the **medial and lateral plantar nerves and vessels** and the **tendons of the flexor digitorum longus** and **flexor hallucis longus.** Attached to the tendon of the flexor digitorum longus are the muscles of the second layer, namely the **quadratus plantae** and the **lumbrical muscles (ATLAS PLATE 424).**

1. The **medial and lateral plantar nerves** course into the foot deep to the abductor hallucis.

The **medial plantar nerve** supplies sensory innervation to the medial three and one-half toes. It also innervates the abductor hallucis, flexor digitorum brevis, flexor hallucis brevis, and the 1st lumbrical muscle. It divides into a **proper digital branch to the great toe** and three **common plantar digital nerves (ATLAS PLATE 425).** The latter split into proper digital nerves that supply the adjacent surfaces of: (a) the great and 2nd toes; (b) the 2nd and 3rd toes, and (c) the 3rd and 4th toes.

The **lateral plantar nerve** crosses the foot to supply the skin of the little toe and the lateral half of the 4th toe through its **superficial branch.** After supplying the muscles of the little toe, the lateral plantar nerve sends its **deep branch** medially and deep with the lateral plantar artery to innervate all of the intrinsic muscles of the foot not supplied by the medial plantar nerve (**ATLAS PLATES 425, 426**).

2. The **medial and lateral plantar arteries** are the terminal branches of the posterior tibial artery (**ATLAS PLATES 425, 426, 428 #428.1**).

The **medial plantar artery** is smaller than the lateral, and it courses along the medial side of the foot accompanying the medial plantar nerve. It divides into a digital branch that supplies the large toe and an anastomosing branch that joins a branch from the lateral plantar artery.

The **lateral plantar artery** crosses the foot to the base of the 5th metatarsal bone, sending a branch to the little toe. It then turns medially and, accompanied by the **deep branch of the lateral plantar nerve,** forms the **plantar arch.** From this arch stem four **plantar metatarsal arteries.** These course between the metatarsal bones to the toes. Each divides into two **digital vessels** that supply the adjacent surfaces of two toes (**ATLAS PLATES 426, 428 #428.1**).

3. **Second layer: tendons and muscles (ATLAS PLATE 424).** The tendons of the flexor hallucis longus and flexor digitorum longus course to the distal phalanges of the toes within the second layer of plantar foot muscles. The tendon of the flexor digitorum longus has attached to it the quadratus plantae and the lumbrical muscles. These assist the long flexor in its action on the lateral four toes.

The **quadratus plantae** arises by two heads from the calcaneus (**ATLAS PLATES 424, 425**). These fuse and insert onto the lateral border of the tendon of the flexor digitorum longus where the main tendon splits into its four digital tendons. The quadratus plantae straightens the traction of the flexor digitorum longus tendon, making it parallel with the long axis of the foot. It is supplied by the lateral plantar nerve.

The **lumbricals** are four small muscles that arise from the digital tendons of the flexor digitorum longus at their division from the main tendon (**ATLAS PLATES 423, 424**). The 1st lumbrical arises from

◄ Grant's 348, 430
Netter's 516, 517, 524
Rohen 501, 502

► Grant's 346, 348
Netter's 516, 517
Rohen 501, 502

◄ Grant's 342, 424, 425, 430
Netter's 516, 517
Rohen 501, 502

► Grant's 561, 567
Rohen 500, 501

◄ Grant's 421
Netter's 516
Rohen 464, 501

► Grant's 346, 424, 425, 430
Netter's 516–518, 523
Rohen 501, 502

► Netter's 516, 517
Rohen 501, 502

◄ Grant's 421
Netter's 516
Rohen 461, 464, 501

► Grant's 421
Netter's 516
Rohen 461, 464

the medial side of the main flexor tendon, but each of the other lumbrical muscles arises from two adjoining digital tendons. The muscles insert distally onto the medial sides of the dorsal hood of the lateral four toes. The most medial (1st) lumbrical is supplied by the medial plantar nerve; the other three are supplied by the deep branch of the lateral plantar nerve. The lumbricals flex the metatarsophalangeal joints and extend the interphalangeal joints.

Trace the medial and lateral plantar nerves and arteries distally. Find small branches of the **medial plantar nerve** entering the deep surface of the abductor hallucis and flexor digitorum brevis muscles (**ATLAS PLATE 425**). Follow also branches of the **medial plantar artery,** which course to the large and 2nd toes. Follow the medial plantar nerve distally and find:

a. its branch to the **flexor digitorum brevis** (a muscle in the 3rd layer),

b. the **proper digital branch** along the medial side of the large toe, and

c. three **common digital branches** near the bases of the metatarsal bones.

Note that each common digital nerve splits into two proper digital branches that supply the adjacent surfaces of two toes: **the first** between the great toe and the 2nd toe, **the second** between the 2nd and 3rd toes, and **the third** between the 3rd and 4th toes (**ATLAS PLATE 425**).

Trace the **lateral plantar nerve** distally as it crosses the foot from medial to lateral with the **lateral plantar artery.** Over the 5th metatarsal bone note that the lateral plantar nerve divides into **superficial and deep branches.** Also at this site the lateral plantar artery turns medially and, accompanied by the deep branch of the lateral plantar nerve, courses deep to the flexor tendons to form the **plantar arterial arch (ATLAS PLATE 426).**

Dissect the **superficial branch of the lateral plantar nerve** and follow it to its division into one branch that supplies the lateral surface of the little toe and a **common digital branch** that divides to supply the adjacent surfaces of the 4th and 5th toes (**ATLAS PLATE 425**).

Identify the heads of the **quadratus plantae,** the **four lumbrical muscles,** and the **tendons of the flexor hallucis longus** and **flexor digitorum longus.** Cut the heads of the quadratus plantae from the calcaneus. Cut the **common tendon** of the flexor digitorum longus and the tendon of the flexor hallucis longus at its entrance point into the plantar foot. Reflect the cut structures and follow the lumbrical muscles to their insertions on the medial side of the four lateral toes.

► Grant's 430, 431
Netter's 516, 517
Rohen 464, 465

D. Third Layer of Plantar Muscles (Figure 23-7). Recall that in the first layer of plantar muscles there were two abductors and one flexor. In the third layer there are two flexors and an adductor (with two heads). These are the **flexor hallucis brevis** medially, the **flexor digiti minimi brevis** laterally, and the **adductor hallucis,** which consists of **oblique and transverse heads.** Deep to the oblique head of the adductor hallucis courses the **plantar arterial arch** and the **deep branch of the lateral plantar nerve (ATLAS PLATES 426, 427).**

◄ Grant's 424, 425, 430
Netter's 517, 518, 523
Rohen 465, 501, 502

1. The **flexor hallucis brevis** arises from the cuboid and lateral cuneiform bones and from the tendon of the tibialis posterior near its insertion. The belly of the muscle divides into medial and lateral parts that attach to the sides of the proximal phalanx of the large toe (**ATLAS PLATE 427**). It is

► Grant's 430
Netter's 517
Rohen 465

a flexor of the large toe and is supplied by the medial plantar nerve.

2. The **flexor digiti minimi brevis** arises from the 5th metatarsal bone and the sheath covering the fibularis longus tendon. It inserts on the lateral side of the base of the proximal phalanx of the little toe (**Figure 23-7**). It flexes the little toe and is supplied by the lateral plantar nerve.

3. The **adductor hallucis** consists of oblique and transverse heads (**ATLAS PLATE 427**). The **oblique head** arises from the bases of the 2nd, 3rd, and 4th metatarsal bones and from the sheath of the tendon of the fibularis longus muscle, and it courses distally and medially toward the large toe. The **transverse head** arises from the joint capsules of the 3rd, 4th, and 5th metatarsophalangeal joints and from the deep transverse metatarsal ligaments. It crosses the foot transversely from lateral to medial and joins the fibers of the oblique head to form a single tendon that inserts on the lateral surface of the proximal phalanx of the large toe (**Figure 23-7**). It adducts the large toe.

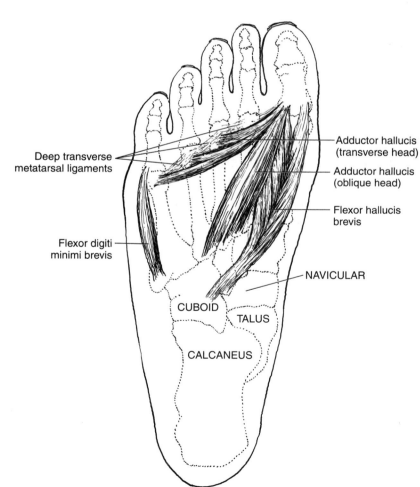

Figure 23-7. The third layer of plantar muscles.

Dissect the **flexor hallucis brevis** and the oblique head of the **adductor hallucis.** Separate them from underlying structures, sever their origins, and turn the muscle bellies distally. Trace the **plantar arterial arch** and the **deep branch of the lateral plantar nerve** crossing the foot deep to the 3rd layer of muscles (**ATLAS PLATE 426**).

Identify one or more **plantar metatarsal arteries,** which branch from the arterial arch and extend between the metatarsal bones along the surface of the interosseous muscles. Note that the metatarsal arteries become **common digital arteries,** and that each of these divide into two **proper plantar digital arteries** that supply the adjacent surfaces of two toes (**ATLAS PLATE 428 #428.1**). Trace the plantar arterial arch to its junction with the **dorsalis pedis artery,** which enters the plantar surface of the foot from the dorsal surface between the 1st and 2nd metatarsal bones (**ATLAS PLATES 411, 426, 428, #428.1**).

Dissect the **flexor digiti minimi brevis** from its origin on the 5th metatarsal bone to its common insertion with the abductor digiti minimi (1st layer) on the lateral side of the little toe (**Figure 23-7**). Sever the origin of the transverse head of the adductor hallucis and reflect it medially to its insertion on the large toe. Now the interosseous muscles should be visible.

▶ Grant's 348, 430, 431
Netter's 517–519, 523
Rohen 465

◀ Grant's 424, 425, 430
Netter's 517, 518, 523
Rohen 465, 501, 502

◀ Grant's 424, 425
Netter's 517, 518
Rohen 501, 502

◀ Grant's 428, 430, 431
Netter's 516, 517
Rohen 464, 465

▶ Grant's 431
Netter's 417–419
Rohen 465

▶ Grant's 431
Netter's 518, 519
Rohen 465

E. **Fourth Layer of Plantar Muscles (Figure 23-8).** This deepest muscle group includes **three plantar and four dorsal interosseous muscles.** They are comparable to the interosseous muscles in the hand. Within the foot, however, the **midline of the 2nd digit is used as the central axis** for movement of the toes, rather than the 3rd digit. All the interossei are supplied by the **lateral plantar nerve.**

1. **Plantar interossei.** The three plantar interossei are located in the three most lateral interosseous spaces and they arise along the medial side of the 3rd, 4th, and 5th metatarsal bones (**ATLAS PLATE 428 #428.2**). Their tendons are inserted distally onto the medial side of the proximal phalanx of the corresponding toes. Because the 2nd digit serves as the central axis in the foot, these muscles **adduct** the 3rd, 4th, and 5th toes and **flex** their proximal phalanges.

2. **Dorsal interossei.** The four dorsal interossei are within the four interosseous spaces (**ATLAS PLATE 428 #428.3**). Each is bipennate and arises by two heads from the adjacent sides of two metatarsal bones. Their tendons insert on the bases of the proximal phalanges and dorsal digital expansions. They **abduct the toes** and **flex the metatarsophalangeal joints.** The first is inserted on the medial side of the 2nd toe, and the others insert on the lateral sides of the 2nd, 3rd, and 4th

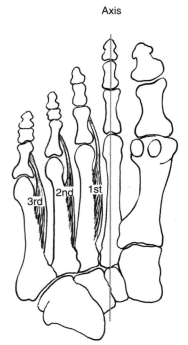

Plantar interossei (adductors)

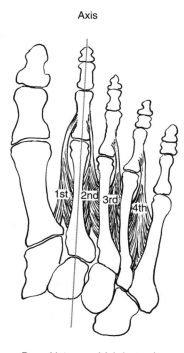

Dorsal interossei (abductors)

Figure 23-8. The plantar and dorsal interosseous muscles.

toes. The 2nd toe receives two dorsal interosseous muscles but no plantar interosseous muscle.

Because each toe must have an abductor and an adductor, 10 muscles are required for these actions. The plantar and dorsal interosseous muscles account for 7, the large toe has its own abductor hallucis and adductor hallucis, and the little toe has its abductor digiti minimi, making 10 in all.

Identify the **deep transverse metatarsal ligaments** interconnecting the distal ends of the metatarsal bones, helping to bind them together (**ATLAS PLATE 455 #455.2**). Cut these ligaments and separate the toes to dissect the interosseous muscles. Detach and reflect the origins of the flexor digiti minimi brevis and the oblique head of the adductor hallucis to expose the intermetatarsal spaces.

◄
Grant's 430
Netter's 510, 518

Trace the three plantar interosseous muscles and note that each arises from a single metatarsal bone. Follow their tendons across the metatarsophalangeal joints to their insertions on the **medial surfaces** of the proximal phalanges of the 3rd, 4th, and 5th toes (**Figure 23-8**).

◄
Grant's 431
Netter's 517–519
Rohen 465

From either the dorsal or plantar surface identify the four dorsal interosseous muscles. Follow the tendons of the medial two dorsal muscles distally to their insertions, one on each side of the **second digit.** Follow the tendons of the 3rd and 4th muscles to their insertions on the lateral sides of the 3rd and 4th digits (**Figure 23-8**).

◄
Grant's 431
Netter's 518–519
Rohen 465

Clinical Relevance

Tibial nerve injury. If the tibial nerve is injured as it enters the posterior compartment of the leg the muscles of this compartment and those in the plantar aspect of the foot become paralyzed. Additionally, sensory innervation on the plantar foot is lost, and the sole of the foot may become ulcerated without the person realizing it.

Medial plantar nerve entrapment. This condition occurs when the medial plantar nerve is compressed by the flexor retinaculum as a result of repetitive sports activities, such as long-distance running and repetitive eversion of the foot. The medial aspect of the plantar foot experiences sensation loss, and some of the muscles of the large toe experience a loss of function.

Arterial occlusive disease. This condition can occur because of an inadequate arterial supply to the muscles of the posterior compartment of the leg. Use of the afflicted limb in walking is limited and the pain is excruciating. Called intermittent claudication, the pain is relieved by resting, but it returns with walking again.

Calcaneal bursitis. This is an inflammation of the bursa deep to the calcaneal tendon on the posterior surface of the calcaneus. It is most often caused by overuse of the lower limb in sports, such as long-distance running, or by trauma sustained by professional basketball players, but it also can occur as a result of wearing overly tight shoes.

Ruptured calcaneal tendon. Rupture of the calcaneal tendon is usually due to a severe contracture of the gastrocnemius-soleus muscle group when a person is not physically in condition. Surgery is required to repair a complete rupture of the tendon; however, a partial rupture may heal without surgery.

Fracture of the calcaneus. This injury can be caused by a person falling from a height and landing on his heels and is most serious when there is a fracture at more than one part of the bone. The talus is driven into the calcaneus to cause the fractures. It is exceedingly painful because the talocalcaneonavicular joint sustains the weight of the body, and fracture of the calcaneus disables this joint.

Plantar fasciitis. Inflammation of the plantar aponeurosis, called plantar fasciitis, is usually the result of sports activities, such as running in uncomfortable shoes. The pain is usually in the posterior heel region and seems to be more painful after a period of rest and then commencing to walk again. It frequently occurs in runners.

Bunions. A bunion can develop on the medial surface of the metacarpophalangeal joint of the large toe. This condition is often seen in women who wear pointed shoes or who wear shoes that are too small for their feet. A movement of the distal part of the large toe toward the lateral side of the foot also develops. Bunions can be painful because they can become inflamed and they may eventually require surgical attention.

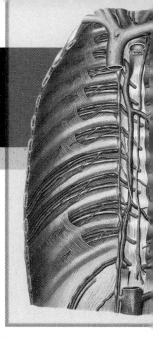

Joints of the Lower Limb

OBJECTIVES

1. Visualize the sacrospinous and sacrotuberous ligaments and the sacroiliac joint posteriorly.

2. Study the symphysis pubis and its ligaments.

3. Dissect the hip joint, anterior and posterior approaches.

4. Dissect the knee joint, anterior and posterior approaches.

5. Visualize the superior, middle, and inferior tibiofibular joints.

6. Dissect the ankle joint.

7. Understand the arches of the foot and dissect the subtalar, talocalcaneonavicular, and calcaneocuboid joints.

8. Visualize the tarsometatarsal joint and study the metatarsophalangeal and interphalangeal joints.

Atlas Key:

Clemente Atlas, 5th Edition = Clemente Plate #

Grant's Atlas, 11th Edition = Grant's Page #

Netter's Atlas, 3rd Edition = Netter's Plate #

Rohen Atlas, 6th Edition = Rohen Page #

The joints of the lower limb include those that articulate the two pelvic bones with the vertebral column, the **sacroiliac joints,** and the two pelvic bones with each other, the **symphysis pubis,** as well as the joints of the free limb. The latter include the **hip, knee,** and **ankle joints;** the **tibiofibular joints;** the **transverse tarsal joint;** the **intertarsal, tarsometatarsal,** and

►
Grant's 290, 291, 294, 295
Netter's 340–342
Rohen 432, 435, 438

intermetatarsal joints; and finally the **metatarsophalangeal** and **interphalangeal joints.**

I. Sacroiliac Joint (ATLAS PLATES 271, 273)

The sacroiliac joints are synovial joints, one on each side of the sacrum. Each joint interconnects the **auricular surface** of the **ilium** with the reciprocally curved surface of the **sacrum.** The sacrum presents its lateral surfaces to form the joints, and the **anterior, interosseous,** and posterior **sacroiliac ligaments** bind the bones together (**Figure 24-1**).

Stability to the sacroiliac articulations also comes from the **sacrotuberous** and **sacrospinous ligaments**

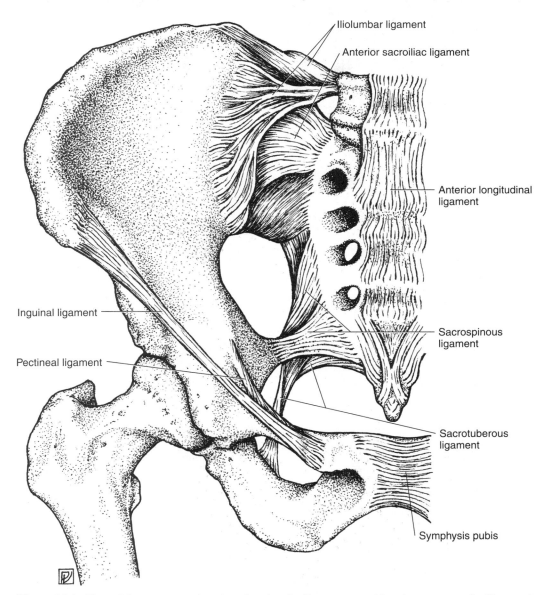

Figure 24-1. The pelvis: anterosuperior view showing the ligaments attaching the sacrum to the ilium and ischium.

inferiorly and the **sacroiliac ligaments** above. Because the sacrum lies inferior to most of the vertebral column, considerable weight is transmitted to it. This pressure tends to rotate the **upper end of the sacrum forward and downward** and its **lower end and the coccyx backward and upward.** Ligaments prevent this displacement **(Figure 24-2).** The ligaments that maintain stability of the joint by **resisting forward motion of the upper end of the joint** are the interosseous and posterior and anterior sacroiliac ligaments **(Figure 24-2).**

The **interosseous sacroiliac ligament** forms the strongest bond between the sacrum and the ilium, and it stretches above and behind the synovial joint **(Figure 24-3).** Overlying the interosseous ligament are the short and

◄ Grant's 298, 299, 372, 376
Netter's 152, 340, 341
Rohen 444, 445

◄ Grant's 294, 298, 372
Netter's 152, 341, 539
Rohen 444, 445

long **posterior sacroiliac ligaments** interconnecting the posterior iliac spines to the sacrum **(ATLAS PLATE 273 #273.1).** The **anterior sacroiliac ligaments** strengthen the joint capsule anteriorly **(ATLAS PLATE 271).**

The ligaments that **prevent backward rotation of the lower end** of the sacrum and coccyx are the two sacrotuberous and sacrospinous ligaments **(Figure 24-2).**

The **sacrotuberous ligaments** are broad and strong and extend on each side between the posterior and lateral surfaces of the sacrum and coccyx down to the ischial tuberosity **(ATLAS PLATE 273 #273.1).** The **sacrospinous ligaments** are thin and triangular. They extend laterally on each side from the margin of the sacrum and coccyx to the spine of the ischium

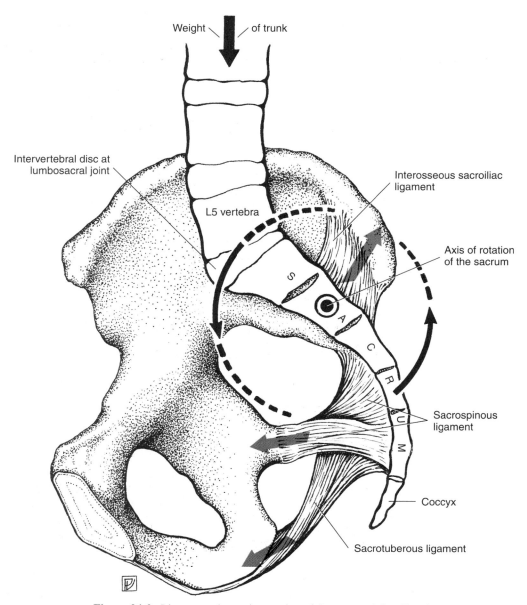

Weight ↘ ↙ of trunk

Intervertebral disc at
lumbosacral joint

L5 vertebra

Interosseous sacroiliac
ligament

Axis of rotation
of the sacrum

S A C R U M

Sacrospinous
ligament

Coccyx

Sacrotuberous ligament

Figure 24-2. Ligaments that resist rotation of the sacrum (after Grant).

(**ATLAS PLATE 272 #272.2**). The sacrotuberous and sacrospinous ligaments convert the greater and lesser sciatic notches into the **greater and lesser sciatic foramina.** Through these foramina, structures leave the pelvis to enter the gluteal region.

On a skeleton study the surfaces that articulate the sacrum to the pelvis, both anteriorly and posteriorly. Note that the curved auricular surfaces of the sacrum fit into reciprocally shaped ridges on the two ilia. **On the cadaver** reflect the medial attachment of the cut gluteus maximus muscle to the sacrum and

◄
Grant's 188, 189,
299, 372, 376
Netter's 152, 340,
341
Rohen 444, 445,
466, 467
►
Grant's 294
Netter's 539

◄
Grant's 370, 372
Netter's 152, 340,
341
Rohen 444

coccyx and identify the **sacrotuberous** and **sacrospinous ligaments.** Note also the **posterior sacroiliac ligament** (**ATLAS PLATE 273**).

Cut the attachments of the lower end of the **erector spinae muscle** and expose the region between the posterior superior iliac spine and the sacrum (**ATLAS PLATE 335**). Deep to this site is located the **interosseous sacroiliac ligament** and the **cavity of the synovial joint.** See **ATLAS PLATE 273 #273.2** or **Figure 24-3** to view a frontal section through the sacroiliac joint.

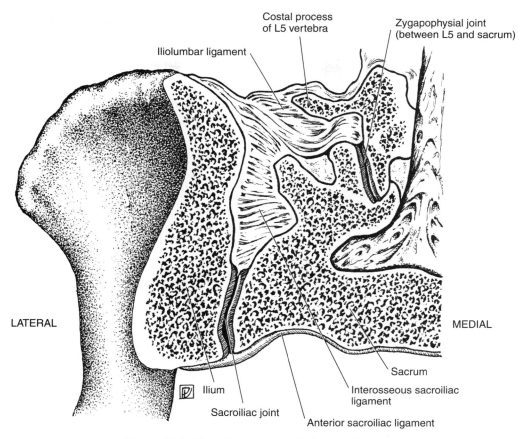

Costal process
of L5 vertebra

Zygapophysial joint
(between L5 and sacrum)

Iliolumbar ligament

LATERAL

MEDIAL

Sacrum

Ilium

Interosseous sacroiliac
ligament

Sacroiliac joint

Anterior sacroiliac ligament

Figure 24-3. Frontal section through the sacroiliac joint.

II. Symphysis Pubis

The symphysis pubis is a midline fibrocartilaginous joint between the medial surfaces of the two pubic bones (**Figure 24-4**). It is bounded superiorly by the **superior pubic ligament** extending between the pubic tubercles and inferiorly by the **arcuate pubic ligament** between the inferior pubic rami. The **interpubic fibrocartilaginous disc** (thicker in women) is interposed between the two bony articulating surfaces.

Posterior to the symphysis pubis are the **retropubic space,** the **prostate** in males, and the anterior surface of the **bladder.** Anterior to the symphysis is the **suspensory ligament of the penis or clitoris** and inferiorly is found the **urogenital diaphragm.** Normally, movements of the symphysis pubis only involve a slight distension of the cartilage, but during pregnancy, the cartilage becomes softer and allows the female pelvis to enlarge during parturition.

◄

Grant's 186, 187, 195, 263, 291
Netter's 240, 341, 342
Rohen 189, 337, 436, 445

◄

Grant's 107, 224, 241, 250, 258
Netter's 242, 335, 348, 352, 361, 377
Rohen 340

OPTIONAL DISSECTION

If the symphysis pubis was removed as a wedge during dissection of the pelvis, study the joint and envision its relationships on an articulated skeleton.

If the symphysis pubis is intact in your cadaver, you may remove a wedge of the pubis that contains the symphysis in the following manner:

1. Cut the attachments of the anterior abdominal muscles along the superior surface of the pubic bones above the symphysis pubis.

2. Clean the inner surface of the symphysis pubis by removing its fascial lining. Retract the bladder from the anterior pelvic surface.

3. Use a probe and locate the inferior border of the symphysis pubis from the pelvic side. Push the probe forward into the perineum just below the symphysis.

4. Cut the soft tissue (suspensory ligament of the penis or clitoris) on the anterior surface of the symphysis down to the probe at the inferior border of the symphysis.

5. With a hand saw, cut through the anterior pubis about 2 cm lateral to the midline on each side and remove a wedge of bone containing the symphysis pubis. Do not cut the bladder within the pelvis or the penis or clitoris within the perineum.

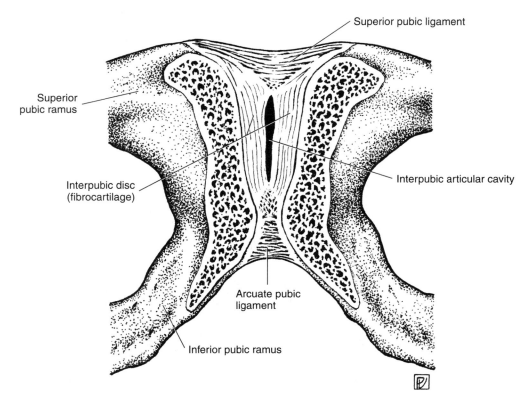

Figure 24-4. Frontal section through the symphysis pubis.

> **6.** Visualize the symphysis by making a frontal saw cut through the bony wedge (**Figure 24-4**). Observe the **superior pubic** and **arcuate pubic ligaments** that define its upper and lower borders and the **interpubic disc** interposed between the pubic surfaces.

III. Hip Joint

The hip joint allows a wide range of movement, yet it is strong and stable and bears the weight of the head, trunk, and upper limbs. It is a ball-and-socket synovial joint in which the **head of the femur** articulates with the **acetabulum** within the deep acetabular fossa (**Figure 24-5**). The acetabulum is formed by the fusion of the three components of the hip bone, the ischium, ilium, and pubis (**ATLAS PLATE 265 #265.2**). The head of the femur is covered with hyaline cartilage, except for a small pit where the **ligament of the head of the femur** is attached.

The cavity of the acetabulum is deepened by a fibrocartilaginous rim called the **acetabular labrum**. The **transverse ligament of the acetabulum** (**ATLAS PLATE 433 #433.3**) crosses the acetabular notch to form a foramen through which vessels and nerves course to supply the joint. Surrounding the joint is a strong and dense **fibrous capsule,** which attaches 2 to 5 mm beyond the labrum of the acetabulum and then,

► Grant's 376, 377, 380
Netter's 469, 475, 486
Rohen 444, 445

◄ Grant's 262, 376–379, 381–383, 405
Netter's 469, 486
Rohen 445

◄ Grant's 378–380, 382, 383
Netter's 469, 486, 494
Rohen 444, 445

► Grant's 187–189, 376, 377
Netter's 469
Rohen 444, 445

like a sleeve, around the neck of the femur (**ATLAS PLATE 432**). Many capsular fibers along the femoral neck, called **reticular fibers,** are reflected upward as longitudinal bands that hug the periosteum. They contain many nutrient vessels that supply the head of the femur, and if the neck of the femur is fractured, these vessels may be destroyed, resulting in necrosis of the femoral head.

The capsule of the hip joint is thickest anteriorly and superiorly where the greatest pressure for standing is exerted and thinner inferomedially and behind. It consists of longitudinally oriented fibers and a zone of circular fibers that form a ringlike cuff around the neck of the femur, called the **zona orbicularis.** The longitudinal fibers are strengthened by the iliofemoral, pubofemoral, and ischiofemoral ligaments.

The **iliofemoral ligament** is strong and triangular and is often described as an inverted Y (**Figure 24-6**). The stem of the Y is attached superiorly to the anterior superior iliac spine, while the two diverging limbs of the Y descend to both ends of the intertrochanteric line of the femur. This ligament is located on the anterior aspect of the joint, and its strength resists and limits extension of the femur.

The **pubofemoral ligament** also is triangular. It attaches above to the obturator crest and superior ramus of the pubis, and inferiorly it strengthens the anteromedial aspect of the capsule, blending with the iliofemoral ligament (**Figure 24-6**).

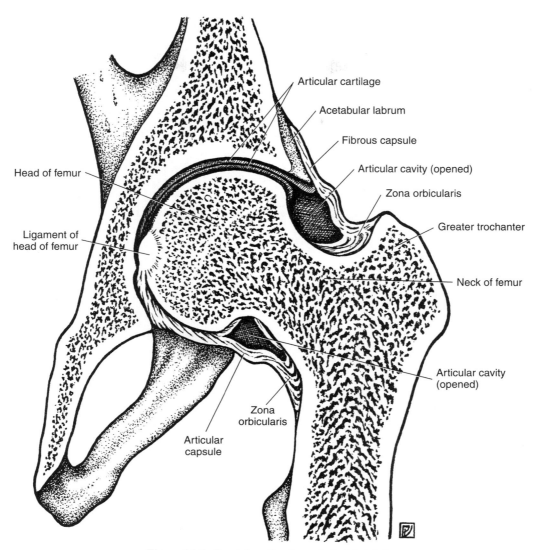

Figure 24-5. Frontal section through the hip joint.

The **ischiofemoral ligament** arises from the ischium and the posterior aspect of the acetabulum (**Figure 24.7**). Its fibers spiral laterally on the posterior aspect of the capsule, some forming the zona orbicularis around the femoral neck and others attaching to the greater trochanter (**ATLAS PLATE 432 #432.2**).

The hip joint is surrounded by muscles. **Anteriorly** are the **pectineus, tendon of the psoas major, iliacus,** and, more laterally, the **straight head of the rectus femoris muscle. Superiorly,** the **reflected head of the rectus femoris** lies adjacent to the medial part of the capsule, and the **gluteus minimus** overlies its lateral part. **Posteriorly,** the capsule is covered by the lateral rotators of the femur: the **piriformis, tendon of obturator internus,** the two **gemelli** above, and the **quadratus femoris** and **obturator externus** below.

▶
Grant's 373, 375, 382, 383
Netter's 486, 494

◀
Grant's 359, 367, 372, 375
Netter's 474, 477, 478
Rohen 452–456

▶
Grant's 359, 376, 382, 383
Netter's 474, 475, 478
Rohen's 452, 453

The **arteries** supplying the joint are the **medial and lateral femoral circumflex,** the **superior and inferior gluteal,** and the **first perforating branch of the deep femoral.** Five nerves supply the hip joint: the **femoral, obturator, accessory obturator** (when present), **superior gluteal,** and the **nerve to quadratus femoris.**

A. Anterior Dissection. Place the cadaver face up (supine) and dissect the hip joint on one side.

1. Cut the origins of the sartorius, rectus femoris, and pectineus muscles and reflect their bellies downward.

2. Sever and reflect the femoral vessels and nerve to expose the iliopsoas muscle and tendon.

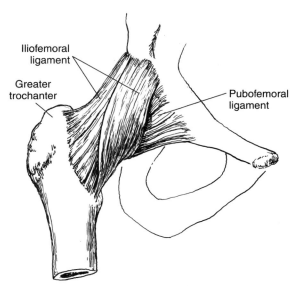

Figure 24-6. The capsule of the hip joint (anterior view).

3. Cut the attachment of the iliopsoas from the lesser trochanter, and identify a large bursa between the tendon and the joint capsule (**ATLAS PLATES 375, 378**).

4. After exposing the capsule, clean its anterior surface by scraping downward along the fibers.

5. Identify the **iliofemoral ligament.** It appears triangular or as an inverted Y. Trace the proximal limb upward to its attachment below the anterior superior iliac spine, and its distal limbs inferiorly to the medial and lateral ends of the intertrochanteric line of the femur (**ATLAS PLATE 432 #432.1**).

6. Clean the medial aspect of the capsule and identify thinner fibers that course inferolaterally from the pubic part of the acetabulum. These form the **pubofemoral ligament.** Note that they cross the lower anterior part of the joint to merge with the medial limb of the iliofemoral ligament (**Figure 24-6**).

7. Cut the joint capsule vertically along a line between the iliofemoral and pubofemoral ligaments. Turn the femoral head within the cavity but do not dislocate the joint at this point (**ATLAS PLATE 433 #433.2**).

B. Posterior Dissection. Turn the cadaver face down (prone) and approach the hip joint posteriorly.

1. Reflect the cut ends of the gluteus maximus. Sever the insertions of the gluteus medius and

▶
Grant's 189, 298, 372, 375, 377
Netter's 469, 477, 485
Rohen 454, 456

▶
Grant's 189, 298, 377
Netter's 469
Rohen 444, 445

▶
Grant's 378, 379, 383
Netter's 469, 486
Rohen 445

◀
Grant's 186, 187, 376, 382, 383
Netter's 469
Rohen 444, 445

◀
Grant's 172, 262, 298
Netter's 469
Rohen 444, 445

gluteus minimus from the greater trochanter. Reflect the muscles and note that bursae underlie their insertions.

2. Sever the piriformis, obturator internus and the two gemelli, the quadratus femoris, and the underlying obturator externus directly adjacent to the joint. Remove these muscles to expose the posterior joint capsule.

3. Clean the fibrous capsule and identify the **ischiofemoral ligament** attached to the back of the ischium. Note that its oblique fibers spiral transversely to the greater trochanter (**Figure 24-7**). Observe that some fibers are continuous with the circular fibers of the zona orbicularis that encircle the femoral neck.

4. Rotate the limb laterally to relax the capsule and make a vertical incision along the middle of the posterior capsule to open the joint.

5. With the cadaver still prone, dislocate the femoral head from the acetabulum by dangling the limb over the edge of the dissection table and rotating the foot (and femur) medially. This will tear the ligament of the head of the femur, and the femoral head will dislocate posteriorly through the opening in the capsule.

6. Examine the acetabulum (**ATLAS PLATE 433 #433.3**). Note the fibrocartilaginous rim called

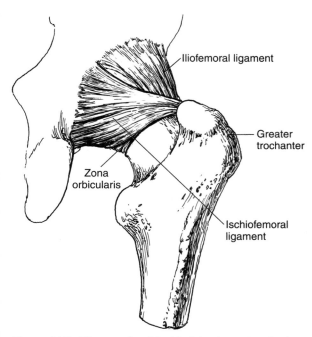

Figure 24-7. The capsule of the hip joint (posterior view).

the **acetabular labrum.** Find the **transverse ligament of the acetabulum** that bridges the acetabular notch. Deep to this ligament is a branch of the obturator artery that helps supply the femoral head (**Figure 24-8**).

7. Within the socket, identify the horseshoe-shaped **lunate surface** and the fat pad covered

Grant's 378–380, 383
Netter's 469
Rohen 444, 445

with synovial membrane in the floor of the acetabulum (**ATLAS PLATE 433 #433.3**).

8. Examine the neck and head of the femur. Note that the femoral head is covered with articular cartilage except for the pit where the ligament of the head of the femur is attached (**ATLAS PLATE 432 #432.3**).

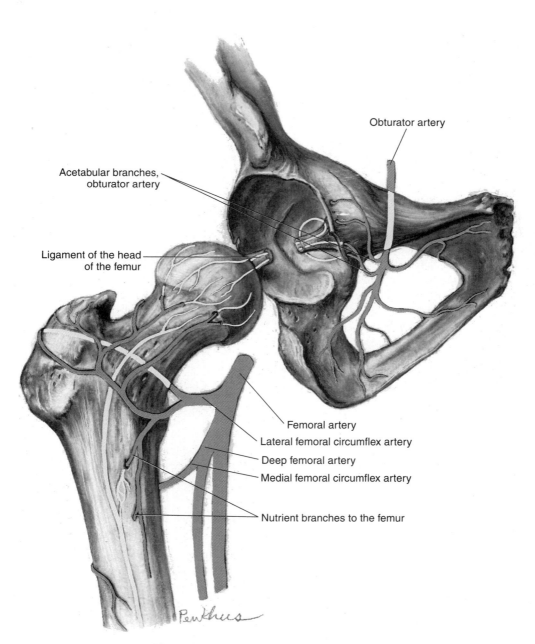

Figure 24-8. Arteries supplying the hip joint.

IV. Knee Joint
(ATLAS PLATES 434–445)

The compound knee joint involves the articulation of the condyles of the femur with the condyles of the tibia. In addition to the tibiofemoral articulation, the patella, a large sesamoid bone within the tendon of the quadriceps femoris muscle, articulates with the patellar surface of the femur. To dissect the joint sequentially, its anterior aspect and sides are dissected before continuing posteriorly.

A. Anterior, Medial, and Lateral Aspects of the Knee Joint. The most prominent anterior feature of the knee joint is the **patella**. On both sides of the patella are located the condyles of the femur and slightly below, the condyles of the tibia, all of which are palpable (**ATLAS PLATES 434, 435**).

1. **Patella.** The patella is located on the anterior patellar surface of the femur, fitting between the two femoral condyles. It is a flat, nearly circular sesamoid bone, with a triangular distal border that comes to an apex inferiorly. Its anterior surface is palpable, and it is embedded in the back of the **quadriceps tendon (ATLAS PLATES 403, 437, 437.2, 440 #440)**. The tendon continues inferiorly as the **patellar ligament** and inserts on the tibial tuberosity. The borders of the patella give attachments to tendinous fibers of the vastus medialis and vastus lateralis.

2. **Bursae (ATLAS PLATES 440, 441).** Of clinical importance are the bursae that are associated with the front of the knee joint because they are subject to inflammation. They include:

   a. A large **subcutaneous prepatella bursa (ATLAS PLATE 434 #434.1).** located between the skin and the lower part of the patella (inflammation of which is often called "housemaid's knee").

   b. A smaller **subcutaneous infrapatellar bursa** located between the skin and the tibial tuberosity (inflammation of which is sometimes called "clergyman's knee").

   c. The **deep infrapatellar bursa** found deep to the patellar ligament. It is interposed between the ligament and the upper part of the tibial tuberosity.

   d. The **suprapatellar bursa,** which is quite large and lies deep to the quadriceps tendon and patella anterior to the distal femur. It extends as far as 5 cm (two inches) above the patella.

Cut the fascia lata vertically and horizontally on the **lateral aspect of the knee** and identify the tendon of the biceps femoris muscle. Free the tendon

► Grant's 391, 393, 397, 401, 406
Netter's 488–493
Rohen 449

◄ Grant's 387–403
Netter's 488–493
Rohen 446–448

► Grant's 367, 390, 393, 394, 401
Netter's 488, 491, 493
Rohen 10, 436, 437, 458

► Grant's 392, 402, 403, 406
Netter 493

◄ Grant's 357, 393, 400, 404
Netter's 488, 491–493
Rohen 441, 447, 448

► Grant's 392, 393, 396, 403
Netter's 489, 491, 493
Rohen 446, 448

◄ Grant's 392, 396, 402, 403
Netter's 493
Rohen 447, 448

► Grant's 393–395, 399, 401
Netter's 488–493
Rohen 446–448

► Grant's 393, 400
Netter's 491
Rohen 446

► Grant's 397, 398, 402, 403
Netter's 493, 499, 500
Rohen 446, 448

to its insertion, and cut the muscle 7 cm above the knee and reflect its distal end. Deep to the biceps tendon locate the cordlike **fibular collateral ligament** attached to the lateral epicondyle above, and to the head of the fibula below (**ATLAS PLATES 435, 436**).

Find the sartorius, gracilis, and semitendinosus on the **medial aspect of the knee.** Cut across these muscles 7 cm above the knee, free their tendons distally, and reflect them downward. Deep to the tendons find the **tibial collateral ligament** and note its attachment to the medial meniscus (**ATLAS PLATE 435 #435.1**).

Make a small incision into the skin covering the anterior patella and open the **prepatellar bursa (ATLAS PLATE 434 #434.1).** Find the tendons of the vastus lateralis and vastus medialis as they join the common quadriceps tendon that attaches to the patella. Make a transverse incision across all the vastus muscles and their tendon 7 cm above the patella. Reflect the quadriceps tendon and the patella downward to open the anterior joint cavity (**Figure 24-9**).

Identify the **infrapatellar synovial fold (ATLAS PLATE 436 #436.1).** Note that this membrane is located in the intercondylar notch of the femur and that it expands laterally into two triangular **alar folds (Figure 24-10).** Place a probe between the lower part of the femur and the deep surface of the quadriceps femoris tendon and explore the large **suprapatellar bursa (ATLAS PLATE 441 #441.2).** Clean the intercondylar notch of the femur by removing the infrapatellar synovial fold and its alar folds and the infrapatellar fat pad. This will expose the **cruciate ligaments** anteriorly.

Probe the **fibular** and **tibial collateral ligaments** and the **lateral and medial menisci.** Note that these semilunar fibrous structures (erroneously often called "cartilages") are attached to the upper surface of their respective tibial condyles.

Cut the fibular collateral ligament and observe that the cruciate ligaments straighten as you medially rotate the femur. Confirm that the **anterior cruciate ligament** attaches to the anterior part of the tibial plateau and that the **posterior cruciate ligament** attaches to the medial condyle of the femur in the intercondylar notch.

B. Posterior Aspect of the Knee Joint. Located behind the knee joint is the **popliteal fossa.** The **upper third** of the floor of the fossa is formed by the popliteal surface of the femur and its **lower third** by the popliteus muscle. The **middle third** of the popliteal floor is the posterior aspect of the capsule of the knee joint (**ATLAS PLATE 418**).

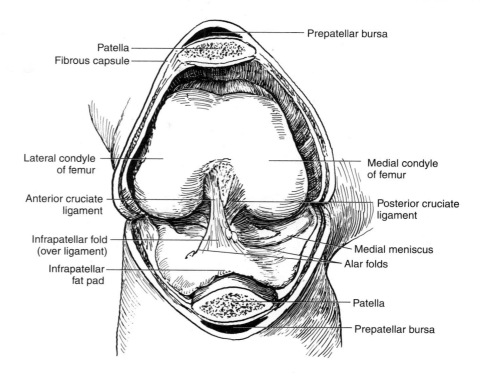

Figure 24-9. The knee joint opened anteriorly (after Grant).

Remove the vessels, nerves, and fat in the popliteal fossa to expose the capsule of the knee joint from behind. Cut the semimembranosus muscle in the thigh 7 cm above the knee. Follow the distal part of the muscle to the tibia, and note that its insertion continues upward and laterally on the posterior aspect of the joint capsule as the **oblique popliteal ligament.** Detach the origins of the two heads of the **gastrocnemius muscle** and the **plantaris muscle** and reflect them downward to expose the **popliteus muscle**.

▶
Grant's 394, 397
Netter's 491
Rohen 446

◀
Grant's 367, 372, 397, 398
Netter's 493, 500
Rohen 448, 458, 460

◀
Grant's 367, 397–399, 418
Netter's 477, 493, 499, 500
Rohen 457, 460

1. **Popliteus muscle.** The popliteus muscle is a flat muscle that forms the floor of the lower part of the popliteal fossa. Inferiorly, it attaches to the posterior surface of the tibia above the soleal line, and its fibers course upward and laterally toward the lateral condyle of the femur. Superiorly, its tendon splits. The lateral half attaches to the lateral condyle of the femur, while the medial half of the tendon attaches to the posterior part of the lateral meniscus (**ATLAS PLATES 418, 431, 440**). When the knee joint is in the hyperextended "locked" position, lateral rotation of the femur must occur before the joint can be unlocked and the leg flexed. **It is the lateral part of the popliteus muscle that initiates this lateral rotation of the femur.** Furthermore, contraction of the **medial part of the popliteus draws the lateral meniscus posteriorly** and protects it from being crushed between the femoral and tibial lateral condyles.

2. **Cruciate ligaments (Figures 24-9 to 24-11).** The anterior and posterior cruciate ligaments are strong fibrous bands that connect the tibia to the femur in a crossed pattern like the letter X. When viewed anteriorly, the anterior ligament attaches to the anterior part of the tibial plateau and the posterior ligament attaches to the medial condyle

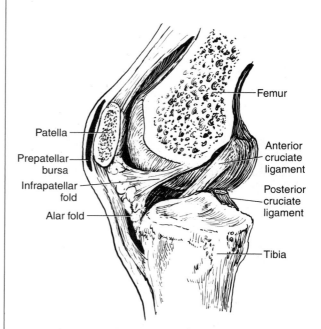

Figure 24-10. Sagittal section of the knee joint, showing the prepatellar bursa and infrapatellar and alar folds.

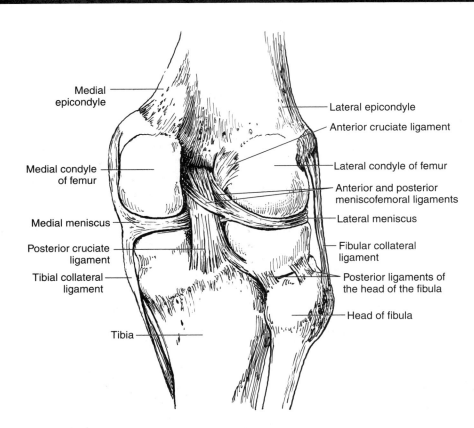

Figure 24-11. The cruciate ligaments (posterior view).

of the femur (**ATLAS PLATE 436 #436.2**). On the **posterior aspect of the joint,** the anterior cruciate ligament attaches to the medial surface of the lateral condyle of the femur, while the posterior cruciate ligament is attached to the posterior intercondylar surface of the tibia (**ATLAS PLATES 438, 440 #440.2, Figure 24-11**).

Extension of the flexed leg at the knee joint is the principal function of the quadriceps muscle, and this action is limited by the anterior cruciate ligament. When the ligament becomes taut, it prevents further extension of the lateral femoral condyle and backward displacement of the femur on the tibia. By limiting extension of the lateral condyle, it causes the femur to rotate medially to the locked (or screw-home) position of full extension. In contrast, the shorter and stronger posterior cruciate ligament prevents the femur from being displaced forward on the tibial plateau during flexion on the leg by its attachment to the lateral surface of the medial femoral condyle.

3. **Menisci.** The menisci are two fibrous, C-shaped plates (formerly called semilunar cartilages) that rest on the tibial condyles and slightly deepen the tibial surface in contact with the femoral condyles.

The **medial meniscus** is semicircular and is attached **anteriorly** to the anterior intercondylar area of the tibia in front of the anterior cruciate ligament and **posteriorly** to

▶
Grant's 394
Netter's 490, 491
Rohen 446

▶
Grant's 397, 398
Netter's 499, 500
Rohen's 457, 460

◀
Grant's 391,
394–397, 400
Netter's 489–493
Rohen 446, 447

the posterior intercondylar area in front of the posterior cruciate ligament (**ATLAS PLATE 443**). Its outer border is connected to the femur and tibia by the fibrous capsule, and it is attached firmly to the tibial collateral ligament.

The **lateral meniscus** is almost a complete ring and is attached to the tibial plateau both anteriorly and posteriorly. Additionally, the posterior border of the meniscus is attached to the medial condyle of the femur by strong bands, the **posterior** and **anterior meniscofemoral ligaments.** The posterior border of the lateral meniscus also receives the insertion of the medial part of the popliteus muscle. The attachments of these ligaments and the popliteus control the mobility of the lateral meniscus and afford it protection from injury.

Cut the attachments of the **popliteus muscle** from the tibia. Reflect it upward and see its medial fibers blending with the capsule of the joint and the lateral meniscus. Then remove the popliteus muscle and open the joint cavity posteriorly. Remove the posterior part of the joint capsule and cut the tendon of the popliteus away from the lateral condyle of the femur.

Identify the cruciate ligaments from behind. Locate the **middle geniculate artery** between these ligaments (**ATLAS PLATE 443 #443.3**). Clean the posterior ends of the cruciate ligaments and observe that the **anterior cruciate ligament** attaches to the medial side of the lateral condyle and the **posterior cruciate ligament** attaches to the posterior intercondylar region of the tibia (**ATLAS PLATES 438 #438.2, 440 #440.2**).

Sever the fibular collateral ligament and rotate the femur medially, thereby untwisting the cruciate ligaments. Cut the anterior cruciate ligament and pull the tibia forward to study the attachments of the menisci. Observe that the **medial meniscus** attaches firmly to the tibia and to the tibial collateral ligament, while the **lateral meniscus** is quite mobile and is **not** attached to the fibular collateral ligament.

Because of the relative immobility of the medial meniscus due to its attachments to the tibia, the joint capsule, and the tibial collateral ligament, it is more frequently injured than the more mobile lateral meniscus.

Injury to the medial meniscus and the tibial collateral and anterior cruciate ligaments occurs frequently in athletes, especially football players. When the foot is firmly fixed on the ground and the tibia is supporting the weight of the body with the leg partially flexed, these three structures are particularly vulnerable if the athlete is hit below the waist from behind ("clipping" in football). Upon impact, the body weight of the victim is thrown medially, and the femur forced into medial rotation. With the foot firmly planted, the tibia is forced into abduction and lateral rotation, and the tibial collateral ligament may become ruptured and the medial meniscus that is attached to it torn. Simultaneously, the anterior cruciate ligament can also be stretched or torn. Injury to the lateral meniscus may also occur, but is less frequent.

V. Tibiofibular Joints (ATLAS PLATE 446 #446.1)

The tibia and fibula articulate at both their upper and lower ends, forming the superior and inferior tibiofibular joints (**Figure 24-12**). Additionally, the shafts of these two bones are interconnected by the crural interosseous membrane, similar to that seen between the bones of the forearm. This is sometimes referred to as the middle tibiofibular joint.

A. The Superior Tibiofibular Joint. This plane or gliding synovial joint is formed by the articulation of the medial surface of the head of the fibula and the lateral condyle of the tibia (**Figure 24-12**). The fibrous joint capsule is strengthened by **anterior and posterior ligaments of the head of the fibula**. The **anterior ligament** consists of transverse bands of fibers extending from the anterior surface of the head of the fibula to the anterior surface of the lateral tibial condyle (**ATLAS PLATE 446 #446.1**). The

◄
Grant's 386, 398, 399
Netter's 491, 499, 500
Rohen 446, 487, 488

◄
Grant's 393–397
Netter's 489–493
Rohen 446–448

◄
Grant's 394, 396, 401, 406
Netter's 491, 493, 495, 496
Rohen 440, 441, 450

►
Grant's 406, 407
Netter's 496, 504, 507

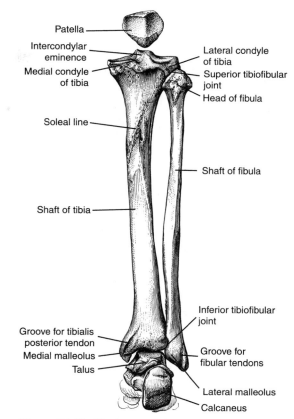

Figure 24-12. The bones of the leg showing the superior and inferior tibiofibular joints (posterior view).

fibers of the **posterior ligament** course vertically from the posterior surface of the head of the fibula to the lateral condyle.

OPTIONAL DISSECTION

With a scalpel scrape the posterior surface of the fibrous capsule of the superior tibiofibular joint and identify the vertical fibers of the posterior ligament of the head of the fibula. Sever the collateral ligaments of the knee (if not already cut) so that the leg can be rotated to visualize the anterior aspect of the joint. Scrape the capsule and define the transverse fibers of the anterior ligament of the head of the fibula. Cut through the ligaments and open the joint to confirm that this joint has a synovial cavity.

B. Crural Interosseous Membrane. Between the interosseous borders of the shafts of the tibia and fibula stretches the tough **crural interosseous membrane (ATLAS PLATE 446 #446.1)**. This strengthens the leg and also serves to separate the anterior and lateral compartments of the leg from the posterior compartment. Some fibers of several muscles take origin from the membrane, and through an opening in its upper part, the **anterior tibial artery** (and its veins) pass between the posterior and anterior compartments.

The interosseous membrane consists of strong oblique fibers oriented downward and laterally from the tibia to the fibula. Its attachments help support the slender fibula, which is subjected to the pull of many muscles acting on the ankle joint and joints of the foot.

OPTIONAL DISSECTION

Expose the interosseous membrane by detaching muscles from its surfaces. Scrape away the attachments of the tibialis anterior and the extensors hallucis longus and digitorum longus on the anterior aspect of the membrane and the tibialis posterior and flexor hallucis longus on its posterior surface. Identify the anterior tibial vessels as they penetrate the upper part of the interosseous membrane.

C. Inferior Tibiofibular Joint. This fibrous joint interconnects the convex medial side of the lower end of the fibula and the concave notch on the lateral side of the lower tibia. There is no synovial cavity, and the joint is bound by the anterior and posterior inferior tibiofibular ligaments and the inferior transverse and interosseous ligaments.

The **interosseous ligament** is a continuation downward of the interosseous membrane of the leg to the distal ends of the tibia and fibula. The joint is strengthened anteriorly by a band of fibers coursing inferolaterally between the tibia and fibula, the **anterior inferior tibiofibular ligament,** and posteriorly by a stronger band also directed inferolaterally, the **posterior inferior tibiofibular ligament (ATLAS PLATES 452, 453).** These ligaments overlie the interosseous ligament and are continuous with the fibrous capsule of the ankle joint below. The lower part of the posterior ligament is a strong band, the **inferior transverse ligament,** which passes across the back of the joint from the lateral malleolar fossa of the fibula nearly to the tibial malleolus.

OPTIONAL DISSECTION

Reflect the muscles and tendons in the three compartments of the leg to expose the inferior tibiofibular joint. Remove the retinacula and remove the tendons by detaching their insertions. Clean the anterior and posterior inferior tibiofibular ligaments by scraping their surfaces with a scalpel. Note that the **anterior ligament** is a flat band between the anterior borders of the two bones.

On the posterior aspect of the joint sever the attachment of the **posterior inferior tibiofibular**

▶
Grant's 412, 413, 432–439, 444
Netter's 495, 496, 505, 506
Rohen 432, 442, 443

▶
Grant's 432–436
Netter's 509
Rohen 449, 450

◀
Grant's 432–434
Netter's 509
Rohen 440, 442, 452, 495

▶
Grant's 433, 435, 436
Netter's 509
Rohen 450

ligament from the lower tibia. Reflect the cut ligament laterally and identify the **inferior transverse ligament** located below and deep to it. Find the strong fibrous bands that compose the **interosseous ligament.** Note that it is continuous above with the interosseous membrane.

VI. Ankle Joint (Talocrural Joint)

The ankle joint is a strong hinge (uniaxial) joint and consists of a three-sided socket formed by the lower malleolar ends of the tibia and fibula and the inferior transverse tibiofibular ligament that overlie the talus **(ATLAS PLATES 448–453).** The talus is cube-shaped, and it fits into the inferior surface of the tibia that is reciprocally shaped **(ATLAS PLATE 453 #453.1).** The lateral surface of the talus articulates with the lateral malleolus of the fibula, while its medial surface articulates with the medial malleolus of the tibia **(Figures 24-12 to 24-15).**

The ankle joint is a synovial joint bound by a **fibrous capsule** that is broad but thin anteriorly and posteriorly. Medially, the capsule is thicker and reinforced by the **deltoid ligament (ATLAS PLATE 453 #453.2),** and laterally it is strengthened by the **anterior** and **posterior talofibular** and the **calcaneofibular ligaments (ATLAS PLATES 449 #449.2, 452 #452.2).** This arrangement affords the joint flexibility and mobility in the sagittal plane in which movement is required. The joint is stable and strong laterally but even stronger medially, where collateral-like ligaments serve as bands between the articulating bones.

A. Remove the retinacula and muscles on the medial aspect of the joint and cut their tendons distally. Upon removing the retinacula, take care not to cut away the fibrous capsule of the joint, which is especially thin.

On the medial side of the joint isolate the **deltoid ligament** (sometimes called the **medial ligament**). It is triangular and consists of three fibrous bands attaching the tibial malleolus to the navicular, calcaneus, and talus bones **(ATLAS PLATE 453 #453.2).** Identify the following parts of the deltoid ligament:

1. The anteriorly directed **tibionavicular fibers** that extend **forward** from the medial malleolus to the tuberosity of the navicular and the plantar calcaneonavicular ligament.

2. The **tibiocalcaneo fibers** in the middle of the ligament. These course **straight downward** from the medial malleolus to the sustentaculum tali of the calcaneus.

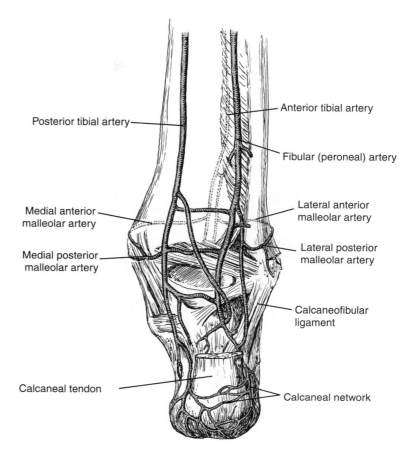

Figure 24-13. Posterior view of the anastomoses around the ankle joint.

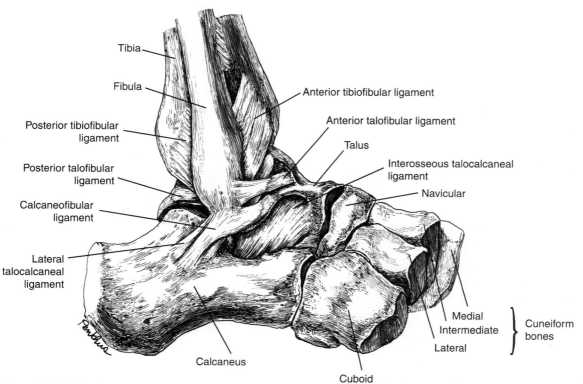

Figure 24-14. The ligaments at the ankle joints. (From Clemente CD. Gray's Anatomy 30th American Edition. Philadelphia: Lea and Febiger 1985.)

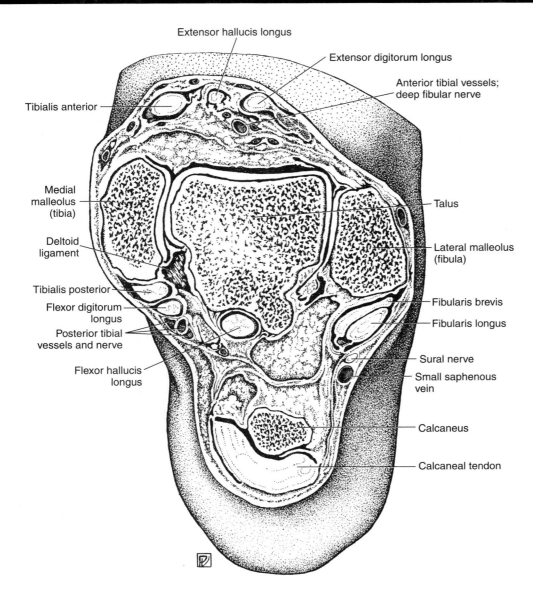

Extensor hallucis longus

Extensor digitorum longus

Anterior tibial vessels;
deep fibular nerve

Tibialis anterior

Medial
malleolus
(tibia)

Deltoid
ligament

Tibialis posterior

Flexor digitorum
longus

Posterior tibial
vessels and nerve

Flexor hallucis
longus

Talus

Lateral malleolus
(fibula)

Fibularis brevis

Fibularis longus

Sural nerve

Small saphenous
vein

Calcaneus

Calcaneal tendon

Figure 24-15. Coronal (vertical) section through the ankle region, showing the talus and the malleoli.

3. The **posterior tibiotalar fibers,** which course **backward** from the medial malleolus to the medial side and tubercle of the talus.

Cut and reflect the **distal** attachments of the tibionavicular, tibiocalcaneal, and posterior tibiotalar parts of the deltoid ligament to expose:

4. The deep part of the deltoid ligament, called the **anterior tibiotalar part.** Its fibers extend from the medial malleolus above to the medial surface of the talus below. Then cut these anterior fibers away from the talus.

B. On the lateral side of the ankle joint expose the lateral malleolus. Define anterior, middle, and posterior fibrous bands, two of which attach the

▶
Grant's 432, 433,
435
Netter's 509
Rohen 450

lateral malleolus to the talus and one to the calcaneus. Trace these lateral ligaments (**ATLAS PLATE 452 #452.2**):

1. The **anterior talofibular ligament.** It extends from the anterior margin of the lateral malleolus forward to the neck of the talus.

2. The **calcaneofibular ligament.** This middle band is a cordlike ligament that passes downward and backward from the lateral malleolus to the lateral side of the calcaneus.

3. The **posterior talofibular ligament.** This strong ligament is best seen on the back of the joint. It courses medially from the lower part of the lateral malleolus to the posterior part of the talus (**ATLAS PLATE 449 #449.2**).

Cut all of the lateral ligaments and the remaining part of the articular capsule to open the ankle joint. Inspect the articular surfaces of the three bones (talus, tibia, and fibula) and note that the socket that receives the talus is broader anteriorly than posteriorly (**ATLAS PLATE 449 #449.1**). Because of this, the talus fits within the socket most tightly when the body is erect and the foot is at a right angle to the leg. When the ankle joint is plantarflexed, the talus is looser, and some movement laterally can occur. Observe that the superior and medial surfaces of the talus articulate with the tibia and medial malleolus, while the lateral surface of the talus is in contact with the lateral malleolus of the fibula (**ATLAS PLATE 448**).

VII. Joints Within the Foot

The joints within the foot include the **intertarsal joints, tarsometatarsal joints, intermetatarsal joints, metatarsophalangeal joints,** and **interphalangeal joints.** Additionally, the arrangement of the bones and joints in the foot results in the formation of the **longitudinal** and **transverse arches of the foot.** This arrangement supports the weight of the body while standing erect and allows leverage for walking, running, and jumping. The arches also provide a concavity that protects the plantar muscles, vessels, and nerves from injury due to pressure.

A. **Arches of the Foot.** The articulated foot presents from medial to lateral a **transverse arch** in the shape of a half dome and, with the two feet together, the shape of a full dome. The rounded medial concavity is rimmed by the two heels. The lateral borders of the two feet and the heads of the metatarsal bases can be seen by impressions made by the soles of wet feet on a dry surface. Additionally, each foot has **longitudinal arches** stretching from heel to toe.

1. **Longitudinal arches.** The longitudinal arrangement of the bones in the articulated foot forms two parallel segments that are referred to as the medial and lateral longitudinal arches. The **medial longitudinal arch** is composed of the **calcaneus, talus, navicular,** the **three cuneiforms,** and the **medial three metatarsals (ATLAS PLATE 459).** The **lateral longitudinal arch** consists of the **calcaneus,** the **cuboid,** and the **lateral two metatarsal bones (Figure 24-16).**

   a. The **medial longitudinal arch** is maintained by ligaments and muscles and not by bony factors. The **plantar aponeurosis** and the **plantar calcaneonavicular ligament** are the most important structures that maintain the integrity of the medial arch (**ATLAS PLATE 459**

▶
Grant's 424, 425, 446, 447
Netter's 510, 514, 518
Rohen 450, 451, 500

◀
Grant's 427, 435–447, 451
Netter's 505–510
Rohen 432, 442, 443, 449–451

▶
Grant's 427, 443, 446, 447
Netter's 505, 506, 510, 518
Rohen 432, 442, 443, 451, 465

◀
Grant's 426, 427
Netter's 505, 506, 510
Rohen 442, 443

◀
Grant's 426, 427
Netter's 510, 514
Rohen 450, 451, 500

#459.3). The ligament supports the head of the talus, which transmits the full weight of the body through the ankle joint to the calcaneus, navicular, the cuneiform bones, and the medial three metatarsals. However important these two structures are, **the muscles and tendons on the plantar surface of the foot are essential in maintaining the medial longitudinal arch.** If support from these muscles and tendons is lost (e.g., if paralyzed) the ligaments alone cannot prevent flattening of the arch. Especially important is the tendon of the flexor hallucis longus, but the tendons of the tibialis posterior, flexor digitorum longus, and tibialis anterior along with the intrinsic plantar muscles all help in maintaining the medial arch.

   b. The **lateral longitudinal arch** is supported by the **plantar aponeurosis,** the **long plantar ligament** that stretches between the calcaneus and the cuboid and metatarsal bones, and the **plantar calcaneocuboid ligament** (short plantar ligament) (**Figure 24-17**). Also important in the support of the lateral arch is the **tendon of the fibularis longus muscle,** which elevates the cuboid bone by its upward pull. The tendons of the flexor digitorum longus to the lateral two toes and the short intrinsic foot muscles of the small toe also assist in maintaining the lateral arch.

2. **Transverse arch.** The transverse arch can best be seen at the tarsometatarsal joints where it is elevated medially across the distal row of tarsal bones. The plantar surfaces of these joints are held together by the **tarsometatarsal ligaments (ATLAS PLATE 455).** The most important factor in maintaining the concave transverse arch of the foot is the **tendon of the fibularis longus muscle.** Its action across the sole of the foot pulls the medial border closer to the lateral border, thereby enhancing the natural concavity on the medial side (**Figure 24-14**).

OPTIONAL DISSECTION

Study an articulated foot (**ATLAS PLATES 450, 451**) and identify:

1. The **medial longitudinal arch** (calcaneus, talus, navicular, three cuneiforms, and the three medial metatarsals).

2. The **lateral longitudinal arch** (calcaneus, cuboid, and the two lateral metatarsals).

3. The dome-shaped **transverse arch** (the three cuneiforms, the cuboid, and the bases of the five metatarsal bones.

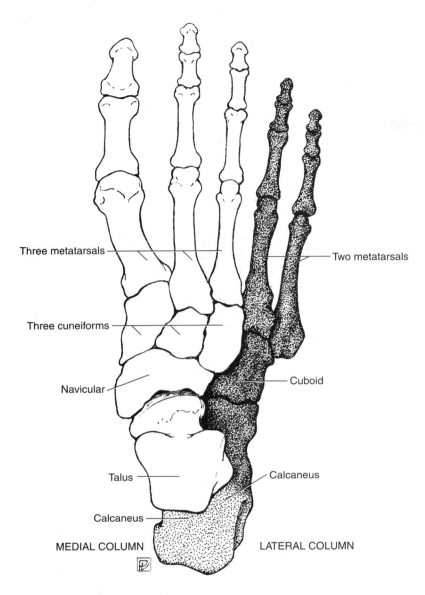

Three metatarsals

Two metatarsals

Three cuneiforms

Navicular

Cuboid

Talus

Calcaneus

Calcaneus

MEDIAL COLUMN   LATERAL COLUMN

Figure 24-16. The tarsal bones that form the medial and lateral longitudinal arches of the foot.

On the cadaver, remove all the muscles, vessels, and nerves from the plantar surface of the foot and expose the plantar ligaments. Find the **long plantar ligament** on the lateral side and the **plantar calcaneonavicular ligament** on the medial side (**ATLAS PLATE 455**). Identify the **tendon of the fibularis longus muscle** in the groove of the cuboid bone. Remove the long plantar ligament to show the attachment of the fibularis longus tendon onto the 1st metatarsal and medial cuneiform bones (**ATLAS PLATE 455 #455.2**).

◄
Grant's 446, 447
Netter's 510
Rohen 449–451

►
Grant's 441
Netter's 505, 506

◄
Grant's 412, 413, 444, 445
Rohen 432, 443, 450, 451, 495

B. Three Important Intertarsal Joints: Subtalar, Talocalcaneonavicular, and Calcaneocuboid Joints

The **subtalar joint** is the articulation between the inferior surface of the talus and the superior surface of the calcaneus (**ATLAS PLATE 453 #453.1**). The **talocalcaneonavicular** joint consists of the rounded head of the talus that fits into a concavity formed by the proximal surface of the navicular bone, the anterior and middle facets on the calcaneus for the talus, and the intervening plantar calcaneonavicular ("spring") ligament (**ATLAS PLATE 454 #454.1**). The **calcaneocuboid joint** is formed by the anterior surface of the calcaneus, which articulates with the proximal surface of the cuboid (**ATLAS PLATE 457 #457.2**).

The talonavicular part of the talocalcaneonavicular joint and the calcaneocuboid joint form a transverse line across the foot and together constitute what is often called the **transverse** (midtarsal) **tarsal joint** (**ATLAS PLATE 457 #457.2**). Although initiation of eversion and inversion of the foot occurs at the transverse tarsal joint, most of these actions occur at the more mobile subtalar joint.

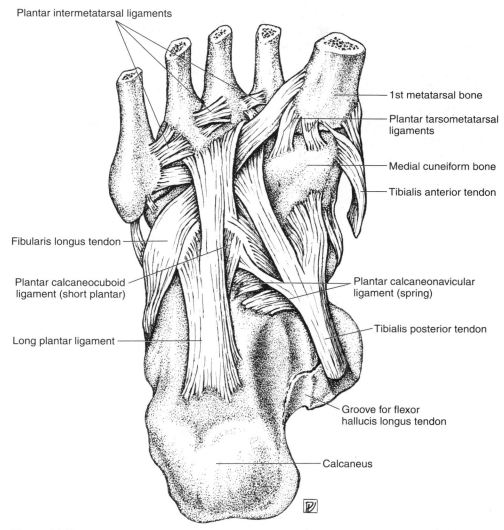

Plantar intermetatarsal ligaments

1st metatarsal bone

Plantar tarsometatarsal ligaments

Medial cuneiform bone

Tibialis anterior tendon

Fibularis longus tendon

Plantar calcaneocuboid ligament (short plantar)

Plantar calcaneonavicular ligament (spring)

Long plantar ligament

Tibialis posterior tendon

Groove for flexor hallucis longus tendon

Calcaneus

Figure 24-17. The plantar ligaments and the insertions of the tendons of the fibularis longus, tibialis posterior, and tibialis anterior (after Grant).

1. **Subtalar joint.** The joints between the talus and the calcaneus have three articular surfaces: anterior, middle, and posterior. The subtalar joint here refers only to the posterior articulation, because the anterior and middle and the talonavicular articulation are considered the talocalcaneonavicular joint.

   A **fibrous capsule** is attached along the margins of the subtalar joint, and medial and lateral talocalcaneal ligaments interconnect the articular surfaces (**ATLAS PLATE 452 #452.2**). The space between the articular surfaces (called the **sinus tarsi**) contains the **interosseous talocalcaneal ligament,** which **tightens during eversion and loosens during inversion of the foot.**

2. **Talocalcaneonavicular joint (ATLAS PLATE 454 #454.1).** This joint consists of the rounded head of the talus resting in a socket formed by three articular surfaces: the anterior and middle

◄
Grant's 427, 436, 442
Rohen 443, 450, 451

►
Grant's 433, 435, 444
Rohen 443, 450

◄
Grant's 445–447
Rohen 443, 450, 451, 495

facets on the underlying calcaneus and the posterior facet of the navicular bone. The floor of the socket is formed by the **plantar calcaneonavicular ligament,** also called the **"spring ligament."** This ligament and the tendons of the tibialis posterior and flexor hallucis longus support the head of the talus to maintain the medial arch of the foot (**ATLAS PLATE 455 #455.2**).

3. **Calcaneocuboid Joint.** This saddle joint permits a gliding movement between the calcaneus and the cuboid that assists in movements of inversion and eversion. The joint is surrounded by an articular capsule and reinforced dorsally by the **calcaneocuboid part of the bifurcated ligament** (**ATLAS PLATE 452 #452.2**) and on its plantar side by the **long plantar ligament** and the **plantar calcaneocuboid ligament** (short plantar ligament) (**ATLAS PLATE 455**).

OPTIONAL DISSECTION

In this dissection the talus is disarticulated from the underlying calcaneus, and the subtalar and talo-calcaneonavicular joints are opened. Remove all soft structures from the dorsum of the foot. Identify and cut the **bifurcated ligament,** which attaches the calcaneus to the cuboid laterally and the navicular medially (**ATLAS PLATE 452 #452.2**). Sever any other ligaments dorsally that attach the talus to the navicular anteriorly and the tibia posteriorly, thereby freeing the talus from above. Laterally, cut the **interosseous talocalcaneal ligament** between the talus and calcaneus and lift the talus from the underlying socket (**ATLAS PLATE 452 #452.2**).

Inspect the articular surfaces for the talus on the calcaneus inferiorly and the navicular anteriorly (**ATLAS PLATE 458**). Within the socket for the head of the talus, push a probe through the **plantar calcaneonavicular ligament** in the floor of the joint and identify the ligament on the plantar surface of the foot (**ATLAS PLATES 454 #454.1, 455**).

Open the **calcaneocuboid joint** by cutting through its articular capsule and note that (a) its synovial cavity is separate from the talonavicular joint and (b) the two joints together compose the **transverse tarsal joint** across the foot (**ATLAS PLATE 457 #457.2**). On its plantar surface, identify the **long plantar ligament** and the **plantar calcaneocuboid ligament** (short plantar) that support this joint and the lateral longitudinal arch (**Figure 24-17**).

◄
Grant's 432, 433, 435, 444–447
Netter's 509
Rohen 450, 451, 495

◄
Grant's 431, 445–447
Netter's 509, 510, 518
Rohen 450, 451

◄
Grant's 412, 413, 442, 444–447
Netter's 505, 506, 510
Rohen 442, 443, 449–451

►
Grant's 448
Netter's 510
Rohen 432, 433, 451

►
Grant's 563
Netter's 510
Rohen 432, 433, 451

C. **Tarsometatarsal Joints.** There are three separate joint cavities between the bases of the five metatarsal bones and the distal row of tarsal bones (the three cuneiform bones and the cuboid) These are:

1. The **medial (1st) tarsometatarsal joint** where the base of the 1st metatarsal bone (large toe) articulates with the medial cuneiform bone by means of a fibrous capsule (**ATLAS PLATE 457 #457.2**). Interosseous ligaments strengthen the capsule.
2. The **intermediate tarsometatarsal joint** where the intermediate and lateral cuneiform bones articulate with the 2nd and 3rd metatarsal bones. Tarsometatarsal ligaments on both the plantar and dorsal aspects of the joint reinforce the joint capsule.
3. The **lateral tarsometatarsal joint** between the cuboid bone and the 4th and 5th metatarsal bones (**ATLAS PLATE 457 #457.2**). Sometimes called the cuboideometatarsal joint, it also is protected by plantar and dorsal tarsometatarsal ligaments.

◄
Grant's 442, 443
Netter's 505, 506
Rohen 449–451

◄
Grant's 432, 433, 442, 446, 447
Netter 510, 518

D. **The Intermetatarsal Joints.** The adjacent surfaces of the **bases** of the four lateral metatarsal bones articulate with each other to form the intermetatarsal joints. These are bound by dorsal, plantar, and interosseous ligaments. More distally, the **heads** of the metatarsal bones are interconnected on their plantar surfaces by the **deep transverse metatarsal ligaments (ATLAS PLATE 455)**.

OPTIONAL DISSECTION

Remove all connective tissue and tendons over the **bases** of the metatarsal bones on the dorsum of the foot to expose the capsules of the three tarsometatarsal joints (**ATLAS PLATE 457 #457.2**). Open these capsules by cutting through their dorsal ligaments. Probe the synovial cavities of these joints and cut the **interosseous metatarsal ligaments** to separate the articular surfaces of these bones.

E. **Metatarsophalangeal Joints.** These five joints are formed by the heads of the metatarsal bones and the concave bases of the proximal phalanges of the toes. Each is surrounded by a **fibrous capsule,** which is thickened at its **sides** to form **collateral ligaments** (**ATLAS PLATE 455**). On the **plantar surface** of each joint is located the long flexor tendon that courses distally to insert on the distal phalanx. The **dorsal surface** of these joints is covered by the **dorsal digital expansions** formed by the extensor tendons and the insertions of the interosseous and lumbrical muscles.

F. **Interphalangeal Joints.** There are nine interphalangeal joints in each foot, two in each of the lateral four toes and one in the large toe. These are hinge joints, similar to those in the hand, and only flexion and extension takes place in them. Each phalanx has a proximal end called the **base** and a distal end called the **head.** The distal end is grooved and fits into the reciprocally curved head of the next phalanx. Each joint has an **articular capsule** strengthened by **collateral ligaments** laterally and medially (**ATLAS PLATE 455 #455.1**).

OPTIONAL DISSECTION

Loosen and lift the extensor digital expansion on the dorsal surface of the middle toe. Note how the tendons of the extensors receive the tendons of the interosseous and lumbrical muscles to form the dorsal expansion. On the sides of the joints note that the capsules are thickened by the **collateral ligaments.** Cut through the lateral aspect of the joint capsules of one metatarsophalangeal and interphalangeal joint to expose the articular surfaces of these relatively simple hinge joints.

Clinical Relevance

Hip joint stability. A stable hip joint depends on a) the gluteus medius and minimus muscles functioning normally; b) the femoral head located normally in the acetabulum; and c) the ligaments that reinforce the joint capsule operating at full strength.

Trendelenburg sign. A patient shows a Trendelenburg sign when the person stands on one leg and the hip descends downward on the other side. This sign occurs when the gluteus medius and minimus are not functioning.

Hip fracture. This fracture often occurs when the thigh at the hip joint twists and the neck of the femur breaks. Older persons with osteoporosis are most prone to this fracture.

Congenital dislocation of the hip joint. This is usually due to the incomplete formation of the superior part of the acetabular labru during development. This allows the femoral head to ride above the acetabulum, resulting in its dislocation superiorly into the gluteal region.

Soft tissue injuries in the knee. These injuries usually include tears of the cruciate ligaments, tears of the menisci, and injury to the collateral ligaments. At times several of these injuries may occur with the same trauma (e.g., tear of the meniscus with a cruciate ligament injury).

Injuries to the ligaments and menisci. These injuries usually happen during sports activities. The medial meniscus is 6 to 7 times more vulnerable to injury than the lateral. This is probably because it is attached to the medial collateral ligament, which does not allow it to move easily within the joint cavity.

Anterior cruciate ligament rupture. These injuries usually occur when the leg is forcibly abducted and twisted in lateral rotation. This injury results in an excessive movement anteriorly of the femur on the tibial plateau.

Dislocation of the patella. This dislocation usually occurs laterally. It is more likely to happen if the lateral condyle of the femur is flat or if the inferior fibers of the vastus medialis are weak and do not prevent the dislocation. The patella can also be dislocated by direct trauma to the vastus medialis at its insertion onto the patella.

Patellar reflex. This reflex tests the L3 segment of the spinal cord by striking the patellar tendon with a reflex (rubber) hammer and noting contraction of the quadriceps.

Arthroscopy of the knee. This is an endoscopic examination of the knee joint cavity and allows removal of damaged tissue, bone chips, or pieces of torn menisci. The arthroscope is inserted through small incisions used as portals to the joint cavity.

Potts ankle fractures. Ankle fractures may involve the fracture of a single bone, such as the lateral malleolus (a first degree fracture). In addition, a 2nd-degree fracture will also involve a break in the medial malleolus. In a 3rd-degree fracture the talus is displaced laterally and the tibial articular surface is fractured ventrally in addition to the fractures of the two malleoli. Sometimes the latter is called a trimalleolar fracture.

Sprained ankle. The lateral ligaments of the ankle joint are those involved in sprained ankle injuries, and these usually occur because of excessive inversion of the foot. Anterior and posterior talofibular and the calcaneofibular ligament are the ligaments most frequently involved. Swelling and pain usually occur.

Flat feet. This occurs when there is a flattening of the medial longitudinal arch. Usually the talocalcaneo-navicular ligament is stretched and weakened and the head of the talus is displaced inferomedially, resulting in the flattening of the medial longitudinal arch. This condition can often be treated with arch supports and foot exercises.

Club feet. In this congenital condition the foot is twisted out of normal position. In the most common type (Talipes equinovarus) the foot is inverted and adducted and the ankle joint is plantarflexed. Frequently, both feet are affected. Surgery can assist these patients to walk without much pain.

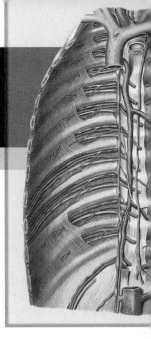

DISSECTION #25

Superficial and Deep Back; Spinal Cord

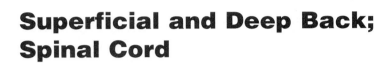

OBJECTIVES

1 Clean and reflect the trapezius and latissimus dorsi muscles **(superficial back muscles).**

2 Understand the source and distribution of the posterior primary rami of the segmental nerves.

3 Dissect and cut the vertebral attachments of the rhomboid muscles; identify the levator scapulae and the superior and inferior posterior serratus muscles **(intermediate back muscles).**

4 Clean the lumbodorsal fascia and separate the three principal columns of muscles that make up the erector spinae muscle **(deep back muscles).**

5 Dissect through the deep back muscles and expose the vertebral column; remove the dorsal laminae of several vertebrae covering the spinal cord.

6 Open the dura mater and study the lower 8 or 10 segments of the spinal cord.

Atlas Key:
Clemente Atlas, 5th Edition = Clemente Plate #
Grant's Atlas, 11th Edition = Grant's Page #
Netter's Atlas, 3rd Edition = Netter's Plate #
Rohen Atlas, 6th Edition = Rohen Page #

The back interacts with the upper and lower limbs and forms the dorsal aspect of the neck, thorax, abdomen, and pelvis. The back also contains the vertebral column, to which are attached many muscles and which encases the spinal cord that gives rise to the 31 pairs of spinal nerves. The superficial, intermediate, and deep muscles of the back will be dissected, and a portion of the vertebral column removed to dissect the lower part of the spinal cord.

►
Grant's 20, 307, 328, 333
Netter's 163, 170, 173, 187
Rohen 226, 229, 231, 234

I. Posterior Primary Rami; Trapezius and Latissimus Dorsi; Rhomboids and Levator Scapulae

The skin over extensor surfaces such as the back is thicker and tougher than that on flexor surfaces because the dermis is thicker. This dorsal skin is supplied with sensory innervation by cutaneous branches of the **posterior primary rami** of segmental nerves (**ATLAS PLATES 326, 327 #327.1**). These are derived from the spinal nerves and course dorsally just beyond the junction of the dorsal and ventral roots. They traverse the deep back muscles, supply them with motor innervation, and continue to the skin of the back. They perforate two large superficial muscles (trapezius and latissimus dorsi) in their course to the skin but they **DO**

NOT supply these superficial muscles with motor innervation (**ATLAS PLATE 338**).

A. Skin Incisions. Incisions must be made to remove the skin and superficial fascia to expose the underlying trapezius and latissimus dorsi muscles.

> Make an incision down the midline of the back from the external occipital protuberance above to the 5th lumbar vertebra (**Figure 25-1: A–B**). Make four other incisions transversely on each side from this midline cut.
>
> 1. From the external occipital protuberance laterally to the mastoid process (**Figure 25-1: A–D**).
>
> 2. Along the superior border of the shoulder to the acromion (**Figure 25-1: C–F**).
>
> 3. From the inferior angle of the scapula laterally to the posterior axillary fold (**Figure 25-1: E–G**).
>
> 4. From the 5th lumbar vertebra laterally along the iliac crest above the gluteus maximus (**Figure 25-1: B–H**).

▶
Grant's 20, 328
Netter's 163, 173, 187, 250
Rohen 229, 230, 231

▶
Grant's 307, 308, 494
Netter's 167, 186, 246, 407

▶
Grant's 307
Netter's 246, 407

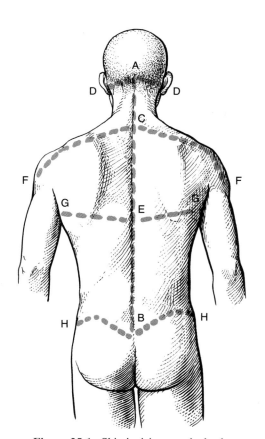

Figure 25-1. Skin incisions on the back.

> Commence reflecting the skin at the corners of the incisions. After reflecting the skin for several inches, make a small incision in the skin flap through which the index finger can be inserted to apply tension on the skin as cutting continues.
>
> Reflect the skin flaps and determine the depth of the superficial fascia by identifying the underlying muscle fibers of the trapezius and latissimus dorsi. As you remove the fascia identify some of the cutaneous nerves of the back that have traversed the muscles. In the upper back probe for these nerves about 2.5 cm lateral to the spinous processes of the vertebrae at successive segmental levels. In the lower thoracic and lumbar levels the nerves penetrate the muscles further laterally (**Figure 25-2**).

B. Posterior (Dorsal) Primary Rami of Spinal Nerves. When a ventral root emerges from the spinal cord, it quickly joins the dorsal root of the same segment just distal to the spinal ganglion to form a **mixed spinal nerve**. The mixed spinal nerve traverses the intervertebral foramen and immediately divides into **anterior** and **posterior primary rami** (**ATLAS PLATE 327 #327.1**).

Each **anterior primary ramus** passes laterally and anteriorly around the body to supply motor and sensory innervation to structures within that segment of the neck or trunk or in the limbs. The **posterior primary ramus** passes posteriorly to supply the deep back muscles and the skin of the posterior neck and trunk (**ATLAS PLATES 326, 332, 333**). There are no structures in the limbs supplied by fibers of posterior primary rami nerves. Upon passing through the back muscles, the cutaneous branches of the posterior primary rami reach the skin where they divide into medial and lateral branches (**ATLAS PLATES 326, 338**).

> After you identify several cutaneous branches of the posterior primary rami coursing through the trapezius and latissimus dorsi muscles, remove the fascia and clean the muscle surfaces from the skull to the iliac crests. Identify the boundaries of two triangles: the **triangle of auscultation** and the **lumbar triangle** (**Figure 25-3**).

The **triangle of auscultation** is bounded superiorly by the trapezius muscle, inferiorly by the latissimus dorsi, and laterally by the medial border of the scapula. When a subject is asked to bend forward with both arms folded across the chest, the interspace between the 6th and 7th ribs becomes subcutaneous within this triangle, and this allows effective auscultation for sounds in the chest with a stethoscope (**Figure 25-3**).

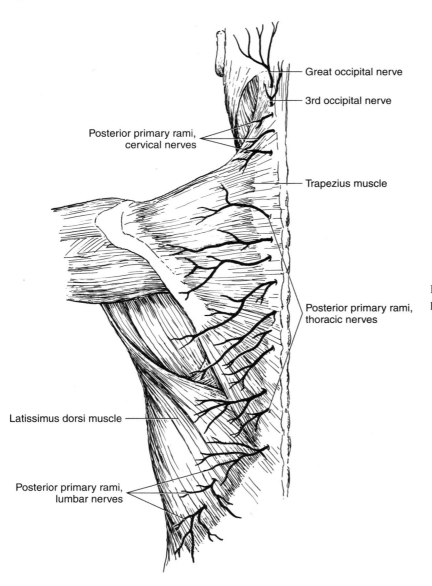

Great occipital nerve

3rd occipital nerve

Posterior primary rami,
cervical nerves

Trapezius muscle

Posterior primary rami,
thoracic nerves

Latissimus dorsi muscle

Posterior primary rami,
lumbar nerves

Figure 25-2. The cutaneous branches of the posterior primary rami.

The **lumbar triangle** (of Petit) is bounded inferiorly by the iliac crest, superiomedially by the latissimus dorsi muscle, and superiolaterally by the external abdominal oblique muscle (**ATLAS PLATES 328, 329**). The floor of this triangle is formed by the internal oblique muscle. On rare occasions this may be the site of an abdominal (lumbar) hernia. More frequently the surgeon approaches the kidney or ureter through this triangle.

C. **Trapezius Muscle (Figure 25-3).** The trapezius muscle is triangular and flat and extends over the back of the neck and upper posterior thorax. It arises **superiorly** from the occipital bone and **medially** from the posterior aspect of the vertebral column, including the ligamentum nuchae and the spinous processes from C7 to T12. From this broad origin its upper fibers descend to the lateral third of the

▶
Grant's 307, 494, 496
Netter's 167, 170, 186
Rohen 226, 227, 234, 405

◀
Grant's 308, 494
Netter's 167, 186, 246

▶
Grant's 509

▶
Grant's 307, 492, 730-732, 820
Netter's 28, 29, 170, 412
Rohen 405, 407, 413

clavicle, its middle fibers course transversely to the acromion, and its lower fibers ascend to the spine of the scapula (**ATLAS PLATE 328**).

The upper fibers of the trapezius, acting with the levator scapulae muscle, **elevate the scapula;** acting with the serratus anterior, it **rotates the scapula counterclockwise,** raising the upper limb above the head; with the rhomboid muscles, the trapezius **retracts the scapula.** When its scapular and thoracic attachments are fixed, the trapezius **pulls the head and neck laterally.**

The trapezius is supplied by the **accessory nerve** after it descends through the posterior triangle of the neck. It courses along the deep surface of the trapezius, accompanied by either the **superficial branch of the transverse cervical artery** or (in cadavers that do not have this vessel) by the **superficial cervical artery.**

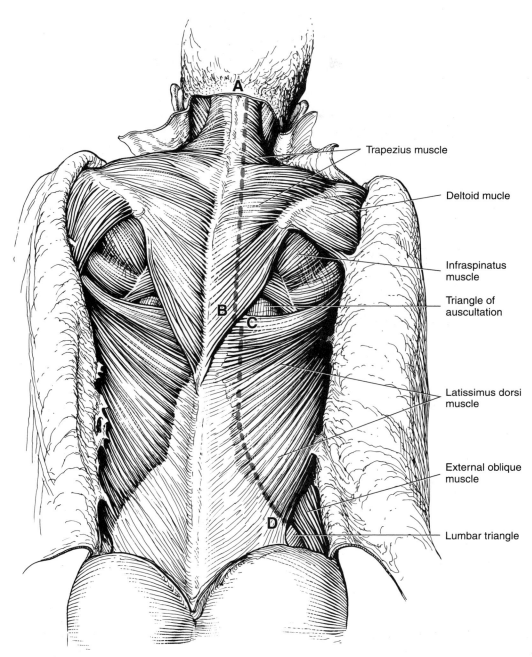

Figure 25-3. The trapezius and latissimus dorsi muscles; lines of incision.

Clean the attachments of the trapezius to the occipital bone superiorly, the ligamentum nuchae and thoracic vertebrae medially, and the scapular spine, acromion, and clavicle laterally. Clean the upper border of the muscle to the clavicle. Manually free the lateral and inferior borders and separate the trapezius from the underlying rhomboid muscles along the vertebral border of the scapula.

Cut the trapezius from below vertically about 2 cm lateral to the vertebrae **(Figure 25-3)**. After

►
Grant's 492, 494, 496
Netter's 170
Rohen 402, 407

cutting upward about 7 or 8 cm, turn the lateral flap over and identify the **accessory nerve** and accompanying vessels on its deep surface **(Figure 25-4)**. Continue the incision superiorly to the upper border of the muscle and reflect both flaps to expose the underlying muscles.

D. Latissimus Dorsi Muscle. The latissimus dorsi muscle is also triangular, and it covers the lumbar region and lower half of the posterior thorax **(ATLAS PLATE 328)**. It takes origin from the lower six

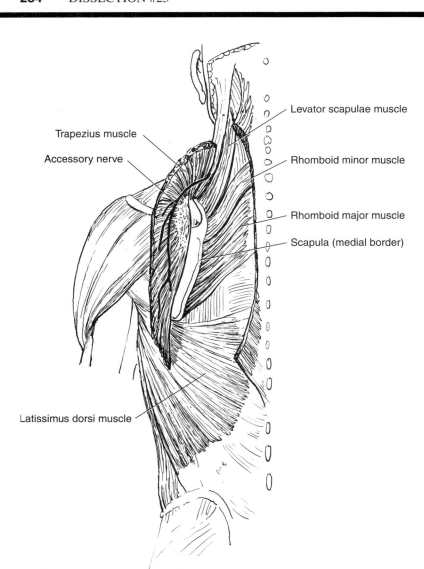

Trapezius muscle

Accessory nerve

Levator scapulae muscle

Rhomboid minor muscle

Rhomboid major muscle

Scapula (medial border)

Latissimus dorsi muscle

Figure 25-4. The deep surface of the reflected trapezius muscle, showing the accessory nerve.

thoracic vertebrae, the lumbodorsal fascia, iliac crest, and the lower three or four ribs. The muscle fibers converge superiorly and laterally, forming a tendon about 6 cm wide that inserts on the humerus (intertubercular sulcus) between the teres major and pectoralis major (**ATLAS PLATES 32, 33**). With the teres major it produces the posterior axillary fold. It adducts, extends, and medially rotates the humerus and swings the arms backward as in swimming. When its insertion is fixed and the arms extended, the latissimus dorsi pulls the trunk forward or upward as in climbing a tree. It is supplied by the **thoracodorsal nerve** (**ATLAS PLATES 19–21**) and receives blood by way of the **thoracodorsal branch of the subscapular artery** (**ATLAS PLATE 16 #16.2**).

Clean the borders of the latissimus dorsi muscle and manually separate its lower part from underlying

◄
Grant's 307, 489, 490, 494, 496
Netter's 167, 170, 186, 246, 409
Rohen 226, 227, 403, 412, 415

►
Grant's 307, 308
Netter's 167, 168, 185, 186
Rohen 227

►
Grant's 308, 494, 496, 732
Netter's 167, 170, 186, 407
Rohen 226, 235, 407

structures. Use a curved incision to cut the muscle from its upper border 5 cm lateral to the midline. Extend the cut below the last rib but above the iliac crest in the region of the lumbar triangle (**Figure 25-3**). Reflect the medial flap, but do not destroy the underlying **serratus posterior inferior.** Separate and reflect the lateral flap from the serratus anterior that arises from the ribs. Identify the **thoracodorsal nerve and artery** coursing along the deep surface of the muscle (**ATLAS PLATES 20, 21**).

E. Rhomboid and Levator Scapulae Muscles (Figure 25-5). Three other muscles attach the shoulder to the vertebral column: (from above downward) the levator scapulae, the rhomboid minor, and rhomboid major (**ATLAS PLATE 328**).

The **levator scapulae** arises from the transverse processes of the upper four cervical vertebrae.

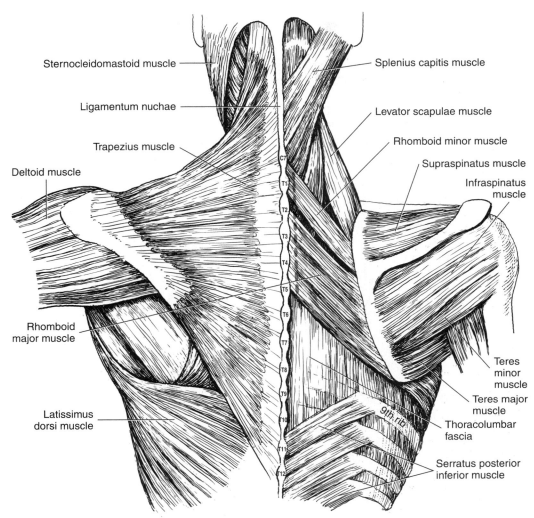

Figure 25-5. The rhomboid and levator scapulae muscles; lines of incision.

This elongated muscle descends in the posterior triangle of the neck to insert along the upper medial border of the scapula (**ATLAS PLATE 332, left side**). It is supplied by fibers from the 3rd and 4th cervical nerves and by the dorsal scapular nerve (C5).

The **rhomboid minor** arises from the lower ligamentum nuchae and the spinous processes of C7 and T1 vertebrae. Its fibers descend to the medial border of the scapula adjacent to the scapular spine (**ATLAS PLATE 328**).

The **rhomboid major** arises from the spinous processes of the 2nd to the 5th thoracic vertebrae. Its fibers also descend laterally below the rhomboid minor to insert along the medial border of the scapula as far as its inferior angle (**ATLAS PLATE 328**). Both rhomboid muscles are supplied by the **dorsal scapular nerve** (C5).

The rhomboid and levator scapulae muscles either stabilize or move the shoulder in concert with other muscles. The rhomboids with the trapezius adduct the

◄
Grant's 307, 308, 492, 496, 509
Netter's 170, 186
Rohen 226, 235, 405

◄
Grant's 494, 496
Netter's 170, 186
Rohen 235, 406

►
Grant's 492, 493
Netter's 413, 460
Rohen 235, 406

scapulas by retracting them closer to the vertebral column, and with the levator scapulae, help rotate the scapula clockwise. The levator scapulae with the trapezius elevates the shoulder when its vertebral end is fixed or bends the neck to the same side when the shoulder is fixed.

After reflecting the trapezius and latissimus dorsi, identify the levator scapulae and the two rhomboids. Separate the rhomboids manually from underlying tissue and identify the **dorsal scapular nerve** descending deep to the muscles. Usually the nerve is accompanied by the **dorsal scapular branch of the transverse cervical artery.** The nerve also helps supply the levator scapulae and most often descends on the medial side of the artery. Sever the rhomboid major and minor from the vertebral column and reflect them laterally. Do not cut the levator scapulae (**Figure 25-6**).

II. Intermediate Muscles of the Back (Figure 25-6)

Two thin sheets of muscle lie deep to the trapezius and latissimus dorsi but superficial to the erector spinae muscle. These are the serratus posterior superior and the serratus posterior inferior. Considered thoracic muscles, they attach medially to the vertebral column and laterally to the ribs (**see ATLAS PLATE 332, left side**). Because they move the ribs, they are also accessory muscles of respiration.

The **serratus posterior superior** attaches medially to the spinous processes of C7, T1–3. It is thin and

►
Grant's 21, 162, 308
Netter's 167, 168, 185
Rohen 226, 227, 228

quadrilateral and inserts inferolaterally by muscular slips to the 2nd, 3rd, 4th, and 5th ribs. Anterior primary rami of T2 to T5 intercostal nerves innervate the muscle.

The **serratus posterior inferior** is also thin and quadrilateral and arises medially from the spines of T11 to L3 vertebrae. Its fibers course superiolaterally to insert onto the lower four ribs (**ATLAS PLATE 332**).

> Sever the serratus posterior superior and posterior inferior medially at their attachments to the vertebral column and reflect the muscles laterally to expose the underlying **thoracolumbar fascia (Figure 25-6)**.

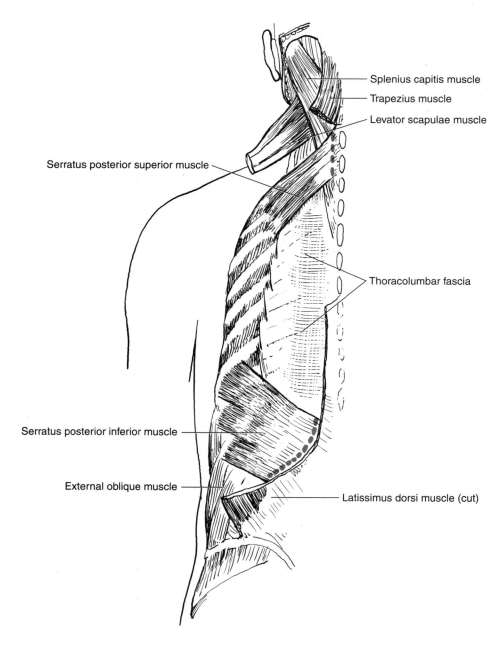

- Splenius capitis muscle
- Trapezius muscle
- Levator scapulae muscle
- Serratus posterior superior muscle
- Thoracolumbar fascia
- Serratus posterior inferior muscle
- External oblique muscle
- Latissimus dorsi muscle (cut)

Figure 25-6. The thoracolumbar fascia and the serratus posterior muscles; lines of incision.

III. Deep Muscles of the Back
(ATLAS PLATES 332, 333, 335)

The deep back muscles are a complex system of longitudinally oriented muscle groups stretching from the pelvis to the skull. They control movements of the vertebral column and, to some extent, the head. They are powerful and, as a group, extend the flexed vertebral column (trunk) to an upright position and also bend the vertebral column laterally. Smaller deep back muscles can rotate the vertebrae. Muscles of the deep back are important in maintaining posture, but their great strength can cause severe painful spasms when they go into tonic contraction. Before addressing these muscle groups study the **thoracolumbar fascia.**

►
Grant's 163–165, 310
Netter's 169, 255, 256, 478
Rohen 282, 335, 453

◄
Grant's 161, 307, 308
Netter's 167, 170, 186, 246
Rohen 226, 227

A. **Thoracolumbar Fascia.** The thoracolumbar fascia (often erroneously called lumbar fascia) extends over the muscle mass of the deep back. In the **thoracic region** it is a thin fibrous layer deep (anterior) to the serratus posterior superior that is attached to the vertebral spines medially and the ribs laterally (**ATLAS PLATE 332**).

In the lumbar region the thoracolumbar fascia divides into posterior and anterior layers that enclose the erector spinae muscle (**Figure 25-7**). The **posterior layer** is a thick aponeurosis attached medially to the spinous processes of the lumbar vertebrae and sacrum and the supraspinous ligaments that interconnect them. It covers the erector spinae muscle posteriorly and is continuous with the aponeurosis from which the latissimus dorsi arises. Superiorly, this posterior layer is continuous with the origin of the serratus posterior inferior and it attaches to the iliac crest inferiorly.

The **anterior layer** is attached medially to the transverse processes of the lumbar vertebrae and the intertransverse ligaments (**ATLAS PLATE 327 #327.2**). It underlies the deep surface of the erector spinae muscle, but fuses laterally with the posterior layer to form an envelope for the erector spinae muscle. This fusion of the two layers gives origin to the upper part of the internal oblique muscle of the anterior wall (**Figure 25-7**).

Deep to the anterior layer of the thoracolumbar fascia is located the **quadratus lumborum muscle (ATLAS PLATE 327 #327.2**), covered on its anterior surface by the thin **fascia of the quadratus lumborum.**

To expose the lower part of the erector spinae muscle, make a vertical incision from the 12th rib to the iliac crest 5 cm from the midline through the posterior layer of thoracolumbar fascia (aponeurosis). At both ends of the vertical incision, cut the aponeurosis medially to the midline and laterally to the border of the erector spinae muscle. Reflect the aponeurosis and lift the lateral side of the erector spinae muscle. Observe the line of fusion between the posterior and anterior layers of the thoracolumbar fascia located at the lateral border of the erector spinae muscle.

Make a vertical cut along the line of fusion and expose the longitudinal fibers of the underlying **quadratus lumborum muscle.** Observe that this muscle extends from the lower border of the 12th rib to the iliac crest. Now, turn your attention to the deep back muscles, starting superiorly with the **splenius capitis** and **splenius cervicis.**

B. **Splenius Capitis and Splenius Cervicis Muscles** (**Figure 25-8**). Located on both sides of the posterior

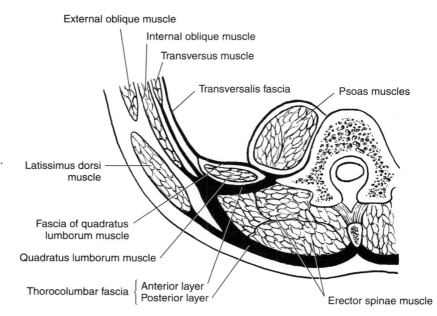

Figure 25-7. The thoracolumbar fascia.

External oblique muscle
Internal oblique muscle
Transversus muscle
Transversalis fascia
Psoas muscles
Latissimus dorsi muscle
Fascia of quadratus lumborum muscle
Quadratus lumborum muscle
Thorocolumbar fascia { Anterior layer / Posterior layer
Erector spinae muscle

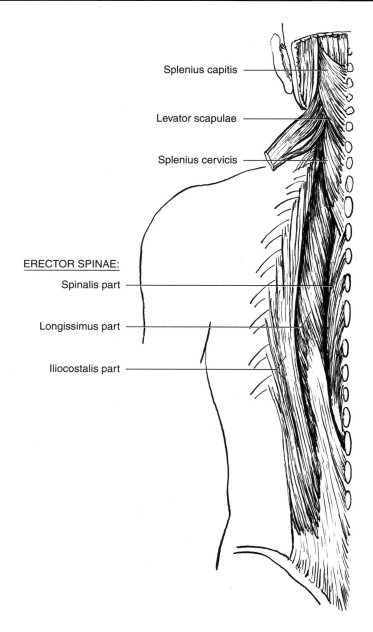

Splenius capitis

Levator scapulae

Splenius cervicis

ERECTOR SPINAE:

Spinalis part

Longissimus part

Iliocostalis part

Figure 25-8. The erector spinae muscle; the splenius muscles.

neck, deep to the trapezius muscles are the splenius capitis muscles and, more inferiorly, the splenius cervicis muscles (**ATLAS PLATE 332**).

The **splenius capitis** arises from the spinous processes of the upper four or five cervical vertebrae. It passes superiorly and laterally as a straight band to insert onto the mastoid process of the temporal bone and the lateral part of the superior nuchal line on the occipital bone. Together, the two splenius muscles form a V (**ATLAS PLATE 332**), and their simultaneous action extends the head posteriorly. Acting separately, each bends the head laterally to that side.

The **splenius cervicis** arises from the spinous processes of the 3rd to 6th thoracic vertebrae (**ATLAS PLATE 332, right side**). Its fibers course superiorly

▶
Grant's 309, 311, 314
Netter's 167, 168
Rohen 226, 227, 228, 235

◀
Grant's 309, 310, 314
Netter's 167, 168, 171, 186
Rohen 226, 234, 235, 383

and laterally to insert on the transverse processes of the upper two or three cervical vertebrae. It assists the splenius capitis in rotating the neck.

Deep to the reflected trapezius, cut the splenius capitis inferiorly at its attachment on the upper four or five cervical spinous processes. Identify and cut the 3rd occipital nerve (dorsal ramus of C3), which pierces the splenius capitis and the trapezius to get to the skin. Sever the attachments of the splenius cervicis from the vertebral spines and reflect the muscle laterally.

Turn your attention to the longitudinal back muscles, collectively called the **erector spinae.**

C. Erector Spinae (Sacrospinalis) Muscle (Figure 25-8). This large muscle mass consists of groups of longitudinally oriented fascicles located lateral to the vertebral column and deep to the thoracolumbar fascia and the serratus posterior, rhomboid, and splenius muscles. The erector spinae muscle groups extend from the sacrum and ilium to the skull and are divided into three longitudinally oriented columns. These columns are the **iliocostalis** (lateral), **longissimus** (intermediate), and **spinalis** (medial) parts of the erector spinae muscle (**ATLAS PLATES 332, 333**).

◄
Grant's 309, 310, 314, 315
Netter's 167, 168
Rohen 222

►
Grant's 309, 310, 314
Netter's 148
Rohen 222

1. **Iliocostalis.** The **iliocostalis column** consists of three ascending parts: the iliocostalis lumborum, iliocostalis thoracis, and iliocostalis cervicis. Inferiorly, the iliocostalis column attaches to the iliac crest and the spines of the lumbar, sacral, and coccygeal vertebrae (**ATLAS PLATE 333**).

◄
Grant's 309, 310, 314
Netter's 168
Rohen 222, 226, 227

   a. **Iliocostalis lumborum.** From its origin inferiorly, the iliocostalis lumborum is directed upward and somewhat laterally and inserts on the inferior borders at the angles of the lower six ribs (**ATLAS PLATE 333**).

   b. **Iliocostalis thoracis.** The iliocostalis thoracis arises from the superior borders of the 6th to 12th ribs, slightly **medial** to the insertions of the iliocostalis lumborum. These fascicles ascend on the posterior chest wall and insert along the superior border of the 1st to 6th ribs and on the transverse process of the C7 vertebra (**ATLAS PLATE 333**).

   c. **Iliocostalis cervicis.** The fibers of the **iliocostalis cervicis** ascend from the 2nd to the 7th ribs to the transverse processes of the 4th, 5th, and 6th cervical vertebrae.

> Lift the cut thoracolumbar fascia and separate the **iliocostalis lumborum** inferiorly. Follow these lateral fascicles upward to their insertions on the inferior borders of the lower six ribs (**ATLAS PLATE 333**).
>
> Identify the origins of the **iliocostalis thoracis** medial to the angles of the **lower six** ribs. Follow these muscular slips upward to their insertions on the **upper six** ribs and on the transverse process of the C7 vertebra (**ATLAS PLATE 333**).
>
> Continue superiorly along this muscular column and identify the origins of the **iliocostalis cervicis** at the angles of the 3rd to 6th ribs, medial to the insertions of the iliocostalis thoracis. Follow these fascicles to the posterior tubercles and transverse processes of the 4th, 5th, and 6th cervical vertebrae (**ATLAS PLATE 333**).

2. **Longissimus.** The **longissimus part** of the erector spinae is the largest and most powerful of the muscle columns in the deep back. Located medial to the iliocostalis part, it also consists of three muscle bundles that ascend successively: the longissimus thoracis, longissimus cervicis, and longissimus capitis (**ATLAS PLATE 333**).

The **longissimus thoracis** is the largest of these three columns, and its lower fibers blend with those of the iliocostalis lumborum. It arises from the aponeurosis of the erector spinae, the lumbodorsal fascia, and the lumbar vertebrae. Some fascicles ascend medially to insert on the transverse processes of all of the thoracic vertebrae, while others ascend more laterally to insert on the lower eight or nine ribs (**ATLAS PLATE 333**).

The **longissimus cervicis** lies medial to the longissimus thoracis. It arises from the transverse processes of the upper four or five thoracic vertebrae and inserts onto the posterior tubercles and transverse processes of the 2nd to the 6th cervical vertebrae.

The **longissimus capitis** arises from the upper four thoracic vertebrae and the lower four or five cervical vertebrae. Its fascicles ascend to insert on the mastoid process of the temporal bone deep to the splenius capitis and sternocleidomastoid (**ATLAS PLATE 333**).

The longissimus thoracis and cervicis extend the vertebral column and, when one side acts alone, bend the vertebral column to that side. The longissimus capitis extends the head and rotates the head (and face) to the same side.

> In the lumbar region, identify the **longissimus thoracis** ascending from the middle of the erector spinae muscle mass. Separate it from the iliocostalis laterally and the more medial spinalis muscles. Follow some fascicles to their insertions on the transverse processes of the thoracic vertebrae and the posterior surfaces of the lower eight ribs (**use ATLAS PLATE 333 as a guide).**
>
> To find the **longissimus cervicis** palpate the upper four ribs and identify the muscle fibers superior and medial to the longissimus thoracis on the transverse processes of the upper four thoracic vertebrae. Follow these fascicles upward to the transverse processes of the 2nd to the 6th cervical vertebrae.
>
> Find the fascicles of the **longissimus capitis** between the longissimus cervicis and the semispinalis capitis. Note that these extend from the articular processes of C4 to C7 and the transverse processes of T1 to T4 superiorly to the mastoid process deep to the splenius capitis and sternocleidomastoid (**ATLAS PLATE 333**).

3. **Spinalis.** The spinalis column of muscles lies medial to the longissimus column, and its parts are often difficult to identify with certainty (**use ATLAS PLATE 333 as a guide**). The **spinalis thoracis** attaches below to the spinous processes of T11 to L2 vertebrae. Its fascicles blend with those of the longissimus thoracis laterally and the semispinalis thoracis on its anterior surface. Superiorly, its fibers extend to the spines of several higher thoracic vertebrae (T1 to T4).

The **spinalis cervicis,** when present, consists of vertically oriented fibers that course upward from the spinous processes of C7, T1, and T2 to the spinous process of the axis (C2). Its fibers are vertical and may be distinguished from the diagonally coursing fibers of the semispinalis cervicis that extend between the transverse processes below to spinous process above.

The fibers of the **spinalis capitis** arise from the spinous processes of cervical vertebrae (C2 to C6) and course vertically to the occipital bone.

◄
Grant's 309, 314, 315
Netter's 168
Rohen 222, 228

►
Grant's 310–312
Netter's 169
Rohen 226, 228

> Do not spend much time dissecting the spinalis muscles unless you have a special interest in their anatomy.

D. **Transversospinalis Muscle Group.** The transversospinalis muscles include the semispinalis, multifidus, rotatores, interspinous, and intertransverse muscles (**ATLAS PLATE 335**). The fascicles of the semispinalis, multifidus, and rotatores are directed upward and medially from the transverse processes of lower vertebrae to the spinous processes of higher vertebrae.

►
Grant's 313–315
Netter's 169
Rohen 226

1. **Semispinalis.** The parts of the semispinalis muscle column are the semispinalis thoracis, semispinalis cervicis, and semispinalis capitis. Fascicles of the **semispinalis thoracis** extend from the T6 to T10 transverse processes to the spinous processes of C6 to T4. The fibers of **semispinalis cervicis** course from the transverse processes of T1 to T6 up to the spinous process of C2 to C5.

The **semispinalis capitis** is a more substantial muscle, located on the posterior aspect of the neck deep to the splenius capitis (**ATLAS PLATES 332, 333, 338**). It can be identified because an incomplete and irregular **tendinous intersection** usually crosses it. The muscle arises from the transverse or articular processes from C4 to T7 vertebrae. It ascends to form a flat belly that inserts on the occipital bone between the superior and inferior nuchal lines, and it will be dissected with the suboccipital region.

The semispinalis thoracis and cervicis extend the thoracic and cervical vertebrae and rotate them to the contralateral side, while the semispinalis capitis extends the head.

◄
Grant's 314, 315
Netter's 168, 169
Rohen 225, 226, 228, 237

►
Grant's 310, 314–316
Netter's 169
Rohen 226

◄
Grant's 309, 311, 314–317
Netter's 167–169, 171
Rohen 222, 226, 235–238

2. **Multifidus.** The multifidus muscle lies deep to the semispinalis muscles and occupies space lateral to the spinous processes of all the vertebrae between the sacrum and axis (**ATLAS PLATES 335, 337**). The parts of the muscle are not named regionally as are other back muscles. **In the sacral region, the multifidus** arises from the dorsal sacrum and dorsal sacroiliac ligaments. **In the lumbar region,** the fasciculi arise from the mamillary processes; **in the thoracic region,** from the transverse processes; and **in the cervical region,** from the articular processes. At each level the fibers pass upward and medially to insert on the spinous process of a higher vertebra. The most superficial fibers extend over four to five vertebrae, while deeper fibers course over two or three vertebrae. The deepest fibers pass only between adjacent vertebrae. The multifidus extends, laterally flexes, and rotates the vertebral column.

3. **Rotatores.** The rotatores lie deep to the multifidus and are located at lumbar, thoracic, and cervical levels (**ATLAS PLATE 335, right side**). Best developed in the thoracic region, the **short rotatores** extend between the transverse process of one vertebra up to the lamina and spinous process of the next higher vertebra. The **long rotatores** extend across two joints. When the rotatores act on one side they rotate the vertebral column to the opposite side, and when they act bilaterally, they extend the vertebral column.

4. **Interspinous and intertransverse muscles** (**ATLAS PLATE 335, 337**). The interspinous muscles are paired short fascicles that extend between the spinous processes of adjacent vertebrae. The intertransverse muscles interconnect adjacent transverse processes. These muscles are best developed in the cervical and lumbar regions and are normally absent or very small in the thoracic region.

> Do not spend time dissecting the transversospinalis muscle groups. If you have a special interest in these muscles, they may be exposed easily upon the removal of the longissimus and spinalis muscle columns. The semispinalis capitis and semispinalis cervicis will be dissected with the suboccipital structures.

IV. Vertebral Canal and Spinal Cord

The spinal cord is best approached by opening the vertebral canal posteriorly. In this dissection, the lower half of the vertebral column is dissected. The occipital bone, the atlas and axis, their joints, and the cervical spinal cord will be studied with the suboccipital triangle.

A. Vertebral Column on an Articulated Skeleton.

Before beginning your dissection make the following observations on the vertebral column in an articulated skeleton.

▶
Grant's 277–279,
286–289
Netter's 147, 148
Rohen 188–191,
197

> Confirm the following points (**ATLAS PLATE 346**):
>
> 1. The vertebral column consists of 33 vertebrae: 7 **cervical,** 12 **thoracic,** 5 **lumbar,** 5 **sacral** (that are fused to form the **sacrum**), and 4 caudal or **coccygeal** (that are also fused, as the **coccyx**).
>
> 2. The cervical, thoracic, and lumbar vertebrae are mobile and allow flexion, extension, lateral flexion, and rotation of the vertebral column.
>
> 3. Examine typical thoracic and lumbar vertebrae (**Figure 25-9**). Note that each consists of an

◀
Grant's 374–376
Netter's 146
Rohen 193

oval, weight-bearing **body** anteriorly and a **vertebral arch** posteriorly. The body and vertebral arch surround the **vertebral canal,** which contains the spinal cord, the meninges, and the vertebral and spinal blood vessels.

4. On an individual vertebra identify the vertical anterior parts of the vertebral arch, called the **pedicles.** Posteriorly are the broader **laminae** that form the roof of the vertebral canal enclosing the spinal cord (**ATLAS PLATES 347, 350**).

5. Note that projecting posteriorly and slanting inferiorly from the vertebral arch is the **spinous process.** Identify the paired **transverse processes** *laterally* and the paired **articular processes** for the adjacent vertebra *superiorly* and *inferiorly.*

6. On the body and transverse processes of thoracic vertebrae identify **costal facets** that

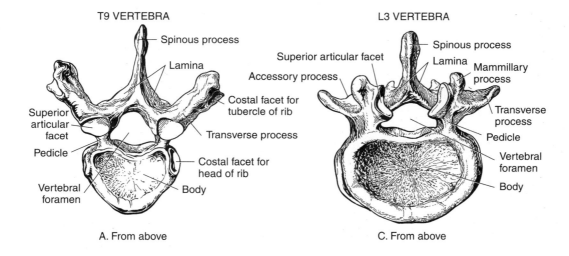

T9 VERTEBRA

- Spinous process
- Lamina
- Superior articular facet
- Pedicle
- Vertebral foramen
- Costal facet for tubercle of rib
- Transverse process
- Costal facet for head of rib
- Body

A. From above

L3 VERTEBRA

- Superior articular facet
- Accessory process
- Spinous process
- Lamina
- Mammillary process
- Transverse process
- Pedicle
- Vertebral foramen
- Body

C. From above

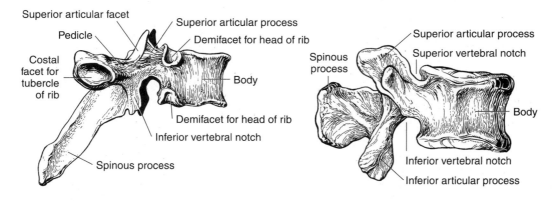

- Superior articular facet
- Pedicle
- Costal facet for tubercle of rib
- Superior articular process
- Demifacet for head of rib
- Body
- Demifacet for head of rib
- Inferior vertebral notch
- Spinous process

B. From the side

- Spinous process
- Superior articular process
- Superior vertebral notch
- Body
- Inferior vertebral notch
- Inferior articular process

D. From the side

Figure 25-9. Typical thoracic and lumbar vertebrae seen from above and from the side.

articulate with the head and tubercle of the ribs (**Figure 25-9, A and B**). Note that the head of each rib articulates on two adjacent vertebral bodies, while the neck of each rib articulates with one transverse process. For example, the head of the 6th rib articulates with the bodies of the T5 and T6 vertebrae, but the tubercle of the 6th rib articulates with the transverse process only of the T6 vertebra (**ATLAS PLATE 347–349**).

7. Realize that in life the bodies of adjacent vertebrae are joined by fibrocartilaginous **intervertebral discs** (**ATLAS PLATES 351, 352**). The highest disc is interposed between the atlas and axis, and the lowest between the 5th lumbar vertebra and the sacrum.

8. Identify the **intervertebral foramina** laterally between the pedicles of adjacent vertebral arches (**ATLAS PLATE 346 #346.1**). Through these foramina course the spinal nerves and vessels.

9. The cervical vertebrae will be studied with the suboccipital dissection.

B. **Vertebral Column in the Cadaver.** To expose and open the vertebral column for the study of the spinal cord within the vertebral canal, proceed as follows:

1. The cadaver should be face down with a wooden block placed under the pelvis, since the spinal cord will be approached posteriorly.

2. Remove all soft tissue of the deep back from the midthoracic region (T5 or T6) to the lower sacrum.

3. Cut away the iliocostalis muscle column and all muscle tissue located between the spinous and transverse processes of the lower six thoracic and five lumbar vertebrae. This will expose the vertebral column.

4. Using bone clippers (or a rongeur), remove the vertebral spines from the vertebrae. In so doing observe the strong **supraspinous ligaments** that interconnect the tips of the spines along the length of the vertebral column (**ATLAS PLATE 348 #348.1**). Also note the **interspinous ligaments** between the sides of the spinous processes. These extend from the supraspinous ligaments to the **ligamenta flava** (**ATLAS PLATE 351 #351.2**). Note also the intertransverse ligaments between adjacent transverse processes.

▶
Grant's 324–327, 332
Netter's 153
Rohen 230, 232

◀
Grant's 239–242, 300, 304, 336
Netter's 148, 151, 152
Rohen 2, 193, 198, 230

▶
Grant's 326
Netter's 163
Rohen 232

◀
Grant's 274, 289, 300, 336
Netter's 16, 148–152
Rohen 193, 197, 198

▶
Grant's 274, 326
Netter's 162, 163, 166
Rohen 230–232

◀
Grant's 299–302, 304, 763
Netter's 151, 152
Rohen 198

▶
Grant's 187, 322, 323, 325
Netter's 103, 162, 163
Rohen 230-232

5. With the spinous processes cut, identify the **ligamenta flava** composed of yellow elastic tissue that interconnect the laminae of adjacent vertebrae. The fibers of these important ligaments allow the laminae a degree of separation during flexion of the vertebral column (**ATLAS PLATES 349 #349.3, 350 #350.4, 351 #351.2**).

6. Remove the laminae of the vertebrae to open the vertebral canal (**Figure 25-10**). With a saw or bone clippers cut through both sides of the dorsal arches of the thoracic vertebrae. Use a chisel and mallet to sever the thicker laminae of the lumbar vertebrae.

7. Upon exposing the spinal cord and its dura mater, note that the **epidural space** between the dura and the bone contains epidural fat, loose areolar tissue, and a plexus of veins (**ATLAS PLATES 163, 360 #360.1**).

C. **Meninges of the Spinal Cord.** The three coverings of the spinal cord are the **dura mater, arachnoid mater,** and **pia mater** (**Figure 25-11**).

1. **Dura mater.** The **dura mater** is a tough inelastic membrane that consists of outer (endosteal) and inner (meningeal) layers (**ATLAS PLATE 360 #360.1**). The dura covering the spinal cord is a loose sac and represents only the inner meningeal layer. The endosteal layer is the periosteum lining the inner surface of the vertebral canal, and between these two layers is the **epidural space.** In addition to fat, also located in the epidural space is the **internal plexus of vertebral veins** that extends the entire length of the vertebral canal (**ATLAS PLATE 361 #361.1**). These veins anastomose superiorly with the venous sinuses in the cranial cavity and drain laterally through segmental intervertebral veins.

The dura mater forms tubular sheaths that are prolonged laterally over the roots of the spinal nerves (**ATLAS PLATE 360 #360.1**). The spinal dura also attaches around the circumference of the foramen magnum superiorly, and it extends downward to the 2nd sacral vertebra, below which it invests the filum terminale to the coccyx.

2. **Arachnoid mater.** The **arachnoid mater** is a membranous network that envelops the spinal cord (and brain) and lies between the dura mater and the pia mater. It is composed of collagen and reticular and elastic fibers, along with flattened cells similar to mesothelial cells. A potential space, the **subdural space,** separates it from the dura mater. The more substantial **subarachnoid**

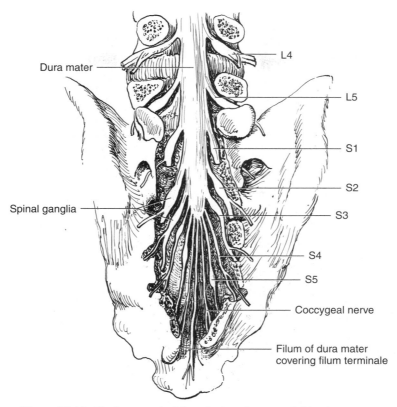

Figure 25-10. The lower end of the spinal cord surrounded by dura mater.

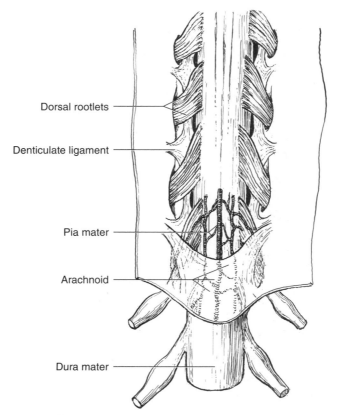

Figure 25-11. The meninges of the spinal cord.

space is located between the arachnoid and the pia mater, and it contains the **cerebrospinal fluid.**

In the lower lumbar region, the arachnoid surrounds the nerves of the cauda equina, and the subarachnoid space enlarges to form a significant pool that contains cerebrospinal fluid. This site is used clinically to secure samples of the fluid or to inject substances into the central nervous system. Lumbar punctures are most often performed between L3 and L4 or L4 and L5 vertebrae.

◄
Grant's 322, 323, 325, 330
Netter's 153, 154
Rohen 230–233

3. **Pia mater.** The **pia mater** is a vascular membrane that closely invests the brain and spinal cord. It contains collagenous, reticular fibers and flat mesothelial-type cells whose basement membrane is enveloped by the end feet of astrocytes (pia–glial membrane). The pia mater contains the arteries and veins of the central neural tissue and is somewhat denser in the spinal cord than in the brain. Below the tapered end of the spinal cord, called the **conus medullaris,** the pia mater forms a long slender filament, the **filum terminale (Figure 25-12).**

◄
Grant's 325, 326, 329
Netter's 153, 154, 162–165
Rohen 230–233

The pia mater also forms a continuous fibrous sheet that courses longitudinally between the dorsal and ventral roots on the two sides of the spinal cord. These two narrow membranous shelves are called **denticulate ligaments** because at 21 points on each side they form toothlike processes that extend laterally (pushing arachnoid with them) to attach to the inner surface of the dura mater (**ATLAS PLATE 358 #358.2**). The most superior attachment of the denticulate ligaments is just above the C1 nerve and the lowest is between the T12 and L1 spinal nerves.

◄
Grant's 325, 329
Netter's 162
Rohen 231

After opening the spinal column, lift the dural sac and cut it longitudinally with sharp scissors. At both ends of the incision, cut the dura laterally to expose the underlying structures.

In the embalmed cadaver the **arachnoid mater will not be seen** as a complete membrane. Instead wisps of the arachnoid network can be identified between the dura and pia (**ATLAS PLATE 358 #358.2**). Realize that in life the arachnoid forms a loose tubular sheath deep to which is the **subarachnoid space** filled with **cerebrospinal fluid.** Note that this fluid serves as a cushion of support for the spinal cord and the nerve roots.

Identify the delicate **pia mater** completely covering the surface of the spinal cord and containing all the blood vessels. Note how it penetrates into the longitudinal sulci within which course spinal

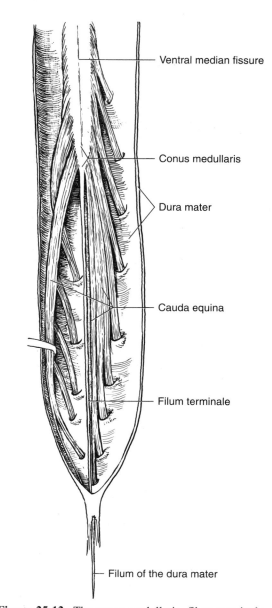

Figure 25-12. The conus medullaris, filum terminale, and cauda equina.

vessels. With fine forceps pick away some pia from the cord surface and see that the enmeshed vessels pull away with the pial layer.

►
Grant's 322, 325
Netter's 153, 154
Rohen 230, 231

◄
Grant's 326, 329
Netter's 162, 165
Rohen 231, 232

D. Spinal Cord and Spinal Roots. The spinal cord is an elongated part of the central nervous system that occupies the upper two thirds of the vertebral canal (about 45 cm). It extends from the foramen magnum to the 2nd lumbar vertebra where it tapers to form the **conus medullaris.** From the lower end of the conus a slender filament, the **filum terminale,** is prolonged to the coccyx (**ATLAS PLATE 359 #359.2**).

Attached to the spinal cord are the **dorsal** and **ventral rootlets** of 31 pairs of spinal nerves: 8 cervical, 12 thoracic, 5 lumbar, 5 sacral, and 1 coccygeal nerve on each side (**ATLAS PLATE 356**). Each spinal nerve is formed at the junction of the sensory dorsal root and the motor ventral root that supplies that segment. The dorsal rootlets at each level collect laterally. They contain an oval swelling, the **dorsal root ganglion,** where the cell bodies of the sensory neurons of that segment are located (**ATLAS PLATE 360 #360.1**). Just distal to the ganglion, the dorsal and ventral roots join to form the mixed **spinal nerve.**

The adult spinal cord does not fill the entire vertebral canal, and its substance ends at the L2 vertebral level. The lower thoracic, lumbar, and sacral spinal roots descend for increasing distances within the dura mater before reaching their corresponding intervertebral foramina. In the lower vertebral canal many spinal roots surround the conus medullaris and filum terminate within the dural sac. This is called the **cauda equina** (**ATLAS PLATES 357–359**).

◄
Grant's 325–328
Netter's 162, 163
Rohen 232

1. Note that the narrow thoracic spinal cord enlarges in the lumbar region (**lumbar enlargement**) because the lumbar and sacral spinal nerves are large and supply a large mass of tissue in the lower limbs.

2. Identify the longitudinal **denticulate ligaments,** one on each side of the cord. With a probe elevate the dorsal rootlets of a thoracic segment and note that the denticulate ligament separates the dorsal roots from the ventral roots (**ATLAS PLATE 358 #358.2**). See how the ligament sends toothlike processes laterally that attach to the dura.

◄
Grant's 325, 327
Netter's 162
Rohen 231

3. Identify the tapered lowest part of the spinal cord, called the **conus medullaris.** Separate it from the surrounding spinal roots and find the slender **filum terminale** extending inferiorly from the conus. Near the middle of the sacrum, note that the filum pierces the dura and continues to the coccyx (**ATLAS PLATE 357 #357.1**).

◄
Grant's 322, 323, 325
Netter's 153, 154
Rohen 230, 231

4. Observe the roots of the spinal nerves as they form the **cauda equina** (horse's tail) around the conus medullaris and filum terminale.

◄
Grant's 322, 323, 325, 330
Netter's 153, 154, 163
Rohen 230

5. Follow a dorsal root to its penetration of the dura mater; cut through the dura at this site, and identify the oval **dorsal root ganglion.** It will be necessary to remove a bit of bone to find the ganglion (**ATLAS PLATE 360 #360.1**).

◄
Grant's 324, 328
Netter's 162, 163
Rohen 230–232

6. Lift the cord slightly and see how the ventral root joins the dorsal root just distal to the ganglion.

Clinical Relevance

Spina bifida. This developmental defect is the result of an incomplete fusion of the posterior arch of a vertebra in the midline. In more serious cases there is a complete lack of fusion at the L5-S1 junction, resulting in a bulging dorsally of the meninges (meningocele) or of the meninges and spinal cord (myelomeningocele).

Scoliosis. This lateral curvature of the spinal column is most frequently located in the thoracic region. The cause is usually either muscular or a bony defect in a vertebra (such as hemivertebra). Often, young or adolescent children who had poliomyelitis or have cerebral palsy develop scoliosis. One shorter lower limb may also cause the condition because the youngster tries to compensate for that abnormality.

Kyphosis. This condition is an abnormal or exaggerated sagittal curvature in the thoracic or cervical vertebral column, producing a "hunchback" deformity. In older adults it can be caused by osteoporosis. It also can result from tuberculosis of the spine in which the bodies of the vertebrae are weakened or degenerated.

Injury to the coccyx. The coccyx can be injured by a direct fall on the lower back or by a painful dislocation of the sacrococcygeal joint. This injury also can also occur to women during childbirth.

Fractures of vertebrae. These fractures can occur anywhere along the vertebral column. The principal danger is the possibility of injuring the spinal cord. Fractures of the cervical vertebrae are the most dangerous because they can result in both paraplegia and interference with the cervical segments that send nerve fibers to the phrenic nerves (C3, C4, and C5), thereby endangering normal breathing.

Laminectomy. This operation on the vertebral column removes the spinous processes and often the vertebral arches of one or more vertebrae in order to access the vertebral canal and spinal cord. This operation is often performed to reduce pressure on the spinal cord or nerve roots (e.g., from a herniated disc).

Lumbar spinal puncture. This procedure, sometimes referred to as a "spinal tap," is done to get a sample of the cerebrospinal fluid (CSF) from the lumbar region of the spinal cord. The CSF is examined to determine if blood or inflammatory cells are present in the fluid. The needle is inserted between the L3 and L4 or, more frequently, between the L4 and L5 vertebrae, with the patient leaning forward or lying on the side with the vertebral column flexed.

Vertebral venous plexus. Frequently called Batson's veins, this venous system is a multivessel pathway by which metastatic tumor cells from cancers in the pelvis may spread to the vertebral column and the cranial cavity. Venous blood may enter this valveless system of veins when intra-abdominal pressure is increased. This route for the return of venous blood from the pelvis explains how cancers of the prostate may spread to the spinal cord and brain even before they are seen in the lungs. Intra-abdominal pressure is increased during defecation, coughing, or sneezing.

Herniated disc. Often called "slipped disc" or "ruptured disc," this condition occurs when the gelatinous part of the intervertebral disc (i.e., the nucleus pulposus) protrudes through the fibrous ring that surrounds the nucleus (annulus fibrosis). Pain results because the herniated material may compress the spinal cord or nerve roots. About 95% of herniated discs occur between L4 and L5 or L5 and S1 vertebrae or the lower cervical region.

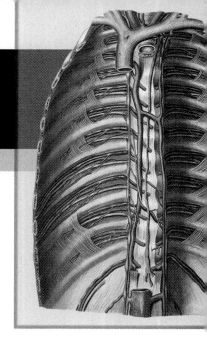

Back of the Neck and the Suboccipital Region

OBJECTIVES

1 Visualize the skeletal features of the posterior skull and upper two cervical vertebrae.

2 Dissect the suboccipital (C1) and greater occipital (C2) nerves and the occipital artery and vein on the posterior scalp.

3 Identify the four muscles that define the suboccipital triangle on each side.

4 Expose the floor of the suboccipital triangle and see the vertebral artery crossing from lateral to medial deep in the triangle.

Atlas Key:

Clemente Atlas, 5th Edition = Atlas Plate #

Grant's Atlas, 11th Edition = Grant's Page #

Netter's Atlas, 3rd Edition = Netter's Plate #

Rohen Atlas, 6th Edition = Rohen Page #

The suboccipital region is located below the occipital bone on the posterior aspect of the neck. Within this region is the important **suboccipital triangle,** which lies deep to the splenius capitis and semispinalis capitis muscles. The borders of this triangle are formed by the suboccipital muscles, and the region contains cervical nerves, the important vertebral artery, and venous channels (**ATLAS PLATE 339**).

◄
Grant's 316–318
Netter's 168, 169, 171
Rohen 35

►
Grant's 592, 764, 765
Netter's 7, 8
Rohen 25, 32, 33

◄
Grant's 280–290, 592, 764, 765
Netter's 12, 15, 17, 18
Rohen 32, 33, 198, 200

I. Posterior Skull and First Two Cervical Vertebrae

The skeletal structures in the suboccipital region are the occipital bone, the atlas, and the axis. The joints are the atlantooccipital and atlantoaxial articulations, and these are specialized for nodding and rotating the head.

On a skeleton with an intact skull and vertebral column observe the following:

A. Two horizontally curved ridges, one above the other, on both sides of the external surface of the occipital bone. These are the superior and inferior nuchal lines (**Figure 26-1**) on which attach muscles of the posterior neck (**ATLAS PLATES 516, 536**).

B. The **external occipital protuberance,** a bony prominence in the midline between the two superior nuchal lines (**ATLAS PLATE 536**). This prominence lies at the upper end of the **external occipital crest** that ends at the foramen magnum and affords attachment for the ligamentum nuchae.

C. Identify the midline junction of the occipital bone with the two parietal bones. This site is the **lambda** and, in the newborn, the location of the **posterior fontanelle** (**ATLAS PLATE 519**

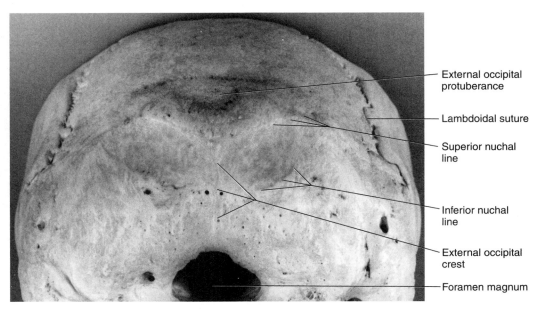

External occipital protuberance

Lambdoidal suture

Superior nuchal line

Inferior nuchal line

External occipital crest

Foramen magnum

Figure 26-1. Photograph of the posterior aspect of the skull, showing the bony processes on the occipital bone.

#519.1). Extending laterally between the occipital and parietal bones is the **lambdoid suture** (**ATLAS PLATES 515, 516**).

D. Identify the articulation of the occipital bone with the temporal (mastoid part) and parietal bones, called the **asterion.**

E. Identify the **atlas.** Observe that it has no true spinous process and that it lacks a body (**ATLAS PLATE 342, Figure 26-2A**). Note also:

1. The delicate **posterior arch** and the groove on its superior surface for the vertebral artery.

2. The **posterior tubercle** of the posterior arch on which attaches the ligamentum nuchae.

3. The **transverse processes** within which are the foramina for the vertebral arteries.

4. The **anterior tubercle** on the curved **anterior arch.** Note that when the atlas and axis are articulated, the **odontoid process** (dens) of the axis projects upward behind the anterior arch. It is maintained there by a strong transverse ligament (**ATLAS PLATE 344 #344.2**).

5. The concave **superior articular facets** located on the superior surfaces of the lateral masses. These receive the **occipital condyles.** Note the two circular **inferior articular facets** on the inferior surface of the lateral masses that articulate with the axis.

◄
Grant's 598, 599
Netter's 7, 11
Rohen 35

◄
Grant's 590

◄
Grant's 285, 291–293
Netter's 15, 17
Rohen 198, 200

►
Grant's 282–285, 320
Netter's 15, 17, 18, 146
Rohen 189, 190, 198, 199

►
Grant's 20, 307, 316, 317
Netter's 163, 170, 173, 250
Rohen 226, 227, 229, 234

F. Identify the axis (C2) and observe that it serves as a pivot on which the atlas and skull rotate (**ATLAS PLATE 342 #342.3, Figure 26-2B**). Note the:

1. **Odontoid process** (dens) that projects upward from the vertebral body. Observe the oval articular facet on the anterior surface of the dens that forms a joint with the posterior aspect of the anterior arch of the atlas.

2. Transverse groove on the posterior surface of the dens across which courses the transverse ligament of the atlas.

3. **Superior** and **inferior articular facets** on the upper and lower surfaces of the body of the axis. These articulate with the atlas and the C3 vertebra.

4. Small **transverse processes** and **foramen** on each side for the vertebral artery.

5. The thick **laminae** and **pedicles** and the large spinous process. Onto the latter attach several muscles that move the head.

II. Dorsal Rami of the Cervical Nerves (ATLAS PLATE 338)

The skin on the back of the neck and the posterior scalp is supplied by sensory fibers in the dorsal primary rami of cervical nerves. These rami course through the deep back muscles and supply them with motor innervation. After

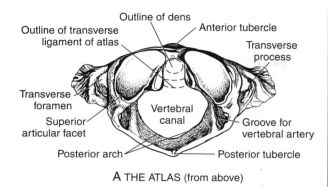

A THE ATLAS (from above)

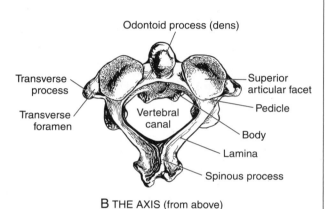

B THE AXIS (from above)

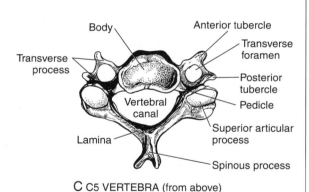

C C5 VERTEBRA (from above)
TYPICAL CERVICAL VERTEBRA

Figure 26-2. Cervical vertebrae seen from their superior aspect. **A.** The atlas. **B.** The axis. **C.** The C5 vertebra.

coursing through the deep back muscles, the dorsal primary rami perforate the trapezius muscle to get to the superficial fascia and skin. They **DO NOT** supply the trapezius with innervation, but simply pass through it to reach the surface.

The **dorsal primary ramus of C1** is called the **suboccipital nerve**. It is principally a motor nerve and

► Grant's 316, 317
Netter's 171
Rohen 236, 237

► Grant 307, 316–318
Netter's 20, 170, 171
Rohen 234–240

► Grant's 316, 320, 607
Netter's 20, 170, 171
Rohen 234–237

► Grant's 307
Netter's 170, 171
Rohen 226, 234, 236, 237

► Grant's 308, 309, 314
Netter's 167, 168, 171
Rohen 235

will be dissected when the suboccipital triangle is exposed (**ATLAS PLATE 339**).

The **dorsal primary ramus of C2** is both motor and sensory and is larger than other cervical dorsal rami. It emerges laterally between the atlas and the axis and gives rise to a small **lateral branch** that supplies motor fibers to the splenius capitis, semispinalis capitis, and longissimus capitis. The larger **medial branch** is the **greater occipital nerve** (**ATLAS PLATES 338, 339, Figure 26-2**). It ascends across the suboccipital triangle, pierces the semispinalis capitis, and emerges superficially, where it is joined by the **occipital artery**, a branch of the external carotid. The nerve and artery divide into terminal branches that supply the skin of the posterior scalp (**ATLAS PLATE 338**).

The **dorsal primary ramus of C3** is a mixed nerve and is found between the axis and the 3rd cervical vertebra. It divides into a lateral branch that often joins C2 and a medial branch that pierces the splenius capitis and trapezius to supply the skin of the lower occipital region as the **3rd occipital nerve** (**Figure 26-3**).

Because the deep fascia on the posterior scalp is dense, it is sometimes difficult to dissect the greater occipital nerve and occipital artery. **Know where to look.**

With skin reflected from the posterior skull, feel for the most prominent point on the external occipital protuberance, the **inion**. Dissect into the deep fascia 3 cm inferior to the inion and 2 cm lateral to the midline to identify the site where the **greater occipital nerve** pierces the semispinalis capitis and trapezius (**ATLAS PLATE 338**).

Carefully detach the **trapezius** from the occipital bone superiorly and the scapula laterally. Reflect the

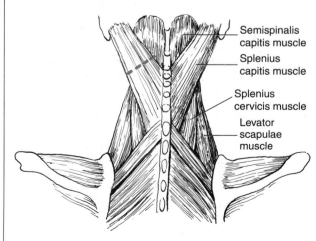

Figure 26-3. Muscles of the posterior neck deep to the trapezius.

muscle medially to the vertebral column. To free the nerve, cut through the trapezius from the site where the greater occipital nerve pierces it to its upper border. Deep to the trapezius is the **splenius capitis muscle.** Transect this muscle midway along its belly, turn back its ends, and identify the occipital artery coursing from lateral to medial deep to the splenius (**Figure 26-3**).

Deep to the splenius capitis detach the **semi-spinalis capitis muscle** from the occipital bone (**Figure 26-4**). This muscle can usually be identified because its fibers are vertical, and it frequently contains a tendinous intersection through its belly (**ATLAS PLATE 333**). To free the nerve, cut through the muscle from the point where the greater occipital nerve penetrates it to its upper border. Now follow the greater occipital nerve and artery along their course on the scalp.

With the trapezius, splenius capitis, and semi-spinalis capitis muscles reflected, the muscles of the suboccipital triangle are exposed (**ATLAS PLATE 335**). Follow the greater occipital nerve downward to the inferior border of the obliquus capitis inferior muscle.

◄ Grant's 308, 309, 311, 314, 316
Netter's 167–169, 171
Rohen 237, 238

III. Suboccipital Triangle (ATLAS PLATES 339–314)

Four small suboccipital muscles on each side deep to the semispinalis capitis are concerned with extension of the head at the atlantooccipital joints and rotation of the head at the atlantoaxial joint. Three of the four muscles bound the **suboccipital triangle.** These are the **rectus capitis posterior major, obliquus capitis superior,**

◄ Grant's 318
Netter's 171
Rohen 236, 237

► Grant's 316, 318
Netter's 171
Rohen 237, 238

► Grant's 316–318
Netter's 168, 169, 171
Rohen 237, 238

◄ Grant's 316–318
Netter's 168, 169, 171
Rohen 237, 238

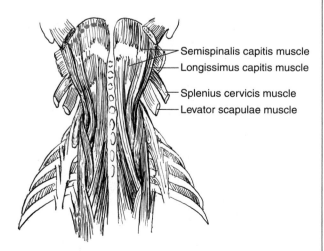

— Semispinalis capitis muscle
— Longissimus capitis muscle

— Splenius cervicis muscle
— Levator scapulae muscle

Figure 26-4. The sacrospinalis and longissimus capitis muscles.

► Grant's 316, 318
Netter's 171
Rohen 237, 238

► Grant's 321, 736, 737, 786
Netter's 28, 29, 67
Rohen 168, 169

and **obliquus capitis inferior.** The 4th muscle, the **rectus capitis posterior minor,** is located just medial to the major (**Figure 26-5**).

The **obliquus capitis inferior** stretches laterally from the spinous process of the axis upward to the transverse process of the atlas. It turns the face toward the same side (**ATLAS PLATES 340 #340.1, 341**).

The **obliquus capitis superior** is a vertical muscle extending from the transverse process of the atlas superiorly to the occipital bone, attaching between the superior and inferior nuchal lines. It extends the head.

The **rectus capitis posterior major** arises from the spinous process of the axis and ascends to insert on the lateral part of the superior nuchal line of the occipital bone. It extends the head and bends it laterally to the same side (**ATLAS PLATE 340 #340.1**).

The **rectus capitis posterior minor** is smaller and lies medial to the major. It arises from the posterior arch of the atlas and inserts on the inferior nuchal line of the occipital bone. It also extends the head.

All four suboccipital muscles are supplied by the posterior primary ramus of C1, called the **suboccipital nerve.** This nerve (**ATLAS PLATES 339, 341**) courses **through** the suboccipital triangle, giving motor branches to the four muscles, and it also sends a branch to the semispinalis capitis.

Remove the fibrous connective tissue and fat deep to the semispinalis and identify the three muscles that form the suboccipital triangle. Find the **obliquus capitis inferior,** the inferior boundary of the triangle, as it extends from the spinous process of the axis to the transverse process of the atlas. Identify the **obliquus capitis superior,** the lateral boundary, attached to the transverse process of the atlas and extending vertically to the occipital bone.

Identify the **rectus capitis posterior major,** the medial boundary of the triangle extending from the spinous process of the axis to the lateral half of the superior nuchal line of the occipital bone. Also identify the **rectus capitis posterior minor** located medial to the major and extending from the posterior tubercle of the atlas to the medial half of the superior nuchal line.

Probe the tissue **within** the suboccipital triangle and find the **suboccipital nerve** (**ATLAS PLATE 341**). This nerve is the posterior primary ramus of C1, and it supplies all four muscles of the suboccipital region.

IV. Vertebral Artery

The vertebral artery is the first branch from the subclavian artery, and it arises from its posterior aspect (**ATLAS PLATES 490, 491**). The **first part** of the vertebral

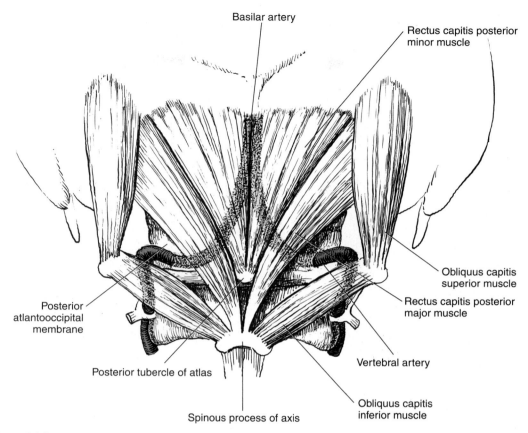

Figure 26-5. The suboccipital triangles, showing the vertebral arteries and their junction to form the basilar artery.

courses superiorly, medially, and deeply between the anterior scalene and longus colli muscles and normally enters the transverse foramen of the C6 vertebra.

The **second part** ascends through the transverse foramina of the upper six cervical vertebrae. It is surrounded by a plexus of veins and sympathetic nerve fibers and reaches the upper surface of the transverse process of the atlas (**ATLAS PLATE 490 #490.1**). The **third part** of the vertebral artery bends 90° medially to lie along a groove on the posterior arch of the atlas. **It is at this site that the vertebral artery crosses the floor of the suboccipital triangle from lateral to medial.** The dorsal ramus of the C1 nerve emerges dorsally between the artery and the posterior arch of the atlas (**ATLAS PLATE 341**).

The **4th part** of the vertebral artery makes another 90° turn superiorly and pierces the posterior atlantooccipital membrane to enter the cranial cavity through the foramen magnum. Ascending medially to the ventral surface of the medulla oblongata, it joins the vertebral artery from the other side to form the **basilar artery** (**Figure 26-5**).

In the neck, the vertebral artery gives off muscular and segmental intervertebral spinal branches. In the

▶
Grant's 622, 624
Netter's 132, 134
Rohen 93, 474

◀
Grant's 318, 321, 736
Netter's 17, 29, 130, 164, 171
Rohen 73, 75, 168, 240

▶
Grant's 329
Netter's 132, 134
Rohen 232

◀
Grant's 622, 624
Netter's 130, 132, 134, 164
Rohen 93, 99, 103

cranial cavity, it gives off the **anterior spinal artery** just below the junction that forms the basilar artery (**ATLAS PLATE 358 #358.1**). The two anterior spinal arteries join and descend along the anterior median fissure of the spinal cord, and they anastomose with segmental spinal branches that enter the cord along the roots. The **posterior inferior cerebellar branch** is the largest branch from the vertebral artery (**ATLAS PLATE 526 #526.2**). It takes a winding course to supply structures in both the medulla and the cerebellum.

The **posterior spinal artery** may branch from the vertebral, but usually it is derived from the posterior inferior cerebellar branch. It descends on the posterolateral surface of the spinal cord just medial to the dorsal roots, and it anastomoses with segmental spinal arteries that enter the cord along the dorsal roots.

Saw through the middle of the clavicle, open the sternoclavicular joint, and mobilize the medial half of the clavicle. Leave the clavicular attachment of the sternocleidomastoid muscle. Separate the internal jugular vein and common carotid artery and locate the **vertebral artery** posterior to them as it branches from the subclavian (**ATLAS PLATES 490, 491**).

Trace the vertebral artery superiorly and medially behind the anterior scalene muscle and in front of the longus colli muscle to the transverse process of the C7 vertebra. Note that the artery enters the transverse foramen of the C6 vertebra and then ascends in the neck through the transverse foramina of the upper six vertebrae (**ATLAS PLATE 491 #491.1**).

Return to the suboccipital triangle and sever the attachments of the inferior oblique and rectus capitis posterior major from the spinous process of the axis. Reflect these muscles, remove the underlying fat, and trace the vertebral artery from lateral to medial. Note that it perforates the posterior atlantooccipital membrane to enter the cranial cavity through the foramen magnum.

◄
Grant's 321, 736
Netter's 28, 29, 130
Rohen 168, 169

◄
Grant's 318, 321, 736
Netter's 130, 171
Rohen 73, 75, 240

Clinical Relevance

Dislocation of cervical vertebrae. Cervical vertebrae are less tightly articulated with each other, and their facets are more horizontal. This makes them more prone for dislocation rather than fracture. Less severe dislocations may not injure the spinal cord; however, severe dislocations can injure the cervical spinal cord, resulting in sensory or motor disabilities in the upper and lower limbs.

Fracture or dislocation of the atlas. The first cervical vertebra is a relatively delicate bony ring with lateral masses interconnected by a transverse ligament. Blows on the top of the head or head-first falls (such as diving in a shallow swimming pool) may compress the lateral masses, thereby fracturing one or both arches. This can result in rupture of the transverse ligament and release the odontoid process of the axis. This endangers the cervical cord with puncture by the pointed dens.

Fracture or dislocation of the axis. The arch of the axis is most frequently fractured when the head is hyperextended on the neck. This fracture is the means by which hanging results in death, and it is sometimes called the "hangman's fracture." The body of the axis is displaced forward from the C3 vertebra, and injury to the brainstem and upper spinal cord results in death.

Cervical disc herniation. Less common than herniation in the lumbar region, herniation of cervical intervertebral discs most frequently occurs between the 5th and 6th cervical vertebrae or between the 6th and 7th vertebrae. Pain is felt in the lower neck and along the peripheral field of the involved nerve. Protrusions of disc substance may compress the spinal cord and compress the blood supply of the cord.

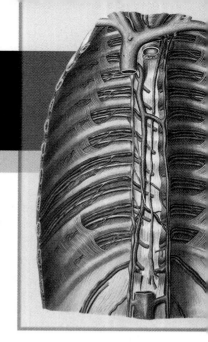

The Superficial Face and Anterior Scalp

OBJECTIVES

1 Examine certain bony landmarks on an articulated skull and study the surface anatomy of the face and forehead.

2 Dissect the muscles of facial expression and the other superficial structures of (a) the lips, mouth, and chin; (b) the external nose; and (c) the anterior orbital region and the eyelids.

3 Dissect the superficial vessels of the face and branches of the trigeminal nerve.

4 Dissect the parotid gland and its duct and the branches of the facial nerve on the superficial face.

Atlas Key:

Clemente Atlas, 5th Edition = Atlas Plate #

Grant's Atlas, 11th Edition = Grant's Page #

Netter's Atlas, 3rd Edition = Netter's Plate #

Rohen Atlas, 6th Edition = Rohen Page #

I. Bony Landmarks and Surface Anatomy of the Face and Forehead

▶
Grant's 588, 589
Netter's 2
Rohen 22, 23, 47

The bones of the skull articulate at suture lines and give the head its general configuration and shape. The soft structures that overlie the facial bones and the cartilages of the nose and ears present identifiable features that we use to recognize one another. Knowledge of facial anatomy is essential for the repair of disfiguring facial injuries and developmental defects. Examine the following on an articulated skull:

A. Front of Skull and Mandible (ATLAS PLATES 514). Note the following:

1. The two **bony orbits.** These cavities contain the eyeballs and other related structures. The upper border of each orbit is called the **supraorbital margin** and is formed by the frontal bone.

2. The **supraorbital foramen** (or **notch**) located about 3 cm lateral to the midline along the supraorbital margin. Through this opening pass the **supraorbital vessels and nerve.**

3. The **infraorbital margin** is formed by the maxilla medially and the zygomatic bone laterally. Identify the **infraorbital foramen** below the infraorbital margin about 3 cm lateral to the midline. Through this opening course the **infraorbital vessels and nerve.**

4. The **anterior nasal aperture** that opens into the nasal cavities. It is bounded laterally and below

by the maxillary bones and above by the nasal bones. Through the aperture can be seen one or more **nasal conchae** laterally and, in living persons, the **nasal septum** in the midline.

5. That below the infraorbital foramen, the root of the canine tooth forms an elevation called the **canine eminence.** This is located between two depressions: the **canine fossa** laterally and the **incisive fossa** medially.

6. That the **mandible** is the largest bone of the face. It has two halves at birth, but the fibrous joint between them anteriorly becomes ossified by the end of the first year. Identify the **mental protuberance** that forms the bony prominence of the chin (**ATLAS PLATE 515**).

7. The curved **body of the mandible** and its **alveolar part** that contains the sockets for the lower teeth. About 3 cm lateral to the midline identify the **mental foramen.** Through this opening the inferior alveolar nerve and vessels emerge. They are then called the **mental vessels and nerve.**

8. Confirm that the supraorbital, infraorbital, and mental foramina, through which pass the principal sensory nerves of the face, are aligned vertically about 3 cm lateral to the midline (**ATLAS PLATE 514**).

B. Lateral Aspect of the Skull and Mandible (**ATLAS PLATE 515**). Note:

1. That the body of the mandible is continued posteriorly on both sides to the **angles of the mandible,** from which the broad **rami** project upward on each side.

2. That the lateral surface of the **mandibular ramus** is flat, and its upper border is marked by the **mandibular notch.** This border is bounded **anteriorly** by the pointed **coronoid process** and **posteriorly** by the rounded articular **condyle of the mandible.**

3. The **mandibular foramen** on the medial surface of the ramus (**ATLAS PLATE 581 #581.2**). The medial border of this foramen is marked by a phlange of bone called the **lingula.** Into this foramen pass the **inferior alveolar vessels and nerves** for the lower teeth.

4. That the **zygomatic bone** forms the prominence of the cheek below and lateral to the orbit (**ATLAS PLATE 515**). Observe that it articulates with an anterior projection of the

◄
Grant's 589
Netter's 2
Rohen 22, 23, 47

►
Grant's 664, 665
Netter's 14
Rohen 54, 55

◄
Grant's 590
Netter's 13, 14
Rohen 52, 54

►
Grant's 591, 654, 655
Netter's 4, 12
Rohen 20, 29, 52

◄
Grant's 589
Netter's 2
Rohen 22, 23

►
Grant's 655, 659, 691, 764–767
Netter's 4, 8, 34, 51, 64
Rohen 24-26, 43, 45, 125

►
Grant's 590, 653, 654, 657
Netter's 4, 12, 23, 26, 49, 55
Rohen 20, 28, 32, 125

►
Grant's 603, 764, 813
Netter's 8, 21
Rohen 26, 32

◄
Grant's 590, 591, 654, 655, 665
Netter's 4, 12–14
Rohen 21, 52, 55

◄
Grant's 590, 591
Netter's 4
Rohen 20–23

temporal bone to form the thin **zygomatic arch.**

5. The **temporomandibular joint (TMJ)** by following the zygomatic arch posteriorly. Posterior to the joint note the opening of the **external acoustic meatus.**

6. The **temporal fossa** medial to the zygomatic arch. This extends upward on the side of the skull to the **superior temporal line.** Within this fossa is located the **temporalis muscle.**

7. The **infratemporal fossa,** inferior to the temporal fossa and behind the maxilla. Observe that it communicates with the temporal fossa.

8. The **lateral pterygoid plate** of the sphenoid bone that is separated from the maxilla by the **pterygomaxillary fissure.** Probe a small inverted pyramidal space behind the orbit, called the **pterygopalatine fossa.** Note that it communicates with the infratemporal fossa through this fissure (**ATLAS PLATE 515 #515.2**).

9. The **mastoid process** of the temporal bone located posterior to the external acoustic meatus. Also identify the slender **styloid process** on the base of the skull anterior to the mastoid process (**ATLAS PLATE 515 #515.1**).

10. The **stylomastoid foramen,** posterior to the base of the styloid process (**ATLAS PLATE 536, right side**). This foramen transmits the **facial nerve** onto the face. The **stylomastoid branch of the posterior auricular artery** enters the foramen on its way to the middle ear.

II. Skin Incisions; Reflections of Skin Flaps (Figure 27-1)

Skin incisions must not be deeper than the epidermal layer or else superficial facial muscles will be removed along with the skin flaps. The skin of the face varies in thickness. It is thin around the eyes, thicker over the forehead, temples, and around the mouth, and thickest over the chin. The muscles of the face are embedded within the connective tissue immediately deep to the skin.

A. Skin Incisions. The cadaver is to be supine (face up) with a wooden block placed under the posterior neck.

1. Make a midline incision on the scalp from the vertex to the forehead, down the middle of the nose to the upper lip (**Figure 27-1: A–B–C**).

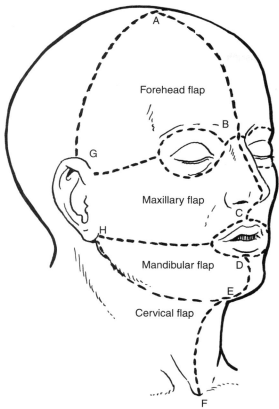

Figure 27-1. Skin incisions on the superficial face.

Continue in the midline from the middle of the lower lip, over the chin, and along the neck to the suprasternal notch (**Figure 27-1: D–E–F**).

2. Make circular incisions from the nose around both orbits to the upper border of the external ear (**Figure 27-1: B–G**).

3. Make another circular incision around the mouth, close to the margin of the lips. Carry this incision laterally on both sides to the lower border of the external ears (**Figure 27-1: C–H**).

4. Make incisions on each side from the lower margin of the chin in the midline, laterally along the lower border of the mandible to the ear lobe (**Figure 27-1: E–H**).

5. Make vertical incisions down the lateral surface of the head from the vertex to the upper border of the external ear (**Figure 27-1: A–G**).

B. Skin Reflections. The incision lines described above create four flaps on each side, as shown in **Figure 27-1.** Remove the flaps by cutting the epidermal layer only to the depth of the **dermal papillae**. These small conical projections of

dermis form a punctated pattern and attach into pits on the deep surface of the epidermis.

1. Remove the **anterior forehead skin flaps** at the bridge of the nose between the eyebrows. Note that the subcutaneous tissue is both dense and thick.

2. Remove the **maxillary skin flaps.** Even though the skin is thinner than on the forehead, use the dermal papillae as your guide. Reflect the flaps laterally to the external ear and remove the skin around the mouth to the margin of the upper lip.

3. Remove the **mandibular skin flaps** next. Cut around the margin of the lower lip and reflect the flaps laterally. Remove the skin from the anterior neck, leaving the underlying **platysma muscle** intact.

III. External Muscles of the Mouth (Figure 27-2)

Several superficial facial muscles attach to the upper and lower lips. These change the shape of the mouth, and their fibers interlace with the circular fibers of the **orbicularis oris** that close the mouth. Blending with the orbicularis oris from below, above, and from the sides, these muscles elevate and depress the lips (**ATLAS PLATES 494, 495**).

▶
Grant's 603, 604
Netter's 22, 50
Rohen 62, 63

A. Expose the oval fibers of the **orbicularis oris muscle** by removing the skin above and below the lips.

B. At the lateral angle of the mouth, define the **depressor anguli oris** and the slightly deeper **depressor labii inferioris** extending upward to the corner of the mouth. Note that these muscles receive fibers from the **platysma muscle** in the neck (**ATLAS PLATE 494**).

C. Identify a series of muscles that converge on the mouth from above. From **lateral to medial,** these include:

1. The **zygomaticus major** and a thin muscle slip above it, the **zygomaticus minor.** These muscles extend from the zygomatic bone to the angle of the mouth, which they draw upward and laterally, as in laughing.

2. The **levator labii superioris** that descends from the lower margin of the orbit to the upper lip. It raises the upper lip.

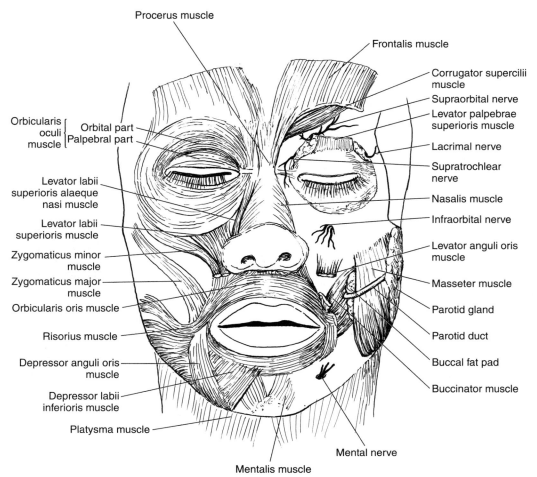

Procerus muscle

Frontalis muscle

Corrugator supercilii muscle

Supraorbital nerve

Levator palpebrae superioris muscle

Orbicularis oculi muscle — Orbital part / Palpebral part

Lacrimal nerve

Supratrochlear nerve

Levator labii superioris alaeque nasi muscle

Nasalis muscle

Infraorbital nerve

Levator labii superioris muscle

Levator anguli oris muscle

Zygomaticus minor muscle

Masseter muscle

Zygomaticus major muscle

Parotid gland

Orbicularis oris muscle

Parotid duct

Risorius muscle

Buccal fat pad

Depressor anguli oris muscle

Buccinator muscle

Depressor labii inferioris muscle

Platysma muscle

Mental nerve

Mentalis muscle

Figure 27-2. The muscles of facial expression.

3. The small **levator labii superioris alaeque nasi,** which passes downward from the medial angle of the eye. It divides into a fascicle that attaches to the alar cartilage of the nose and a more lateral slip that blends with the levator labii superioris.

D. At the lateral angle of the mouth, find the small **risorius muscle** that courses horizontally superficial to the platysma fibers. It is the "grinning" muscle.

E. Upon dissecting the **levator anguli oris** and **buccinator, do not cut the facial artery** that ascends superficial to these muscles.

1. On one side of the face cut the origins of the zygomaticus major and minor and turn them downward. Deep to these find the facial artery, and then use forceps to remove the buccal fat

◄
Grant's 600, 603
Netter's 56, 117
Rohen 76–79

pad from a small fossa anterior to the masseter muscle (**ATLAS PLATE 495**).

2. Find the **levator anguli oris** deep to the levator labii superioris and buccal fat pad (**ATLAS PLATE 494**). It arises from the canine fossa of the maxilla and descends to the angle of the mouth.

3. Realize that the **buccinator muscle** forms the lateral wall of the oral cavity. Place a finger into the mouth and press the cheek outward. The buccinator lies between the mandible and maxilla (**Figure 27-3**).

IV. External Nose (ATLAS PLATE 558)

The external nose is formed by a framework of bone and hyaline cartilage. It is pyramidal in shape, and the framework is covered by delicate muscle fibers and skin. Superiorly, the **root** of the nose is continuous with the forehead. It extends downward and anteriorly as the **dorsum** of the nose. Inferiorly, the **base** of the nose over the upper lip is perforated by apertures called the **nostrils** or **external nares.**

A. On an articulated skull note that the nasal bones form sutures with each other in the midline and with the frontal bone above and the maxilla laterally (**ATLAS PLATE 558 #558.1**). Look into the nasal cavities through the anterior aperture and observe that bone does not form the anterior part of the nose and nasal septum (**ATLAS PLATE 514 #514.1**).

B. Visualize the nasal cartilages (**ATLAS PLATES 558, 560 #560.1**). These include the **septal cartilage** in the midline, the **lateral cartilages,** and the **major** and **minor alar cartilages.** Observe that the lateral cartilages are expansions of the midline septal cartilage and are located on both sides of the nose inferior to the nasal bone (**ATLAS PLATE 560 #560.1**).

◄
Grant's 680
Netter's 32
Rohen 49, 56

C. Remove the skin of the nose, starting superiorly. Note that deep to the skin are thin muscle fibers that form the **transverse** (compressor) and **alar** (dilator) **parts of the nasalis muscle.** Identify the **external nasal nerve** at the lower border of the nasal bone (**ATLAS PLATES 501, 512, 513**).

◄
Grant's 600, 603
Netter's 20, 22, 32, 41, 50
Rohen 62, 63, 72, 77, 78, 80

This sensory nerve is the continuation of the **anterior ethmoid nerve** from V3. It supplies the lateral skin (**ala**), the tip (**apex**), and the skin around the nostril (**vestibule**).

V. Anterior Orbital Region

The orbit is a pyramidal space surrounded by bones. It houses the eyeball and the muscles, vessels, and nerves essential for normal vision. At this time only the surface anatomy and superficial muscles of the anterior orbit will be considered.

A. Surface Anatomy. Use a mirror on yourself, or observe the following features on a friend:

1. The globe of the eye is protected anteriorly by **eyelids** onto which are attached short, rather rigid hairs, the **eyelashes** (**ATLAS PLATE 538**).

2. The upper eyelid is larger than the lower, and it can be elevated and lowered voluntarily. The **palpebral fissure** is the opening between the two eyelids.

3. The two eyelids meet at the medial and lateral sides to form the **medial and lateral angles of the fissure** (**ATLAS PLATE 538**).

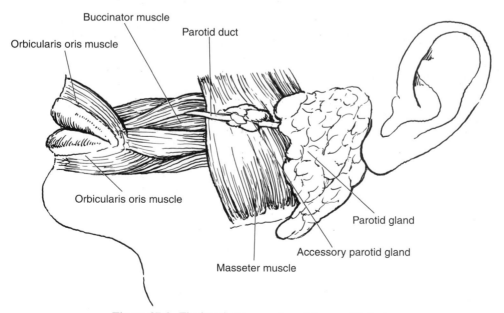

Figure 27-3. The buccinator muscle and the parotid duct.

4. Each eyelid contains a fibrous plate called the **tarsus.** These are attached to bone at the orbital angles by **medial and lateral palpebral ligaments.** Palpate the medial palpebral ligament as a **horizontal cord** by rubbing a fingertip between the medial angle of the eye and the nose (**ATLAS PLATE 542**).

5. The white region of the anterior eyeball is the **sclera,** and it is covered by a membrane, the **bulbar conjunctiva.** The membrane continues over the inner surface of the two eyelids as the **palpebral conjunctiva** (**ATLAS PLATE 538**).

6. Pull down the lower eyelid and see the reflection of the palpebral and bulbar conjunctivae, called the **conjunctival fornix** (**ATLAS PLATE 538 #538.3**). Observe that the palpebral conjunctiva is highly vascular. This diminishes over the sclera and ceases where the white sclera joins the transparent cornea overlying the colored iris (the **sclerocorneal junction**).

7. The **iris** is the colored anterior part of the eyeball, visible through the **cornea.** Note its radial striations and the opening in its center, the **pupil.**

8. The diameter of the pupil varies, depending on the amount of light that enters the eye. This can be demonstrated in a darkened room by flashing a light into the eye and observing that the pupil constricts and then dilates when the light is removed. This action is due to the circular **sphincter of the pupil** (under parasympathetic control) and the radially oriented **dilator of the pupil** (under sympathetic control) (**ATLAS PLATES 554, 557 #557.1**).

9. The medial angle of the eyelid overlies a small, reddish region called the **lacrimal caruncle.** It contains sebaceous glands and is bounded laterally by a semilunar fold of conjunctiva called the **plica semilunaris** (**ATLAS PLATE 538**).

B. Superficial Muscles of the Orbit (Figures 27-2, 27-6). The superficial muscle around the orbit is the **orbicularis oculi,** and it is used to close the orbital opening voluntarily. Also in this region is the small **corrugator supercilii** and the broad frontal belly of the **occipitofrontalis muscle** on the forehead (**ATLAS PLATE 539 #539.2**).

The orbicularis oculi muscle consists of orbital and palpebral parts. The **orbital part** arises medially from the medial palpebral ligament and the frontal and

◄
Grant's 604
Netter's 77, 79
Rohen 142

►
Grant's 600, 602, 603, 645
Netter's 22, 50, 77, 117
Rohen 56–61, 76–79, 81

◄
Grant's 640, 641, 645
Netter's 77, 79, 83–86
Rohen 133, 134, 142

►
Grant's 600, 602, 603
Netter's 22, 50, 77
Rohen 58, 59, 142

◄
Netter's 77
Rohen 130, 146

►
Grant's 604, 645
Netter's 77
Rohen 142

◄
Grant's 641, 648, 650
Netter's 77, 79, 84–86
Rohen 133, 134

◄
Netter's 84, 115, 126

◄
Grant's 641
Netter's 77, 78

maxillary bones. Its fibers form a concentric ring that surrounds the orbit, and it overlies the bony orbital margin. The **palpebral part** is thin and also arises from the medial palpebral ligament (**ATLAS PLATE 539 #539.2**). Its fibers pass over both eyelids and interlace laterally at the lateral palpebral raphe.

With the forehead skin removed, dissect the oval fibers of the **orbital part of the orbicularis oculi muscle.** Note that a branch of the facial nerve enters the muscle laterally to supply it (**ATLAS PLATES 539 #539.1, #791**).

Dissect the **palpebral part of the orbicularis oculi** by removing the skin from the eyelids. Note that the delicate muscle fibers overlie the fibrous orbital septum. Identify the **medial palpebral ligament** from which some of the palpebral fibers arise (**ATLAS PLATE 539 #539.2**).

Note the fibrous orbital septum deep to the palpebral muscle fibers. It attaches to the margins of the bony orbit, and its central part is thickened to form the fibrous **tarsal plates** that give the eyelids their firmness (**ATLAS PLATES 542**). Note that the upper tarsus is larger than the lower, being about 1 cm high at its center.

Realize that the inner surface of the upper tarsus contains the **tarsal glands** and that their secretions open onto the palpebral margin.

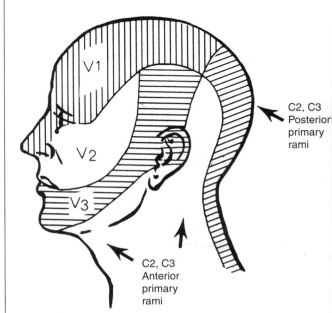

Figure 27-4. Cutaneous fields innervated by the trigeminal nerve and the posterior rami of C2 and C3 nerves.

VI. Superficial Vessels and Nerves of the Face (Figures 27-5, 27-7)

The **arteries** that supply the superficial face and scalp are branches of the external carotid that ascend to the face from the neck. Other branches of deeper vessels in the head reach the face through foramina in the facial bones. The **sensory nerves** of the face are branches from the three divisions of the trigeminal nerve. All reach the face through foramina in bones except the **auriculotemporal nerve,** a branch of the mandibular nerve that supplies the skin of the temple. This latter nerve is seen in another dissection.

A. **Facial Artery and Vein.** The **facial artery** arises in the neck from the external carotid, just superior to the origin of the lingual artery (**ATLAS PLATES 506, 510**). In 20% of cases it arises by a common stem with the lingual artery. The facial artery courses over the lower border of the mandible and

▶
Grant's 600, 601, 734, 736
Netter's 19, 32, 36, 65, 81
Rohen 76, 78, 79, 82, 83, 168–170

▶
Grant's 600, 667, 710
Netter's 19, 66, 81
Rohen 78, 79, 170, 173

▶
Grant's 600, 734, 736
Netter's 19, 65, 66
Rohen 78, 79, 166, 167

enters the face anterior to the masseter muscle. It continues superiorly in a tortuous course to the angle of the mouth, where it gives off **labial branches.** Ascending along the side of the nose, it reaches the medial angle of the orbit as the **angular artery** (**ATLAS PLATE 512**), anastomosing with the dorsal nasal branch of the ophthalmic artery.

The **facial vein** normally descends adjacent to the facial artery. It lies deep to the zygomaticus major and courses superficial to the masseter muscle near its anterior border. Inferior to the mandible the facial vein joins the anterior division of the **retromandibular vein** before entering the **internal jugular vein (ATLAS PLATE 500).**

Identify the tortuous **facial artery** as it crosses the mandible just anterior to the masseter muscle. Find the **facial vein** 1 cm posterior to the artery. Follow the vessels superiorly to the angle of the mouth,

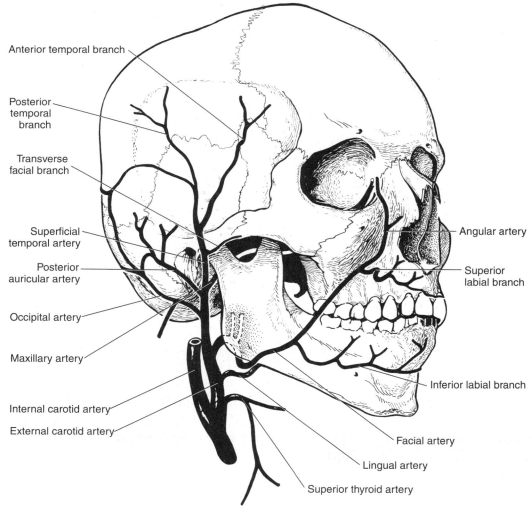

Anterior temporal branch

Posterior temporal branch

Transverse facial branch

Superficial temporal artery

Posterior auricular artery

Occipital artery

Maxillary artery

Internal carotid artery

External carotid artery

Angular artery

Superior labial branch

Inferior labial branch

Facial artery

Lingual artery

Superior thyroid artery

Figure 27-5. The external carotid artery and its branches.

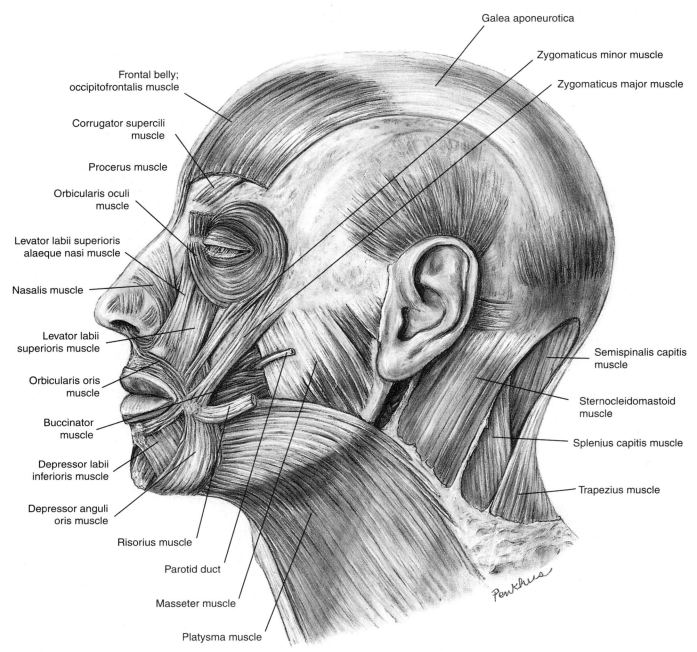

Figure 27-6. Lateral view of facial and upper cervical muscles. (From Clemente CD. Gray's Anatomy. 30th American Edition. Philadelphia: Lea and Febiger, 1985)

where **inferior** and **superior labial branches** are given off to the lips (**ATLAS PLATE 501**). Probe the vessels superiorly along the side of the nose to the medial angle of the eye where they anastomose with vessels that course in the orbit.

B. Orbital Vessels and Nerves That Supply the Face and Scalp. Superficial neurovascular structures

▶
Grant's 604, 646,
647, 806, 807
Netter's 19, 20, 32,
41, 67, 81, 82, 116
Rohen 77, 79, 82,
84, 134, 142

from the orbit include the **supraorbital and supratrochlear vessels** and nerves (V1), the **infratrochlear** (V1) and **external nasal** (V1) **nerves,** and the **dorsal nasal vessels.** Laterally, the **lacrimal nerve** (V1) and artery along with two small cutaneous nerves, the **zygomaticotemporal** (V2) and **zygomaticofacial** (V2), supply small areas of skin on the upper eyelid, temple, and cheek (**ATLAS PLATES 500, 501, 510**).

V2

Zygomaticotemporal nerve

Zygomaticofacial nerve

Infraorbital nerve

V1

Supraorbital nerve

Supratrochlear nerve

Lacrimal nerve

Infratrochlear nerve

External nasal nerve

V3

Auriculotemporal nerve

Buccal nerve

Mental nerve

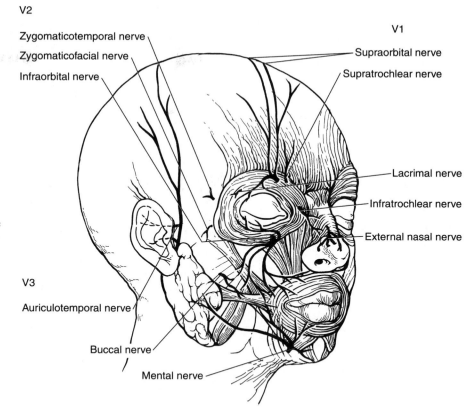

Figure 27-7. Cutaneous branches of the trigeminal nerve.

Make a 5-cm incision as deep as the bone across the forehead, 4 cm above the supraorbital margin (**Figure 27-8**). Then make two vertical incisions from the horizontal incision: one in the midline down to the bridge of the nose, and the other down to the lateral angle of the orbit. Scrape the flap away from the underlying frontal bone with the handle of a scalpel and **reflect it down to the supraorbital margin.** Identify the following on the inner surface of the flap:

1. The **supraorbital nerve and vessels** emerging from the supraorbital foramen (or notch) 3 cm lateral to the midline. They pierce the occipitofrontalis muscle and supply the scalp. Medial and slightly inferior to these, find the **supratrochlear nerve and vessels.** These branches of the ophthalmic vessels and nerve are also studied when the orbit is dissected (**ATLAS PLATES 500, 501, 510**).

2. The small **corrugator supercilii muscle** medially on the flap (**ATLAS PLATE 494**). It passes laterally to the skin of the eyebrow, which it wrinkles as in frowning.

▶
Grant's 600, 604
Netter's 22, 32, 50
Rohen 79

▶
Grant's 600, 603, 605
Netter's 20, 32, 39
Rohen 72

◀
Grant's 604, 608, 806
Netter's 19, 20, 32, 41
Rohen 77, 79, 82, 142

▶
Grant's 604, 677, 806
Netter's 19, 20, 32, 36, 41, 77, 79, 81
Rohen 67, 68, 79, 81–83, 142

◀
Grant's 600, 604
Netter's 22, 50
Rohen 60

3. The vertical fibers of the **frontalis part** of the **occipitofrontalis muscle.** Its fibers blend with those of the small **procerus muscle,** the corrugator supercilii, and the oval fibers of the orbicularis oculi (**Figure 27-2**).

Probe the dorsum of the nose where the nasal bone meets the upper border of the lateral nasal cartilage and identify the **external nasal branch** of the anterior ethmoid nerve (V1; **ATLAS PLATE 501**).

C. **Infraorbital Nerve and Artery.** The superficial branches of the **infraorbital nerve** reach the face through the infraorbital foramen, located 1 cm below the inferior margin of the orbit and 3 cm lateral to the midline. Its exit is in line vertically down from the supraorbital foramen (**Figure 27-9**). The infraorbital nerve is derived from the maxillary division of the trigeminal nerve (V2). In its course along the floor of the orbit, the nerve is joined by the infraorbital branch of the maxillary artery, and together they emerge from the foramen onto the anterior face. The infraorbital nerve supplies the lower eyelid, the side of the nose, the anterior face below the orbit, and the upper lip.

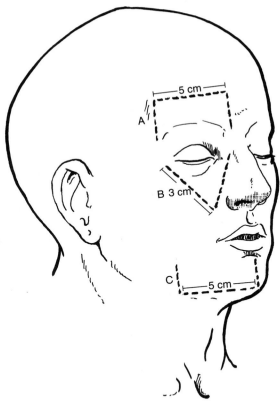

Figure 27-8. Incisions used to locate the 3 divisions of the trigeminal nerve on the face: **A,** for supraorbital and supratrochlear branches; **B,** for infraorbital branch; **C,** for mental branch of mandibular nerve.

To locate the infraorbital nerve, make a **V-shaped** incision deep to the bone below the lower eyelid, as shown in **Figure 27-8B**. The point of the V should be 3 cm lateral to the midline, at the level of the inferior margin of the nostril. The two vertical arms of the V should be directed upward toward the medial and lateral angles of the eye. **Do not cut the facial artery medially.** Lift the cut tissue upward off the bone, starting inferiorly at the point of the V, until the infraorbital foramen and its nerve and vessels are reached.

D. Mental Nerve (V3). The mental branch of the mandibular nerve emerges through the mental foramen on the anterior surface of the mandible below the lower 2nd premolar tooth (**Figures 27-7, 27-9**). It is the terminal branch of the inferior alveolar nerve that supplies all of the lower teeth. The mental nerve is sensory to the skin of the chin and the lower lip.

To dissect the mental nerve, make two vertical incisions on the chin, deep to the bone over the mandible. The medial incision, 1 cm lateral to the

▶
Grant's 600, 603,
652, 812
Netter's 19, 21, 32,
56, 57, 65, 68, 119
Rohen 76, 77

▶
Grant's 600, 601,
656, 668
Netter's 21, 50, 57
Rohen 68, 78, 153,
169

◀
Grant's 605, 677,
806, 810
Netter's 20, 42, 67,
116
Rohen 72, 73, 79,
82

▶
Grant's 600, 601,
652, 656, 658, 766
Netter's 21, 50, 51,
57
Rohen 58, 60, 167

midline, should extend up to the lower lip. The second vertical incision should be parallel and 5 cm lateral to the first. Cut horizontally along the mandible, interconnecting the lower ends of the vertical incisions to form a flap, as shown in **Figure 27-8C**. Elevate the flap upward from the underlying bone with a scalpel handle until the mental nerve and small vessels are located at the foramen.

VII. Superficial Structures on the Lateral Face

Located inferior and anterior to the external ear on the lateral aspect of the face is the **parotid gland,** the largest salivary gland. Its surface is covered by the dense **parotid fascia,** through which emerge the **parotid duct** and the branches of the **facial nerve** that supply the muscles of facial expression (**ATLAS PLATES 495, 498–501**). Anterior to the ear and coursing superiorly over the temporal region are the **superficial temporal artery and vein.** Slightly deep to these vessels ascends the **auriculotemporal branch** of the mandibular nerve, which is sensory to the temporal region (**ATLAS PLATES 510, 511**). The **transverse facial branch** of the superficial temporal artery crosses the face superficial to the masseter muscle. It is usually accompanied by one or two branches of the facial nerve (**ATLAS PLATE 501**).

Comment. The dense fascia over the parotid gland and masseter muscle makes this dissection difficult. Because the parotid duct and the superficial vessels and nerves course transversely, the fascia should always be probed and cut in that same direction (i.e., across the face) and **NEVER VERTICALLY.**

A. The skin should be removed from the side of the face, if this has not already been done. Identify the contours of the **masseter muscle** and its fascia attaching to the zygomatic arch superiorly and the ramus of the mandible inferiorly.

B. Find the **parotid duct** coursing along an imaginary line across the face from the ear lobe to the region midway between the upper lip and the nose (**ATLAS PLATE 498 #498.1**). Upon isolating the duct (2.5 cm below the zygomatic arch), follow it around the anterior border of the masseter muscle, where it penetrates the **buccinator muscle** and opens into the oral cavity opposite the upper 2nd molar tooth (**Figure 27-3**). Remove the **buccal fat pad** located anterior to the masseter muscle and superficial to the buccinator.

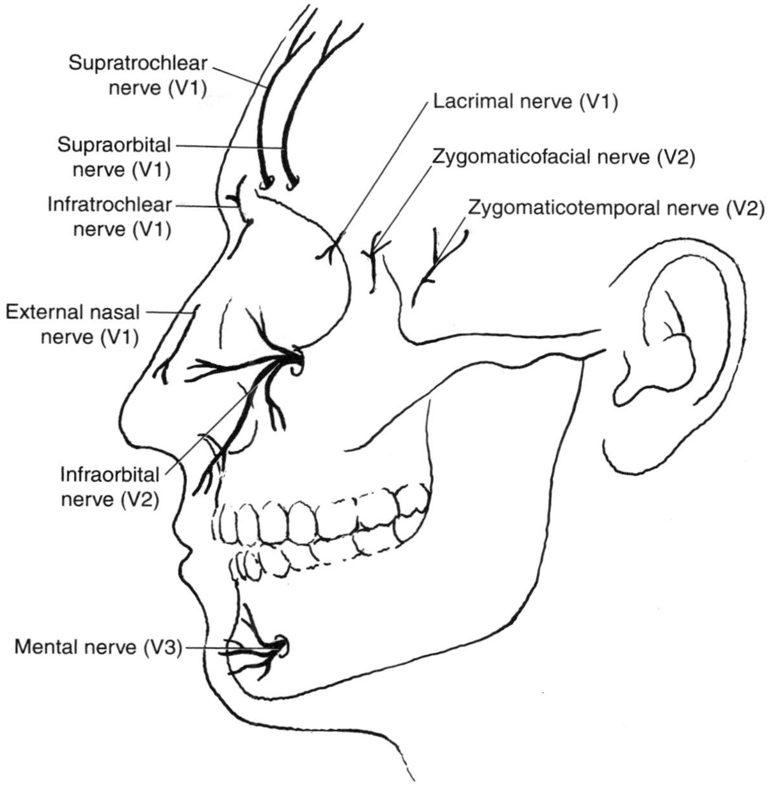

Figure 27-9. Sensory branches of the trigeminal nerve on the anterior face.

Labels on figure:
- Supratrochlear nerve (V1)
- Supraorbital nerve (V1)
- Infratrochlear nerve (V1)
- External nasal nerve (V1)
- Lacrimal nerve (V1)
- Zygomaticofacial nerve (V2)
- Zygomaticotemporal nerve (V2)
- Infraorbital nerve (V2)
- Mental nerve (V3)

C. Carefully dissect above and below the duct to locate branches of the **facial nerve** that course across the face parallel to the duct (**ATLAS PLATES 500, 501**).

D. After finding one or more branches of the facial nerve, dissect them back to the parotid gland, remove pieces of the gland with forceps, and probe until other branches of the nerve are found emerging from two or more common trunks.

E. Identify the following branches of the facial nerve (**Figure 27-10**):

1. The **temporal branch,** ascending anterior to the ear along the side of the head.

2. One or more **zygomatic branches** that cross the zygomatic bone to the lateral angle of the eye.

3. The **buccal branch** passing across the face to the region of the cheek and mouth.

4. The **mandibular branch** coursing below the angle of the mandible and along its lower border toward the chin.

5. The **cervical branch** descending from the lower part of the parotid gland to the neck under the platysma muscle which it supplies.

◄
Grant's 603, 652, 812, 813
Netter's 21, 27, 117
Rohen 74, 76–78, 80

►
Grant's 600, 601, 652, 710, 810
Netter's 19, 20, 27, 36, 42, 57, 65–67
Rohen 76–78, 80, 82, 178

◄
Grant's 603, 812, 813
Netter's 27, 117
Rohen 74, 78

F. Continue removing pieces of the parotid gland to identify the main trunk of the facial nerve emerging from the stylomastoid foramen.

G. Dissect the **superficial temporal artery and vein** anterior to the ear. Follow the vein downward behind the ramus of the mandible, where it becomes the **retromandibular vein** after it receives the maxillary vein. Probe behind and deep to the superficial temporal vessels and find the **auriculotemporal branch of the mandibular nerve** (**ATLAS PLATES 501, 510, 511**). It supplies the side of the head with sensory innervation.

Clinical Relevance

Cuts and incisions on the side of the face. Fibers of facial muscles are most often continuous with adjacent or underlying connective tissue. Thus, facial cuts or lacerations have a tendency to gape. In their repair, attention should be paid to the natural lines of cleavage to prevent excessive scarring.

Philtrum. This region of the face lies below the nose and above the upper lip, and it is bounded by two slightly elevated vertical ridges. Here the maxillary

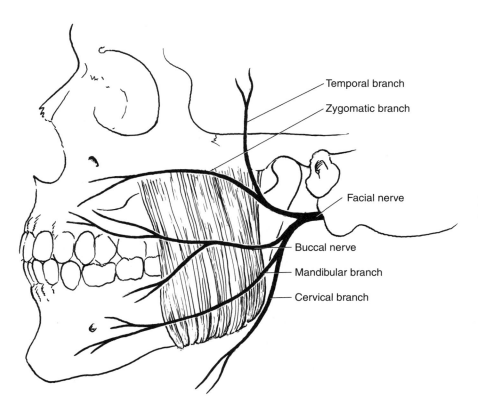

Temporal branch
Zygomatic branch
Facial nerve
Buccal nerve
Mandibular branch
Cervical branch

Figure 27-10. Branches of the facial nerve over the lateral and anterior face.

processes meet the frontonasal process during development of the face. Failure of this junction results in the condition called "hair lip" or cleft upper lip. This condition may occur unilaterally or bilaterally.

Wounds of the scalp. The edges of wounds of the scalp are held adjacent to each other because of the strength and integrity of the epicranial aponeurosis. If the aponeurosis is cut as in deep transverse or coronal wounds of the scalp, the edges of the wound separate or gape because of the pull of the frontalis and occipitalis bellies of the occipitofrontalis muscle. A rich arterial blood supply to the scalp is principally responsible for the healing of scalp wounds, but it also accounts for the fact that scalp wounds bleed profusely. Local pressure applied to the scalp helps stop bleeding. Healing, even of extensive scalp injuries, can be expected if these sources of blood are retained.

Scalp infections. A loose connective tissue layer is located deep to the galea aponeurotica. Infections can spread easily in this layer and even pass by way of emissary veins into the cranial cavity and involve the meninges. This layer of the scalp is frequently called the "dangerous area," and it is here that an intracranial venous sinus thrombosis can begin to form. Scalp infections can spread anteriorly to the eyelids and nose, but attachments of the epicranial aponeurosis prevent spread posteriorly and laterally. The extravasation of blood often results in "black eyes" because of the loose connective tissue in the eyelids.

Facial nerve palsy. This is usually referred to as Bell's palsy, and its overt symptoms relate to the fact that the muscles supplied by the facial nerve are paralyzed. Lesions anywhere along the course or origin of the nerve result in obvious effects on the muscles of facial expression. If lesions are in the brain or near the geniculate ganglion, both motor (including autonomic) and sensory functions are affected. However, if the lesion is at or near the exit of the nerve from the stylomastoid foramen or on the side of the face, only the facial musculature is affected. The ipsilateral face sags and there is a loss of facial expressions on the denervated side. At times the nerve is injured at birth by forceps delivery.

Mumps. This is an acute infection of the parotid and submandibular glands. Because of the tough, tight-fitting, and richly innervated fascia over these glands, any edema that causes pressure on the fascial covering results in extreme pain upon opening and closing of the mouth.

Infraorbital nerve anesthesia. The repair of wounds on the face below the orbit or on the upper lip, or the repair of the incisor teeth in the maxilla, requires a local anesthesia of the infraorbital nerve. The anesthesia is best achieved by raising the upper lip and, simultaneously, gently feeling for the infraorbital foramen. The needle is then passed superiorly (aspirating first to be sure it is not in a vessel) and then delivering the anesthetic slowly and carefully to prevent any passage of the fluid into the orbit.

Trigeminal neuralgia. This condition (sometimes called *tic douloureux*) affects the sensory root of the trigeminal nerve. It characteristically involves sudden and extremely painful attacks at which a person expresses a motor reaction (or tic) to the excruciating pain. The cause has not yet been determined, but some believe that an aberrant blood vessel presses the nerve in the cranial cavity, whereas others believe that some pathologic cause exists in the trigeminal ganglion of the central pathway of the nerve. Surgical treatment may involve making a lesion in one or another aspect in the course of the trigeminal nerve, either intracranially or extracranially.

Laceration of the facial artery. Cuts on the face that sever the facial artery or one of its branches bleed profusely. Applying pressure over the vessel as it crosses the mandible may reduce the bleeding. Anastomoses across the midline, however, may only partially suppress the bleeding, and, at times, pressure on both sides may be required for acute care.

Because of this excellent blood supply, wounds on the face heal rapidly.

The "danger area" on the face. Infections in a "butterfly-shaped" region below the orbits (including the nose and upper lip) can be dangerous because of the anastomosis of the facial vein with the cavernous sinus within the cranial cavity. This valveless venous interconnection extends from the facial veins through the inferior orbital veins to the cavernous sinus. It can be a pathway for the passage of infectious material from pimples or boils in this part of the face to the intracranial sinuses.

Fractures of the mandible. A fracture of the mandible from a blow on the side of the face frequently involves a second fracture on the opposite side. A fracture of the neck of the mandible may also fracture the opposite body of the mandible. This is because the mandible is, in effect, a ringlike bone, and a strong impact on one side is also transmitted to the opposite mandibular side away from the trauma.

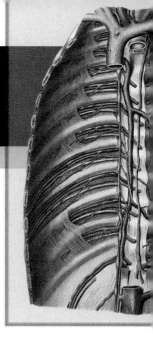

DISSECTION #28

Temporal and Infratemporal Regions (Deep Face)

OBJECTIVES

1 Visualize the veins of the temporal region, deep face, and retromandibular region.

2 Dissect the muscles of mastication and understand their actions.

3 Dissect the maxillary artery and its branches and the mandibular division of the trigeminal nerve and its branches.

4 Dissect the temporomandibular joint and understand its structure and movements.

Atlas Key:

Clemente Atlas, 5th Edition = Atlas Plate #

Grant's Atlas, 11th Edition = Grant's Page #

Netter's Atlas, 3rd Edition = Netter's Plate #

Rohen Atlas, 6th Edition = Rohen Page #

The deep face includes the **temporal region** anterior to the external ear and the **infratemporal region** deep to the zygomatic arch and ramus of the mandible. The muscles insert on the mandible and are the **muscles of mastication.** Most of the nerves are branches of the **mandibular division of the trigeminal** and are both sensory and motor in function. The arteries are derived from the **maxillary branch of the external carotid.**

I. Veins of the Temporal and Retromandibular Regions

To visualize the anatomy of the deep face, certain superficial facial structures must be removed. Observe

◄
Grant's 658, 661, 668
Netter's 36, 50, 51, 65–67
Rohen 52, 58, 59, 80–83

►
Grant's 607, 610, 734
Netter's 27, 66

◄
Grant's 600, 734, 738
Netter's 19, 27, 57, 66
Rohen 74, 76, 78, 178

that the veins of the temporal region and the face drain inferiorly and posteriorly to larger veins in the neck. The venous pattern that often is found has the **superficial temporal vein** receiving the smaller **transverse facial vein** and joining the **maxillary vein** to form the **retromandibular vein (Figure 28-1).** This latter vessel descends within the substance of the parotid gland, and about 3 cm below the earlobe, it divides into **anterior** and **posterior branches.**

The **anterior branch of the retromandibular vein** courses forward to join the facial vein. This vessel then crosses the external and internal carotid arteries to join the **internal jugular vein** near the greater horn of the hyoid bone.

The **posterior branch of the retromandibular vein** receives the **posterior auricular vein** to form the **external jugular vein (ATLAS PLATE 477).** Descending along the anterior surface of the sternocleidomastoid muscle, the external jugular flows into the **subclavian vein (Figure 28-1).**

Identify the **facial vein** along the anterior border of the masseter muscle (**ATLAS PLATES 500, 510**). Find the **superficial temporal vein** anterior to

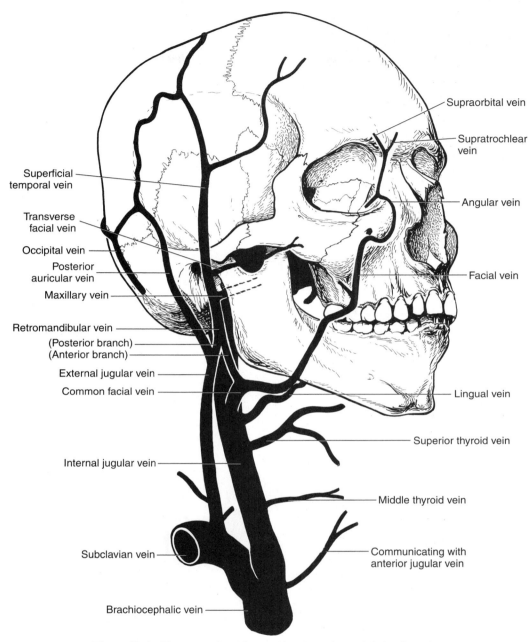

Figure 28-1. The external and internal jugular veins and their tributaries.

the ear as it is formed by the junction of the **anterior** and **posterior temporal veins.** Preserve the facial and superficial temporal veins. Remove the parotid gland piecemeal until the **maxillary vein** and artery are identified coursing deep to the posterior border of the ramus of the mandible. Follow the maxillary vein as it joins the superficial temporal vein to form the **retromandibular vein (ATLAS PLATES 508, 511).**

Continue to remove more parotid tissue and follow the retromandibular vein inferiorly to the angle of the

◄
Grant's 607, 610, 734
Netter's 19, 66
Rohen 78, 170, 171, 178

►
Grant's 710, 734
Netter's 27, 66

mandible, where it usually divides into **anterior** and **posterior branches (Figure 28-1).** Trace the facial vein from the masseter muscle to the **anterior division of the retromandibular vein,** where it forms the **common facial vein.**

Identify the **posterior auricular vein** descending behind the ear and follow it to its junction with the **posterior division of the retromandibular vein.** This usually occurs about 3 cm below the earlobe, near the anterior border of the sternocleidomastoid muscle **(Figure 28-1).**

Trace the anterior division of the retromandibular vein to its junction with the **internal jugular vein** near the greater horn of the hyoid bone. Follow the posterior division of the retromandibular vein to the external surface of the sternocleidomastoid muscle, where it descends as the **external jugular vein**.

II. Masseter and Temporalis Muscles (ATLAS PLATES 498, 499)

The four muscles of mastication are attached to the lower jaw, and they move the mandible for the purposes of chewing and talking. These muscles are the **masseter,**

►
Grant's 600, 656, 668
Netter's 50, 51
Rohen 58, 78, 169

temporalis, and the **medial** and **lateral pterygoids.** Two of the muscles are located more superficially on the face, whereas the two pterygoid muscles lie deep to the mandible in the infratemporal region (**ATLAS PLATES 498, 499, 502, 503**). All four muscles are innervated by the mandibular division of the trigeminal nerve.

A. **Masseter Muscle (Figure 28-2).** The masseter muscle is powerful and arises from the zygomatic arch and descends to cover the coronoid process and ramus of the mandible (**ATLAS PLATE 498**). Most of its fibers insert onto the angle and ramus of the mandible, but some deep fibers insert onto the coronoid process of the mandible. Its action is to elevate the mandible to occlude the teeth during chewing.

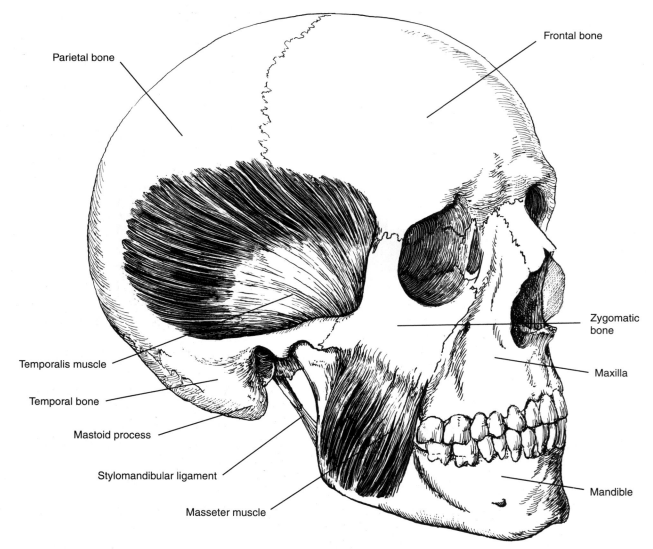

Figure 28-2. Lateral view of the skull showing the masseter and temporalis muscles and the stylomandibular ligament. (From Clemente CD. Gray's Anatomy. 30th American Edition. Philadelphia: Lea and Febiger, 1985.)

B. Temporalis Muscle (Figure 28-2). The temporalis muscle is fan shaped and arises in the temporal fossa on the side of the skull. Its fibers converge and pass downward **behind** the zygomatic arch to insert on the coronoid process and the anterior border of the mandibular ramus (**ATLAS PLATE 499**). The temporalis elevates the mandible and closes the mouth. Its posterior fibers also retract the protruded mandible, and it helps in side-to-side grinding movements.

◄ Grant's 656, 657, 668
Netter's 42, 50
Rohen 58, 59, 79

Remove the fascia superficial to the masseter muscle, and note the direction of its fibers. Detach the posterior half of its origin from the zygomatic arch. Reflect these fibers downward and identify the **masseteric nerve and artery,** which pass through the mandibular notch located between the condyloid and coronoid processes (**ATLAS PLATE 510**). Note that the nerve is a branch of the mandibular nerve and the artery a branch of the maxillary.

To study the temporalis muscle, the masseter muscle must be reflected downward. Do the following:

1. Clean the fascia from the surface of the zygomatic arch.

2. Pass the handle of a pair of forceps or a probe deep to the zygomatic arch to protect the underlying structures.

3. **SAWCUT #1:** Make an oblique sawcut through the zygomatic bone as far anteriorly as possible (**Figure 28-3**).

4. **SAWCUT #2:** Saw through the zygomatic process of the temporal bone posteriorly, anterior to the temporomandibular joint (**Figure 28-3**).

5. Reflect the cut zygomatic arch downward with the attached masseter muscle. It will be necessary to cut the masseteric nerve and vessels that enter the muscle on its deep surface.

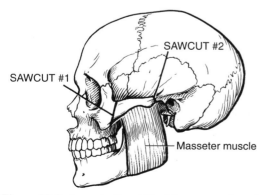

Figure 28-3. Sawcuts (1 and 2) of the zygomatic arch.

6. Strip the masseter muscle away from most of the mandible, leaving it attached inferiorly on the lower margin of the mandible.

7. This exposes the thick **temporal fascia** that overlies the temporalis muscle. Remove the fascia to expose the fan-shaped muscle arising from the temporal fossa and inserting onto the coronoid process and anterior border of the mandible (**ATLAS PLATE 499**).

III. Infratemporal Fossa and Its Contents

The infratemporal fossa lies deep to the ramus of the mandible. Within the fossa are located the **lateral and medial pterygoid muscles,** the **maxillary vessels and their branches,** and the **branches of the mandibular nerve** below the foramen ovale. The ramus of the mandible must be removed to dissect the infratemporal fossa.

Make the following three additional sawcuts:

1. Insert a probe behind the coronoid process that extends from the lower margin of the mandibular notch downward and forward midway along the anterior border of the mandibular ramus.

2. **SAWCUT #3:** Protect the soft structures behind the mandible. Make an oblique sawcut that separates the coronoid process (onto which inserts the temporalis muscle) from the rest of the mandible (**Figure 28-4**).

3. Reflect the coronoid process and the attached temporalis muscle upward, and identify the **deep temporal vessels and nerves** that enter the muscle (**ATLAS PLATE 512**).

4. Before removing the mandibular ramus, place the handle of a scalpel medial to the mandible to protect the deep soft structures.

5. **SAWCUT #4:** Saw through the **neck of the mandible** just below the temporomandibular joint (**Figure 28-5**).

6. **SAWCUT #5:** Before cutting across the mandibular ramus, pass a pair of forceps or scalpel handle **behind the mandibular ramus** 1 cm above the mandibular arch and the lower teeth. This will save the **inferior alveolar nerve and vessels** that enter the mandibular foramen on the medial surface of the ramus. Make the sawcut (**Figure 28-5**) and remove the ramus and any remaining bony fragments.

► Grant's 600, 653,
Netter's 41, 42, 50
Rohen 63, 65, 80

◄ Grant's 657
Netter's 50
Rohen 79

► Grant's 658–661, 668
Netter's 36, 51, 80–84
Rohen 59, 63, 80-84

► Grant's 658-660
Netter's 36, 42, 65, 67
Rohen 63, 80–82, 84

► Grant's 658-660, 810
Netter's 36, 65, 67
Rohen 63, 72, 73, 80–83

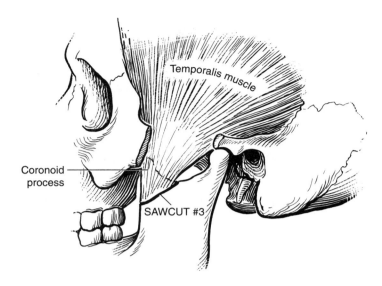

Figure 28-4. Sawcut (3) at the coronoid process.

7. Probe the fatty tissue within the infratemporal region, and identify vessels, nerves, and the pterygoid muscles.

A. Maxillary Artery and Vein (ATLAS PLATES 506–513, Figure 28-6). The maxillary artery enters the infratemporal region by coursing medially behind the mandible about 2 cm below the temporomandibular joint. The artery is best studied in three parts: the **mandibular** (or first) part, the **pterygoid** (or second) part, and the **pterygopalatine** (or third) **part.**

1. **Mandibular (or first) part of the maxillary artery.** The first part of the maxillary artery courses from the mandibular ramus to the lateral pterygoid muscle. It gives rise to four branches. Two small branches course **upward and backward** toward the ear (**deep auricular and anterior**

◄
Grant's 658-660, 810
Netter's 36, 65, 67, 130
Rohen 65, 80–83, 166, 169

►
Grant's 613, 710, 734
Netter's 66

◄
Grant's 659–660, 668
Netter's 36, 65
Rohen 80, 82

►
Grant's 658, 659, 810
Netter's 36, 67
Rohen 63, 72, 73, 80–83

►
Grant's 661, 811, 813
Netter's 36, 42, 67, 125
Rohen 72, 73, 81, 82, 84, 151

►
Grant's 658–661, 810, 811
Netter's 36, 42, 67
Rohen 63, 72, 73, 80, 81, 83

tympanic), the third vessel **ascends** to the dura mater **(the middle meningeal),** and the fourth vessel **descends** to the mandibular foramen to enter the mandibular canal **(inferior alveolar branch; ATLAS PLATE 512).** At times, an **accessory meningeal artery** may arise directly from the maxillary, but more frequently it ascends as a branch of the middle meningeal.

Maxillary Vein and Inferior Alveolar Nerve. The lateral part of the infratemporal fossa also contains the **maxillary vein** and the **pterygoid venous plexus,** located both lateral to and between the pterygoid muscles **(ATLAS PLATE 511).** The maxillary vein courses with the first part of the maxillary artery and joins the superficial temporal vein to form the retromandibular vein.

Accompanying the inferior alveolar branch of the maxillary artery and vein is the **inferior alveolar nerve (ATLAS PLATE 512).** From this branch of the mandibular nerve (V3) arises the **mylohyoid nerve,** just above the mandibular foramen **(ATLAS PLATE 513).** The delicate mylohyoid nerve supplies two muscles, the **anterior belly of the digastric** and the **mylohyoid muscle,** both located in the suprahyoid region.

On the lateral surface of the medial pterygoid muscle is located the important **lingual nerve (ATLAS PLATE 513),** also a branch of the mandibular nerve (V3). The lingual nerve is sensory to the anterior two-thirds of the tongue, and it also carries taste fibers and preganglionic parasympathetic fibers that join it from the **chorda tympani** nerve.

Pick away the fatty tissue in the infratemporal fossa, and find the branches of the first part of the **maxillary artery** and the **inferior alveolar** and **lingual nerves.** Identify the **maxillary vein** coursing

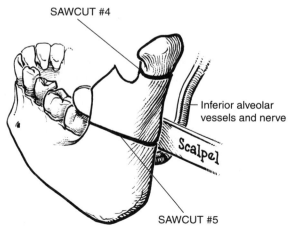

Figure 28-5. Sawcuts at the neck (4) and ramus (5) of the mandible.

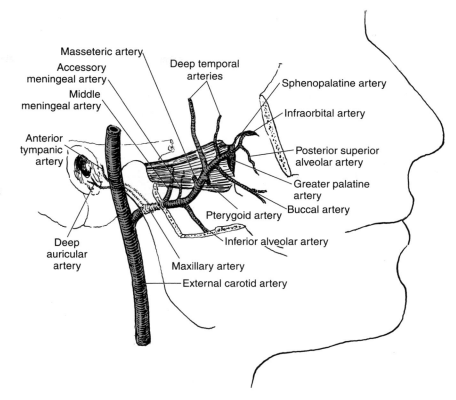

Masseteric artery
Accessory meningeal artery
Middle meningeal artery
Anterior tympanic artery
Deep temporal arteries
Sphenopalatine artery
Infraorbital artery
Posterior superior alveolar artery
Greater palatine artery
Buccal artery
Pterygoid artery
Inferior alveolar artery
Deep auricular artery
Maxillary artery
External carotid artery

Figure 28-6. The maxillary artery and its branches (after Grant's).

with the maxillary artery (**ATLAS PLATE 511**). Remove the vein and its tributaries and concentrate on the arteries and nerves.

Find the small **deep auricular** and **anterior tympanic** branches of the maxillary artery just below the temporomandibular joint. These course posteriorly to supply the wall of the external auditory meatus and the tympanic membrane (**ATLAS PLATE 512**). Identify the **middle meningeal branch** of the maxillary artery. Note that it courses vertically, deep to the lateral pterygoid muscle, to the foramen spinosum (**ATLAS PLATES 506, 513**).

Dissect the **inferior alveolar branch** from the maxillary artery as it descends with the **inferior alveolar nerve**. Find these structures as they traverse the mandibular foramen (**ATLAS PLATE 512**). The inferior alveolar nerve is the sensory nerve of the lower teeth. Accompanied by blood vessels, this nerve sends branches into each of the sockets and roots of the lower teeth. Confirm that the inferior alveolar vessels and nerve become the **mental nerve and vessels** beyond the mental foramen on the chin (**Figure 28-7**).

Turn your attention to the pterygoid muscles.

◄
Grant's 660
Netter's 36, 65
Rohen 63, 82

►
Grant's 660-662, 665
Netter's 36, 42, 51
Rohen 59, 80, 81

◄
Grant's 658, 659, 677, 810
Netter's 36, 42, 65, 67
Rohen 63, 72, 79–83

►
Grant's 658, 659, 810, 811
Netter's 36, 42, 51
Rohen 67, 80, 81

Lateral Pterygoid Muscle (**Figure 28-8**). The lateral pterygoid is a short, thick muscle, and it consists of upper and lower heads. Its fibers course transversely, unlike those of the masseter, temporalis, and medial pterygoid, which are essentially vertical (**ATLAS PLATE 502**). The smaller **upper head** arises from the greater wing of the sphenoid bone, while the **lower head** arises from the lateral pterygoid plate. The two heads converge posteriorly and insert onto the neck of the mandible and the capsule of the temporomandibular joint. The lateral pterygoid muscles open the mouth by pulling the condyle and articular disc forward, and they also protrude the mandible. When one muscle acts singly, it protrudes the mandible on that side. The two sides acting alternately results in grinding of the lower jaw.

Medial Pterygoid Muscle (**Figure 28-8**). The medial pterygoid muscle is the deepest muscle of mastication, and it arises from the lateral pterygoid plate of the sphenoid bone and the pyramidal process of the palatine bone. Its fibers pass inferiorly, posteriorly, and laterally, nearly parallel to those of the masseter muscle, to insert on the **medial surface** of the ramus and angle of the mandible (**ATLAS PLATES 502, 503**). The medial pterygoid and the masseter form a sling for the mandible. The two medial pterygoids elevate and protract the mandible. When the medial and lateral pterygoids of one side act alternately with those

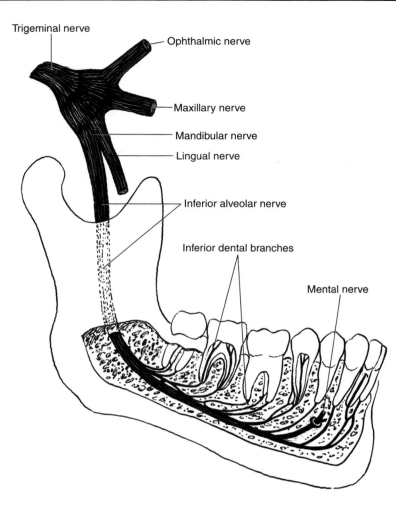

Trigeminal nerve

Ophthalmic nerve

Maxillary nerve

Mandibular nerve

Lingual nerve

Inferior alveolar nerve

Inferior dental branches

Mental nerve

Figure 28-7. The inferior alveolar branch of the mandibular nerve.

of the other side, they produce the side-to-side grinding movements during chewing.

After the first part of the maxillary artery is dissected, see if that vessel continues superficial (56%) or deep (44%) to the lower head of the lateral pterygoid muscle (**ATLAS PLATE 512**). Identify and clean the two heads of the lateral pterygoid muscle. Separate the two heads and find the **buccal branch of the mandibular nerve** between them (**ATLAS PLATES 512, 513**).

Even though the **buccal nerve** supplies a small motor twig to the lateral pterygoid, it is principally a sensory nerve to the skin over the buccinator muscle, the mucous membrane on the inner surface of the cheek, and the buccal surface of the gums.

To dissect the second and third parts of the maxillary artery, the **lateral pterygoid muscle must be removed.** Detach the posterior part of the **upper head** from the capsule of the temporomandibular joint. Remove its fibers piecemeal with forceps and

◄
Grant's 604, 658,
659, 810, 811
Netter's 20, 42, 67
Rohen 63, 72, 80,
82, 83

►
Grant's 658, 659,
661, 810, 811
Netter's 36, 42, 67
Rohen 72, 73, 80,
81, 83

►
Grant's 658, 660
Netter's 36
Rohen 63, 80–82

scissors. Remove the **lower head** of the lateral pterygoid by first severing its insertion on the mandible posteriorly. Then, use the handle of a scalpel to detach its fibers from the lateral pterygoid plate.

Inferiorly, identify the **lingual** and **inferior alveolar nerves** as they descend between the mandible and the medial pterygoid muscle (**ATLAS PLATE 512**).

2. **Second part of the maxillary artery.** The second (pterygoid) part of the maxillary artery supplies the muscles of the deep face. It may pass superficial to both heads of the lateral pterygoid or deep to the lower head (33%) on its course to the pterygopalatine fossa.

Follow the second part of the maxillary artery, and note its muscular branches: the **deep temporal branches** to the temporalis muscle, the **masseteric branch** (already cut), and the **pterygoid branches** to those two muscles. See also the slender **buccal artery** that courses with the buccal nerve (**ATLAS PLATE 512**).

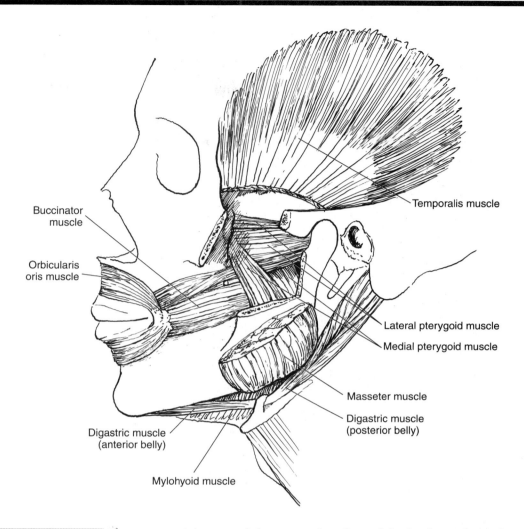

Figure 28-8. The pterygoid and buccinator muscles with the masseter and temporalis muscles cut.

Temporalis muscle

Buccinator muscle

Orbicularis oris muscle

Lateral pterygoid muscle

Medial pterygoid muscle

Masseter muscle

Digastric muscle (posterior belly)

Digastric muscle (anterior belly)

Mylohyoid muscle

Visualize the medial pterygoid muscle as it descends to the mandible and how it forms a sling with the masseter muscle for that bone. Keep the medial pterygoid intact (**ATLAS PLATES 503, 513**).

Mandibular Nerve and Its Branches. The mandibular nerve descends from the cranial cavity to the uppermost part of the infratemporal fossa. It traverses the foramen ovale, where the sensory root is joined by the motor root to form a mixed nerve. Below the foramen ovale, the mandibular nerve divides into anterior and posterior divisions. The **anterior division** of the mandibular nerve is principally motor to the muscles of mastication, but it also gives rise to the buccal nerve, essentially a sensory nerve (see above). The **posterior division** is predominantly sensory and gives rise to the auriculotemporal, inferior alveolar, and lingual nerves.

The **auriculotemporal nerve** is formed by two small roots that encircle the middle meningeal artery and then rejoin (**ATLAS PLATES 563 #563.1**). As its name implies, it supplies sensory fibers to the auricle of the

► Grant's 601, 652, 658, 806, 817
Netter's 20, 36, 42, 57, 67
Rohen 63, 73, 78–80, 82, 169

◄ Grant's 659, 661, 806, 810
Netter's 42, 67, 125
Rohen 68, 72, 83, 84

► Grant's 659, 671, 806, 810
Netter's 42, 67, 116, 125
Rohen 63, 72, 80, 81

ear and the temporal surface of the head anterior and superior to the ear (**ATLAS PLATES 501, 510**). **The otic ganglion is located just medial to the mandibular nerve.** Postganglionic secretomotor parasympathetic nerve fibers leave the otic ganglion and course along the auriculotemporal nerve on their way to the parotid gland (**ATLAS PLATE 563 #563.1**).

The **inferior alveolar nerve** (**Figure 28-7**) courses inferiorly from the mandibular nerve trunk and is joined by the inferior alveolar vessels above the mandibular foramen. It is the largest branch from the posterior division, and as it descends, it passes between the two pterygoid muscles. Initially, it is a mixed nerve, but before entering the mandibular foramen it gives off the **mylohyoid nerve,** which carries motor fibers to the mylohyoid and anterior digastric muscles (**ATLAS PLATES 512, 513**). The inferior alveolar nerve courses within the mandibular canal and is sensory to all of the lower teeth on that side. It emerges from the mental foramen on the anterior aspect of the chin to supply the skin in that region.

The **lingual nerve** supplies the anterior two-thirds of the tongue, the mandibular gums, and the floor of the mouth with fibers of general sensation. All of the **trigeminal fibers** within the lingual nerve are sensory; however, high in the infratemporal fossa the lingual nerve is joined by the slender **chorda tympani nerve** derived from the facial nerve (**ATLAS PLATE 512**).

The **chorda tympani nerve** arises from the facial nerve within the facial canal of the temporal bone, posterior to the tympanic cavity, about 7 mm above the stylomastoid foramen (**ATLAS PLATES 626, 629**). It enters the tympanic cavity through a small foramen in its posterior wall (posterior canaliculus) and arches forward across the malleus on the medial surface of the tympanic membrane. Anteriorly, it traverses another small foramen (anterior canaliculus) to reach the superior part of the infratemporal fossa (**ATLAS PLATES 513, 607**). Continuing anteriorly the chorda tympani nerve joins the sensory fibers of the lingual nerve from behind (**ATLAS PLATES 607, 626, 629**).

The chorda tympani nerve contains **preganglionic** parasympathetic facial nerve fibers to the submandibular ganglion. **Postganglionic** secretomotor fibers from the submandibular ganglion supply the submandibular and sublingual glands. The chorda tympani nerve also carries special sensory **taste fibers** from the anterior two-thirds of the tongue back to the facial nerve. The cell bodies of these taste fibers are in the **geniculate ganglion,** the sensory ganglion of the facial nerve, located at the **genu of the facial nerve** in the temporal bone (**ATLAS PLATE 626 #626.2**).

With the lateral pterygoid muscle removed, identify again the inferior alveolar nerve and vessels. Just superior to the mandibular foramen, find the slender **mylohyoid branch of the inferior alveolar nerve.** Follow this nerve to the floor of the mouth below the mandible. It contains motor fibers to the mylohyoid and anterior digastric muscles (**ATLAS PLATE 512**).

With bone-cutting forceps (or a chisel, mallet, and bone forceps) open the mandibular canal from the **outer surface** of the mandibular ramus. Follow the mandibular nerve branches into one or more sockets of the lower teeth (**ATLAS PLATE 580 #580.1**).

Find the **lingual nerve** as it descends from the mandibular nerve trunk. Note that its course is parallel but anterior and medial to the inferior alveolar nerve. It supplies general sensory trigeminal fibers to the mucous membrane covering the floor of the mouth and to the anterior two-thirds of the tongue. Trace the lingual nerve superiorly to the site where it is crossed by the maxillary artery.

Locate the delicate **chorda tympanic nerve** medial to the middle meningeal artery. Trace it forward as it loops to join the posterior aspect of the lingual nerve

◄
Grant's 658, 659, 744, 810
Netter's 36, 42, 67, 125
Rohen 72, 73, 80–83, 151

◄
Grant's 661, 806, 813
Netter's 42, 67, 125
Rohen 72, 73

►
Grant's 688, 690, 808
Netter's 4, 12, 36
Rohen 37, 63

◄
Grant's 721, 813
Netter's 42, 117, 125
Rohen 74, 83, 124, 151

►
Grant's 658-660
Netter's 36, 37, 65
Rohen 63, 80–83

►
Grant's 658-660
Netter's 36, 65
Rohen 63, 80–82

◄
Grant's 658, 659
Netter's 36, 42, 67, 125
Rohen 72, 73, 81, 183

►
Grant's 658-660
Netter's 36, 65
Rohen 63, 80–82

►
Grant's 659, 660
Netter's 36, 37, 48, 65
Rohen 63, 146

◄
Grant's 658, 659, 744, 810
Netter's 36, 42, 67, 125
Rohen 72, 73, 80–83, 151

►
Grant's 659, 660, 683
Netter's 36, 37, 48, 65
Rohen 63, 80, 146

(**ATLAS PLATE 512**). Know that the chorda tympani nerve carries preganglionic parasympathetic fibers (V11) to the submandibular ganglion, and special sensory taste fibers from the anterior two-thirds of the tongue to the facial nerve.

3. **Third part of the maxillary artery; pterygopalatine fossa.** In the most medial region of the deep face is located a cleft between bones called the **pterygopalatine fossa** (**ATLAS PLATES 515 #515.2, 541**). It is bounded anteriorly by the rounded infratemporal surface of the **maxilla,** behind by the pterygoid process of the **sphenoid bone,** and medially by the perpendicular plate of the **palatine bone** (**ATLAS PLATE 541**).

The fossa communicates **anteriorly** with the orbit through the inferior orbital fissure; **posteriorly** are the foramen rotundum and the pterygoid canal, which communicate with the middle cranial fossa and the foramen lacerum; **medially,** the fossa communicates with the nasal cavity through the sphenopalatine foramen; **inferiorly,** the fossa narrows to form the greater palatine canal to the oral cavity; and **laterally,** the fossa opens into the infratemporal region (**ATLAS PLATE 563 #563.2**).

As the third part of the maxillary artery enters the pterygopalatine fossa it quickly divides into several branches that course to other parts of the head through these communications (**ATLAS PLATE 512, Figure 28-6**).

Medially, the **sphenopalatine branch** traverses the sphenopalatine foramen in the palatine bone along with nasal nerves to reach the nasal cavity (**ATLAS PLATE 562**).

Anteriorly, the **infraorbital branch** enters the orbit by way of the infraorbital fissure to join the infraorbital nerve. Also the **posterior superior alveolar branch** courses anteriorly with accompanying branches of the maxillary nerve and divides into smaller vessels that supply the upper molar and premolar teeth (**ATLAS PLATES 563 #563.2, 580 #580.1**).

Inferiorly, the **greater palatine branch** accompanies the palatine nerves. It descends through the greater palatine canal to the oral cavity, where it divides to supply both the soft and hard palates (**ATLAS PLATE 562 #562.2**).

Another branch, the **artery of the pterygoid canal,** will be seen when the nasal cavity is dissected. At that time the nerve of the pterygoid canal and the pterygopalatine ganglion will also be identified (**ATLAS PLATE 562 #562.2**).

Follow the maxillary artery medially in the infratemporal region to the pterygopalatine fossa, and note that it divides into several branches. Trace the main trunk medially through the sphenopalatine foramen where it enters the nasal cavity as the **sphenopalatine artery (ATLAS PLATE 513)**. Probe gently into the foramen and then downward from the pterygopalatine fossa into the greater palatine canal. Find the **greater palatine artery** descending from the maxillary artery, but do not dissect it into the oral cavity, since this is more easily done when the nasal cavity is opened.

Look for the **infraorbital branch** of the maxillary artery that courses anteriorly and superiorly. It enters the infraorbital canal and joins the infraorbital nerve (**ATLAS PLATE 512**). Finally, look for a branch that courses anteriorly and inferiorly on the infraorbital surface of the maxilla. This is the **posterior superior alveolar artery** to the upper molar and premolar teeth.

Turn your attention to the temporomandibular joint.

▶
Grant's 653, 657,
664, 665
Netter's 14, 36, 51
Rohen 54–57, 79

◀
Grant's 658-660
Netter's 36, 65
Rohen 63, 81

▶
Grant's 658-660,
811
Netter's 14, 36, 81
Rohen 54, 55

IV. Temporomandibular Joint (ATLAS PLATES 504, 505)

A. **Structure of the Temporomandibular Joint.** The temporomandibular joint (TMJ) is a condylar joint consisting of upper and lower parts, each containing a complete synovial cavity (**Figure 28-10**). The two parts are separated by an articular disc, and the joint is surrounded by a fibrous articular capsule. Strengthening the capsule is the **lateral temporomandibular ligament (Figure 28-9).** It attaches superiorly to the articular tubercle on the zygomatic arch and inferiorly onto the neck of the mandible (**ATLAS PLATE 504 #504.1**). The TMJ interconnects this tubercle and the anterior rim of the mandibular fossa superiorly with the condyle of the mandible inferiorly.

Crossing the medial aspect of the TMJ is the **sphenomandibular ligament,** extending from the spine of the sphenoid to the lingula of the mandible (**ATLAS PLATE 504 #504.2**). It is an embryologic remnant of the sheath of Meckel's cartilage, but it does not add to the strength of the joint. Neither does the **stylomandibular ligament** stretching from the apex of the styloid process to the angle of the mandible (**ATLAS PLATE 504 #504.2**).

B. **Movements at the TMJ.** The mandible can be **depressed** (opening the mouth), **elevated** (closing the mouth), **protracted** (pushing the lower jaw forward), and **retracted** (pulling the lower jaw backward). Protracting and retracting the jaw alternatively by the two TMJs swings the chin from side to side. When this is combined with elevation and depression of the jaw, the grinding action used for chewing occurs. Food grinding can be performed on one side of the mouth by the unilateral action of the pterygoids on that side. If the jaw is in a position of rest, the heads of the

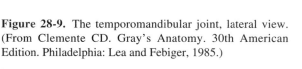

Figure 28-9. The temporomandibular joint, lateral view. (From Clemente CD. Gray's Anatomy. 30th American Edition. Philadelphia: Lea and Febiger, 1985.)

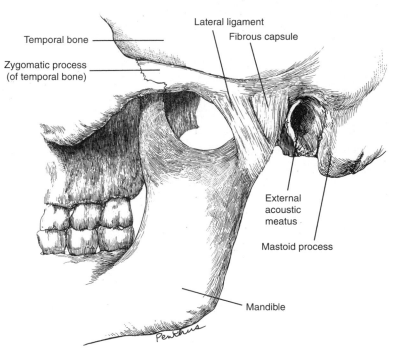

Temporal bone

Zygomatic process (of temporal bone)

Lateral ligament

Fibrous capsule

External acoustic meatus

Mastoid process

Mandible

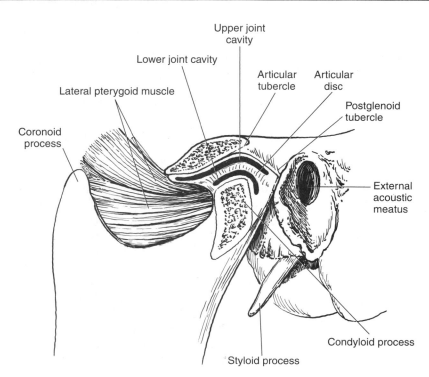

Figure 28-10. Sagittal section: left temporomandibular joint

condyles and the articular discs lie completely within the mandibular fossae.

1. **Opening and closing.** When the mouth is opened **passively,** as in sleep, there is a hingelike movement of the mandible downward, the transverse axis of which is between the two mandibular condyles. When the mouth is opened **actively,** as in chewing, the articular discs and the heads of the mandible glide forward to lie below the articular tubercles of the temporal bones (**ATLAS PLATE 505**). At the same time, the mandible rotates downward in a hingelike movement. There are simultaneous gliding and hinge movements of the mandible and disc. In closure, or jaw elevation, the movements are just reversed.

2. **Protraction and retraction.** In **protraction,** the condyles and discs of both sides also slide forward on the surface of the temporal bones, but the mouth remains closed, and the hinge movement of the mandible does not occur. **Retraction** is simply the reversed action, returning the discs and condyles to the rest position.

3. **Side-to-side movements.** The grinding action of the jaw can occur on one side only or in an alternating pattern, on one side and then the other. This action involves both protraction of the jaw and a hingelike action of the mandibular condyle. Grinding on one side only occurs by the simultaneous action of the two pterygoids on that one

▶
Grant's 659, 664
Netter's 4, 12–14
Rohen 21, 53, 54

▶
Grant's 665, 764, 765
Netter's 4, 8, 9, 14
Rohen 26, 32, 52, 54

side. Opening the mouth results from the action of the lateral pterygoids and the digastric muscles, whereas closure of the jaw occurs by the combined action of the masseters, temporalis, and medial pterygoid muscles.

ON A SKULL (ATLAS PLATES 504 #504.1, 515 #515.1): Before dissecting the TMJ, identify the curved **mandibular notch** between two prominent processes along the superior border of the mandible. Note the pointed, triangular **coronoid process** anteriorly, which serves for the insertion of the temporalis muscle. **It is not a part of the TMJ.** Posterior to the mandibular notch, identify the **condylar process.** It consists of the smooth mandibular **head** that serves as the inferior articular surface of the TMJ and a narrowed region below the head, called the **neck.**

Also on a skull, identify the zygomatic process projecting forward anteriorly from the temporal bone. Find an oval depression, the **mandibular fossa,** just anterior to the external auditory meatus (**ATLAS PLATE 603 #603.1**). On the inferior surface of the zygomatic process find the rounded **articular tubercle** just anterior to the mandibular fossa. Realize that in life a fibrous oval **articular disc** is interposed between the head of the mandible and the mandibular fossa and articular tubercle above, creating two joint cavities (**ATLAS PLATE 505**).

ON THE CADAVER: Remove the fibrous capsule from the lateral surface of the TMJ. Note that the TMJ consists of upper and lower joint cavities separated by a fibrous articular disc (**Figure 28-10**). Probe the upper synovial cavity and, with a scalpel, cut the attachments of the articular disc. Disarticulate the condyle of the mandible and probe the lower joint cavity. Observe how the articular disc accommodates the shapes of the bony structures forming the TMJ.

◀
Grant's 652, 653, 664, 665
Netter's 14, 36, 51
Rohen 54, 57, 79

Clinical Relevance

Skull fracture at the pterion. This injury on the side of the skull can become serious because the anterior branch of the middle meningeal artery courses along the dura mater immediately deep to the pterion. The pterion is the site of articulation of the frontal, parietal, temporal (squamous part), and sphenoid (greater wing) bones. Thus, a hard blow to the side of the head could cause a hemorrhage of the underlying artery, resulting in pressure on the brain that might be transmitted to the vital centers of the medulla and result in death.

LeFort fractures. These fractures of the maxilla usually result from severe trauma to the face. They are classified as LeFort I, II, and III.

LeFort I: A horizontal maxillary fracture where the tooth-bearing portion of the maxilla is separated from its attachments. Inferior to the fracture are the upper teeth and maxillary dental arch, the palate, inferior parts of the pterygoid processes, and part of the wall of the maxillary sinuses.

LeFort II: An injury in which the entire maxilla and nasal bones are separated from their attachments. Essentially the central region of the face is separated from the rest of the skull.

LeFort III: An injury in which the maxilla, nasal bones, and both zygomatic bones are separated from their attachments to the rest of the skull.

Surgical removal of the parotid gland. This operation, called parotidectomy, is performed to remove the site of a primary carcinoma of the parotid gland. Removal of the superficial part of the gland reveals the facial nerve that must be preserved to retain the function of the ipsilateral muscles of facial expression. Deep to the facial nerve is the more substantial part of the gland that lies behind the angle of the mandible and the mastoid process. Removal of the gland alters the smooth contour anterior and inferior to the earlobe, revealing the protrusion of the ramus and angle of the mandible just deep to the skin and a hollow region posterior to the mandible.

Parotid tumors. A parotid gland tumor puts pressure on the retromandibular vein and the superficial temporal artery that course posterior to the gland. The thick and tough parotid fascia does not allow significant anterior protrusion of an enlarged gland. Usually the branches of the facial nerve coursing through the gland become involved, and a facial paralysis on the ipsilateral side may develop. At times pain is referred to the temporomandibular joint by the fibers of the auriculotemporal nerve that ascends anterior to the ear and posterior to the joint.

Dislocation of temporomandibular joint. At times during the sudden contraction of the lateral pterygoid muscle (e.g., during a wide yawn), the two heads of the mandible and the articular discs dislocate anteriorly beyond the articular tubercles of the temporal bone. If this occurs the mandible remains open and the person is unable to close the mouth. Dislocation of the mandible on one side can occur if the opened jaw is struck by a blow (as in boxing). Reduction of the dislocated jaw is achieved by using both thumbs within the opened mouth and pressing down on the lower molar teeth on both sides, thereby overcoming the actions of the jaw-opening muscles and the contractures of the lateral pterygoid muscles.

Frey's syndrome. After a significant amount of time following a wound to the side of the face that injures the parotid gland, a patient may exhibit perspiration from the skin over the gland when eating or chewing gum. This occurs because of the regeneration of parasympathetic in the auriculotemporal nerve that were injured by the wound. These find their way into branches of the great auricular nerve and then innervate sweat glands in the field of that nerve.

Blockage of the parotid duct. If the parotid duct is blocked, the build-up of saliva in the gland causes painful inflammation and swelling of the gland. Usually such a blockage is due to a small calcified stone. Visualization of the parotid duct can be achieved by injecting a radiopaque fluid through the opening of the duct in the oral cavity. This technique is called sialography, and the stone that can block the duct is called a sialolith.

Posterior Triangle of the Neck

OBJECTIVES

1 Remove the skin from the posterior triangle of the neck and identify the strands of the platysma muscle.

2 Dissect the accessory nerve; external jugular vein; and the lesser occipital, great auricular, transverse cervical, and supraclavicular sensory nerves.

3 Identify the omohyoid, splenius capitis, levator scapulae, and the scalene muscles.

4 Remove the middle third of the clavicle; dissect the subclavian vessels and the thyrocervical trunk and its branches.

5 Dissect the trunks of the brachial plexus; find the suprascapular, phrenic, dorsal scapular, and long thoracic nerves.

Atlas Key:

Clemente Atlas, 5th Edition = Atlas Plate #

Grant's Atlas, 11th Edition = Grant's Page #

Netter's Atlas, 3rd Edition = Netter's Plate #

Rohen Atlas, 6th Edition = Rohen Page #

473, 477). Dissection of this region will focus on neurovascular structures in the neck that descend beneath the clavicle into the axilla. These include the **subclavian artery,** which continues as the axillary artery, and the **roots and trunks of the brachial plexus,** which become the cords of the plexus in the axilla. Additionally, **cutaneous branches of the cervical plexus** become superficial in the posterior triangle, and the **spinal accessory nerve** (XIth cranial nerve) crosses the floor of the triangle.

I. Boundaries of the Posterior Triangle; Skin Incisions

The posterior triangle (**Figure 29-1, ATLAS PLATE 471 #471.1**) located posterolaterally in the neck is bounded **inferiorly** by the middle third of the clavicle, **posteriorly** by the anterior border of the trapezius muscle, and **anteriorly** by the posterior border of the sternocleidomastoid muscle (**ATLAS PLATES**

◄
Grant's 724, 729, 731
Netter's 23
Rohen 178

A. Skin Incisions (Figure 29-2). Make one skin incision from the mastoid process to the suprasternal notch, roughly corresponding to the anterior border of the sternocleidomastoid muscle (**Figure 29-2 A–B**). **DO NOT CUT INTO THE SUPERFICIAL FASCIA** to avoid severing the external jugular vein and the great auricular and transverse cervical nerves.

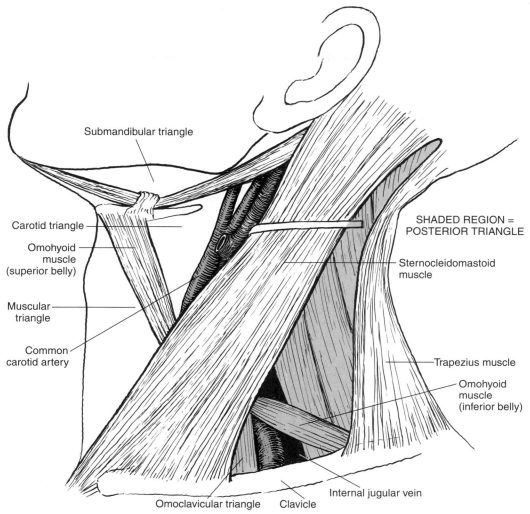

Figure 29-1. The posterior triangle and its muscular floor.

Make a second incision between the mastoid process and the external occipital protuberance on the back of the skull (**Figure 29-2 A–C**). The incision along the clavicle (**Figure 29-2 B–D**) was made when the pectoral region was dissected. Reflect and elevate the skin as far as the midline on the back of the neck, but leave it attached posteriorly in the midline (between C and D, **Figure 29-2**).

Note that the thin superficial fascia in this region contains strands of the **platysma muscle** (**ATLAS PLATES 472, 476**), whereas the dense underlying **investing layer of deep cervical fascia** stretches between the trapezius and sternocleidomastoid muscles, both of which it invests (**ATLAS PLATE 474**).

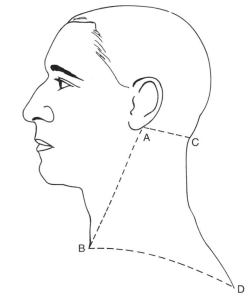

Figure 29-2. Skin incisions to open the posterior triangle.

Labels in Figure 29-1:
- Submandibular triangle
- Carotid triangle
- Omohyoid muscle (superior belly)
- Muscular triangle
- Common carotid artery
- Omoclavicular triangle
- Clavicle
- Internal jugular vein
- SHADED REGION = POSTERIOR TRIANGLE
- Sternocleidomastoid muscle
- Trapezius muscle
- Omohyoid muscle (inferior belly)

II. Superficial Vessels and Nerves (Figures 29-3 and 29-4)

Within the superficial fascia and in the underlying investing fascia, find the accessory nerve, the superficial veins, and the cutaneous nerves in this region.

These latter nerves (**Figure 29-4**) are derived from the C2, C3, and C4 cervical segments. They emerge from behind the posterior border of the sternocleidomastoid muscle to enter the posterior triangle and include the **lesser occipital, great auricular, transverse cervical,** and **supraclavicular nerves.**

A. Spinal Accessory Nerve. To expose the **accessory nerve,** dissect in the posterior triangle

along an imaginary line interconnecting the earlobe, when the face is anterior, and the acromion where it articulates with the clavicle (**ATLAS PLATE 476**). The accessory nerve descends initially deep to the sternocleidomastoid muscle; then, it enters the posterior triangle a bit above the midpoint of that muscle. Traversing posteroinferiorly through the triangle, it courses under the anterior border of the trapezius approximately 2 inches above the clavicle (**ATLAS PLATES 476-480**). It supplies both the sternocleidomastoid and trapezius muscles.

B. External Jugular Vein (Figure 29-4). Dissect the external jugular vein in the superficial fascia

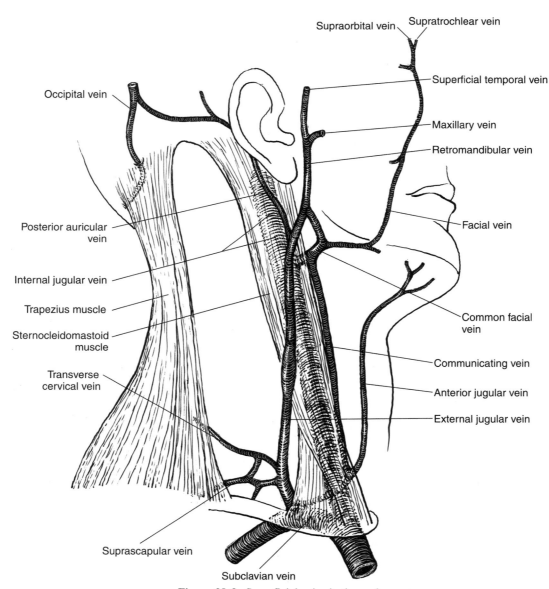

Figure 29-3. Superficial veins in the neck.

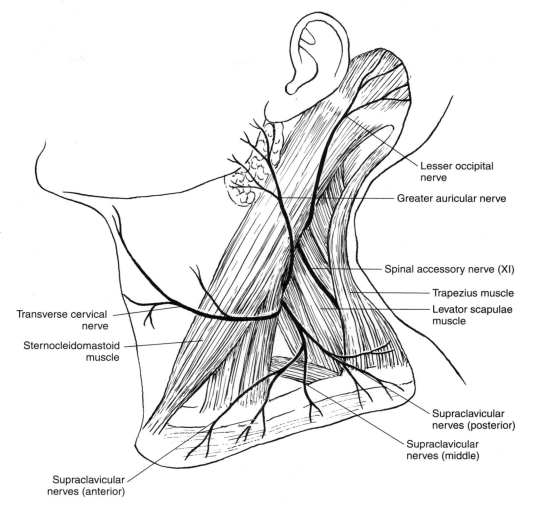

Figure 29-4. Sensory nerves of the cervical plexus and the spinal accessory nerve.

Labels in figure:
- Lesser occipital nerve
- Greater auricular nerve
- Spinal accessory nerve (XI)
- Trapezius muscle
- Levator scapulae muscle
- Supraclavicular nerves (posterior)
- Supraclavicular nerves (middle)
- Supraclavicular nerves (anterior)
- Sternocleidomastoid muscle
- Transverse cervical nerve

as the vessel descends obliquely across the external surface of the sternocleidomastoid muscle. The vein commences near the angle of the jaw where typically it is formed by the junction of the posterior auricular and retromandibular veins (**ATLAS PLATE 447**). Inferiorly, the vein pierces the deep fascia to flow into the subclavian vein or the internal jugular vein near its junction with the subclavian vein (**ATLAS PLATES 482, 483**).

C. Lesser Occipital Nerve (C2). To find this nerve, dissect along the posterior border of the upper one third of the sternocleidomastoid muscle. It emerges near the accessory nerve and ascends toward the scalp behind the ear near the mastoid process (**ATLAS PLATE 477**).

D. Great Auricular Nerve (C2, C3). Identify this nerve as it ascends from behind the posterior border of the sternocleidomastoid muscle and crosses obliquely over the external surface of

◄
Grant's 730, 732
Netter's 27, 28
Rohen 179, 180

that muscle toward the ear (**ATLAS PLATES 476, 477**). It is often found posterior and parallel to the external jugular vein.

E. Transverse Cervical Nerve (C2, C3). This nerve and its branches emerge behind the sternocleidomastoid muscle and course horizontally across the surface of that muscle to supply most of the skin over the anterior triangle of the neck (**ATLAS PLATE 477**).

F. Supraclavicular Nerves (C3, C4). These cutaneous nerves descend in the posterior triangle from behind the sternocleidomastoid to the skin over the clavicle. They include **medial, intermediate,** and **lateral supraclavicular** branches and supply skin over the acromion and the upper two intercostal spaces (**ATLAS PLATE 477**).

After dissecting the superficial veins and nerves, remove the remainder of the dense fascia that covers the muscles of the posterior triangle.

III. Omohyoid and Other Posterior Triangle Muscles

The muscles located more deeply in the posterior triangle include the inferior belly of the **omohyoid** and the muscles that form the floor of the triangle. These include (from above following downward) the **splenius capitis; levator scapulae;** and the **posterior, middle, and anterior scalene muscles.**

The omohyoid muscle divides the posterior triangle into two triangles. The upper **occipital triangle** contains the **occipital vessels, accessory nerve, roots of the brachial plexus,** and the floor muscles. The lower **omoclavicular (subclavian) triangle** contains the **subclavian vessels** and their branches as well as the continuation of the **trunks of the brachial plexus** that pass laterally from between the anterior and middle scalene muscles.

A. **Omohyoid Muscle.** Remove the fat from the posterior triangle and identify the small, ribbon-like **inferior belly** of the **omohyoid muscle** crossing the posterior triangle obliquely just above the clavicle (**ATLAS PLATE 478**). This is the lower part of a muscle containing two thin bellies interconnected by a tendon, and it extends between the hyoid bone to the upper border of the scapula (**ATLAS PLATE 479**).

B. **Other Muscles.** Clean the surface of the **splenius capitis** and **levator scapulae** muscles (**ATLAS PLATES 473, 475**), and again identify the accessory nerve descending over them to the trapezius muscle. Locate the **anterior** and **middle scalene muscles** and observe how the roots and trunks of the brachial plexus and, somewhat lower, the subclavian artery emerge between them (**ATLAS PLATES 473, 491 #491.1**). Identify the more deeply placed posterior scalene.

IV. Expose the Subclavian Vessels and Brachial Plexus By Removing the Middle Third of the Clavicle

Confirm that the anterior and middle scalene muscles attach onto the 1st rib (**ATLAS PLATE 491 #491**). When you resect the middle one third of the clavicle, **BE CERTAIN THAT YOU PRESERVE THE ANTERIOR SCALENE MUSCLE** to retain its important relationship to the vessels and nerve trunks in the region.

A. **Exposure of Structures Deep to the Clavicle.** On one side, cut away the clavicular attachment of the sternocleidomastoid muscle and reflect it

▶
Grant's 732, 733
Netter's 412
Rohen 182-184

◀
Grant's 731, 732
Netter's 23, 26
Rohen 181, 182, 185

▶
Grant's 762, 736, 737
Netter's 29, 412
Rohen 168, 184, 185

medially to expose the medial two thirds of the clavicle. Identify the anterior scalene muscle behind the clavicle and the **phrenic nerve** (C3, C4, and C5) that courses along its anterior surface.

B. **Remove the Middle Portion of the Clavicle.** With a handsaw, cut through the clavicle approximately 2 inches medial to the acromion. Make a second sawcut 1 inch lateral to the sternoclavicular joint. Remove the isolated intermediate portion of the clavicle (see **ATLAS PLATE 481**) by freeing it from the underlying subclavius muscle. Identify the **subclavian vein,** which lies **IN FRONT OF THE ANTERIOR SCALENE MUSCLE,** in contrast to the **subclavian artery and the trunks of the brachial plexus,** which course **BETWEEN THE ANTERIOR AND MIDDLE SCALENE MUSCLES (ATLAS PLATE 481).**

V. Subclavian Vessels

The axillary vein becomes the **subclavian vein** as it passes over the 1st rib. It joins the **internal jugular vein** to form the **brachiocephalic vein** on each side. The **external jugular vein** flows either into the internal jugular or the brachiocephalic vein (**ATLAS PLATES 482, 483**).

The **subclavian artery** passes laterally through the base of the posterior triangle deeper and slightly superior to the subclavian vein (**Figure 29-5**). With the artery course the trunks of the brachial plexus (**ATLAS PLATE 481**). The anterior scalene muscle lies in front of the subclavian artery and partially obscures the vessel (**ATLAS PLATE 488**). The muscle divides the artery into three segments, the 1st is medial to, the 2nd behind, and the 3rd lateral to the muscle.

A. **Subclavian Vein (Figure 29-3).** Identify the subclavian vein in the soft tissue deep to the clavicle. Find the transverse cervical and suprascapular veins that often flow across the omoclavicular (subclavian) triangle into the external jugular (**Figure 29-3**). Find the smaller anterior jugular vein (**ATLAS PLATE 482**).

B. **Subclavian Artery.** Dissect the lower portions of the trunks of the brachial plexus and find the subclavian artery that courses anterior to them. The third part of the artery (lateral to the anterior scalene muscle) (**ATLAS PLATES 481, 488, 491 #491.1**) courses downward and laterally over the

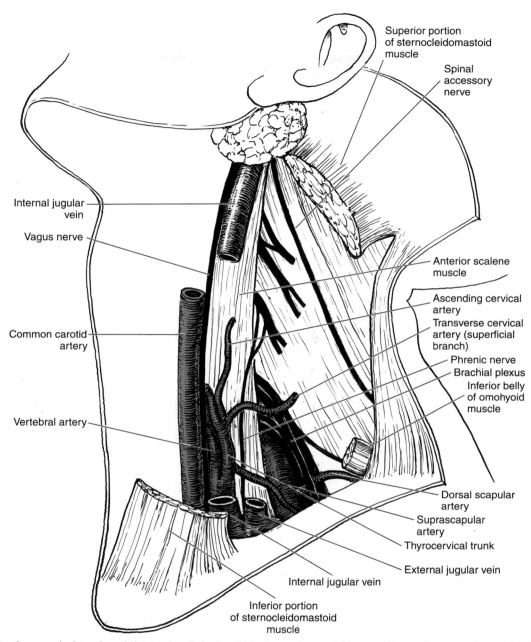

Figure 29-5. The thyrocervical trunk and the trunks of the brachial plexus. Sternocleidomastoid muscle removed; carotid sheath removed to expose common carotid artery, internal jugular vein, and vagus nerve.

cervical pleura to the 1st rib (**ATLAS PLATE 483**). Pull aside the inferior belly of the omohyoid muscle and look for the **suprascapular artery** and, more superiorly, the **transverse cervical artery** (**Figure 29-6A**). These vessels usually cross the external surface of the anterior scalene muscle superficial to the subclavian artery.

1. Suprascapular artery. Determine if the suprascapular artery arises as a branch from

the **thyrocervical trunk** (**Figure 29-6A**). This trunk is a short vessel that branches from the first part of the subclavian artery. If the suprascapular artery does not arise from the thyrocervical trunk, it will arise as a separate branch directly from the 3rd part of the subclavian artery (**Figure 29-6B**).

From either origin, follow the suprascapular artery laterally and downward (behind and

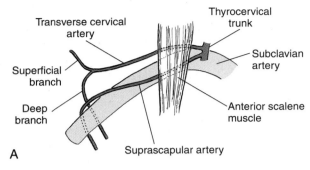

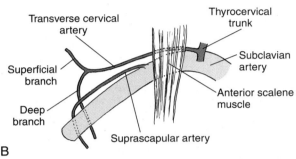

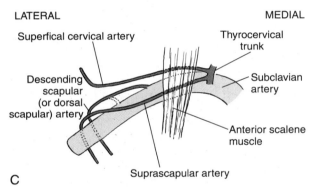

Figure 29-6. Vascular patterns related to the suprascapular and transverse cervical arteries.

A. The transverse cervical arises from the thyrocervical trunk and divides into a superficial and deep branch and the suprascapular artery also branches from the thyrocervical trunk.

B. The transverse cervical is similar to that seen in **A;** however, the suprascapular artery arises from the subclavian distal to the anterior scalene muscle.

C. The suprascapular artery arises from the thyrocervical trunk, but the superficial branch of the transverse cervical artery is replaced by the superficial cervical artery. The deep branch of the transverse cervical artery is replaced by the descending scapular (or dorsal scapular) artery.

parallel to the clavicle) toward the suprascapular notch (**ATLAS PLATE 481**). Note that the suprascapular artery is accompanied by the **suprascapular nerve.** At the suprascapular notch or "foramen" (formed by **the superior transverse scapular ligament),**

follow the artery **OVER** the ligament to enter the supraspinatus fossa, where the nerve courses **DEEP** to the ligament (**ATLAS PLATE 25**).

► Grant's 470, 731–733 Netter's 29, 410, 412 Rohen 168, 169, 180, 184

2. **Transverse Cervical Artery.** Look for the **transverse cervical artery.** In slightly more than 50% of cadavers, this vessel arises from the thyrocervical trunk and courses laterally in the posterior triangle superior to the suprascapular artery and superficial to the anterior scalene muscle, subclavian artery, and trunks of the brachial plexus. When present, the artery divides into a **superficial branch,** which **ascends** in the neck deep to the trapezius and a **deep branch,** which **descends** deep to the levator scapulae and rhomboid muscles.

If such a pattern for the transverse cervical artery is not found, look for the superficial cervical artery from the thyrocervical trunk. It crosses the posterior triangle and disappears beneath the levator scapulae and trapezius muscles **without** giving off a deep branch. In these cases, another vessel called the descending scapular or dorsal scapular artery will arise directly from the subclavian and descend along the medial margin of the scapula (**Figure 29-6C**).

Although other vascular patterns might exist, the most common are illustrated in the three diagrams of **Figure 29-6.**

VI. Cervical Part of the Brachial Plexus

The **brachial plexus** commences in the neck through the union of the anterior primary rami of the lower four cervical (C5, C6, C7, and C8) and first thoracic (T1) nerves. The 5th and 6th cervical roots join to form the **upper (superior) trunk,** the 7th forms the **middle trunk,** and the 8th cervical and 1st thoracic join to form the **lower (inferior) trunk.**

A. **Brachial Plexus (in the neck).** Separate the trunks of the brachial plexus by probing through the fascia surrounding the large nerve bundles. Trace the trunks medially to the cervical and thoracic roots and laterally where they split **into anterior and posterior divisions** beneath the middle portion of the clavicle (which has been removed).

B. **Suprascapular Nerve (C5, C6).** Locate the **suprascapular nerve** branching from the upper trunk of the brachial plexus near the junction of the anterior primary rami of C5 and C6 (**ATLAS PLATE 481**). Follow the nerve posteriorly and inferiorly in front of the middle scalene muscle toward the superior border of the scapula, where it is joined by the suprascapular vessels.

C. Phrenic Nerve (C3, C4, C5). Identify the phrenic nerve (**Figure 29-5**) coursing obliquely across the external surface of the anterior scalene muscle (**ATLAS PLATES 479–481**). It can be easily isolated by gently probing the superficial surface of the muscle.

D. Nerve to the Subclavius Muscle (C5, C6). This slender nerve may have been destroyed when the midportion of the clavicle was removed. If intact, it can be found to arise from the upper trunk of the brachial plexus, descend vertically across the third part of the subclavian artery, and end in the subclavius muscle.

E. Dorsal Scapular and Long Thoracic Nerves. Separate the anterior and middle scalene muscles and expose the uppermost parts of the brachial plexus at its roots. Identify the **dorsal scapular nerve** (C5) (also called the **nerve to the rhomboids**), which pierces through the middle scalene muscle and descends deep to the levator scapulae and trapezius to reach the vertebral border of the scapula (**ATLAS PLATE 339**).

Trace the **long thoracic nerve** (C5, C6, C7) superiorly to the neck from the lateral surface of the serratus anterior muscle in the axilla (**ATLAS PLATES 20, 21, 481**). Confirm that it arises from the C5, C6, and C7 before the trunks of the plexus are formed.

◀
Grant's 491, 732, 733, 762
Netter's 28, 183, 185, 412, 413
Rohen 182, 183, 185, 187

Clinical Relevance

Congenital torticollis. This condition is caused by a contraction of the neck muscles on one side causing the neck to twist and the head to slant to that side. During delivery of a difficult birth, excessive stretching of the sternocleidomastoid muscle can result in a hematoma followed by the formation of a fibrous scarring in the muscle. Subsequently, tilting of the head to the affected side occurs, with the face directed upward to the opposite side.

Spasmodic torticollis. This condition is caused by repeated chronic contractions of lateral neck muscles such as the sternocleidomastoid and trapezius.

Sustained tilting of the head eventually can become involuntary and may even have a psychological basis.

Lesions of the spinal accessory nerve. These lesions are not common, but they can occur from stab wounds or from inadvertent injury during surgery in the posterior triangle of the neck. Tumors of the cervical lymph nodes can invade the nerve, resulting in its diminished function. Patients present with a weakness in elevating and turning the head to the opposite side, which indicates sternocleidomastoid muscle weakness. Retraction of the scapula is lost and elevating the shoulder is affected. Injury to the accessory nerve usually results in a drooping of the ipsilateral shoulder.

Injury to the phrenic nerve. If the phrenic nerve is severed, a loss of contraction of the ipsilateral half of the diaphragm can result. At times the nerve is blocked temporarily for certain surgical procedures in the thorax, or it may be crushed in the repair of diaphragmatic hernias. Because the phrenic nerve is derived from motor fibers of C3, C4, and C5, irritation of the diaphragm may be referred to the supraclavicular region that is supplied by sensory fibers of the supraclavicular nerves, also from C3, C4, and C5.

Testing the accessory nerve. To test this nerve the patient should be asked to rotate the head (against resistance) to activate the sternocleidomastoid muscle of the opposite side. Additionally, to test the trapezius muscle, the patient is asked to retract both scapulae toward the midline of the back.

Posterior triangle sensory nerve block. Surgery in the posterior triangle requires local anesthesia of the cervical plexus. Sensory nerves (great auricular, lesser occipital, transverse cervical, and supraclavicular nerves) all emerge along the posterior border of the sternocleidomastoid muscle. This procedure also blocks the phrenic nerve. It is not used in persons with cardiac or pulmonary disease.

Suprascapular nerve injury. The suprascapular nerve might be injured when the middle third of the clavicle is fractured. This denervates the supraspinatus and infraspinatus muscles that are lateral rotators of the humerus at the shoulder joint. Because the medial rotators are intact, the upper limb is rotated medially with the hand projecting backward in a "waiter's tip" position. Denervation of the supraspinatus also results in the loss of the initiation of abduction of the humerus (i.e., the first 20° of abduction).

The interscalene triangle. The sides of this triangle are the anterior and posterior scalene muscles and, inferiorly, the first rib. This region is important because the subclavian artery and the trunks of the brachial plexus course through the triangle. Crossing over the triangle are the subclavian vein and the suprascapular and transverse cervical arteries. The phrenic nerve descends along the anterior surface of the anterior scalene muscle. This region is clinically significant when the structures within the triangle (subclavian artery and brachial plexus) are compressed by a cervical rib, by accretions on the first rib, or by contracture of the scalene muscles.

Pleura and lung injury at the root of the neck. The apex of the lung and the cervical extension of the pleura (Sibson's fascia) ascend superiorly into the root of the neck above the clavicle. Penetrating wounds superior to the medial half of the clavicle can puncture the lung and cause it to collapse. The location of the apex of the lung must be considered when puncture of the subclavian vein is made in this region.

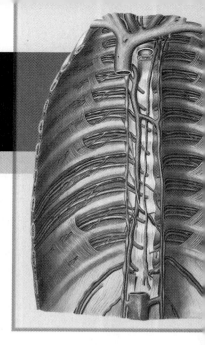

DISSECTION #30

Anterior Triangle of the Neck

OBJECTIVES

1 Examine the surface anatomy of the anterior neck; learn the boundaries of the triangles of the neck.

2 Dissect the superficial veins, platysma muscle, and cutaneous nerves on the anterior neck.

3 Dissect the infrahyoid muscles, the ansa cervicalis, and the muscular triangle.

4 Dissect the thyroid gland, its blood vessels, and the recurrent laryngeal nerves, and the parathyroid glands.

5 Dissect the carotid sheath and the carotid triangle, the superior laryngeal nerve, and branches of the external carotid artery.

6 Dissect the submandibular triangle and submandibular gland; locate the hypoglossal and glossopharyngeal nerves.

7 Dissect the subclavian artery and other structures at the root of the neck.

8 Dissect the submental triangle and the mylohyoid and hyoglossus muscles.

The anterior triangles of the neck are located anterior to the sternocleidomastoid muscles. Among other structures, they contain the thyroid and parathyroid glands; great arteries and veins of the neck and head; infrahyoid muscles and their innervation; four cranial nerves (IX, X, XI, XII); cervical extension of the sympathetic trunk; cervical plexus of nerves; superficial and deep cervical lymph nodes; suprahyoid muscles; submandibular gland; and submandibular and submental lymph nodes.

Within this region of the neck also are located the larynx and trachea and the pharynx and esophagus. These structures are studied in other dissections.

I. Surface Landmarks and Triangles of the Neck

The anterior region of the neck is located anterior to the cervical vertebrae and the cervical spinal cord. It is an exposed and vulnerable region and contains many vital structures. It is clinically useful to identify certain anterior neck landmarks and visualize their relationship to other cervical structures and to vertebral levels of the spinal column.

A. Surface Landmarks. The key surface landmarks on the anterior neck are the **sternocleidomastoid muscles** laterally and the **hyoid bone, trachea, and larynx** in the midline (**ATLAS PLATES 468, 470**). Commence your study of the surface anatomy of the neck by observing and palpating cervical structures on a lab partner.

1. Visualize the anterior border of the sternocleidomastoid muscle by turning the head to the opposite side and slightly depressing the chin.

2. Palpate the two tendons of insertion of the sternocleidomastoid muscle inferiorly; between them is the small **lesser supraclavicular fossa.** Deep to this fossa course the common carotid artery and internal jugular vein. Follow the anterior border of the sternocleidomastoid muscle superiorly to its attachment on the **mastoid process** behind the ear (**ATLAS PLATES 471 #471.1, 473**).

3. With your finger, outline the boundaries of the anterior triangle of the neck on one side:
   a. Anteriorly: the midline
   b. Posteriorly: anterior border of sternocleidomastoid muscle
   c. Superiorly: the inferior border of the mandible and a line continued upward to the mastoid process

4. Palpate the midline depression superior to the manubrium of the sternum, called the **jugular** (or **suprasternal notch**). Palpate the trachea deep to this site and realize that its subcutaneous location allows access to the respiratory airway (tracheotomy) for relief of respiratory distress (**ATLAS PLATE 471 #471.2**).

5. Palpate the **supraclavicular fossa (ATLAS PLATE 468)** above the clavicle lateral to the insertion of the sternocleidomastoid muscle. Feel the pulsations of the **subclavian artery** in this fossa by pressing this site with your fingers.

6. Elevate the chin and palpate the **laryngeal prominence** (Adam's apple) in the midline of the neck. This is the anterior edge of the large thyroid cartilage. Feel the pulsations of the **common carotid artery** lateral to this site where it divides into **internal** and **external carotid arteries (ATLAS PLATE 470)**.

7. Note that on the lateral surfaces of the thyroid cartilage are found the lobes of the **thyroid**

► Grant's 745, 755, 778, 779, 789
Netter's 12, 23–25, 27, 64
Rohen 63, 150, 157, 175

◄ Grant's 750–752, 754
Netter's 24, 25, 27
Rohen 175

► Grant's 749, 752, 757, 778, 779
Netter's 12, 70, 73, 198
Rohen 158, 161

◄ Rohen 157

◄ Grant's 724, 726, 738–741
Netter's 23, 24
Rohen 156, 157

◄ Grant's 2, 479, 725
Netter's 24, 174, 178
Rohen 157

◄ Rohen 157

► Grant's 738–740
Netter's 24, 25, 27
Rohen 175

◄ Grant's 748, 752, 779
Netter's 28, 30, 67, 73
Rohen 169, 184

◄ Grant's 749–757
Netter's 27, 65, 70–72
Rohen 175, 274, 277

gland. Lobes of the **normal gland** are difficult to palpate specifically from other neck structures (**ATLAS PLATE 483**).

8. Palpate the **hyoid bone** about 1 cm above the laryngeal prominence. It can be felt in the neck about 5 cm (2 inches) behind the tip of the chin. Swallow and feel the hyoid bone elevate.

9. Palpate the anterior surface of the **cricoid cartilage** inferior to the laryngeal prominence and 5 cm (2 inches) above the suprasternal notch. The isthmus of the thyroid gland that interconnects the lateral lobes overlies this cartilage.

10. Understand the relationship of anterior neck structures to the vertebral column.
    a. The hyoid bone lies at the level of the 3rd cervical vertebra.
    b. The thyroid cartilage: 4th and 5th cervical vertebrae.
    c. The cricoid cartilage: 6th cervical vertebra.
    d. Inferior to the cricoid cartilage there are 5 cm (2 inches) of trachea in the neck: at the levels of the 7th cervical and 1st thoracic vertebrae.
    e. 5 cm (2 inches) of trachea in the chest: 2nd and 3rd thoracic vertebrae.
    f. The trachea bifurcates: 4th thoracic vertebra.

B. Triangles of the Neck (ATLAS PLATE 471 #471.1, Figure 30-1). There are **anterior and posterior triangles** on both sides of the neck. The two anterior triangles lie medially, and each is flanked by a posterior triangle laterally. Dissection #29 describes the posterior triangle of the neck.

Each **anterior triangle** is further subdivided into three smaller triangles by the anterior and posterior bellies of the digastric muscle and the superior belly of the omohyoid muscle. These are the **submandibular triangle** superior to the hyoid bone and the **carotid** and **muscular triangles** inferiorly. Below the chin and superior to the hyoid bone is the unpaired midline **submental triangle.** The borders of these triangles are as follows:

1. **Anterior triangle**
   a. **Medial border:** Anterior midline of the neck
   b. **Posterior border:** Sternocleidomastoid muscle
   c. **Superior border:** Inferior margin of the mandible

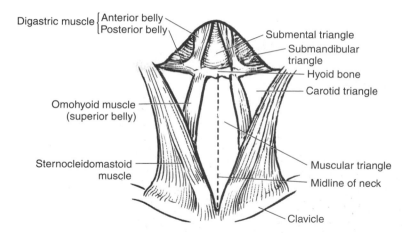

Digastric muscle { Anterior belly / Posterior belly

Submental triangle
Submandibular triangle
Hyoid bone
Carotid triangle

Omohyoid muscle (superior belly)

Sternocleidomastoid muscle

Muscular triangle
Midline of neck
Clavicle

Figure 30-1. Triangles of the neck, anterior view.

2. **Submandibular triangle,** containing the submandibular gland
   a. **Anterior border:** Anterior belly of digastric
   b. **Posterior border:** Posterior belly of digastric
   c. **Superior border:** Inferior margin of the mandible

3. **Carotid triangle,** containing the bifurcation of the common carotid artery, several branches of the external carotid artery, the roots of the ansa cervicalis, and other vessels and nerves
   a. **Superior border:** Posterior belly of the digastric and the stylohyoid muscle
   b. **Posterior border:** Anterior border of the sternocleidomastoid
   c. **Inferior border:** Superior belly of omohyoid

4. **Muscular triangle,** containing three infrahyoid muscles (sternohyoid, sternothyroid, and thyrohyoid), the anterior jugular vein, the thyroid gland, larynx, and trachea
   a. **Medial border:** Midline of the neck
   b. **Posterior superior border:** Superior belly of omohyoid
   c. **Posterior inferior border:** Anterior margin of sternocleidomastoid muscle

5. **Submental triangle,** a single midline triangle that contains important lymph nodes. Its floor is the mylohyoid muscle.
   a. **Inferior border:** the hyoid bone
   b. **Two lateral borders:** the anterior bellies of the right and left digastric muscles

II. Superficial Anterior Cervical Structures

The Jugular Veins (ATLAS PLATES 482, 483).

The **external, anterior,** and **internal jugular veins** of the neck return venous blood from the face,

◄
Grant's 738, 740, 741
Netter's 23, 30, 34, 49
Rohen 181–184

◄
Grant's 738, 739, 741
Netter's 24
Rohen 179, 182

◄
Grant's 739, 741
Netter's 23, 24
Rohen 173, 179

◄
Netter's 24, 25, 27
Rohen 174, 175

►
Grant's 722
Netter's 22
Rohen 58, 77

◄
Grant's 710, 730, 734
Netter's 27
Rohen 170, 174, 179

neck, and cranial cavity, including the brain. The **external jugular** drains the superficial and deep face and descends obliquely on the surface of the sternocleidomastoid muscle. It receives the anterior jugular, transverse scapular veins and it drains into the subclavian vein.

The **anterior jugular vein** commences near the hyoid bone and descends superficially over the strap muscles. The veins of both sides communicate across the midline and they drain into the external jugular or (at times) subclavian vein **(Figure 30-2)**.

The **internal jugular vein** commences just below the jugular foramen. It is directly continuous at the base of the skull with the intracranial sigmoid sinus. In its descent in the neck it is accompanied initially by the internal carotid artery and somewhat lower by the common carotid artery and vagus nerve. The artery, vein, and nerve are surrounded by connective tissue called the carotid sheath. Inferiorly, the internal jugular vein joins with the subclavian vein to form the brachiocephalic vein. The two brachiocephalic veins join to form the superior vena cava, which drains into the right atrium.

The skin (epidermis only) of the anterior and lateral neck should be removed, if not already done. If already completed, review your dissection of the posterior neck region (Dissection #29). In addition to exposing the cutaneous nerves of the **cervical plexus,** removal of the skin of the anterior neck will uncover the **platysma muscle** and the **anterior jugular veins (ATLAS PLATES 472, 482).**

Within the superficial fascia of the anterior neck identify fibers of the **platysma muscle.** Note that this superficial muscle crosses both the mandible and the clavicle. Identify the **cervical branch of the facial nerve** that descends to the platysma.

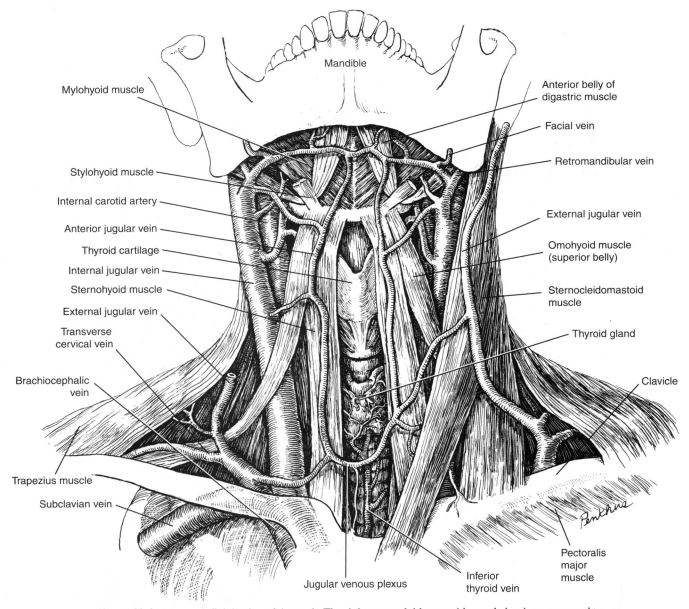

Figure 30-2. The superficial veins of the neck. The right sternocleidomastoid muscle has been removed to reveal the internal jugular vein. (From Clemente CD. Gray's Anatomy. 30th American Edition. Philadelphia: Lea and Febiger, 1985.)

Find the **anterior jugular veins** near the midline on both sides. Note that they descend from the submental region to the jugular notch (**ATLAS PLATE 482**). Quite variable and often unequal in size, these veins communicate across the midline.

Find the **external jugular vein** as it descends across the surface of the sternocleidomastoid muscle. Dissect the vein inferiorly where it pierces the deep fascia and joins the subclavian vein (**ATLAS PLATE 482**).

Detach the insertion of the sternocleidomastoid muscle and reflect the muscle laterally. Note that the **trans-**

◄
Grant's 710, 734
Netter's 27
Rohen 170, 174
►
Grant's 734, 739
Netter's 66
◄
Grant's 710, 730
Netter's 27
Rohen 179
►
Grant's 730
Netter's 20
Rohen 178, 179

verse cervical and **anterior jugular veins** usually flow into the external jugular deep to the sternocleidomastoid muscle (**ATLAS PLATE 483**). Review the following cutaneous branches of the cervical plexus dissected with the posterior triangle (**Figure 30-3**):

1. **Lesser occipital nerve** (C2). It ascends behind the ear along the posterior border of the sternocleidomastoid muscle.

2. **Great auricular nerve** (C2, C3). It ascends obliquely forward toward the ear and parotid region.

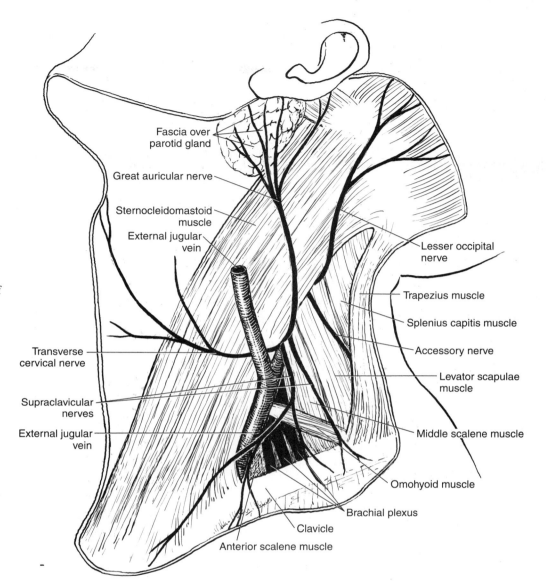

Figure 30-3. Cutaneous nerves of the cervical plexus.

The figure labels: Fascia over parotid gland, Great auricular nerve, Sternocleidomastoid muscle, External jugular vein, Transverse cervical nerve, Supraclavicular nerves, External jugular vein, Lesser occipital nerve, Trapezius muscle, Splenius capitis muscle, Accessory nerve, Levator scapulae muscle, Middle scalene muscle, Omohyoid muscle, Brachial plexus, Clavicle, Anterior scalene muscle

3. **Transverse cervical nerves** (C2, C3). These course around the posterior border of the sternocleidomastoid muscle to supply skin on the anterolateral neck.

4. **Supraclavicular nerves** (C3, C4). These descend posterior to the sternocleidomastoid muscle as medial, intermediate, and lateral branches. These supply the skin over the length of the clavicle.

III. Infrahyoid Strap Muscles; the Ansa Cervicalis

The infrahyoid strap muscles and their innervation (derived from the ansa cervicalis) are best dissected an-

► Grant's 738, 739, 741
Netter's 23–25, 27, 28
Rohen 183

teriorly in the muscular triangle (**ATLAS PLATES 470, 478–480**). Several strap muscles will be detached to expose the thyroid gland, its vessels, and the recurrent laryngeal nerves.

A. **Infrahyoid Muscles (Figure 30-4).** There are four infrahyoid muscles. Two are more superficial: the **sternohyoid** and the **omohyoid** (its superior belly in the muscular triangle and its inferior belly in the posterior triangle). Two others are located deep to these: the **sternothyroid** and the **thyrohyoid**.

1. The narrow **sternohyoid muscle** arises from the medial end of the clavicle and the posterior surface of the manubrium. It passes upward to be inserted along the inferior border of the hyoid bone. It is adjacent medially to the superior belly of the omohyoid muscle (**ATLAS PLATES 470, 478**).

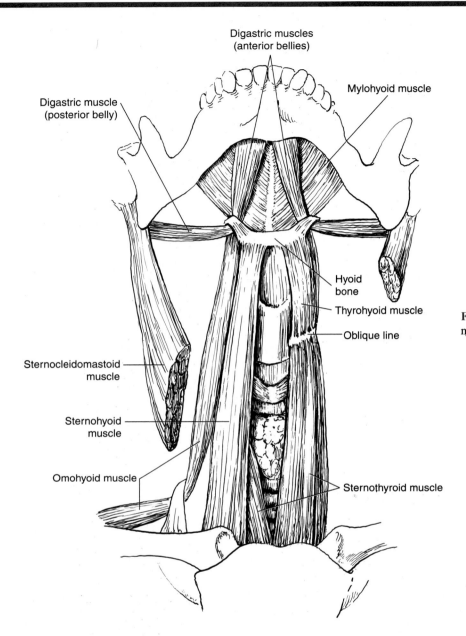

Digastric muscles
(anterior bellies)

Digastric muscle
(posterior belly)

Mylohyoid muscle

Hyoid
bone

Thyrohyoid muscle

Oblique line

Sternocleidomastoid
muscle

Sternohyoid
muscle

Omohyoid muscle

Sternothyroid muscle

Figure 30-4. Strap muscles and the digastric and mylohyoid muscles, anterior view.

2. The **omohyoid muscle** consists of two bellies joined by a tendon between them. The **superior belly** attaches above to the hyoid bone just lateral to the sternohyoid muscle. The **inferior belly** is attached along the superior border of the scapula just medial to the scapular notch. The tendon between the two bellies and its fascial attachment are located anterior to the internal jugular vein (**ATLAS PLATE 470**).

3. The **sternothyroid muscle** is shorter than the sternohyoid and lies deep to it. Attached to the posterior surface of the manubrium, it extends superiorly to the lamina of the thyroid cartilage (**ATLAS PLATE 470**).

▶
Grant's 739, 741,
760
Netter's 25, 27
Rohen 157, 182

4. The **thyrohyoid muscle** is a small quadrilateral muscle between the thyroid cartilage to the greater horn of the hyoid bone. It lies deep to the upper part of the sternohyoid and might appear to be an upward extension of the sternothyroid muscle (**ATLAS PLATE 586**).

The omohyoid and sternohyoid depress the hyoid bone or help stabilize it. The sternothyroid depresses the larynx, while the thyrohyoid either elevates the larynx or depresses the hyoid bone during different stages of swallowing.

Remove the fascia covering the infrahyoid muscles, but be careful not to sever the small nerves that supply them. At the level of the laryngeal prominence (Adam's apple), identify the most medial of the strap muscles, the **sternohyoid.** Pass the handle of your scalpel between it and the underlying cartilage and sternothyroid muscle. Separate the two muscles down to the sternum. Detach the sternohyoid inferiorly and reflect it upward to the hyoid bone. This exposes the **sternothyroid** and, more superiorly, the **thyrohyoid.** Lateral to the severed sternohyoid identify the **superior belly of the omohyoid.**

Turn your attention to the **ansa cervicalis** and the innervation of the infrahyoid muscles.

B. Ansa Cervicalis (Figure 30-5). The ansa cervicalis is a nerve formation composed of fibers from the first three cervical nerves (C1, C2, C3). In this formation a branch of the anterior primary ramus of C1 courses forward high in the posterior neck and **enters the sheath of the hypoglossal nerve trunk.** Many of these C1 fibers leave the hypoglossal nerve to form the **superior root of the ansa cervicalis.** This descends deep to the sternocleidomastoid muscle, anterior to the common carotid artery (**ATLAS PLATE 480**). Other fascicles of C1 fibers leave the hypoglossal nerve to supply the thyrohyoid and geniohyoid muscles.

The **inferior root of the ansa cervicalis** is a delicate nerve formed by the junction of branches from the 2nd and 3rd cervical nerves. It descends lateral to the internal jugular vein, then crosses anterior to the vein and

◄
Grant's 748–750, 752
Netter's 22–25, 27
Rohen 175, 182, 183

►
Grant's 739
Netter's 28
Rohen 182, 184

◄
Grant's 738, 739, 741
Netter's 27, 28, 30
Rohen 181–183, 184

►
Grant's 749–757
Netter's 27, 66, 70–72
Rohen 157, 162, 175, 244, 266, 271

►
Grant's 744, 751, 757
Netter's 29, 30, 65, 70–72
Rohen 84, 162, 169, 185

joins the superior root to form the loop of the ansa cervicalis (**ATLAS PLATE 479**). All of the strap muscles are innervated from the ansa and its roots except the thyrohyoid, which gets fibers only from C1.

Reflect the cut lower end of the sternocleidomastoid muscle. To find the **inferior root** of the ansa cervicalis, probe the fascia of the carotid sheath lateral to the internal jugular vein at the level of the bifurcation of the common carotid artery. Follow the root inferiorly and then anterior to the vein, where it joins the **superior root** to form the loop of the ansa cervicalis adjacent to the common carotid artery (**ATLAS PLATE 479**). Look for delicate nerve branches to individual strap muscles.

The nerve to the superior belly of the omohyoid usually branches from the superior root as it descends toward the ansa. The sternohyoid, sternothyroid, and inferior belly of the omohyoid often get their branches directly from the loop formation. The delicate C1 filament to the thyrohyoid muscle enters the muscle along its lateral border.

IV. Thyroid Gland; Superior and Inferior Thyroid Arteries; Recurrent Laryngeal Nerves; Parathyroid Glands

A. Thyroid Gland. The highly vascular thyroid gland, located in the lower anterior neck, consists of conical right and left lobes (**ATLAS PLATE 483**). Situated anterior to and at the sides of the trachea, the lobes extend from the 5th or 6th tracheal ring inferiorly to the oblique line on the thyroid cartilage superiorly. They are interconnected by a narrow transverse isthmus overlying the upper three tracheal rings. In 30% of cadavers a **pyramidal process** extends upward from the isthmus and may reach the hyoid bone. This process and other nodules of thyroid tissue may persist as remnants of the **thyroglossal duct,** which descends from the tongue to the neck during development. The hormones secreted by the thyroid gland stimulate and increase the rate of cellular metabolism (thyroxin) and lower the blood calcium level (calcitonin).

The thyroid gland is supplied (a) from above by the **superior thyroid artery** (Figure 30-6), off the external carotid, and (b) from below by the **inferior thyroid artery,** off the thyrocervical trunk (**ATLAS PLATES 592, 595**). Importantly, as the branches of the inferior thyroid artery enter the thyroid gland, they are crossed by the recurrent laryngeal nerve, which is ascending to supply muscles in the larynx. The recurrent laryngeal nerve may cross anterior to, posterior to, or between the branches of the inferior thyroid artery (**ATLAS PLATE 595**).

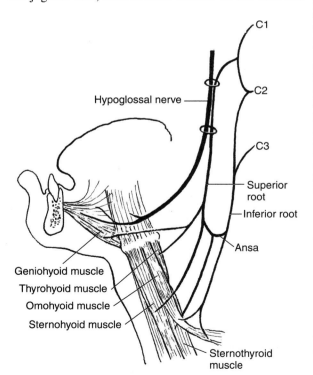

C1

C2

C3

Hypoglossal nerve

Superior root

Inferior root

Ansa

Geniohyoid muscle
Thyrohyoid muscle
Omohyoid muscle
Sternohyoid muscle

Sternothyroid muscle

Figure 30-5. Roots and branches of the ansa cervicalis.

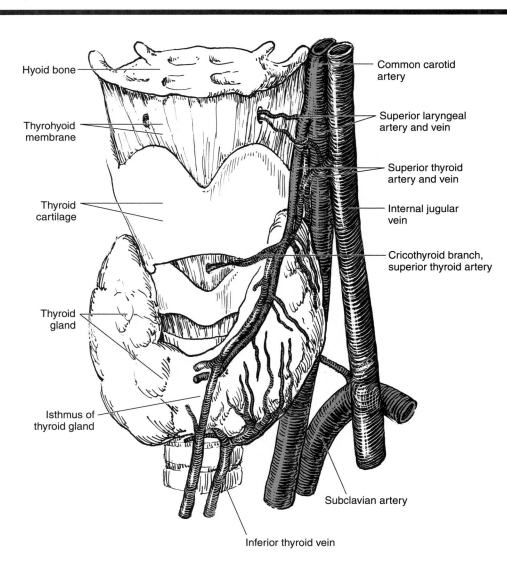

Figure 30-6. Thyroid gland and superior thyroid vessels, anterior view.

Sever the insertions of both sternothyroid muscles from the thyroid cartilage. Detach the superior bellies of both omohyoid muscles from the hyoid bone and reflect all four muscles downward to expose the thyroid gland. On both sides find the **superior thyroid artery** that descends from the external carotid to the **apex of the lateral lobe** of the gland (**ATLAS PLATE 483**).

Identify the isthmus that connects the two lobes across the trachea and sever it in the midline. On each side elevate the cut isthmus and separate the thyroid lobe laterally from the trachea.

Pull the thyroid lobe laterally and probe deeply along the medial border of the gland (**Figure 30-7**). Find the **recurrent laryngeal nerve** ascending in the groove between the trachea and esophagus. Dissect the lower posterior surfaces of the lateral lobes and find the branches of the **inferior thyroid arteries.** They will cross the recurrent nerves upon entering the gland (**ATLAS PLATE 595**).

◄
Grant's 751, 752, 757
Netter's 65, 70–72
Rohen 169, 185

►
Grant's 769, 780
Netter's 71, 72

◄
Grant's 751, 756, 757, 768
Netter's 29, 71, 72
Rohen 162, 168, 169

These nerves are in a vulnerable position when a thyroidectomy is performed. Because all but one pair of muscles of the larynx are supplied by the recurrent laryngeal nerves, injury to them during ligation of the inferior thyroid vessels will result in serious laryngeal dysfunction.

B. Parathyroid Glands. The parathyroid glands are small oval structures that usually are located within the pretracheal fascia posterior to the lateral lobes of the thyroid gland. Although they vary in number and size (**ATLAS PLATE 484 #484.2**), there are usually four parathyroid glands, two on each side, and they measure about 6 mm in length, 3 mm in width and 2 mm in thickness.

The location of the superior parathyroid glands behind the upper half of the lateral lobes is more constant than that of the inferior glands (**Figure 30-7**). The latter may be within the pretracheal fascia near the lower pole of the gland, or they may be within the capsule of the gland, or embedded within thyroid tissue. Their blood

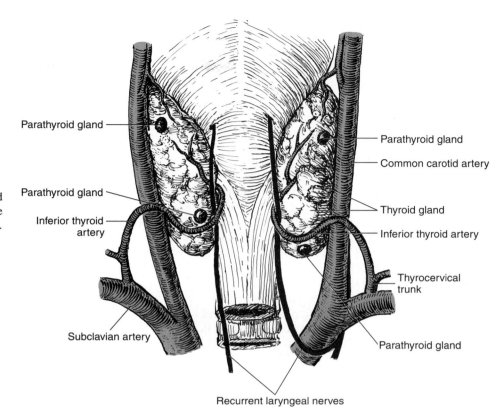

Figure 30-7. Thyroid and parathyroid glands, the inferior thyroid arteries, and the recurrent laryngeal nerve (posterior view).

Parathyroid gland

Parathyroid gland

Inferior thyroid artery

Subclavian artery

Parathyroid gland

Common carotid artery

Thyroid gland

Inferior thyroid artery

Thyrocervical trunk

Parathyroid gland

Recurrent laryngeal nerves

supply comes from the same vessels that supply the thyroid gland, and they produce a hormone important for the metabolism of calcium and phosphorus.

> Positive identification of the parathyroid glands in the gross anatomy laboratory is difficult because of their small size and variability in location. Their yellowish-brown color also makes it hard to distinguish them from surrounding tissue. You may look for the superior parathyroid glands posterior to the lateral lobes of the thyroid gland within the pretracheal fascia. They are most often found behind the upper half of the lateral lobes and may be close to their upper poles.

V. Structures Within or Adjacent to the Carotid Triangle

The carotid triangle is bounded by the **posterior belly of the digastric,** the **superior belly of the omohyoid,** and the **anterior border of the sternocleidomastoid muscle** (Figure 30-1). It is a small region in the upper neck where many important structures are found (**ATLAS PLATES 478–480**). Among these are the following:

Internal jugular vein and several tributaries

Trunks of the **vagus (X), accessory (XI),** and **hypoglossal (XII) nerves**

The **superior laryngeal branch of the vagus** (which

◄
Grant's 739, 741, 744, 745
Netter's 23, 24, 27, 28
Rohen 156, 157, 171, 173

►
Grant's 738, 739, 741
Netter's 27, 66
Rohen 170–173

divides into internal and external laryngeal branches) and the **pharyngeal branch of the vagus**

The roots of the **ansa cervicalis** (already dissected)

Bifurcation of the common carotid artery into **internal and external carotid branches**

The **carotid sinus nerve**

Superior thyroid, lingual, and **ascending pharyngeal** branches of the external carotid artery

Facial, occipital, and **posterior auricular** branches of the external carotid artery, which arise slightly higher but will also be considered at this time

A. **Internal Jugular Vein (ATLAS PLATES 482, 483).** The internal jugular vein forms at the base of the skull and descends in the neck adjacent to the common carotid artery. It is crossed by the posterior belly of the digastric muscle and lies deep to the lower part of the sternocleidomastoid muscle. Coursing superficial and lateral to the carotid arteries, it receives the **facial, lingual,** and **superior thyroid veins** and, slightly lower, the **middle thyroid vein.**

> Retract the sternocleidomastoid muscle and probe the carotid sheath at the level of the laryngeal prominence. Separate the **internal jugular vein** from the **common carotid artery** and identify its **facial, lingual,** and **superior thyroid** venous tributaries (**ATLAS PLATE 483**).

B. Vagus (X), Accessory (XI), and Hypoglossal (XII) Nerves (ATLAS PLATES 479–481). The vagus and accessory nerves emerge from the skull through the jugular foramen, as does the glossopharyngeal nerve. At this foramen the **sigmoid sinus** in the cranial cavity becomes the internal jugular vein in the neck. The hypoglossal nerve enters the neck through the hypoglossal canal of the occipital bone.

In the neck the **vagus nerve** courses within the carotid sheath posterior to the internal jugular vein and common carotid artery. The **accessory nerve** descends in the neck initially deep to the posterior belly of the digastric muscle. At the level of the hyoid bone it pierces the deep surface of the sternocleidomastoid muscle, supplies it, and then crosses the posterior triangle of the neck to supply the trapezius muscle (**ATLAS PLATES 479–481**).

The **hypoglossal nerve** is the great motor nerve of the tongue. High in the carotid triangle it lies between the internal jugular vein and the internal carotid artery (**ATLAS PLATES 479, 480**). Near the lower border of the posterior belly of the digastric muscle, the nerve turns 90° forward and courses anteriorly and superiorly between the hyoglossus and mylohyoid muscles to enter the oral cavity (**ATLAS PLATE 492 #492.1**).

1. To find the trunk of the **vagus nerve**, separate the common carotid artery and internal jugular vein at the level of the laryngeal prominence. Probe deeply, using vertical strokes, between the vein and artery, and separate the trunk of the vagus nerve from the connective tissue of the carotid sheath.

2. Locate the **accessory nerve** by lifting and separating the sternocleidomastoid muscle from the underlying fascia nearly to its attachment on the mastoid process. Stroke the upper deep surface of the muscle with a probe and isolate branches of the nerve. Note that it descends to the trapezius muscle across the posterior triangle.

3. Find the **hypoglossal nerve** by using the posterior belly of the digastric muscle as a landmark (**ATLAS PLATES 479, 480**). Probe deeply along the lower border of the digastric muscle, slightly above the hyoid bone. Isolate the nerve trunk as it turns anteriorly and crosses the external carotid artery (and its lingual branch) to the border of the mylohyoid muscle. Follow the nerve deep to the mylohyoid and superficial to the hyoglossus muscle. Note that the nerve enters the oral cavity between these two muscles (**ATLAS PLATE 492 #492.1**).

▶
Grant's 783, 818, 819
Netter's 71, 72, 76, 124
Rohen 84, 151, 162

◀
Grant's 762, 767–769
Netter's 28, 30, 65, 67
Rohen 73, 75, 179, 181

▶
Grant's 741, 766, 767, 783–785
Netter's 67, 70, 76
Rohen 162

◀
Grant's 739, 753, 766–769
Netter's 28, 30, 65, 67
Rohen 75, 81, 84, 151, 183

◀
Grant's 751, 752, 754, 756, 786
Netter's 28, 65, 67
Rohen 75, 162 169, 181, 183, 272

◀
Grant's 730–732, 739, 820
Netter's 28, 30, 121, 123
Rohen 163–165, 179, 184, 235

▶
Grant's 769, 818, 819
Netter's 67, 119, 120, 124
Rohen 165

◀
Grant's 739, 743, 744
Netter's 28, 29, 55, 65–67, 122
Rohen 75, 84, 152, 162, 173

C. Superior Laryngeal and Pharyngeal Branches of the Vagus Nerve

1. The **superior laryngeal branch of the vagus nerve** courses inferiorly and anteriorly from the vagal nerve trunk. High in the neck it descends posterior and then medial (or deep) to the internal and external carotid arteries toward the upper part of the larynx. Deep to the arteries it divides into a larger **internal laryngeal** branch and a delicate **external laryngeal** branch.

The **internal branch** pierces the thyrohyoid membrane as do the superior laryngeal vessels (**ATLAS PLATES 594, 595**). It is the sensory nerve to the internal surface of the upper half of the larynx and is the important sensory nerve for the cough reflex.

The **external branch** descends deep to the sternothyroid muscle and is the motor nerve to the cricothyroid muscle of the larynx (**ATLAS PLATE 589**).

Identify the **internal branch** and trace it back to the superior laryngeal nerve behind the carotid arteries. To do this, probe the surface of the thyrohyoid membrane near the lateral border of the thyrohyoid muscle. Isolate the internal branch piercing the membrane slightly above the superior laryngeal vessels (**ATLAS PLATES 594, 595**). Carefully dissect the nerve laterally until you reach the point where it and the external branch come off the superior laryngeal nerve.

Trace the delicate **external branch** inferiorly to the cricothyroid muscle. It accompanies the superior thyroid artery posterior to the sternothyroid muscle and lateral to the inferior constrictor muscle (**ATLAS PLATE 588**). Note that it gives off a small twig to the superior constrictor before it enters the cricothyroid muscle.

2. The **pharyngeal branch of the vagus** arises slightly superior from the vagal trunk than the superior laryngeal nerve. It is the **principal motor nerve to the pharynx** (**ATLAS PLATE 588**). The motor fibers of the pharyngeal branch are derived from the cranial root of the accessory nerve (XI), which emerge from the medulla oblongata and become part of the vagus nerve (X). In the neck the pharyngeal branch joins with sensory fibers from the glossopharyngeal nerve (IX) and with sympathetic fibers to form the **pharyngeal plexus**. From this plexus motor fibers supply the three pharyngeal constrictor muscles and all of the muscles of the soft palate except the tensor palati. Think of their innervation as XI via X.

Probe the region **between the external and internal carotid arteries** high in the neck behind the posterior belly of the digastric muscle to find the pharyngeal branch of the vagus. The nerve curves parallel but inferior to the glossopharyngeal nerve and descends to the posterior surface of the middle constrictor muscle, where it helps form the **pharyngeal plexus (ATLAS PLATE 588).** If you cannot identify this nerve now, you will have another opportunity when the posterior pharynx is dissected.

D. Bifurcation of the Common Carotid Artery, the Carotid Sinus Nerve

The **common carotid artery** arises from the brachiocephalic artery on the right side and from the arch of the aorta on the left side (**ATLAS PLATES 152, 155**). Both vessels ascend within the anterior triangle of that side, each accompanied by the internal jugular vein and vagus nerve within the carotid sheath. Normally, there are no branches off the common carotid artery before it bifurcates into the **internal** and **external carotid arteries** at the upper border of the thyroid cartilage. Near this division two visceral receptor sites, the **carotid sinus** and the **carotid body,** are located within the vessels.

The **carotid sinus** is a baroreceptor located in the wall of the most proximal part of the internal carotid artery. It appears as a slight dilatation in the vessel. The **carotid body** is a chemoreceptor site found in the posterior wall of the common carotid artery at its point of bifurcation. Its chemosensitive cells respond to changes in O_2 and CO_2 levels in the blood, and this results in changes in breathing patterns.

The carotid sinus and carotid body are innervated by the **carotid sinus nerve.** It contains visceral afferent fibers of the glossopharyngeal nerve and has communicating branches from the vagus nerve and superior cervical ganglion.

Follow the common carotid artery to its point of bifurcation. Separate the internal and external carotid arteries superiorly to the ramus of the mandible. Look for the small carotid sinus plexus at the bifurcation. Twist the vessels and probe gently between them to identify the delicate **carotid sinus nerve** (often double). It ascends on the lower anterior surface of the internal carotid artery and then courses posteriorly to join the glossopharyngeal and vagus nerves.

E. Branches of the External Carotid Artery (Figure 30-8).
The external carotid artery at the bifurcation lies anterior to the internal carotid, but as it ascends, it gradually courses lateral to the internal carotid. At this point in the dissection six branches of the external carotid should be identified. These are the **superior thyroid, ascending pharyngeal, lingual, facial, occipital,** and **posterior auricular arteries (ATLAS PLATE 506).**

▶
Grant's 736, 741, 744, 750, 751
Netter's 30, 65, 70–72, 130
Rohen 84, 168, 169, 175, 184

◀
Grant's 736, 739, 768, 769
Netter's 30, 65, 67, 124
Rohen 169, 179, 184

▶
Grant's 653, 769
Netter's 30, 36, 65, 130
Rohen 146, 153

▶
Grant's 671, 741, 745, 746
Netter's 30, 65, 130
Rohen 152, 153, 168

◀
Grant's 816–819
Netter's 124
Rohen 164

▶
Grant's 319, 652, 736, 742
Netter's 19, 30, 32, 65
Rohen 80, 81, 168–170, 183

◀
Grant's 816–819
Netter's 119, 124, 125
Rohen 63, 164

▶
Grant's 307, 316, 736, 741
Netter's 19, 30, 65, 66
Rohen 76, 168, 235–237

◀
Grant's 736, 739, 741
Netter's 30, 65, 124
Rohen 168–170, 184

1. Identify the **superior thyroid artery** arising from the anterior aspect of the external carotid near the bifurcation. Follow its descent along the lateral border of the thyrohyoid muscle to the superior pole of the thyroid gland (**ATLAS PLATE 483**). Identify its **superior laryngeal branch** piercing the thyrohyoid membrane with the internal laryngeal nerve.

2. Find the slender **ascending pharyngeal artery** by probing just above the bifurcation anterior and medial to the internal carotid artery along the side of the pharynx. It ascends vertically from its origin on the **posterior surface** of the external carotid. Its principal branches supply the pharynx, but small twigs also go to the middle ear and dura mater (**ATLAS PLATE 589**).

3. Identify the **lingual artery,** arising from the external carotid at the level of the greater horn of the hyoid bone. It usually is the second branch from the anterior aspect of the external carotid (**ATLAS PLATES 492 #492.1, 510, 513**). Its origin may be difficult to find because (a) it may lie deep to the posterior belly of the digastric or (b) in about 20% of cases the lingual and facial arteries arise as a common stem. Follow the lingual artery as it loops superiorly and then passes **anteriorly deep to the hyoglossus muscle to enter the oral cavity.**

4. Find the **facial artery** arising from the external carotid about 1 cm superior to the lingual artery or from a common facial–lingual trunk (**ATLAS PLATES 480, 493 #493.1, 506**). Probe above the greater horn of the hyoid bone and follow the artery deep to the posterior belly of the digastric muscle and then anteriorly along the border of the submandibular gland. From this site the facial artery courses over the mandible onto the face.

5. Identify the **occipital artery** arising posteriorly from the external carotid opposite or slightly superior to the facial artery (**ATLAS PLATE 506**). Follow it posteriorly adjacent to the posterior belly of the digastric muscle. Lift the sternocleidomastoid muscle, identify the underlying splenius muscle, and realize that the occipital artery courses to the back of the scalp deep to the splenius.

OPTIONAL DISSECTION

6. If time permits, find the smaller **posterior auricular artery** arising posteriorly from the

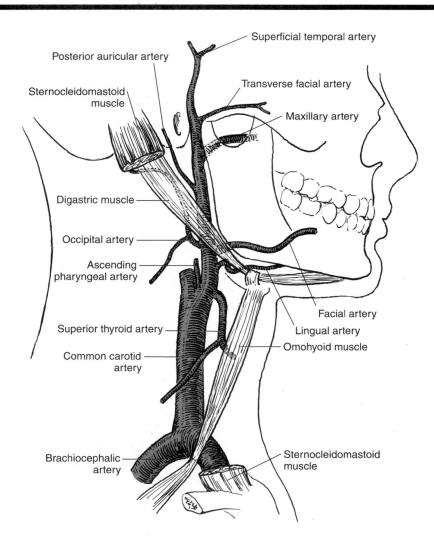

Figure 30-8. External carotid artery and its branches.

external carotid just above the posterior belly of the digastric (**ATLAS PLATES 506, 510**). Follow it behind the external ear between the parotid gland and the styloid process of the temporal bone. Note that its branches include the **stylomastoid artery,** which leaves the stylomastoid foramen with the facial nerve, an **auricular branch** to the skin of the ear, and an **occipital branch** to the scalp behind the ear (**ATLAS PLATE 506**).

VI. Suprahyoid Region (ATLAS PLATES 492, 493, 570)

The **suprahyoid region** lies above the hyoid bone and below the mandible. Within this region on both sides are located the submandibular triangles laterally, and between them, a single submental triangle (**Figure 30-1**).

Each **submandibular triangle,** bounded by the anterior and posterior bellies of the digastric muscle and the

▶
Grant's 724, 732, 738, 743
Netter's 23, 24, 28, 30, 49, 55
Rohen 81, 84, 151, 152, 157, 166

◀
Grant's 600, 652, 704, 706
Netter's 19, 30, 65, 130
Rohen 78, 80

▶
Grant's 724, 747
Netter's 19, 30, 32, 65
Rohen 156, 157

inferior border of the mandible, contains the **submandibular gland.** Through each triangle course the facial and lingual vessels and the hypoglossal nerve. Additionally, located here are a number of lymph nodes that drain the parotid and submandibular glands as well as the scalp posterior to the external ear (**Figure 30-9**). Along with the **digastric muscle,** the **stylohyoid** and, more deeply, the **hyoglossus muscles** are found within the submandibular triangle. The latter muscle extends from the greater horn of the hyoid bone to the base of the tongue (**ATLAS PLATE 492 #492.1**).

The **submental triangle** is in the midline and is bordered on both lateral sides by the anterior bellies of the two digastric muscles and inferiorly by the hyoid bone. The roof of this triangle is formed by the **mylohyoid muscles,** which join as a raphe in the midline and serve as the floor of the oral cavity (**ATLAS PLATE 571 #571.1**).

The **submental lymph nodes** that drain the central part of the lower lip, the tip of the tongue, and the floor of the mouth are located in the superficial fascia of this triangle (**Figure 30-9**).

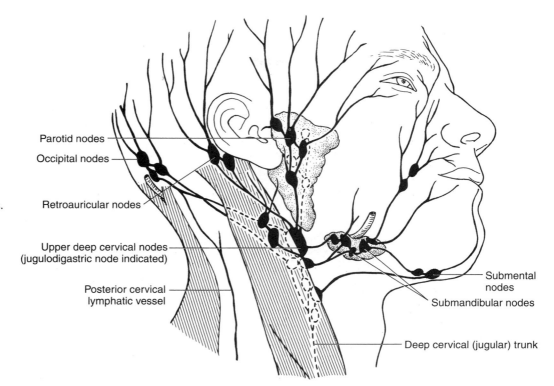

Figure 30-9. Lymph nodes of the face and upper neck regions.

Parotid nodes

Occipital nodes

Retroauricular nodes

Upper deep cervical nodes (jugulodigastric node indicated)

Posterior cervical lymphatic vessel

Submental nodes

Submandibular nodes

Deep cervical (jugular) trunk

Expose the anterior belly of the digastric muscle medially and the submandibular gland and posterior belly of the digastric muscle laterally. Mobilize the superficial part of the gland by loosening the fascia around it and identify the **facial vein** and **cervical branch of the facial nerve,** which cross superficial to the gland. Dissect the **facial artery** along the deep surface of the gland, where it may even be embedded in the gland. Follow the artery across the lower border of the mandible (**ATLAS PLATE 493 #493.1**).

Pull the submandibular gland laterally and identify the intermediate tendon between the two bellies of the digastric muscle. Note the fascial sling that attaches the tendon to the hyoid bone (**ATLAS PLATE 492 #492.1**).

Identify the **stylohyoid muscle** descending along the superior surface of the posterior belly of the digastric muscle. At its insertion on the hyoid bone, note that it splits to surround the intermediate tendon of the digastric muscle. Branches of the facial nerve supply both the stylohyoid and posterior digastric muscles.

Define the **hyoglossus muscle,** which attaches along the greater horn of the hyoid bone and ascends to the tongue. Identify again the hypoglossal nerve and follow it forward along the superficial surface of the hyoglossus muscle until it disappears between the hyoglossus and mylohyoid muscles. The nerve

◄
Grant's 738, 741
Netter's 65
Rohen 183

►
Grant's 739, 743
Netter's 23–25, 27, 28, 49, 64
Rohen 60, 151, 156, 157, 175

►
Grant's 658, 659, 671
Netter's 36, 42, 56, 65, 67
Rohen 63, 72, 73, 152, 169, 183

◄
Grant's 739, 740, 742, 766, 767
Netter's 23–25, 30, 42, 49, 55
Rohen 57, 60, 63, 81, 151, 166

◄
Grant's 741, 744, 821
Netter's 25, 30, 49, 55
Rohen 61, 166, 167

courses between these two muscles to enter the oral cavity and supply the tongue muscles.

Clean the two **anterior bellies of the digastric muscle** and define the **submental triangle.** Remove the fascia covering the floor of the triangle to expose the two **mylohyoid muscles** and the raphe formed by their junction in the midline (**ATLAS PLATE 571**). You now see the floor of the oral cavity from below.

Find the **submental artery,** a branch of the facial artery. It courses anteriorly after the facial artery curves around the base of the mandible (**ATLAS PLATE 493 #493.2**). Mobilize the submandibular gland away from the mandible and find the delicate **mylohyoid nerve** as it enters the suprahyoid region from the oral cavity. To locate this nerve, probe along the lower border of the body of the mandible near its middle. Note that the nerve joins the submental artery and courses anteriorly to supply the mylohyoid muscle and the anterior belly of the digastric.

VII. Deep Structures at the Root of the Neck (Figure 30-10)

Several structures should be dissected in the deep lower neck region lateral to the trachea and esophagus. Referred to as the root of the neck, the structures of importance lie deep to the inferior part of the sternocleido-

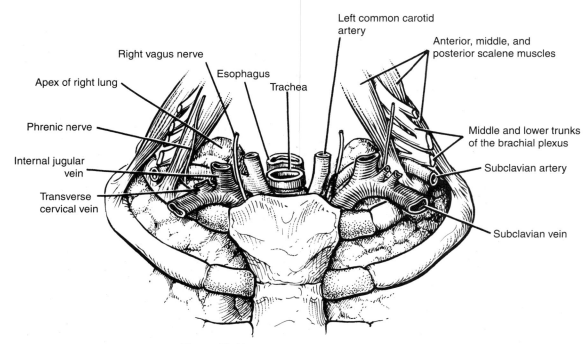

Right vagus nerve

Apex of right lung

Phrenic nerve

Internal jugular vein

Transverse cervical vein

Esophagus

Trachea

Left common carotid artery

Anterior, middle, and posterior scalene muscles

Middle and lower trunks of the brachial plexus

Subclavian artery

Subclavian vein

Figure 30-10. Structures at the root of the neck.

mastoid muscle. The vessels in the region include the **common carotid artery,** the **subclavian artery and its branches,** the **junction of the internal jugular vein with the subclavian vein,** and the **thoracic duct** near this junction (**ATLAS PLATE 483**). The root of the neck also contains the **trachea,** upper **esophagus,** and the **vagus nerves** and their **recurrent laryngeal branches.** More deeply is the cervical extension of the **sympathetic trunk** and its **stellate ganglion** (**ATLAS PLATES 18 #18.1, 165**).

Dissect on the left side. Detach the subclavius muscle from the clavicle, saw through the middle of the clavicle, and disarticulate the sternoclavicular joint. Remove the medial half of the clavicle. Open the field further by cutting the common carotid artery and internal jugular vein about 2 cm above the clavicle and reflect these vessels upward.

Remove the left lobe of the thyroid gland. Identify the left subclavian vein lying superficial to the anterior scalene muscle and the left subclavian artery that courses deep to this muscle (**ATLAS PLATES 481, 488**). Remove the subclavius muscle and seek the branches of the subclavian artery.

Identify first the **internal thoracic artery** descending from the subclavian posterior to the first rib. Find the **thyrocervical trunk** ascending from the subclavian opposite the origin of the internal thoracic (**ATLAS PLATE 491, #491.1**). Expose the thyrocervical trunk completely and identify its **inferior**

◄
Grant's 737, 756–758, 761, 762
Netter's 24, 25, 28–30, 65, 70
Rohen 168–172, 184, 185, 187

►
Grant's 736, 737
Netter's 29, 130
Rohen 168

►
Grant's 65–67, 751, 756, 761
Netter's 29, 67, 124, 190, 194, 260
Rohen 162, 269, 272, 275, 277

◄
Grant's 470, 492, 736, 737
Netter's 29, 67, 70, 71, 130, 131
Rohen 162, 168, 169, 277, 396

thyroid, suprascapular, and **transverse cervical** branches. Medial to the origin of the thyrocervical trunk find the **vertebral artery** (**ATLAS PLATES 490, 491**). Follow this branch superiorly and medially between the anterior scalene and longus colli muscles to the transverse process of the C6 vertebra.

If time permits, identify the **costocervical trunk,** which arises from the posterior surface of the subclavian and quickly divides into the superior intercostal and deep cervical branches.

Locate again the **recurrent laryngeal nerve** in the groove between the esophagus and the trachea, just above the sternum (**ATLAS PLATES 162, 481**), and the **phrenic nerve** descending along the anterior surface of the anterior scalene muscle.

Clinical Relevance

Horner's syndrome. This syndrome usually the results from a lesion of the sympathetic trunk in the neck, although it can also develop if an injury occurs in the spinal cord or in the T1 to T4 nerve roots that course to the sympathetic trunks. The symptoms include: a) **constriction of the pupil** (since the dilator is denervated); b) **ptosis** (drooping of the eyelid, since the tarsus muscle is denervated); c) **ipsilateral anhidrosis** (lack of sweating) on the face because the sweat glands are denervated; and d) less constantly, a sink-ing of the eyeball in the orbit **(enophthalmos),** because the orbitalis muscle at the apex of the orbit is denervated. This syndrome often occurs if there is cancer at the apex of the lung that spreads to the stellate ganglion or in persons with a cervical rib on the C7 vertebra.

Injury to the recurrent laryngeal nerves. The recurrent laryngeal nerve may be injured by tumors of the thyroid gland or during thyroidectomy. The resultant effect is paralysis of the laryngeal muscles on the side of injury. If one nerve is injured, hoarseness of the voice results. Care must be taken during ligation of the inferior thyroid artery, because the nerve ascends either anterior or posterior (or between) the branches of the artery where it is in danger of being contused or severed.

Thyroidectomy. Surgical removal of the thyroid gland (with some gland left behind) is a common procedure for nodular goiter, and removal of the gland for malignant growths is often necessary. When possible, surgeons leave the posterior parts of the lobes, thereby preserving the parathyroid glands.

Goiter. This is a nonspecific and common disorder of the thyroid gland due to a nodular enlargement of the gland. It most often is caused by a deficiency in iodine in the diet. If the enlargement is significant (presenting as a visible mass in the neck) it can extend into the thorax. A goiter can also put pressure on the trachea (causing respiratory problems) or on the jugular vein (causing venous compression).

Ludwig's angina. This inflammatory condition in the submandibular triangle is usually caused by infections of lower molar teeth. Often the jugulodigastric lymph node may be infected and can be palpated and tender to the touch adjacent to the angle of the mandible.

Tracheostomy. This important operation is performed to create an opening in the trachea in a person with upper airway obstruction, thereby allowing ventilation to occur in the lungs. Often it is a life-saving procedure if the patient has aspirated a foreign body, has an edema within the larynx, or has suffered a severe trauma to the head or neck. Today a cricothyroidotomy is often preferred to a tracheostomy. For a tracheostomy, an incision is made above the jugular notch and between the infrahyoid muscles. The isthmus of the thyroid gland is retracted and the trachea is cut between the 1st and 2nd tracheal rings (or between the 2nd and 3rd), and a tracheostomy tube is inserted into the trachea and secured into position. Care must be taken not to sever vessels on the trachea.

Central venous line placement. The subclavian veins are often used to insert a catheter into the venous system for the purpose of administering nour-

ishing fluids or to measure venous pressure in the right atrium. Another venous line approach is to puncture the internal jugular vein and advance the catheter into the right brachiocephalic vein to the superior vena cava and then into the right atrium. Care must be taken not to puncture the pleura and apex of the lung (avoiding a pneumothorax) and also not to insert the needle too deeply into the subclavian or common carotid arteries.

Endarterectomy of the internal carotid artery. The internal carotid artery may develop plaques or atherosclerotic thickenings on its internal surface that diminish or obstruct arterial blood flow. Symptoms such as loss of orientation or dizziness can result, which may last for about a day or so (called transient ischemic attack or TIA). Other symptoms of a minor stroke can result as well. A narrowing of the internal carotid artery can be treated by stripping the internal surface of the carotid of its attached atherosclerotic plaque (a procedure called endarterectomy).

Esophageal cancer. Difficulty in swallowing (dysphagia) is frequently the presenting symptom of a person who has developed cancer of the esophagus. The patient often describes experiencing chronic esophagitis after lying down to sleep shortly after the evening meal. Enlargement of cervical lymph nodes and hoarseness due to pressure of the tumor on the recurrent laryngeal nerve are also seen in these patients.

Thyroglossal duct cysts. The thyroid gland begins development by the thyroglossal duct that is directed inferiorly from the foramen cecum on the dorsum of the tongue. The gland proliferates from this duct, passing anterior to the hyoid bone to its final position over the larynx. Usually this duct disappears; however, if it does not, a thyroglossal duct cyst may remain at any site along the original pathway from the tongue to the neck. These cysts can readily be removed surgically.

Tracheoesophageal fistula. One of the common esophageal anomalies is a fistula between the trachea and the esophagus. Most frequently the upper portion of the esophagus ends as a closed blind pouch with the lower part communicating with the trachea. Other variations of this anomaly exist. The infant develops respiratory problems because it aspirates mucous. These fistulas are caused by an incomplete separation of the two organs by the tracheoesophageal septum.

Thyroid ima artery. In addition to the superior and inferior thyroid arteries, the thyroid gland may receive (in 10% of cases) a small unpaired thyroid ima artery from the brachiocephalic trunk (or from its main branches or from the aortic arch). When present, the vessel ascends to the gland on the anterior surface of the trachea and must be considered when a tracheostomy is performed.

Parathyroid glands. These small glands are vitally important in the regulation of calcium metabolism. They are usually located within the capsule of the thyroid gland and are in danger of being excised or damaged during the removal of the thyroid gland. They are supplied by the superior and inferior thyroid arteries, and one or more glands must be spared during thyroid surgery.

The carotid pulse. The carotid pulse can be palpated in the carotid triangle just lateral to the hyoid bone. At this site the external carotid artery becomes superficial and emerges from under the sternocleidomastoid muscle.

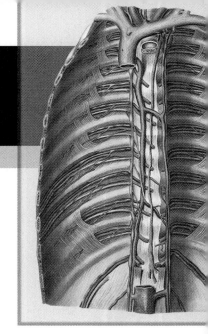

DISSECTION #31

The Scalp; the Floor of the Cranial Cavity; the Base of the Brain

OBJECTIVES

1 Understand the layers of the scalp; learn the blood supply and cutaneous innervation of the scalp.

2 Remove the calvaria (skull cap) and a wedge of occipital bone to expose the meninges and the brain.

3 Learn and then cut the reflections of dura mater; remove the brain from the cranial vault.

4 Study the internal surface of the base of the skull and identify structures that pass through the foramina of the three cranial fossae.

5 Identify the major dural venous sinuses.

6 Learn the arterial supply of the brain; dissect the circle of Willis and other vessels along the ventral surface of the brain.

To study the contents of the cranial cavity and remove the brain for inspection, the scalp must be reflected, the bony skull cap (the calvaria) removed, and the reflections of dura mater surrounding the brain must be cut and opened.

I. The Scalp (ATLAS PLATE 520 #520.2)

◄
Grant's 608, 610
Netter's 19, 20, 22
Rohen 77–79, 81, 85

A. Layers of the Scalp (Figure 31-1). The soft tissues of the scalp cover the skull from the eyebrows to the

superior nuchal lines on the occipital bones. The scalp extends laterally between the inferior temporal line on both sides of the skull. It is composed of three fused layers: (a) the **skin;** (b) a layer of **dense subcutaneous connective tissue;** and (c) the bellies of the occipitofrontalis muscle interconnected by a strong, broad aponeurosis called the **galea aponeurotica.** Some descriptions include two layers deep to the aponeurosis, a layer of **loose connective tissue** and the **periosteum** of the bones of the cranial vault.

Students often learn these layers with the following letter-word association:

S – skin

C – connective tissue (dense)

A – aponeurosis

L – loose connective tissue

P – periosteum or pericranium

353

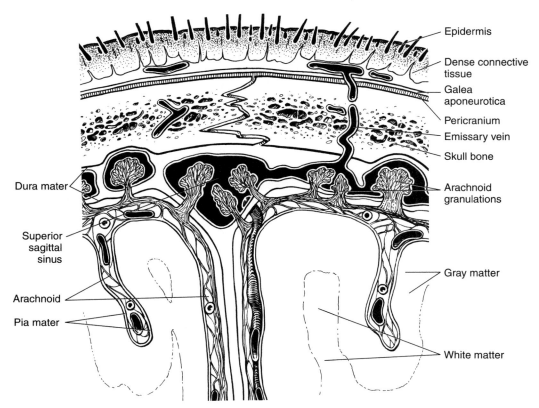

Figure 31-1. The scalp, skull, meninges, and brain.

B. Vessels of the Scalp (ATLAS PLATES 501, 506).
The scalp is richly supplied with blood, and it
bleeds profusely when severely injured. Its arteries
are derived from both the external and internal
carotid arteries. From the **external carotid artery**
it receives blood by way of the large **superficial
temporal** and **occipital arteries** and the smaller
posterior auricular artery. These vessels supply
the lateral and posterior parts of the scalp (**ATLAS
PLATE 506**).

From the **internal carotid artery,** two terminal
branches of the ophthalmic artery emerge from the orbit
to supply the anterior half of the scalp. These are the
supraorbital and **supratrochlear arteries,** and they
anastomose with the superficial temporal and occipital
arteries (**ATLAS PLATE 501**).

The veins accompanying the arteries not only drain
the scalp but also the calvaria by way of the **diploic
veins.** Venous blood draining the scalp in the facial,
superficial temporal, and occipital veins flows into both
internal and **external jugular veins (ATLAS PLATES
482, 501).**

C. Nerves of the Scalp. The anterior part of the scalp is
supplied with sensory innervation by the **supraorbital** and **supratrochlear** branches of the **frontal
nerve (V1).** The lateral scalp receives sensory fibers

◄
Grant's 600, 608
Netter's 19, 65
Rohen 78, 79, 85

◄
Grant's 608
Netter's 94, 96
Rohen 30, 34, 87,
88

◄
Grant's 604, 605,
608
Netter's 20, 28,
123
Rohen 76, 85

by way of the **zygomaticotemporal** (V2) and **auriculotemporal** (V3) nerves.

The posterior scalp is supplied by the **greater
occipital** and **3rd occipital nerves (ATLAS PLATES
388, 341**), and the scalp behind the ear by the **lesser
occipital nerve.** Motor innervation to the frontalis and
occipitalis muscles comes from the facial nerve (VII).

Firmly press your opened hand on top of your
head and move the layers of the scalp forward and
backward. The portion of the scalp that moves with
your hand includes the skin, dense connective tissue,
and the galea aponeurotica. These layers glide over
the bones because loose connective tissue lies deep to
the aponeurosis. Accidents that result in shearing
injuries of the scalp occur because the outer three
layers separate from the pericranium along this loose
connective tissue layer. Infections also can spread
widely throughout the scalp within this loose layer.
Learn the blood supply and innervation of the scalp,
but do not spend time dissecting these vessels and
nerves.

**Skin Incisions. Support the head by placing a
block under the posterior neck with the cadaver
supine (face up).** To remove the scalp make a

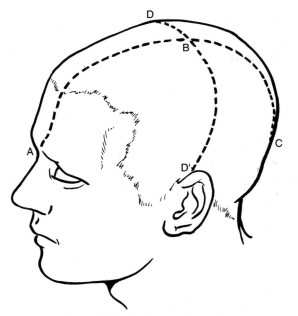

Figure 31-2. Incisions of the scalp.

sagittal incision in the midline of the skull cap from the bridge of the nose to the external occipital protuberance (**Figure 31-2, A–B–C**). Make a second incision coronally across the vertex of the skull from ear to ear (**Figure 31-2, D–B–D**). Separate the scalp deep to the aponeurosis along the loose connective tissue layer and reflect four flaps downward (**Figure 31-3**).

▶
Grant's 590–592
Netter's 2, 4, 8
Rohen 20, 22, 29

Remove any remaining tissue from the outer surfaces of the frontal, parietal, and the upper parts of the temporal and occipital bones.

Identify the following (**ATLAS PLATES 515 #515.1, 516**):

1. **Coronal suture,** between the posterior border of the frontal bone and the anterior borders of the parietal bones.

2. **Sagittal suture,** between the two parietal bones in the midline.

3. **Lambdoid suture,** between the posterior borders of the two parietal bones and the squamous part of the occipital bone (**ATLAS PLATE 515 #515.1**).

4. **Squamosal suture,** between the superior borders of the temporal bone and the parietal bone (**ATLAS PLATE 515 #515.1**).

5. **Bregma,** the intersecting site of the coronal and sagittal sutures. In the newborn infant, it is the membranous **anterior fontanelle (ATLAS PLATE 519 # 519.1).**

6. **Lambda,** the point where the sagittal and lambdoid sutures meet. In the newborn infant, it is the site of the smaller membranous **posterior fontanelle (ATLAS PLATE 519).**

Figure 31-3. Sutures of the skull and the line for the circular saw cut.

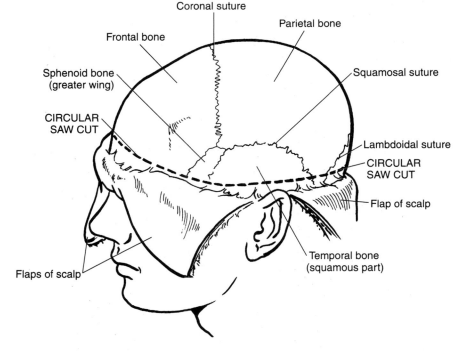

II. Removal of Skull Cap and Wedge of Occipital Bone

A. Removal of Skull Cap. One objective in removing the skull cap is to retain an intact dura mater on the inner surface of the calvaria. It can be separated completely from the bone and observed as a continuous sac of fibrous tissue enclosing the brain. Realize that the frontal and occipital bones are somewhat thicker than the temporal and parietal bones.

◀
Grant's 608–612
Netter's 95
Rohen 88

Be certain that all scalp tissue has been removed. Scrape away the attachments of the temporalis muscles on the skull to the level of the zygomatic arch. Remove **all muscle attachments** on the posterior skull.

Use a glass marking pencil on the dry skull to outline the skull cap that will be removed: **anteriorly,** on the forehead 2 cm above the supraorbital margins; **laterally,** on the squama of the temporal bone 2.5 cm superior to the external auditory meatus; **posteriorly,** 2.5 cm superior to the occipital protuberance (**Figure 31-3**).

Make saw cuts in the bones along the lines encircling the calvaria. Avoid cutting too deeply, and be cautious when the bone dust becomes reddish brown because the **outer table** of bone has been cut and the marrow cavity entered. Now use a chisel within the saw cuts and stroke it gently with a mallet to split the **inner table** of bone. Try not to sever the dura mater that underlies the inner table.

With the inner table cut around the entire skull, pry the underlying dura away from the inner surface of the skull cap. Gradually remove the calvaria leaving the dural sac that covers the superior and lateral surfaces of the brain intact (**ATLAS PLATE 521**). Be gentle—use your fingers and the handle of a scalpel because tearing the dura will damage the brain.

B. Removal of an Occipital Bone Wedge. Removing a wedge from the posterior part of the skull will further open the cranial cavity and expose the dura mater covering the occipital lobes and the cerebellum (**Figure 31-4**).

Turn the cadaver face down (prone). Identify the lower part of the lambdoid sutures as they extend posterolaterally below the cut edge of the skull. Identify the posterolateral rim of the foramen magnum. With the suboccipital muscles reflected, identify and cut the posterior atlantooccipital membrane but do not sever the vertebral arteries.

Draw a line on both sides from the point where the cut edge of the skull crosses the lambdoid suture to the posterolateral edge of the foramen magnum. Saw along these two lines and then use a chisel and mallet, as was done in removing the skull cap (**Figure 31-4**).

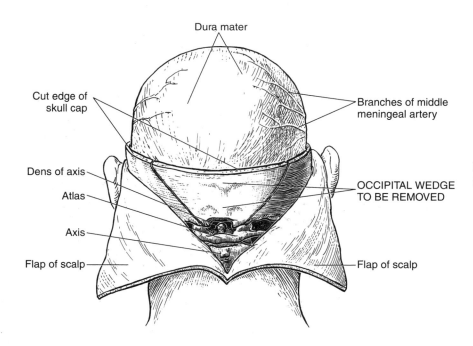

Dura mater

Cut edge of skull cap

Branches of middle meningeal artery

Dens of axis

Atlas

Axis

OCCIPITAL WEDGE TO BE REMOVED

Flap of scalp

Flap of scalp

Figure 31-4. The occipital wedge that is to be cut after the skull cap s been removed.

Separate the dura mater from the inner surface of the occipital wedge. Study the inner surface of the skull cap and the occipital wedge (**ATLAS PLATE 517**).

1. On the inner surface of the skull cap, observe:
   a. The **sagittal, coronal,** and **lambdoid sutures.** At times these are difficult to see. In older persons sutural joints may become ossified.
   b. The **sulcus for the superior sagittal sinus**.
   c. Small pits in the bone for **arachnoid granulations.** Called **granular foveolae,** they are found on both sides of the midline sulcus (**ATLAS PLATE 517**).
   d. The **frontal crest,** a bony projection in the midline of the frontal bone. On it attaches the falx cerebri of the dura mater.
   e. The sulci on both sides for the **middle meningeal arteries** and their branches (**ATLAS PLATE 517**).

2. On the inner surface of the occipital wedge, identify:
   a. The **grooves for the transverse sinuses,** extending laterally from the midline. Also, note a depression for the **confluence of sinuses.**
   b. The **cerebellar fossae** that houses the cerebellum.

III. Meninges; Removal of the Brain

A. Meninges. Three membranes surround the brain and spinal cord. These are the meninges, and from outside inward they are the **dura mater,** the netlike **arachnoid,** and the vascular **pia mater.** The cranial dura mater is considered here.

1. **Dura mater.** This thick, dense outer membrane within the cranial cavity is composed of two layers: an inner **meningeal layer** and an outer **endosteal layer** closest to the bones. The two layers are completely fused **except** where they separate to form the walls of the **venous sinuses,** where they form **dural sacs** for the pituitary gland and the trigeminal ganglion and where they form **tubular sheaths** for the cranial nerves emerging through foramina at the base of the skull.
   a. **Dural folds or septa.** Four septa are formed by inward duplications of the meningeal layer of dura. These divide the cranial cavity into spaces that accommodate different parts of the brain. The four septa are:

► Grant's 610–613
Netter's 96, 97
Rohen 86, 87, 139

◄ Netter's 4

► Grant's 611–613, 616
Netter's 98, 100, 137
Rohen 64, 67, 69, 87

► Grant's 612, 613
Netter's 97
Rohen 86

► Grant's 612, 619, 620
Rohen 64
◄ Grant's 610, 611
Netter's 94–96
Rohen 85

► Grant's 611
Netter's 94, 95

► Grant's 612, 613
Netter's 98
Rohen 85, 98, 114

1) The **falx cerebri.** This sickle-shaped vertical dural sheet projects inferiorly between the cerebral hemispheres (**ATLAS PLATE 522**). It is narrow anteriorly and attached to the crista galli of the ethmoid bone. The falx broadens posteriorly and is attached in the midline to the upper surface of the tentorium cerebelli. The convex superior margin of the falx attaches longitudinally on both sides of the sagittal suture to enclose the **superior sagittal sinus.** Its concave inferior margin contains the **inferior sagittal sinus.** Where this latter margin attaches along the superior surface of the tentorium cerebelli courses the **straight sinus (Figure 31-5).**

2) The **tentorium cerebelli (ATLAS PLATE 532)** is a crescent-shaped sheet of dura mater that covers the cerebellum transversely and underlies the occipital lobes of the cerebral cortex. Its anterior border encircles the midbrain, and its edges attach to the anterior clinoid processes of the sphenoid bone. Its posterior border is attached around the inner surface of the temporal and occipital bones.

3) The **falx cerebelli** is a small vertical reflection of dura mater located in the midline below the tentorium that extends between the two cerebellar hemispheres. It is attached superiorly to the tentorium, posteriorly to the internal occipital crest, and inferiorly to the margin of the foramen magnum.

4) The **diaphragma sellae** is a circular, horizontal fold of dura mater that forms the roof of the hypophyseal fossa (**ATLAS PLATES 525 #525.1, 533 #533.2**). It covers the pituitary gland except for a small opening through which courses the pituitary stalk. Dura also lines the sella turcica and completes a close-fitting sac for the pituitary gland (**ATLAS PLATES 525 #525.1, 533 #533.2**).

With the calvaria and occipital wedge removed, examine the dura mater and identify:

The **middle meningeal vessels** and their branches (**ATLAS PLATE 521**). These vessels may rupture from a head injury, resulting in an epidural hematoma (blood between the skull and the dura mater). This serious problem causes pressure on the brain and could be fatal if not relieved.

The **arachnoid granulations.** These projections of arachnoid mater cells are found mostly along the sides of the superior sagittal sinus (**ATLAS**

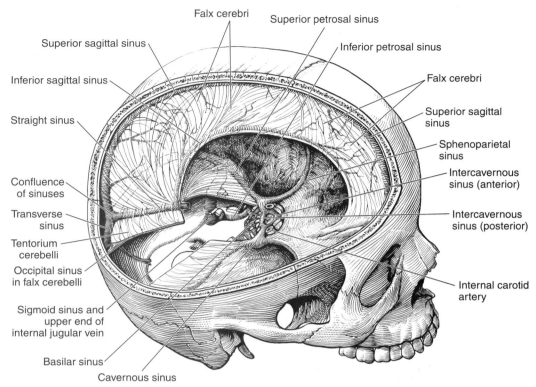

Figure 31-5. The intracranial dural reflections and the dural sinuses (after Sobotta).

PLATE 521). Tufts of arachnoid deep to the dura are adjacent to the endothelium of the venous sinuses, and this allows the passage of cerebrospinal fluid into the venous system from the subarachnoid space.

Keep the cadaver prone for the next procedure.

B. Removal of the Brain. To remove the brain from the cranial cavity *in one piece,* the dura mater must be reflected on both sides of the cortex, the tentorium cerebelli cut along its peripheral attachment, and the medulla oblongata severed at the foramen magnum.

1. Identify the **superior sagittal sinus** extending in the midline longitudinally within the dura mater the entire length of the brain **(Figure 31-6)**.

2. With forceps and sharp scissors, make a longitudinal opening in the dura mater **lateral to the superior sagittal sinus.** Extend the opening lateral to the sinus along the length of the cerebrum from frontal to occipital poles. Make a similar longitudinal cut on the other side of the sinus **(Figure 31-6)**.

▶
Grant's 612–614
Netter's 6, 9, 35
Rohen 30, 86, 87
◀
Grant's 610–612
Netter's 94–97
Rohen 87

▶
Grant's 616
Netter's 98
Rohen 87, 97

3. Make transverse cuts laterally in the dura across the cerebrum on both sides from the midpoint of the longitudinal incisions to the margins of the skull above the ears.

4. This results in a median longitudinal strip of dura that contains the superior sagittal sinus and four triangular flaps of dura. Upon reflecting the flaps over the cut skull, you will encounter a few attachments to the underlying meninges or even small vessels; these may be severed.

5. Lift the frontal lobes gently and sever the attachment of the median longitudinal strip of dura from the **crista galli** anteriorly. As you lift the central strip, sever any attachments the dura might have with the cerebral cortex. This releases the sickle-shaped **falx cerebri** from its location between the cerebral hemispheres **(ATLAS PLATE 522)**. Pull the falx backward as far as possible and note that it is still attached posteriorly and inferiorly to the tentorium cerebelli.

6. Gently elevate the right occipital lobe and visualize the underlying tentorium cerebelli **(ATLAS PLATE 532)**. With a sharp scalpel,

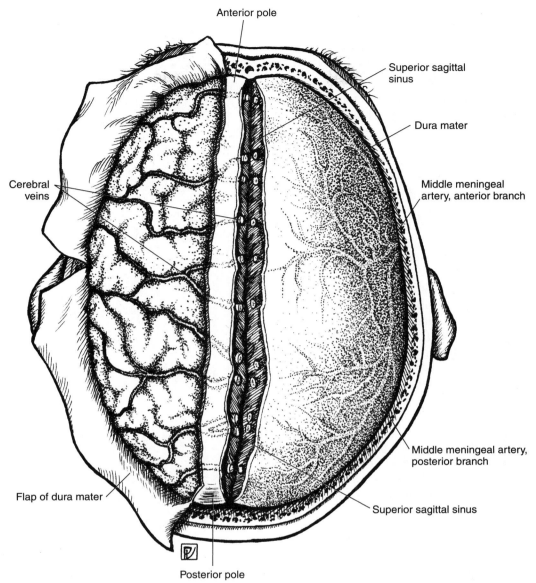

Figure 31-6. The dura mater and the opened superior sagittal sinus. On the *left side* the dura has been opened and the dural flaps reflected.

sever the attachment of the tentorium anteriorly from the clinoid process. Extend this incision posteriorly and laterally immediately adjacent to the inner surface of the temporal bone and then posteriorly in front of the transverse sinus.

Repeat the procedure by lifting the left occipital lobe and severing the attachments of the tentorium on that side. Next detach the **falx cerebelli** from the **inferior** surface of the tentorium.

7. The cerebellum is now free of its dural attachments. Mobilize it slightly forward and visualize the foramen magnum from within the cranial cavity.

▶
Grant's 612, 620
Netter's 98
Rohen 97

◀
Grant's 612, 613
Netter's 97, 137
Rohen 86

▶
Grant's 616, 618
Netter's 98
Rohen 97

8. With the brain unrestrained by dura, commence its removal by elevating the frontal lobes and the olfactory bulbs and tracts. Sever the **optic nerves, internal carotid arteries, pituitary stalk,** and **oculomotor nerves.** Cut the delicate **trochlear nerves** (if not already cut), the large **trigeminal nerves,** and medially and deep in the middle cranial fossa, the **abducent nerves (ATLAS PLATE 532).**

9. Elevate the cerebrum, brainstem, and attached cerebellum from the base of the skull. On the surface of the temporal bone, sever the **facial** and **vestibulocochlear nerves** near the internal

acoustic meatus. Next, cut the **glossopharyn-geal, vagus,** and **accessory nerves** proximal to the jugular foramen. Most deeply, cut the **hypoglossal nerves** and the **vertebral arteries** and sever the **brainstem** just above the foramen magnum (**ATLAS PLATE 532**). Cut away any remaining filaments attached to the skull and remove the brain from the cranial cavity in one piece.

IV. Base of Skull: Bony Markings; Foramina (Figure 31-8)

Before studying the floor of the cranial cavity in the cadaver, identify the foramina in the floor of a dry skull.

A. Internal Surface of the Base of a Dry Skull. The internal surface of the floor of the cranial cavity is marked by three fossae: the **anterior, middle,** and **posterior cranial fossae** (**ATLAS PLATE 536**). On the bony structures forming the floor of these fossae rest the **frontal** and **temporal lobes** of the cerebrum as well as the **brainstem and cerebellum.**

1. **Anterior cranial fossa (ATLAS PLATE 537).** Identify:
   a. Both orbital plates of the frontal bone.
   b. The **cribriform plate of the ethmoid bone,** located between the two orbital plates. Note the many foramina in the cribriform plate.
   c. The **crista galli.** Onto this anterior midline process attaches the anterior end of the falx cerebri. Note the **foramen cecum.**
   d. The **lesser wings of the sphenoid bone** projecting laterally from the body of the sphenoid bone. The medial ends of their posterior borders form the **anterior clinoid processes.**

2. **Middle cranial fossa (ATLAS PLATE 537).** Identify:
   a. The **greater wings of the sphenoid bone** laterally and the **body of the sphenoid bone** medially. The latter contains the **sella turcica** for the pituitary gland. Note the **posterior clinoid processes.**
   b. The **squamous** (lateral) and the **petrous** (posterior) parts of the temporal bone.
   c. The **arcuate eminence.** Deep to this elevation on the petrous part of the temporal bone is the **anterior semicircular canal** of the inner ear.

   d. Locate the following foramina:
      1) **Optic foramen**
      2) **Superior orbital fissure**
      3) **Foramen rotundum**
      4) **Foramen ovale**
      5) **Foramen spinosum**
      6) **Foramen lacerum**

3. **Posterior cranial fossa (ATLAS PLATE 537).** Identify:
   a. The **petrous** and **mastoid** parts of the **temporal bone** posterior to the arcuate eminence.
   b. The posterior part of the body of the sphenoid bone.
   c. The **squamous, basilar,** and **condylar parts** of the **occipital bone.**
   d. Locate the following foramina:
      1) **Internal acoustic meatus**
      2) **Jugular foramen**
      3) **Hypoglossal canal**
      4) **Foramen magnum**

B. Internal Surface of the Base of the Skull in the Cadaver. With the brain removed, study the base of the skull and identify the severed nerves and vessels that traverse the foramina.

1. Identify again the **superior sagittal sinus** along the convex upper surface of the falx cerebri. Note the smaller **inferior sagittal sinus** along the concave lower free margin of the falx (**ATLAS PLATE 522**). Observe that the superior sagittal sinus usually empties into the **right transverse sinus** on the right side of the internal occipital protuberance.

2. Follow the inferior sagittal sinus posteriorly to its site of junction with the **straight sinus** (**ATLAS PLATE 522**). Note that the straight sinus extends posteriorly along the junction of the falx cerebri and the tentorium cerebelli. It flows most often into the **left transverse sinus.**

3. Cut any attachments and remove the falx cerebri and tentorium cerebelli. Turn your attention to the floor of the cranial cavity.

4. Identify the **anterior cranial fossa** in front, posterior to it at a lower level, the **middle cranial fossa,** and posterior and inferior to this, the **posterior cranial fossa.** Note that the **frontal and temporal lobes** rest in the anterior and middle cranial fossae. Posteriorly, the **cerebellum** and **brainstem** (the

▶
Grant's 614, 615, 618
Netter's 8, 9
Rohen 26, 30, 34

◄
Grant's 614, 616
Netter's 9, 10
Rohen 30

▶
Grant's 610–613, 616
Netter's 94, 96–98
Rohen 86, 87, 121

◄
Grant's 614, 615
Netter's 6, 35
Rohen 30, 34

▶
Grant's 613, 616
Netter's 97, 98, 137, 138
Rohen 67, 145

◄
Grant's 614, 615
Netter's 9, 10
Rohen 26, 30, 34

▶
Grant's 614, 615, 618–622
Netter's 9, 10, 99–101
Rohen 26, 30, 34, 65, 66, 100

rhombencephalon) occupy the posterior cranial fossa (**ATLAS PLATES 532, 534**).

5. In the floor of the posterior fossa, identify the curved **sigmoid sinus.** It is the extension of the transverse sinus and terminates at the jugular foramen.

6. Identify the **superior petrosal sinus** along the superior border of the petrous part of the temporal bone (**ATLAS PLATES 522, 523**). It extends from the lateral aspect of the body of the sphenoid bone at the **cavernous sinus** and courses laterally and posteriorly to the transverse sinus (**Figure 31-7**).

7. Remove the dural covering from the **cavernous sinus.** Note that within this sinus

▶
Grant's 616, 620, 621
Netter's 98
Rohen 87

◀
Grant's 613, 614, 616
Netter's 97, 98
Rohen 87, 120

◀
Grant's 613, 616
Netter's 97, 98, 130, 133
Rohen 87

▶
Grant's 613
Netter's 97, 98
Rohen 69–73, 83

◀
Grant's 613, 616
619–621
Netter's 98
Rohen 64, 69

are delicate interlacing threads of fibrous tissue that form intercommunicating "caverns." Identify the **oculomotor, trochlear,** and **abducent nerves;** the **ophthalmic** and **maxillary divisions of the trigeminal nerve;** and the **internal carotid artery,** all of which traverse the sinus (**Figure 31-8**).

8. Posterior and anterior to the cavernous sinuses, note the **anterior** and **posterior intercavernous sinuses** crossing the midline (**ATLAS PLATES 523, 532**).

9. Posterior to the sphenoid bone, open the dural covering over the **trigeminal cave.** Identify the roots of the three divisions of the **trigeminal nerve** and the **trigeminal ganglion** (**ATLAS PLATE 532**).

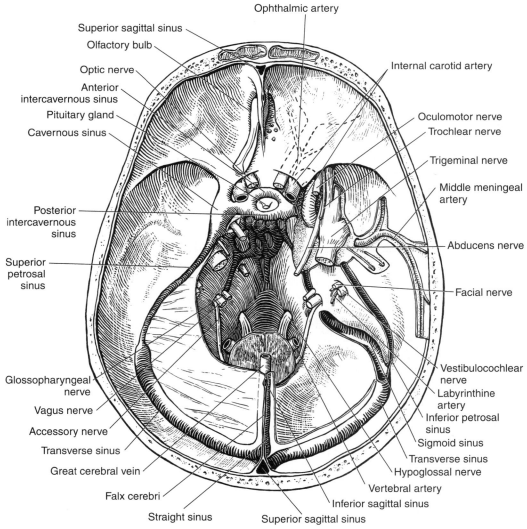

Figure 31-7. The dural sinuses and severed cranial nerves at the base of the skull (after Sobotta).

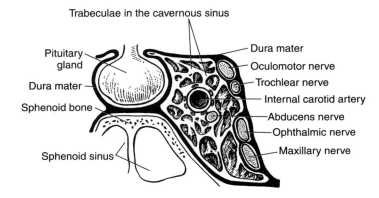

Figure 31-8. Frontal section through the pituitary gland and cavernous sinus.

10. Identify the stalk (infundibulum) of the pituitary gland (hypophysis) traversing a small opening in the **diaphragma sellae** that covers the hypophyseal fossa (**ATLAS PLATE 533 #533.2**).

11. Identify the foramina and the severed cranial nerves and vessels that traverse them.

a. Try to identify filaments of the **olfactory nerve (I)** that enter the cranial cavity through the small foramina in the cribriform plate (**ATLAS PLATES 531, 564, 565**).

b. Identify the **optic nerves (II)** medial to the anterior clinoid processes and the **internal carotid arteries** just lateral to these nerves.

c. In the **middle cranial fossa,** find the **oculomotor (III)** and delicate **trochlear nerves (IV)** just lateral to the diaphragma sellae. Note that these two nerves course anteriorly to the orbit through the superior orbital fissure (**ATLAS PLATE 532**).

d. Identify the divisions of the **trigeminal nerve (V)** within the trigeminal cave. Note that the **ophthalmic division (V1)** passes along the lateral wall of the cavernous sinus and through the superior orbital fissure. The **maxillary division (V2)** courses in the floor of the cavernous sinus to the **foramen rotundum,** while the **mandibular division (V3)** courses inferiorly to the **foramen ovale.**

e. Lateral to the mandibular nerve find the **foramen spinosum** and the middle meningeal artery entering the middle cranial fossa (**Figure 31-7**).

f. In the **posterior cranial fossa,** identify the cut end of the **abducent nerve (VI),** located medially. It ascends to the superior orbital fissure. Find the **facial (VII)** and **vestibulocochlear (VIII) nerves** together at the

◄ Grant's 612, 619, 620
Rohen 64

► Grant's 615, 616, 618, 816–821
Netter's 8, 98, 119–122
Rohen 67, 73, 75, 99

◄ Grant's 616, 617, 619, 622, 800–803
Netter's 38, 39, 113
Rohen 143

◄ Grant's 609, 616, 734
Netter's 98
Rohen 64, 68, 69

◄ Grant's 616, 620, 806–811
Netter's 41, 42, 82, 98, 125
Rohen 68, 72, 73

► Grant's 616, 622–624
Netter's 98, 124, 130, 132–134
Rohen 64, 69, 87, 93, 99, 103

◄ Grant's 614, 616, 618
Netter's 9, 10, 65, 67, 95, 125
Rohen 30, 34, 38

◄ Grant's 616, 618
Netter's 130, 132–134, 136
Rohen 69, 97

internal acoustic meatus (**ATLAS PLATE 532**). Also identify (if possible) the delicate **labyrinthine artery.**

g. Posterior and medial to the internal acoustic meatus, find the **jugular foramen.** Identify the most anterior nerve filaments in the foramen as the **glossopharyngeal (IX) nerve (Figure 31-7**). The most posterior filaments at the foramen are the spinal fibers of the **accessory (XI) nerve.** These ascend through the foramen magnum and then descend through the jugular foramen into the neck. Between the IXth and XIth nerves are the filaments of the **vagus (X) nerve.** Note also that the **sigmoid sinus** courses through the jugular foramen to become the internal jugular vein below the skull.

h. Medial and inferior to the jugular foramen, find the **hypoglossal nerve (XII)** traversing the **anterior condyloid canal (ATLAS PLATE 532**). The rootlets that form this nerve can usually be found behind the cut vertebral artery.

V. Arterial Blood Supply to the Brain

Two pairs of arteries enter the cranial cavity to supply blood to the brain: the **internal carotid** and **vertebral arteries.** The **internal carotid artery** enters the carotid canal on the inferior surface of the temporal bone. It ascends vertically, curves forward and medially, and then leaves the carotid canal to course across the foramen lacerum. Traversing the cavernous sinus (**Figure 31-8**), it curves in an S-shaped manner to enter the floor of the cranial cavity just lateral to the optic chiasma (**ATLAS PLATES 525, 526, 532**). Within the cranial cavity, it gives off the **ophthalmic, anterior cerebral, middle**

cerebral, posterior communicating, and **anterior choroid branches.**

The **vertebral artery** arises from the first part of the subclavian artery and courses superiorly, medially, and dorsally to enter the transverse process foramen of the C6 vertebra (**ATLAS PLATES 490, 491**). It ascends through similar foramina of the upper five cervical vertebrae and turns 90° medially along a groove on the upper surface of the atlas. It then perforates the posterior occipitoatlantal membrane to enter the skull through the foramen magnum. The two vertebral arteries join to form the **basilar artery,** but before this junction, they give rise to the **anterior and posterior spinal arteries** and the **posterior inferior cerebellar arteries (ATLAS PLATES 526, 527).**

The arterial **circle of Willis** is formed by the anterior and middle cerebral branches of the internal carotid arteries and the two posterior cerebral branches of the basilar artery. These vessels are interconnected anteriorly by an **anterior communicating artery** between the two anterior cerebral vessels and a **posterior communicating artery** on each side that connects the posterior cerebral with the internal carotid. The circle of Willis surrounds the optic chiasma and the hypophyseal stalk (**Figure 31-9**).

▶
Grant's 329,
622–624
Netter's 131–134,
164
Rohen 94, 98, 99
◀
Grant's 616, 618,
622–624, 736
Netter's 130,
132–134
Rohen 73, 75, 93,
99, 103, 168

◀
Grant's 622–624
Netter's 132, 133
Rohen 93, 99
▶
Grant's 622–624
Netter's 132, 133
Rohen 93, 94, 99

Identify the cut internal carotid and vertebral arteries on both sides (**ATLAS PLATE 526**). Observe how the two vertebral arteries, often unequal in size, join near the midline to form the basilar artery. Identify the **posterior spinal artery.** This descends along the posterior surface of the spinal cord and arises from each vertebral artery or, more frequently, from its **posterior inferior cerebellar branch.** This latter tortuous branch ascends to the posterior part of the cerebellum. Find small branches that arise from each vertebral artery and unite to form the important **anterior spinal artery.** This vessel descends in the anterior median fissure of the spinal cord (**ATLAS PLATE 358 #358.1**).

Observe that the **basilar artery** forms by the union of the two vertebral arteries near the lower border of the pons. From it, **pontine branches** penetrate the brainstem. The **labyrinthine branch** enters the internal acoustic meatus, but may be difficult to identify.

Note successively (**Figure 31-9**):

The **anterior inferior cerebellar arteries** coursing to the cerebellum.

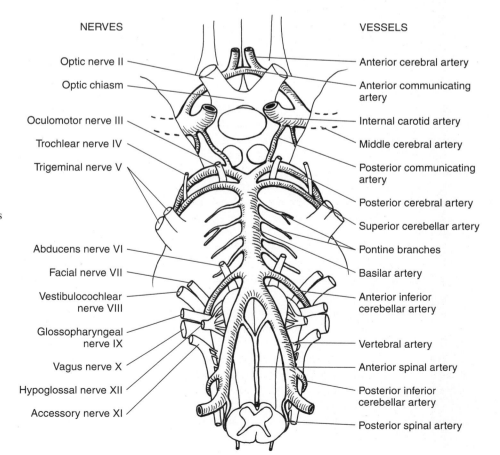

Figure 31-9. The arteries and cranial nerves at the base of the brain.

NERVES

Optic nerve II
Optic chiasm
Oculomotor nerve III
Trochlear nerve IV
Trigeminal nerve V
Abducens nerve VI
Facial nerve VII
Vestibulocochlear nerve VIII
Glossopharyngeal nerve IX
Vagus nerve X
Hypoglossal nerve XII
Accessory nerve XI

VESSELS

Anterior cerebral artery
Anterior communicating artery
Internal carotid artery
Middle cerebral artery
Posterior communicating artery
Posterior cerebral artery
Superior cerebellar artery
Pontine branches
Basilar artery
Anterior inferior cerebellar artery
Vertebral artery
Anterior spinal artery
Posterior inferior cerebellar artery
Posterior spinal artery

The **superior cerebellar arteries** located just posterior to the oculomotor nerves.

The **posterior cerebral arteries,** the terminal branches of the basilar, found immediately anterior to the oculomotor nerves.

The **posterior communicating arteries** between the posterior cerebral and the internal carotid arteries.

Dissect the internal carotid arteries by separating the frontal and temporal lobes. Identify the **middle cerebral branch** of the internal carotid artery along the lateral (sylvian) sulcus (**ATLAS PLATE 526 #526.2**). Separate the inferior surfaces of the two frontal lobes and find the two **anterior cerebral branches** of the internal carotids passing forward between the two hemispheres. Spread the frontal lobes about 1 cm, and observe the transversely coursing **anterior communicating artery** between the two anterior cerebral branches (**ATLAS PLATES 526.2 #526.2, 527**).

Review the vessels that form the **circle of Willis:**

2 posterior cerebrals

2 posterior communicating

2 internal carotids

2 anterior cerebrals

1 anterior communicating

◄
Grant's 622, 624
Netter's 133
Rohen 93, 94, 99

Clinical Relevance

Occlusion of cerebral veins. Cerebral veins may be occluded by thrombi or from the growth of a cerebral tumor. At the base of the skull the veins most often blocked are the transverse, sigmoid, and cavernous sinuses. Additionally, the superior sagittal sinus can be blocked dorsally or posteriorly. Infections or thrombophlebitis of the facial veins on or around the nose in the so-called "butterfly area" of the upper lip and zygomatic process can readily throw off thrombi that achieve the cavernous sinus by way of anastomoses through the superior ophthalmic vein. These infections can affect the cranial nerves traversing the cavernous sinus and develop into generalized meningitis.

Brain tumors. The nature and origin of a tumor within the cranial vault must be determined. Very frequently these are metastatic growths from a primary tumor elsewhere in the body, such as cancers of the lung, breast, or organs in the pelvis. Primary malignant tumors also arise from neuroglial cells or from the secretory cells of the choroid plexus. These tumors are often aggressive and have a dim prognosis. Other tumors arise from the meninges and are most often seen in relation to the intracranial dural reflections, such as the falx cerebri and the tentorium cerebelli, as well as to tumors along the vestibulocochlear nerve (acoustic tumors). Meningeal tumors often have a better prognosis because surgery can successfully remove them.

Meningitis. This condition is an infection of the pia mater and arachnoid layers of the meninges and it most often occurs by the spread of infective matter via the bloodstream. These infections are usually bacterial and in most instances are transmitted from an infected nasal cavity up through the cribriform plate of the ethmoid bone. Virulent infections can lead to brain edema and death, but the infections usually respond well to antibiotic therapy.

Epidural hematoma. Injury to the side of the head can result in tearing of the anterior division of the middle meningeal artery. Blood can extravasate and then clot between the skull and the dura mater, forming an epidural hemotoma. The clot can produce pressure on the motor region of the precentral gyrus, resulting in symptoms related to motor functions of the limbs or speech.

Fracture of the calvaria. Hard blows to the head can result in a depressed fracture of a part of one of the bones covering the brain. These fractures can occur at the site where the blow was received, but fractures may radiate in more than one direction from the point of impact. In some instances a blow to the head does not fracture the bone at the site of trauma; however, a fracture can occur on the skull at the site opposite to the point of impact. These are called *"contrecoup"* fractures and are common.

Herniation of the tentorium cerebelli. The tentorium cerebelli is a reflection of dura mater between the cerebellum and the occipital lobes of the cerebral cortex. It attaches anteriorly on both sides of the sphenoid bone. An opening between these attachments called the tentorial notch surrounds the midbrain. When tumors invade the cerebrum superior to the tentorium, increased intracranial pressure will often force the temporal lobes to herniate through the opening and cause the lateral part of the temporal lobe to be contused or lacerated. Injury to the adjacent oculomotor nerve results in ophthalmoplegia (paralysis of the 3rd cranial nerve).

Tumors of the pituitary gland. Pituitary tumors force an upward bulging of the diaphragma sellae and cause pressure on the overlying hypothalamus with accompanying endocrine disorders. The adjacent optic chiasma is often injured, affecting the crossed fibers from the nasal half of the two retinas.

Anosmia. The cribriform plate of the ethmoid bone transmits the neural fibers from the primary receptors for the sense of smell. Serious trauma to the forehead (such as hitting the head on the windshield in an auto accident) can shear these delicate fibers. This injury can result in the loss of the olfactory sense (called anosmia).

Subdural hemorrhage or hematoma. These injuries are usually caused by trauma to the forehead or occipital region that results in a slow hemorrhage from cerebral veins that drain into the superior sagittal sinus. Blood accumulates deep to the dura mater and can cause increased intracranial pressure. At times acute symptoms develop, but often a slower bleeding results in a chronic condition. Surgical relief is achieved by trephining burr holes in the skull and removing the blood clot.

Stroke. Stroke is a general term to describe a neurologic condition resulting from a cerebral or subarachnoid hemorrhage or from the release of an atherosclerotic plaque that obstructs a cerebral artery. Most of these emboli derive from plaques near the carotid bifurcation, and the blocked branch of the internal carotid artery quickly results in the formation of a degenerated region of brain called a cerebral infarct.

Intracerebral aneurysms. Most intracerebral aneurysms develop at the base of the brain from vessels forming the circle of Willis. A frequent site is the branching of the internal carotid artery. Other sites include the branching of the anterior and posterior communicating arteries and the branching of the basilar artery into the two posterior cerebral arteries. Often without warning, acute symptoms result if an enlarged aneurysm ruptures. Surgical procedures may be used to "clip" or ligate the aneurysm once its location is established, or the aneurysm may be sealed by microcoils inserted radiographically through catheters that are guided to the lesion site from the femoral artery up to the cerebral circulation.

Fractures within the middle cranial fossa. Weakened by numerous foramina sulci, sinuses, and canals, the bones in the floor of the middle cranial fossa are subject to more fractures than those in the anterior and posterior cranial fossae. Fractures in the middle fossa can affect any of the cranial nerves from the 3rd through the 8th, presenting symptoms relating to the functions of these nerves peripherally. These breaks in the floor of the skull result in leakage of cerebrospinal fluid (CSF).

Fractures in the anterior cranial fossa. These fractures often involve the cribriform plate of the ethmoid bone and result from trauma to the forehead, such as might be sustained in an auto accident. In these instances there may be a tearing of the dura mater deep to the olfactory bulb, resulting in leakage of CSF into the nasal cavity. This condition is called cerebrospinal rhinorrhea, and the symptom is dripping of CSF from the anterior nasal openings (anterior nares). High levels of glucose in the CSF differentiates this fluid from fluid that results from an upper nasal infection or a "runny nose."

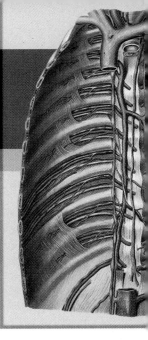

DISSECTION #32

The Orbit: Superior and Anterior Dissections

OBJECTIVES

1 Study the bony walls of the orbit on a skull; identify the foramina for the orbital vessels and nerves.

2 Dissect the orbit from above and visualize the periorbita, extraocular muscles, ophthalmic artery and its branches, ophthalmic division of the trigeminal nerve and branches, and the trochlear, oculomotor, and abducens nerves.

3 Visualize the optic nerve, ciliary ganglion, and the delicate vessels and nerves around the optic nerve.

4 Dissect the orbit from an anterior approach; study the eyelids, conjunctiva, bulbar fascia, the insertions of the extraocular muscles, and the lacrimal apparatus.

Atlas Key:

Clemente Atlas 5th Edition = Atlas Plate #

Grant's Atlas 11th Edition = Grant's Page #

Netter's Atlas 3rd Edition = Netter's Plate #

Rohen Atlas 6th Edition = Rohen Page #

Within the orbital cavities are located the eyeballs, the optic nerves, the muscles that move the eyeball and elevate the upper eyelid, and the vessels and nerves that supply these structures. Additionally, each orbital cavity contains a lacrimal gland, two small lacrimal canals, and a lacrimal sac.

I. The Bony Orbit
(ATLAS PLATES 514, 540)

Each orbital cavity serves as the bony socket for the eyeball. The socket is shaped like a four-sided pyramid

▶
Grant's 640, 641
Netter's 2
Rohen 23

◄
Grant's 589, 640
Netter's 2–4
Rohen 20, 21,
44–47

and formed by parts of seven bones: the **maxilla, zygomatic, frontal, lacrimal, sphenoid,** and **ethmoid** bones and a small part of the **palatine bone.** Before dissection, study the inner walls of the orbit and know that the bones are lined by a layer of periosteum, called the **periorbita.**

A. Bones of the Orbit (ATLAS PLATE 514). Study the orbit on a skull from an anterior orientation. Do the following:

1. Palpate the **anterior rim of the orbit** and identify the **frontal bone** above, the **zygomatic bone** laterally, and the **maxilla** inferiorly and medially.

2. Note that the **roof of the orbit** is formed by the orbital plate of the **frontal bone** and the lesser wing of the **sphenoid bone.**

3. Note that the **floor of the orbit** is thin. It consists of the orbital surfaces of the **maxilla** and

zygomatic bone and, posteriorly, the small orbital process of the **palatine bone.**

4. Feel the thin **medial wall of the orbit.** Identify the frontal process of the **maxilla,** the orbital lamina of the **ethmoid bone,** the lesser wing of the **sphenoid bone,** and, anteromedially, the **lacrimal bone.**

5. Note that the thicker **lateral wall** is formed by the orbital surface of the **zygomatic bone** and the greater wing of the **sphenoid bone.**

B. Observe the following:

1. That the roof of the orbit separates the orbital structures from the frontal lobe of the brain.

2. That the floor of the orbit forms the roof of the large **maxillary sinus.** It is subject to fractures **(ATLAS PLATE 540 #540.2).**

3. That the thin medial wall separates the orbit from the ethmoid sinuses. It also is subject to fractures.

C. Identify the following openings and foramina and learn the structures that traverse them (ATLAS PLATES 531, 532, 534):

1. **The optic canal,** located in the lesser wing of the sphenoid bone. It transmits the optic nerve and ophthalmic artery **(Figure 32-1).**

2. **The superior orbital fissure (ATLAS PLATE 532).** This lies between the greater and lesser wings of the sphenoid bone. It transmits the following **(Figure 32-1):**
   a. Oculomotor nerve
   b. Trochlear nerve

► Grant's 640
Netter's 2, 41, 79
Rohen 23, 47, 132

◄ Grant's 689, 690, 692
Netter's 41, 44, 45
Rohen 47, 130, 147

◄ Grant's 640
Netter's 2, 10, 79
Rohen 47, 134–135

► Grant's 615, 640, 643
Netter's 2, 10
Rohen 46, 47

◄ Grant's 615, 620, 621, 640
Netter's 2, 10, 79
Rohen 23, 30, 34, 47

c. Frontal, lacrimal, and nasociliary branches of the ophthalmic nerve
   d. Abducens nerve
   e. Ophthalmic veins
   f. Two small arteries: the orbital branch of the middle meningeal and a recurrent dural branch of the lacrimal
   g. Sympathetic (postganglionic) nerve fibers

3. **The inferior orbital fissure (ATLAS PLATE 514, 541).** This cleft lies between the floor (maxilla) and the lateral wall (great wing of the sphenoid bone) of the orbit. It transmits:
   a. The infraorbital branch of the maxillary nerve
   b. A small vein that interconnects the inferior ophthalmic vein with the pterygoid plexus of veins
   c. The infraorbital artery and vein
      Note: the infraorbital groove and canal are anterior extensions of the infraorbital fissure. The canal opens below the eye at the infraorbital foramen.

4. Find the **anterior and posterior ethmoidal** foramina along the suture line between the roof and medial wall of the orbit **(ATLAS PLATES 540, 541 549).** Through these foramina pass the **anterior and posterior ethmoidal** vessels and nerves, branches of the ophthalmic vessels, and nasociliary nerve.

II. The Orbit From Above (ATLAS PLATES 546–549)

Dissection of the orbit from above allows the student to study most of the important orbital structures from the

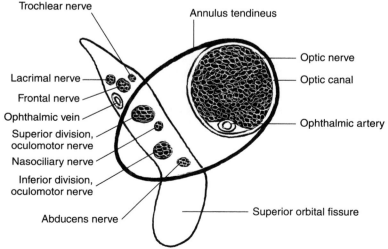

Figure 32-1. Diagram of the oval annulus tendineus, showing the structures that enter the orbit within the annulus. Note that the trochlear, lacrimal, and frontal nerves and ophthalmic vein traverse the superior orbital fissure outside the annulus.

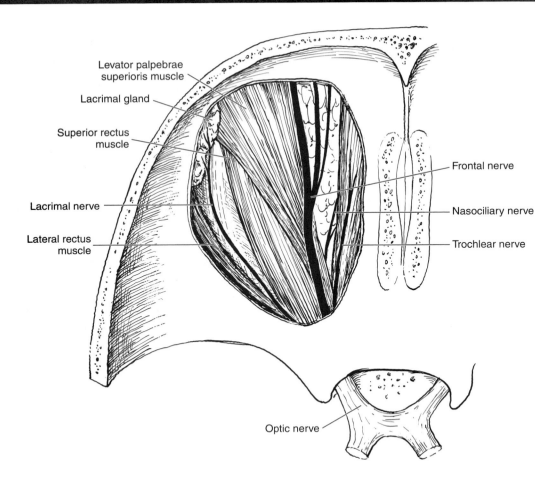

Figure 32-2. Left orbit. Dissection from above, stage I.

apex of the orbit posteriorly to the anterior end of the orbital cavity. In this dissection the muscles, vessels, and nerves are studied in dissection stages.

A. Stage I, Superior Approach (Figure 32-2). The order of structures to be seen in stage I are the **periorbita**, the **frontal nerve, supraorbital artery, lacrimal nerve and artery, trochlear nerve**, the **superior oblique muscle**, the **levator palpebrae superioris muscle**, and the **superior rectus muscle.**

◄
Grant's 642–646
Netter's 80–82
Rohen 68, 69, 72, 73, 140

Dissect either right (**ATLAS PLATE 546**) or left (**Figure 32-2**) orbit from above; the other orbit will be dissected anteriorly.

1. Strip the dura mater from the floor of the anterior cranial fossa. With mallet and chisel, break through the center of the thin orbital plate of the frontal bone. Carefully chip away the entire orbital plate piecemeal but retain the underlying periorbita (periosteum) intact. Carry this procedure anteriorly into the frontal sinus and medially into the ethmoid air cells.

►
Netter's 79, 80, 82
Rohen 135, 141

2. At the apex of the orbit, insert a probe between the lesser wing of the sphenoid bone and the periorbita through the superior orbital fissure. Carefully chip away the roof of the superior orbital fissure (i.e., the lesser wing of the sphenoid bone). Do not injure the nerves that pass through the fissure and **especially be careful NOT to destroy the delicate trochlear nerve near the medial end of the fissure.**

3. Identify the optic canal and insert a probe through it. Remove the bone that forms the roof of this canal and expose the **annulus tendinous (ATLAS PLATES 550, 551, 553).** From this tendinous ring at the apex of the orbit arise several extraocular muscles **(Figure 32-1).**

4. With the orbital plate removed and the apex of the orbit exposed, open the periorbita by severing it both longitudinally and transversely. Cut away the four flaps at the orbital margins.

5. Identify the **frontal nerve** coursing forward in the middle of the orbit lying on the superior surface of the levator palpebrae superioris muscle (**ATLAS PLATE 546**). Remove orbital fat lateral and medial to the muscle in a piecemeal manner. Follow the frontal nerve forward to its division anteriorly into the more medial **supratrochlear** and **supraorbital** branches. The supraorbital nerve further divides into medial and lateral branches.

6. Identify the **supraorbital artery** by picking away fat medial to the levator palpebrae muscle (**ATLAS PLATE 546**). The vessel eventually joins the supraorbital nerve on the surface of the muscle.

7. Pick away fat lateral to the levator palpebrae muscle. Identify the **lacrimal nerve** and tortuous **lacrimal artery.** These course anteriorly along the lateral side of the orbit to the lacrimal gland (**ATLAS PLATES 546–548**).

▶
Grant's 620, 643, 804, 805
Netter's 80, 82, 98, 115
Rohen 13, 68, 69, 135, 140
◀
Grant's 642, 644, 806
Netter's 41, 82
Rohen 69, 73, 140
◀
Grant's 605, 606, 642, 647
Netter's 81
Rohen 134
▶
Grant's 692, 694, 803–805
Netter's 77, 79, 82, 115
Rohen 140–142
◀
Grant's 642–644, 690, 807
Netter's 41, 81, 82
Rohen 68, 69, 72, 74, 136, 140, 141

8. Identify the delicate **trochlear nerve** on the dorsomedial side of the orbit. Follow it to the upper surface of the **superior oblique muscle,** which it supplies (**ATLAS PLATES 546, 547, 551**).

9. Note that the superior oblique muscle passes forward on the medial side of the orbit (**ATLAS PLATE 551**). Dissect its tendon anteriorly and then around a fibrocartilaginous loop called the **trochlea.** Cut the **frontal nerve** near the apex of the orbit and reflect its anterior end forward.

10. Clean the **levator palpebrae superioris muscle** and note that it inserts onto the upper eyelid (**ATLAS PLATES 545–547, 551**). Verify that it elevates the upper eyelid by gently pulling the muscle. Cut the muscle near its anterior end and reflect its belly posteriorly (**Figure 32-3**).

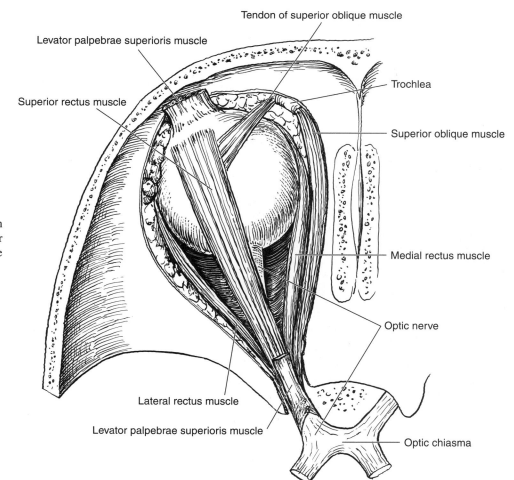

Figure 32-3. Left orbit. Dissection from above, showing the extraocular muscles following transection of the levator palpebral superioris.

Tendon of superior oblique muscle

Levator palpebrae superioris muscle

Trochlea

Superior rectus muscle

Superior oblique muscle

Medial rectus muscle

Optic nerve

Lateral rectus muscle

Levator palpebrae superioris muscle

Optic chiasma

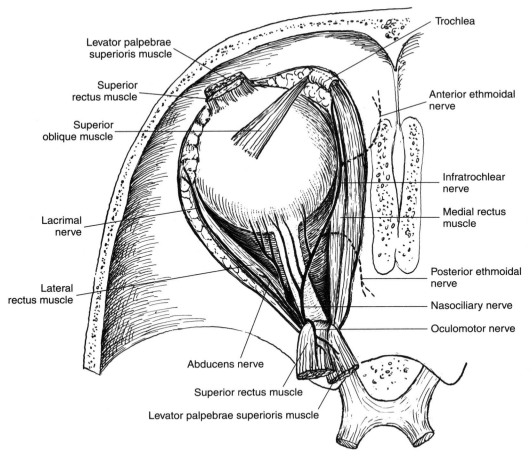

Figure 32-4. Left orbit. Dissection from above, showing the oculomotor, nasociliary, and abducent nerves. Note also the superior oblique muscle and its trochlea.

11. Clean the exposed **superior rectus muscle.** Follow the muscle anteriorly to its insertion on the upper part of the eyeball (**ATLAS PLATES 545–547, 551**). Sever the superior rectus muscle close to the eyeball and reflect it posteriorly. Note that both the superior rectus and the levator muscles are innervated by branches of the oculomotor nerve. A branch usually penetrates through the superior rectus to reach the levator (**ATLAS PLATE 547**).

B. Stage II, Superior Approach (ATLAS PLATE 547). In the second stage of dissection the order of structures to be seen is the **lateral rectus muscle, abducens nerve, nasociliary nerve, ophthalmic artery, superior ophthalmic vein, posterior and anterior ethmoid vessels and nerves, infratrochlear nerve,** and the **superior division of the oculomotor nerve.**

1. On the lateral side of the orbit, find the lacrimal nerve and artery, cut them near the apex, and

◄
Grant's 642, 645, 648, 649, 804
Netter's 79, 80, 82, 115
Rohen 68, 69, 135, 136, 140

►
Grant's 643, 646, 803–805
Netter's 81, 82
Rohen 69, 140, 141

◄
Grant's 642–644
Netter's 80–82
Rohen 140, 141

◄
Grant's 569, 572, 573, 712–714
Netter's 79–82
Rohen 69, 135, 136, 140, 141

reflect them anteriorly. Pick away the fat deep to these cut structures and expose the **lateral rectus muscle** along the lateral wall (**Figure 32-3**).

2. Gently probe the **medial surface** of the lateral rectus muscle and identify the **abducens nerve** (**ATLAS PLATES 547, 548**). It courses along the medial surface of the muscle before entering it (**Figure 32-4**).

3. Continue removing fat and expose the **optic nerve.** Find the **nasociliary nerve, ophthalmic artery,** and **superior ophthalmic vein** (**ATLAS PLATE 548**). Note that these structures **cross the superior surface of the optic nerve from lateral to medial** (**Figure 32-5**).

4. Follow the ophthalmic artery and nasociliary nerve medially and anteriorly and identify their **posterior** and **anterior ethmoidal branches.** These leave the orbit medially

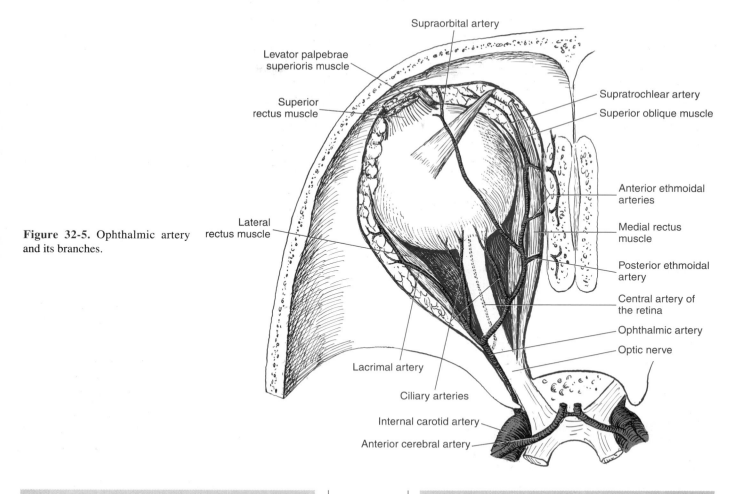

Figure 32-5. Ophthalmic artery and its branches.

through their respective foramina (**ATLAS PLATES 548, 549**).

5. Trace the nasociliary nerve anteriorly beyond the anterior ethmoid branch, where it now becomes the **infratrochlear nerve** (**ATLAS PLATE 548**). It leaves the orbit anteriorly just below the trochlea of the superior oblique muscle.

6. With the superior rectus and levator muscles reflected posteriorly, identify the **superior division of the oculomotor nerve** entering the muscles from below (**ATLAS PLATE 547**). Locate the main trunk of this nerve at the apex of the orbit between the optic nerve and the lateral rectus muscle (**ATLAS PLATE 549**).

C. Stage III, Superior Approach (**ATLAS PLATE 548**). In the third stage of dissection the order of structures to be seen is the **optic nerve, long ciliary nerves** and **arteries, ciliary ganglion,** and **short ciliary nerves and arteries.**

1. Expose the **optic nerve** completely from the optic canal to the eyeball. Note that it has

◄
Grant's 643, 807
Netter's 41, 81, 82
Rohen 141

◄
Grant's 642, 643
Netter's 41, 82

◄
Grant's 642, 644,
646, 804
Netter's 81, 82,
115, 125, 126
Rohen 68, 69, 72,
140, 141

►
Grant's 642–644,
804
Netter's 41, 82,
115, 125, 126
Rohen 68, 69, 72,
73, 83, 136, 141

◄
Grant's 642–644,
647
Netter's 81, 82
Rohen 68, 69, 72,
134, 136, 141

numerous **short** and **long ciliary vessels and nerves** coursing with it. Preserve these delicate structures.

2. **From the nasociliary nerve,** find two delicate branches that course along the optic nerve and reach the eyeball, one on the medial side of the nerve and the other above it. These are the **long ciliary nerves** (**ATLAS PLATE 548**). **Note:** they are accompanied by delicate and tortuous **long ciliary arteries.**

3. To find the ciliary ganglion, stroke the fatty tissue lateral to the optic nerve near the apex of the orbit. The ganglion is the size of a large pinhead and has delicate branches attached to it (**ATLAS PLATE 548**).

4. Identify several **short ciliary nerves from the ganglion.** They accompany **short ciliary arteries** along the optic nerve to the eyeball. Know that:
   a. The **long** ciliary nerves carry
      1) **Sensory fibers** from the **ciliary body, iris, and cornea**

  2) Postganglionic sympathetic fibers to the **dilator of the pupil**
  b. The **short** ciliary nerves carry
  1) Sensory fibers from the sclera and other eyeball structures
  2) Postganglionic sympathetic fibers to blood vessels that supply the eyeball
  3) Postganglionic parasympathetic fibers to the ciliaris muscle and sphincter of the pupil

D. Stage IV, Superior Approach (ATLAS PLATE 549). In the fourth stage of dissection the order of structures to be seen is the **optic nerve** and **dural sheath, central retinal artery,** insertion of the **inferior oblique muscle, inferior rectus muscle, medial rectus muscle, inferior division of the oculomotor nerve,** and the **infraorbital nerve and artery.**

  1. Open the apex of the orbit and expose the optic nerve. Cut the dural sheath around the optic nerve longitudinally from the apex to the eyeball. Sever the optic nerve intradurally, immediately behind the eyeball. Lift the posterior stump **(Figure 32-7)** and identify the **central artery.** It is the small darkened site in the center of the cut nerve **(ATLAS PLATES 549, 556).**

▶ Grant's 647, 650, 651
Netter's 81
Rohen 135, 136

◀ Grant's 643–651, 803–805
Netter's 80–82, 115
Rohen 68, 135, 136, 141

▶ Grant's 644, 803–805
Netter's 41, 115
Rohen 141

◀ Grant's 644, 647, 650, 651
Netter's 81, 83, 86
Rohen 133, 134

  2. Try to find the origin of the central retinal artery from the ophthalmic artery inferior to the optic nerve. Note that it pierces the dural sheath and enters the nerve about 1.25 cm behind the eyeball.

  3. Remove the optic nerve and its sheath completely. Elevate the posterior part of the eyeball and identify the insertions of the **superior and inferior oblique muscles (Figure 32-7).** Find the **inferior rectus muscle** near the floor of the orbit. On the medial side of the orbit identify the **medial rectus muscle** inferior to the superior oblique muscle **(Figure 32-7).**

  4. Above the inferior rectus muscle identify the **inferior division of the oculomotor nerve.** It supplies the inferior oblique and the medial and inferior rectus muscles **(ATLAS PLATE 549).**

  5. Pierce the periorbita and open the infraorbital canal on the lateral side of the floor of the orbit, inferior to the lateral rectus muscle. It may be necessary to probe through some thin bone to find the **infraorbital nerve** (V2) and the **infraorbital artery** that course along this canal to the infraorbital foramen on the face **(ATLAS PLATE 549).**

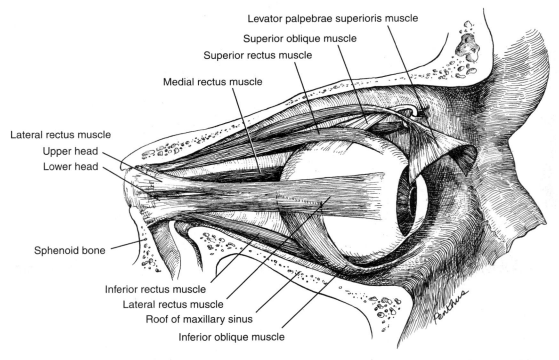

Figure 32-6. Muscles of the right orbit, lateral view. (From Clemente CD. Gray's Anatomy. 30th American Edition. Philadephia: Lea and Febiger, 1985.)

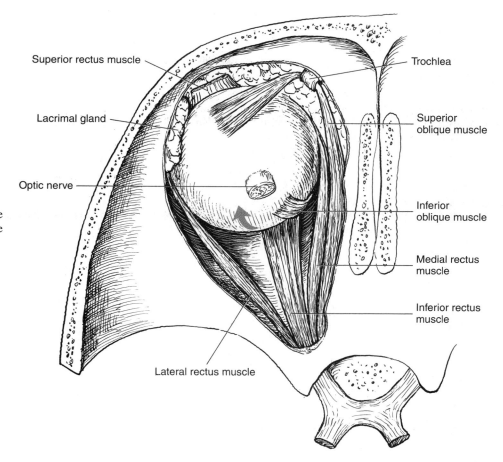

Superior rectus muscle

Trochlea

Lacrimal gland

Superior oblique muscle

Optic nerve

Inferior oblique muscle

Medial rectus muscle

Inferior rectus muscle

Lateral rectus muscle

Figure 32-7. Muscles of the orbit with the optic nerve cut and the posterior pole of the eyeball elevated.

III. The Orbit From the Anterior Approach (ATLAS PLATES 539, 542–545)

Structures in the orbit are surgically approached from an anterior direction. The structures to be seen in this anterior dissection include the **palpebral ligaments, orbital septum** and **tarsal plates; conjunctiva,** insertion of the **levator palpebrae superioris, bulbar fascia** and **suspensory** and **check ligaments; trochlea** of the **superior oblique muscle,** the **lacrimal gland, lacrimal canaliculi, lacrimal sac;** the **insertions of the four rectus muscles,** and the **inferior oblique muscle.**

A. Palpebral Ligaments, Orbital Septum, and Tarsal Plates. The palpebral and orbital parts of the orbicularis oculi muscle were dissected with other structures of the superficial face. Many fibers of the orbicularis oculi muscle attach to the **medial** and **lateral palpebral ligaments** (ATLAS PLATE 542).

Deep to the orbicularis oculi muscle is the **orbital septum.** This thin fibrous membrane attaches to the margin of the orbit, where it is continuous with the peri-

◄
Grant's 604, 640, 641
Netter's 77–80
Rohen 142

►
Grant's 604, 645
Netter's 77
Rohen 132, 142

►
Grant's 604, 645
Netter's 77
Rohen 142

◄
Grant's 604
Netter's 77
Rohen 142

►
Grant's 604
Netter's 77
Rohen 142

◄
Grant's 604, 645
Netter's 77

orbita (**ATLAS PLATE 542 #542.1**). It is perforated by nerves and vessels that emerge from the orbital cavity above the eye to supply the forehead, scalp, and nose (supraorbital, supratrochlear, infratrochlear, and lacrimal).

The **tarsal plates** are thin condensations of fibrous connective tissue located in each eyelid to strengthen their structure (**ATLAS PLATE 542**). The upper plate is semioval, narrow at the sides, and 1 cm high. The lower plate is smaller, narrower, and 0.5 cm high.

1. Pick away the fibers of the orbital and palpebral parts of the orbicularis oculi muscle. Do not destroy the underlying **orbital septum** or the vessels and nerves that perforate the septum (**ATLAS PLATE 542 #542.1**).

2. Identify the strong **medial,** and the more deeply placed **lateral, palpebral ligaments** located at the medial and lateral angles of the orbit. Observe that many of the fibers of the orbicularis oculi muscle attach to the medial ligament. Note also that the tarsal plates are anchored to these ligaments.

3. Dissect the upper eyelid and identify its **tarsal plate** (**ATLAS PLATE 542**). Note that it is larger than the tarsus of the lower lid. Confirm that the tarsal plates attach to the palpebral ligaments.

B. Conjunctiva, Insertion of the Levator Palpebrae Superioris, Bulbar Fascia, Suspensory and **Check Ligaments.** The conjunctiva is a transparent membrane lining the inner surface of each eyelid (palpebral part). It is then reflected over the anterior surface of the sclera and cornea (ocular part). The line of reflection between palpebral and ocular parts is called the **superior fornix** for the upper eyelid and the **inferior fornix** for the lower eyelid (**ATLAS PLATE 538**).

The tendon of the levator palpebrae superioris expands into a wide aponeurosis anteriorly, and it attaches to the upper eyelid. Its insertion splits into three layers: a **superficial layer** that blends into the dermis of the upper eyelid and the orbital septum; a **middle layer** that includes a smooth muscle (**superior tarsal muscle**) and attaches to the upper margin of the superior tarsus; and a **deep layer** that attaches to the superior fornix of the conjunctiva (**ATLAS PLATE 545 #545.1, Figure 32-8**).

▶
Netter's 79

◀
Grant's 604, 645
Netter's 77
Rohen 121, 132, 142

◀
Grant's 640, 641, 645
Netter's 77, 79
Rohen 132, 133, 142

◀
Grant's 645
Netter's 77

▶
Grant's 640, 641, 645
Netter's 77, 79
Rohen 132, 133

The **bulbar fascia** (Tenon's capsule) is a thin, fibrous sheath that surrounds the posterior five-sixths of the eyeball (**ATLAS PLATES 545 #545.1, 553 #553.2**). It extends from the optic disc posteriorly to the cornea anteriorly. The bulbar fascia thickens anteriorly and forms a sling or hammock inferiorly, called the **suspensory ligament** (of Lockwood), on which the eyeball rests. At both its medial and lateral sides the suspensory ligament forms the **medial** and **lateral check ligaments.** These attach to the lacrimal bone medially and the zygomatic bone laterally.

The bulbar fascia is pierced posteriorly by the optic nerve and the ciliary vessels and nerves (**ATLAS PLATE 553 #553.2**). The tendons of the extraocular muscles also pierce this fascia to insert onto the underlying sclera. A potential space between the sheath and the eyeball allows freedom of movement of the eyeball when the muscles contract.

1. Probe the inner surface of the eyelids and observe the glistening layer of **palpebral conjunctiva** that covers it. Confirm that the conjunctiva is continuous at the fornices with the **ocular conjunctiva** covering the eyeball. Note that over the sclera the conjunctiva is **loosely**

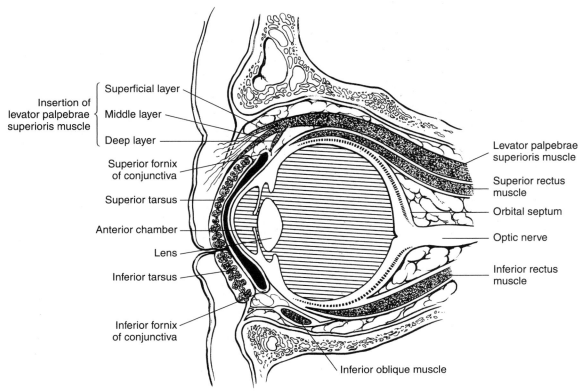

Figure 32-8. Sagittal section of the orbit, showing the insertion of the levator palpebral superioris.

attached to the eyeball. However, it becomes **firmly adherent** to the cornea where it is continuous with the corneal epithelium.

2. Dissect the insertion of the **levator palpebrae superioris** into the upper eyelid (**ATLAS PLATES 545 #545.1, 551 #551.1**). Probe the upper margin of the superior tarsus and note the tendinous fibers of the levator as they descend to attach onto the tarsus (**Figure 32-8**). Place your probe behind the tendon and note that it expands from its narrow muscular belly as it attaches to the tarsus.

3. Expose the anterior surface of the eyeball by cutting through the lateral junction of the eyelids to the bony margin of the orbit. Cut away the upper eyelid. Start laterally and continue medially only to the upper border of the triangular caruncula. Similarly, cut away the lower eyelid to the lower border of the caruncula. Save the **caruncula** and the **lacrimal canaliculi** at the medial canthus. **DO NOT CUT AWAY THE MOST MEDIAL PARTS OF THE EYELIDS (ATLAS PLATES 538, 543, 544).**

4. With the anterior eyeball exposed, pick up the loosely attached conjunctiva over the sclera.

▶
Grant's 640, 645
Netter's 77, 79
Rohen 135, 136

◀
Grant's 604, 644, 645, 804
Netter's 77, 80, 115
Rohen 142

▶
Grant's 643–645, 648, 649
Netter's 79, 80, 82, 115
Rohen 68, 135

◀
Grant's 604, 640
Netter's 77, 79
Rohen 142

With scissors, cut the conjunctiva and the bulbar fascia by making a circular incision about 3 to 5 mm posterior to the sclerocorneal junction. The tendons of the four rectus muscles and two oblique muscles need to penetrate this bulbar fascia to insert onto the sclera (**ATLAS PLATES 545, 553, #553.2**).

C. **Insertions of extraocular muscles (Figures 32-6, 32-9, 32-11) and the Lacrimal Apparatus**

1. **Insertions of extraocular muscles.** The **four rectus muscles** are inserted onto the sclera 0.5 cm behind the cornea. The tendons of the medial and lateral rectus muscles attach slightly more anteriorly than those of the superior and inferior rectus muscles (**Figure 32-10**). In contrast, both oblique muscles insert more posteriorly (**ATLAS PLATE 552**).

Beyond the trochlea, the tendon of the **superior oblique muscle** turns posterolaterally to insert on the **upper** lateral quadrant of the posterior half of the eyeball. The **inferior oblique** muscle arises on the orbital surface of the maxilla. It courses laterally below the inferior rectus in the floor of the orbit and inserts on the **lower** lateral quadrant of the posterior half of the eyeball (**Figure 32-11**).

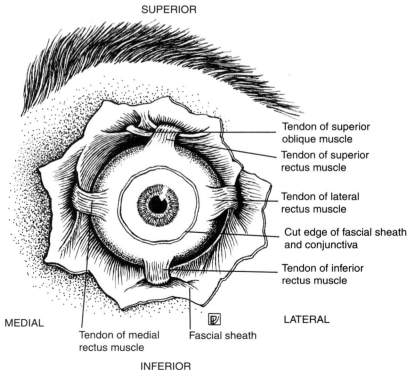

Figure 32-9. Anterior view of the left orbit showing the insertions onto the sclera of the tendons of the four rectus muscles.

RIGHT EYE

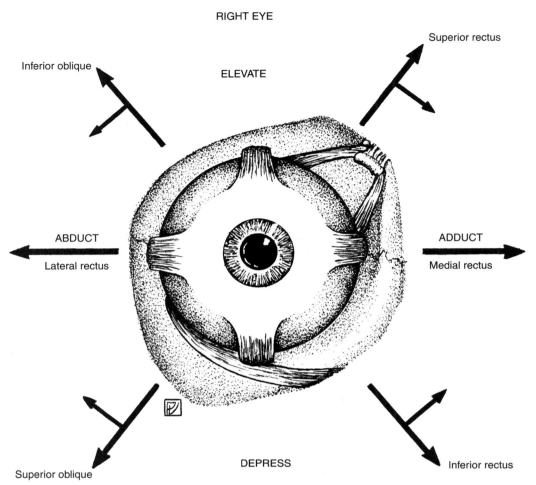

Figure 32-10. Right eye, showing the extraocular muscles from an anterior view of the orbit. Arrows indicate the directions of movements of the extraocular muscles.

To see the insertions of the four rectus muscles from this anterior view, it is best to identify their tendons as they penetrate the bulbar fascia just before reaching the sclera of the eyeball. The insertions of the oblique muscles are best seen from the posterior direction.

◄
Grant's 642, 643, 645, 647, 648
Netter's 80
Rohen 135, 136

2. **Lacrimal apparatus.** The lacrimal apparatus consists of the lacrimal gland, lacrimal canaliculi, lacrimal sac, and nasolacrimal duct (**Figure 32-12**).

►
Grant's 641
Netter's 77, 78
Rohen 142

The **lacrimal gland** consists of orbital and palpebral parts (**ATLAS PLATE 542**). The **orbital part** is larger and lies within a shallow fossa of the frontal bone at the upper lateral aspect of the orbit. The smaller **palpebral part** (about one-third the size) is continuous with the posterior portion of the orbital part. It extends laterally around the free edge of the aponeurosis of the levator muscle to lie within the upper eyelid. The entire gland has 12 to 15 delicate ducts

◄
Grant's 641–644
Netter's 78, 82
Rohen 68, 72, 83, 142

►
Grant's 641
Netter's 78
Rohen 142

that open onto the conjunctiva along the lateral aspect of its superior fornix.

Lacrimal fluid courses downward and medially over the anterior surface of the eyeball and enters two small openings, one in each eyelid, called **puncta lacrimali.** These external openings of two delicate ducts are called the **lacrimal canaliculi,** which are each 1 cm long and lead to a **lacrimal sac (Figure 32-12)**. The lacrimal sac is the upper closed end of the **nasolacrimal duct.** When an excess of lacrimal fluid is produced (as during crying) and cannot be accommodated by the duct system, tears overflow the lower eyelid.

The nasolacrimal duct is a membranous canal between the lacrimal sac and the nasal cavity. It lies within an osseous canal and opens onto the inferior meatus in the lateral wall of the nasal cavity (**ATLAS PLATE 544**).

Initially, visualize the orbital part of the lacrimal gland from above and then the orbital and palpebral parts anteriorly. From anterior, open the upper lateral

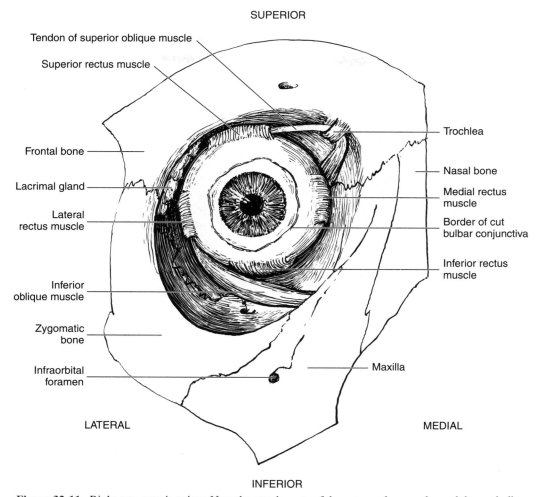

SUPERIOR

Tendon of superior oblique muscle

Superior rectus muscle

Frontal bone

Lacrimal gland

Lateral
rectus muscle

Inferior
oblique muscle

Zygomatic
bone

Infraorbital
foramen

Trochlea

Nasal bone

Medial rectus
muscle

Border of cut
bulbar conjunctiva

Inferior rectus
muscle

Maxilla

LATERAL

MEDIAL

INFERIOR

Figure 32-11. Right eye, anterior view. Note the attachments of the extraocular muscles and the cut bulbar conjunctiva.

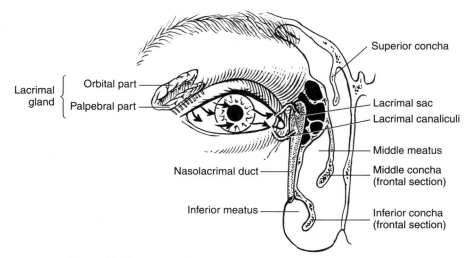

Lacrimal
gland { Orbital part
Palpebral part

Superior concha

Lacrimal sac
Lacrimal canaliculi

Nasolacrimal duct

Middle meatus

Middle concha
(frontal section)

Inferior meatus

Inferior concha
(frontal section)

Figure 32-12. Lacrimal gland and lacrimal apparatus, seen anteriorly.

part of the orbital septum and expose the orbital part of the lacrimal gland and, slightly inferior, the palpebral part of the gland (**ATLAS PLATE 542 #542.1**).

At the medial angle of the eye identify the curved fold of conjunctiva called the **plica semilunaris** (**ATLAS PLATE 538**). Medial to the plica find the small conical body (red in the living eye) called the **lacrimal caruncle.** It contains both sweat and sebaceous glands.

Evert the medial ends of each eyelid, above and below the caruncle. On the inner surface of each lid find a small papilla on which is located a minute opening called the **lacrimal punctum** (**ATLAS PLATE 544**). If a delicate wire or bristle is available, penetrate each of the two punctae and thereby traverse the upper and lower **lacrimal canaliculi** that course medially into the **lacrimal sec.** Dissect behind the medial palpebral ligament to find the lacrimal sac. Finally, open the lacrimal sac and insert a probe down the **nasolacrimal duct** into the nasal cavity (**Figure 32-12**).

◄
Grant's 641
Netter's 77, 78
Rohen 142

Clinical Relevance

Orbital tumors. Malignant tumors of the mucosa in the sphenoid and ethmoid sinuses can spread into the orbit and exert pressure on the optic nerve and other orbital structures. These tumors are often highly malignant and result in a bulging of the eyeball (exophthalmos). Surgery can for a time relieve the bulging, but usually the prognosis is not good.

"Blowout fractures" of the orbit. Although the bones that form the anterior rim of the orbit are quite strong, the inferior and medial walls within the orbital cavity are made of relatively thin bone. Thus, the orbital floor is especially vulnerable, and direct trauma anteriorly can fracture the floor of the orbit, causing orbital fat and other structures to "blow out" into the maxillary sinus inferiorly. The inferior rectus muscle may become entrapped as well, thereby limiting upper gaze. Additionally, the infraorbital nerve may be injured resulting in the loss of sensation to the upper lip and cheek.

"Bloodshot" eyes. When the blood vessels over the anterior aspect of the eyeball become hyperemic and congested, the condition is often called "bloodshot" eyes. This can be caused by smoke or smog in the atmosphere or from dust or any other environmental irritant. Normally the conjunctiva is clear and colorless.

Detachment of the retina. When the retina becomes detached, it occurs between the pigmented layer of the retina (which is firmly fused to the choroid [uvea]) and the neural layer. Fluid often accumulates between the neural and pigmented layers. This complication may develop slowly and not be fully realized for days after the trauma that may have initiated the process. Reattachment is possible today by the use of laser therapy.

Pupillary light reflex. This reflex results in a constriction of the pupil when the retina is exposed directly to a bright light. Afferent impulses from the retina course along the optic nerve, while the motor pathway courses from the parasympathetic Edinger-Westphal nucleus to the ciliary ganglion. Here postganglionic fibers course forward to stimulate the constrictor of the pupil in the iris. Both pupils constrict even though only one retina is stimulated. This is called the consensual light reflex.

Injury to nerves of the orbit. Important nerves to structures around the eye can alter the efficiency of ocular function. The **facial nerve** supplies the orbicularis oculi muscle. Denervation of this muscle results in an inability to close the eyelid completely, which can result in a drooping of the lower lid and a drying of the conjunctiva. The **oculomotor nerve** supplies the levator palpebrae superioris (along with other extraocular muscles). Denervation of the levator may occur from head injury, and this results in a drooping of the upper eyelid (ptosis) in addition to ophthalmoplegia. A lesion along the **sympathetic pathway** to the orbit denervates the superior tarsal muscle in the insertion of the levator palpebrae superioris. This results in ptosis of the upper lid along with constriction of the pupil (Horner's syndrome).

Glaucoma. In this condition, increased intraocular pressure results from a diminished reabsorption of aqueous humor. This causes visual impairment and can even result in blindness from compression of the innermost layer of the eyeball, the visual retina. To save vision in these cases it is imperative to reduce aqueous humor production.

Cataracts. As people age the lens of the eye often becomes opaque, which results in a loss of transparency through the lens. The opaque regions are called cataracts. In recent years ophthalmologists have been able to excise these aged lenses and replace them with newly manufactured clear lenses, a procedure that greatly increases vision in these patients.

"Black eye." Injury to the orbital region from anterior trauma, such as that often encountered in boxing, will injure the skin above or below the orbit. This allows blood to accumulate in the subcutaneous tissue and causes the eyelids and the anterior periorbital region to become edematous and discolored.

Accommodation reflex. Accommodation is a reflexive constriction of the pupil when a person tries to focus on a nearby object after having focused on an object in the distance. This reflex involves parasympathetic fibers that, at the same time, constrict the pupil and stimulate the ciliary muscle fibers, causing a relaxation of the suspensory ligaments of the lens. This results in a more rounded lens required for nearby focusing.

Papilledema. This condition is often the result of increased intracranial pressure and is visualized with an ophthalmoscope as a swelling at the optic disc. The bulging at the disc is accompanied by an increase in CSF pressure around the optic nerve at the back of the eyeball. Congestion in the central retinal vessels can deprive the retina of its arterial supply or its venous drainage.

Inflammation of the tarsal glands. This condition manifests either as cysts of sebaceous glands (called chalasia) or as an inflammation and obstruction of ducts of the ciliary meibomian glands in the eyelid (called styes). The latter are painful, whereas the former can irritate the eyeball when the person blinks. This is especially true if the cyst is on the inner surface of the eyelid and protrudes inwardly.

Corneal reflex. This reflex is elicited by stroking the surface of the cornea with a delicate wisp of cotton. Normally the patient will blink, but a lack of blinking indicates either a lesion of the ophthalmic division of the trigeminal nerve or the inability to close the eye (facial nerve supply to the orbicularis oculi muscle). Physicians must also be certain that the patient is not wearing contact lenses.

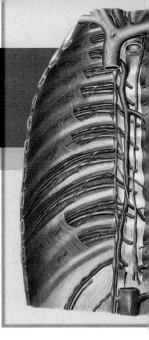

DISSECTION #33

Craniovertebral Joints and Prevertebral Region

OBJECTIVES

1 Examine the base of the occipital bone and study the anatomy of the atlas and axis.

2 Dissect the median and lateral atlantoaxial joints and the atlantooccipital joints and their ligaments.

3 Disarticulate the atlantooccipital joints and separate the head and attached pharynx and larynx anteriorly from the vertebral column along the prevertebral fascial plane.

4 Study the prevertebral muscles and other structures on the anterior aspect of the vertebral column.

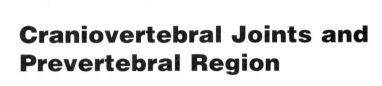

Atlas Key:

Clemente Atlas, 5th Edition = Atlas Plate #

Grant's Atlas, 11th Edition = Grant's Page #

Netter's Atlas, 3rd Edition = Netter's Plate #

Rohen Atlas, 6th Edition = Rohen Page #

By studying the craniovertebral joints and then disarticulating the atlantoaxial joints, the head and attached pharynx and larynx can be separated from the vertebral column along the prevertebral fascial plane. This procedure is necessary to study the pharynx, which will be opened posteriorly in the next dissection.

I. Basilar Part of the Occipital Bone; the Atlas and Axis

The basilar part of the occipital bone rests on the first cervical vertebra, the **atlas,** at the atlantooccipital joints.

►
Grant's 594, 595
Netter's 8, 10
Rohen 25, 27, 32, 33
◄
Grant's 280, 282–285
Netter's 8, 12, 15, 16, 146
Rohen 4, 32, 33, 200

The second cervical vertebra, the **axis,** articulates superiorly with the atlas by way of the median and lateral atlantoaxial joint (**ATLAS PLATE 343 #343.1 and #343.2**). The reciprocal shapes of the occipital condyles and the superior articular facets of the atlas allow the atlantooccipital joints flexion and extension of the head (**as in nodding the head while saying "yes"**) and some lateral bending of the head. Movement at the median and lateral atlantoaxial joints occurs simultaneously and consists of rotation of the atlas and the attached skull upon the axis (**as in shaking the head while saying "no"**).

On a skeleton study the bony structures that form the craniovertebral joints.

A. Occipital Bone (ATLAS PLATE 516 #516.2). Identify the following on the inferior aspect of the occipital bone:

1. The **foramen magnum,** through which the brainstem is continuous with the spinal cord. It also transmits the **vertebral arteries** from the neck and the **spinal parts of the accessory nerves.**

2. The **occipital condyles** located at the sides of the foramen magnum. Note that they are oval, are convex from side to side, and articulate with the atlas.

B. The Atlas. Note that the atlas is a ring of bone with enlarged lateral masses. Identify (**see ATLAS PLATE 342 #342.1 and #342.2**):

1. The curved **anterior arch** with its **anterior tubercle** externally and the **fovea** (or facet) for the **dens of the axis** internally.

2. The larger posterior arch, its posterior tubercle, and the groove for the vertebral artery along its superior surface.

3. The lateral masses of the atlas. Each contains a concave superior articular facet that forms a joint with the corresponding occipital condyle. Note also the flatter inferior articular facets that form lateral atlantoaxial joints with the 2nd cervical vertebra.

4. The transverse processes, each of which contains the transverse foramen that transmits a vertebral artery.

C. The Axis. This 2nd cervical vertebra is the pivot on which the atlas and skull rotate.

1. Identify the body and its unique vertical projection, the **odontoid process** or **dens** (**see ATLAS PLATE 342 #342.3 and 342.4**).

  a. Note that the dens represents the displaced body of the atlas and that it fits superiorly behind the anterior arch of the atlas.

  b. Observe a groove posteriorly on the dens for the **transverse ligament of the atlas**. Also note a small articular facet anteriorly, where it articulates with the anterior atlantal arch (**ATLAS PLATE 344 #344.4**).

  c. Realize that superiorly the dens is also held in position by the **apical and alar ligaments** that attach it to the occipital bone. These limit rotation of the head (**ATLAS PLATE 344 #344.3**).

2. Find the two large oval **superior articular facets** located lateral to the dens. These articulate with the inferior articular surfaces of the atlas. Also identify the two **inferior articular facets** on the inferior surface of the dorsal laminae. These articulate with the 3rd cervical vertebra (**ATLAS PLATE 343 #343.4**).

3. Examine the small transverse processes, each containing its transverse foramen that transmits the vertebral artery (**ATLAS PLATE 342 #342.3**).

◄ Grant's 282–285, 618
Netter's 15, 17, 18, 146
Rohen 188, 200

► Grant's 282, 283, 285, 320, 321
Netter's 18
Rohen 165, 200, 202

► Grant's 320, 321
Netter's 18
Rohen 200, 202

◄ Grant's 282–285, 320, 321
Netter's 15, 18, 146
Rohen 193, 200, 202, 369

► Grant's 320, 321
Netter's 18
Rohen 200

◄ Grant's 282–285
Netter's 15
Rohen 200, 202

4. Note that the large spinous process usually is bifid.

II. Median and Lateral Atlantoaxial Joints; Atlantooccipital Joints

A. The median atlantoaxial joint. The median atlantoaxial joint is a pivot joint in which the dens of the axis articulates anteriorly with the anterior arch of the atlas and posteriorly with the transverse ligament of the atlas (**ATLAS PLATE 344 #344.4**). It can be considered a double joint because there are two separate synovial cavities involved. The anterior surface of the dens and the posterior surface of the anterior arch of the atlas are surrounded by a small fibrous capsule lined on its inner surface by a synovial membrane (**ATLAS PLATE 345 #345.1**). Similarly, the posterior surface of the dens is separated from the transverse ligament of the atlas by a slightly larger synovial cavity.

The ligaments related to the median atlantoaxial joint include:

1. Tectorial membrane. This strong, longitudinally oriented band within the vertebral canal is the superior extension of the posterior longitudinal ligament of the vertebral column (**Figure 33-1**).

2. Transverse ligament of the atlas. This strong ligament attaches to the medial surface of the lateral mass of the atlas on both sides. It becomes broader in the midline as it crosses the posterior surface of the dens. Extending both superiorly to the basilar part of the occipital bone and inferiorly to the body of the axis by longitudinal bands, it resembles a cross. Thus, the entire structure is called the **cruciform ligament of the atlas** (**ATLAS PLATE 344 #344.2**).

3. Alar ligaments. These two powerful ligaments attach the sides of the upper part of the dens to the medial sides of the condyles of the occipital bone. They diverge superiorly and laterally and secure the skull to the axis, and they limit rotation of the head (**ATLAS PLATE 344 #344.3**).

4. Apical ligament of the dens. This thin, rather weak bond stretches from the apex of the dens to the anterior margin of the occipital bone (**Figure 33-3**).

Place the cadaver in the prone (face down) position and, in the suboccipital region, sever any remnants of skin and fascia that may still be connecting the posterior skull and the posterior and lateral neck regions. Cut and reflect downward all muscles that attach the posterior and lateral aspects of the skull to the vertebral column. These include

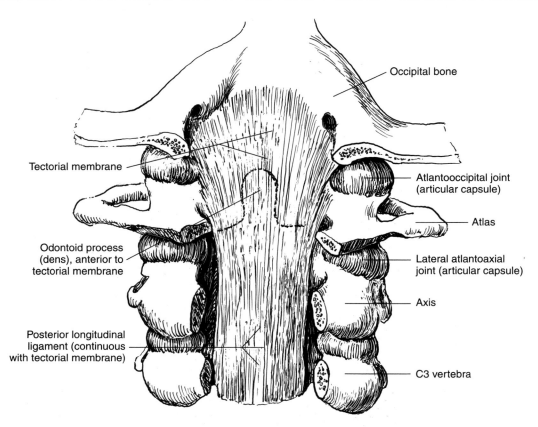

Occipital bone

Tectorial membrane

Atlantooccipital joint
(articular capsule)

Atlas

Odontoid process
(dens), anterior to
tectorial membrane

Lateral atlantoaxial
joint (articular capsule)

Axis

Posterior longitudinal
ligament (continuous
with tectorial membrane)

C3 vertebra

Figure 33-1. Tectorial membrane and posterior longitudinal ligament (posterior view).

the trapezius, splenius capitis, semispinalis capitis, and longissimus capitis (**ATLAS PLATES 328, 330–333**).

Expose the posterior atlantooccipital region by removing the following suboccipital muscles (**see ATLAS PLATES 340, 341**): rectus capitis posterior major and minor and the obliquus capitis superior and inferior. (Some of these may already have been detached when the wedge of the occipital bone was removed.)

Identify the **vertebral arteries** and remove the posterior atlantooccipital membrane that these vessels pierce (**ATLAS PLATE 490 #490.1**). With a pair of bone cutters, resect the posterior arch of the atlas and the laminae and spinous process of the axis to expose the central canal of the vertebral column and the dura mater surrounding the spinal cord.

Identify the origin of the **spinal part of the accessory nerve** (**ATLAS PLATE 357 #357.2**). Open the dura mater, cut the roots of the upper two cervical nerves, and sever the spinal cord at the level of the 3rd cervical vertebra. Remove the cut cord and its surrounding dura mater to expose the **tectorial membrane** which covers the dens and the body of the axis (**ATLAS PLATE 344 #344.1, Figure 33-1**). Note that this glistening

▶
Grant's 320, 321
Netter's 18
Rohen 200, 202

◀
Grant's 320, 321
Netter's 17, 18
Rohen 200, 202

◀
Grant's 318, 794, 795, 820
Netter's 18, 121
Rohen 67, 73, 75, 163

▶
Grant's 285, 320, 618
Netter's 17, 18
Rohen 200, 202

membrane is the superior extension of the posterior longitudinal ligament.

Carefully cut through the tectorial membrane over the dens and reflect the cut ends to expose the **cruciform ligament.** Define the transverse part of the cruciform ligament, and clean the superior and inferior longitudinal extensions (**Figure 33-2**).

Remove the upper extension of the cruciform ligament. This exposes the **apical ligament of the dens** and the two strong **alar ligaments** (check ligaments). These extend superiorly and laterally from the sides of the dens to the occipital bone (**Figure 33-3**).

Cut through the apical ligament of the dens and the alar ligaments and note that the head can now be rotated around the odontoid process more easily.

B. **Lateral atlantoaxial joints.** At these two synovial joints the inferior articular facets of the atlas articulate with the superior articular facets of the axis. Classified as plane joints, they are surrounded by thin, rather loose fibrous capsules. The joints are strengthened posteromedially by two **accessory atlantoaxial ligaments,** one on each side. These attach superiorly to the lateral mass of the atlas and inferiorly to the sides of the dens near its base (**Figure 33-2**).

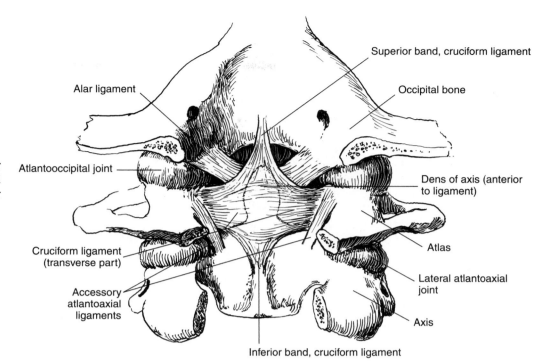

Figure 33-2. Cruciform and alar ligaments at the atlantooccipital and atlantoaxial joints (posterior view).

Superior band, cruciform ligament

Occipital bone

Alar ligament

Atlantooccipital joint

Dens of axis (anterior to ligament)

Atlas

Cruciform ligament (transverse part)

Lateral atlantoaxial joint

Accessory atlantoaxial ligaments

Axis

Inferior band, cruciform ligament

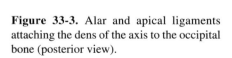

Some fibers of the accessory atlantoaxial ligaments may extend superiorly beyond the lateral mass of the atlas and attach to the occipital bone along the margin of the foramen magnum. Sever these extensions to the occipital bone if they occur in your cadaver.

◄
Grant's 318, 320, 321, 618
Netter's 17, 18, 59–61
Rohen 200, 202

C. The Atlantooccipital Joints. The articulation between the occipital bone and the atlas consists of

two synovial joints, one on each side. In these, the condyles of the occipital bone fit within the superior articular facets on the lateral masses of the atlas (**ATLAS PLATE 343 #343.3 and #342.4**). These joints, surrounded by loose **fibrous capsules** and the **anterior and posterior atlantooccipital membranes,** allow flexion and extension and some side-to-side bending of the head, but not head rotation. Maintaining the head on the vertebral column does

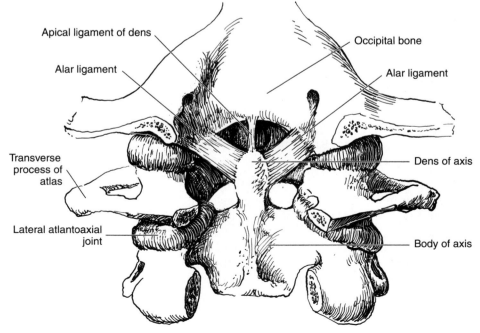

Figure 33-3. Alar and apical ligaments attaching the dens of the axis to the occipital bone (posterior view).

Apical ligament of dens

Occipital bone

Alar ligament

Alar ligament

Transverse process of atlas

Dens of axis

Lateral atlantoaxial joint

Body of axis

not depend on the fibrous capsules or the atlantooccipital membranes around this joint. Stability depends on the alar and cruciform ligaments and the tectorial membrane, which bind the occipital bone and atlas to the axis.

Sever the anterior atlantooccipital membrane and be certain that no structures remain attached to the foramen magnum. Sever the capsules surrounding the atlantooccipital joints. Disarticulate these joints by prying between the bones with a chisel, and enlarge the space between the articular surfaces as much as possible. **Turn the cadaver over to the supine position (face up) to approach the joint anteriorly.**

III. Separation of the Head and Cervical Viscera From the Vertebral Column

The next step in this dissection is to sever any remaining attachments of the vertebral column to the skull. This includes muscles and any other structures in the anterior and lateral vertebral regions.

Cut and reflect the two sternocleidomastoid muscles close to the skull. Manually separate the viscera of the neck (larynx–trachea, pharynx–esophagus, large vessels, and cranial nerves) from the deep back muscles and vertebral column. Do this from the base of the skull to the thorax along the prevertebral fascial plane behind the pharynx and esophagus.

Identify and dissect the **sympathetic trunk** as it extends upward to the large **superior cervical ganglion** within the prevertebral fascial layer (**ATLAS PLATE 589**). Feel for the transverse processes and anterior arch of the atlas superiorly, and cut the **rectus capitis lateralis** muscles on both sides between the atlas and the occipital bone. Anteriorly, cut both **longus capitis** and **rectus capitis anterior muscles** just below the occipital bone (**ATLAS PLATE 488**).

Identify again the atlantooccipital joints by bending the head from side to side. Sever any remaining attachments between the articular surfaces. You should now be able to pull the head, cervical viscera, large cervical vessels, and cranial nerves anteriorly away from the vertebral column along the prevertebral fascial plane. Leave the sympathetic trunk and cervical nerve roots behind with the prevertebral muscles.

▶
Grant's 758,
760–762
Netter's 26, 28
Rohen 184, 185

▶
Grant's 761
Netter's 26

◀
Grant's 751, 754,
758, 761
Netter's 26, 64–67
Rohen 156, 165,
185

▶
Grant's 733, 758,
761, 762
Netter's 26, 28
Rohen 184–186
◀
Grant's 754, 758,
760, 761, 768, 769
Netter's 26, 124,
125
Rohen 167, 185

◀
Grant's 761, 766,
768
Netter's 26, 64
Rohen 166, 167

▶
Grant's 760–762
Netter's 67, 124,
125
Rohen 184, 185

IV. The Prevertebral Region

The prevertebral region contains muscles that flex the head and neck at the atlantooccipital joints and at the cervical intervertebral joints. These muscles lie anterior to the vertebral column and include the longus colli, longus capitis, rectus capitis anterior, and rectus capitis lateralis (**ATLAS PLATE 488**). Coursing on each side through the lateral processes of the cervical vertebrae is the vertebral artery, surrounded by the vertebral venous plexus. Extending inferiorly and laterally from the cervical vertebrae are the scalene muscles, the roots of the cervical nerves, the branches of the cervical plexus, and the subclavian artery (**ATLAS PLATES 483, 488**). These latter structures were dissected in the posterior triangle of the neck.

Pull the skull (detached at the atlantooccipital joints) and the cervical viscera inferiorly, to expose the prevertebral fascia covering the longus capitis and longus colli muscles. Remove the fascia and identify the **longus capitis muscle.** It attaches inferiorly to the transverse processes of the 3rd to the 6th cervical vertebrae and extends upward to the base of the skull (**ATLAS PLATE 488**). Note that above the atlas it overlies the **rectus capitis anterior muscle** and that both muscles have been severed from the skull.

Dissect the more medially placed **longus colli muscle** and observe that its fibers extend inferiorly from the atlas and bodies of the cervical vertebrae to the transverse processes and bodies of lower vertebrae as far as T3 (**ATLAS PLATES 488, 489**).

Identify the anterior and middle scalene muscles inferolaterally, and separate the **trunks of the brachial plexus** and the **subclavian artery** emerging between these two muscles (**ATLAS PLATES 479, 483**). Find the **vertebral artery** as it branches from the subclavian and courses superiorly and medially toward the 6th cervical vertebra (**ATLAS PLATES 490, 491**). Remove fibers of the longus colli and intertransverse muscles to expose the artery and its accompanying veins more completely.

Follow the **sympathetic trunk** from the **superior cervical ganglion** to the thorax. Note other enlargements along the trunk that may indicate sites of other cervical ganglia. Try to find the **cervicothoracic (or stellate) ganglion,** which is the fused inferior cervical and the first (and second) thoracic sympathetic ganglia (**ATLAS PLATES 18, 162, 164, 168**). Note that **gray rami** emerge from the cervical ganglia to join the segmental cervical nerves.

Clinical Relevance

Dislocation of cervical vertebrae. Adjacent cervical vertebrae are not interlocked as they are in the thoracic and lumbar regions. Their articular surfaces are oriented horizontally, which means that they can be dislocated more easily instead of sustaining vertebral fractures. Slight dislocations can even reduce themselves without injuring the spinal cord, but more extensive dislocations with fractures can produce serious spinal cord injury. These are best visualized with magnetic resonance imaging.

Sympathectomy in the cervical region. Cutting the sympathetic nerves that supply the upper limb is usually performed in the neck or through the axilla. This procedure is done to prevent gangrene of the fingers in Raynaud's disease (insufficient blood supply to the fingers). These sympathetic fibers leave the spinal cord in the upper thoracic region and synapse in the stellate or middle cervical ganglion. The postganglionic fibers then course with the roots of the brachial plexus to get to structures in the upper limb.

Fracture and dislocation of the atlas. Injury to the atlas can occur from a blow to the top of the head or from diving into a shallow swimming pool. Such a trauma can compress the lateral processes of the atlas, forcing them laterally and fracturing one or both anterior and posterior arches. If the transverse ligament of the atlas is also ruptured, serious injury to the spinal cord can occur.

Fracture of the axis. The vertebral arch of the axis is one of the more frequent sites of fracture in the cervical vertebrae. These fractures usually occur at the superior and inferior articular processes as a result of hyperextension of the head on the neck. This is the so-called "hangman's fracture." Other serious injuries of the C2 vertebra include the dislocation of the C2 vertebra with respect to the C3 vertebra and the fracture of the odontoid process, which can happen from a blow to the side of the head.

Fracture of the dens. Fracture of the dens accounts for approximately 40% of fractures of the axis, and these usually occur at the base of the process. These fractures are difficult to heal because they are complicated by a loss of blood supply to the dens or by the transverse ligament of the atlas that gets intersected between the fractured parts.

Cervical vertebrae. These are the smallest of the vertebrae and they bear less weight than the others. Their intervertebral discs are thick, relatively speaking, when one considers the size of the vertebral bodies they interconnect. These vertebrae contain a foramen in the transverse processes (except the C7 vertebra) for the passage of the vertebral arteries. Laterally, the tubercles on the transverse processes afford attachment of the levator scapulae muscle and the scalene muscles. The first two vertebrae, the atlas and axis, differ in shape from the lower cervical vertebrae. The atlas bears the weight of the skull, whereas the axis, the strongest cervical vertebra, allows the atlas and the skull to rotate from side to side in a manner of a person shaking the head indicating the word "no."

Cervical zygapophysial joints. Zygapophysial joints are synovial articulations between the superior and inferior articular processes of adjacent vertebrae. In the cervical region these joints are oriented on a slope and are higher anteriorly than posteriorly. This structure facilitates flexion and extension of the cervical vertebrae. In contrast, these joints in the thoracic region allow limited flexion and extension but facilitate rotation. Joints in the lumbar region limit rotation, but flexion and extension are still allowed. The zygapophysial joints are clinically important because of their proximity to the intervertebral foramina and the segmental nerves. In aging patients they may develop osteoarthritis and cause pain or limited muscle function in the affected dermatome.

Compression of the C2 ganglion or nerve. This is a painful condition that on one side may be brought about by rotating the head to the opposite side, while simultaneously over-extending the head. By this action the C2 nerve and ganglion may be compressed between the C1 and C2 vertebrae.

Ligamentum nuchae. This ligament extends from the external occipital protuberance to the spinous process of the C7 vertebra in the midline posteriorly. Although it lies dorsal to the vertebral bodies, it helps to support the head and resists flexion of the cervical vertebrae.

Cervical lymph node infections. These infections occur as a result of infections in the head or neck. The jugulodigastric node located just inferior to the angle of the mandible is the most common cervical node to become enlarged from pharyngeal or other head or neck infections.

Cervical ribs. This is an enlarged costal process of the C7 vertebra which usually is a small part of the transverse process. These anomalies can present problems because they can put pressure on the subclavian artery and the inferior trunk of the brachial plexus. This latter condition forms the principal pathology of the "thoracic outlet syndrome," a problem that usually requires surgery for relief.

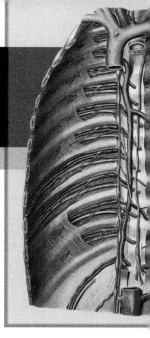

DISSECTION #34

The Pharynx: External and Internal Dissections

OBJECTIVES

1. Understand the structure of the pharynx and its relationship to surrounding structures.

2. Identify the superior laryngeal and pharyngeal branches of the vagus nerve.

3. Dissect the pharyngeal fasciae, stylopharyngeus muscle, and glossopharyngeal nerve.

4. Dissect the pharyngeal constrictor muscles and the vessels that supply the pharynx.

5. Open the pharynx posteriorly and study its three parts: nasopharynx, oropharynx, and laryngopharynx.

6. Identify certain features on the internal aspect of the three parts of the pharynx.

Atlas Key:

Clemente Atlas, 5th Edition = Atlas Plate #

Grant's Atlas, 11th Edition = Grant's Page #

Netter's Atlas, 3rd Edition = Netter's Plate #

Rohen Atlas, 6th Edition = Rohen Page #

I. Structure and Relationships of the Pharynx; Vagus and Glossopharyngeal Nerves (ATLAS PLATE 589)

▶
Grant's 739–745,
768, 769, 816–821
Netter's 28, 30, 65,
67, 119–122
Rohen 75, 84, 164,
165, 183, 184
◀
Grant's 766–771,
774–777
Netter's 59–64
Rohen 164, 167

▶
Grant's 766–769
Netter's 59, 61, 63
Rohen 164, 167

The pharynx is a muscular tube located posterior to the nasal cavities, the mouth, and the larynx. It extends from the base of the skull to about the 6th cervical vertebra and measures 12 to 14 cm in length (5 to 6 inches). It is widest superiorly (3.5 cm) and narrowest inferiorly (1.5 cm), where it becomes continuous with the esophagus (**ATLAS PLATE 589**). The pharynx serves both digestive and respiratory functions, since it communicates superiorly with the nasal and oral cavities and inferiorly with the larynx and esophagus.

Lateral to the pharynx descending into the neck from the jugular foramen in the skull are the **glossopharyngeal, vagus,** and **accessory nerves** and the **internal jugular vein** (**ATLAS PLATE 589**). Adjacent also are the **internal** and **external carotid arteries,** branches from the external carotid, and the **hypoglossal nerve** (**ATLAS PLATE 492 #492.1**). The slender, pointed styloid process and its attached muscles are located superiorly and laterally.

The pharynx is bounded **superiorly** by the body of the sphenoid bone and the basilar part of the occipital bone and **inferiorly** by the esophagus. It is separated from the cervical vertebrae, the anterior vertebral muscles, and the prevertebral fascia by loose areolar connective tissue (**ATLAS PLATES 587, 588**).

A. The Carotid Arteries and the Vagus Nerve. The common carotid artery bifurcates into internal and external carotid branches at the level of the superior thyroid notch on the thyroid cartilage. Adjacent to these two vessels is the vagus nerve and its **superior laryngeal** and **pharyngeal branches (ATLAS PLATE 589).**

Identify the following:

1. **Internal carotid artery.** Find the internal carotid artery and follow its ascent from the bifurcation to the carotid canal at the base of the skull. Use a probe to separate it from the external carotid just above the bifurcation (**ATLAS PLATES 479, 480**).

2. **External carotid artery.** Find the external carotid artery ascending anterior to the internal carotid. Locate its small **ascending pharyngeal branch,** which is long and slender and arises from the posterior aspect of the external carotid near the bifurcation (**ATLAS PLATES 506, 589**). It courses superiorly on the lateral side of the pharynx.

3. **Vagus nerve.** Identify the vagus nerve again, and locate its **superior laryngeal** and **pharyngeal** branches that were identified in the anterior triangle of the neck (Dissection 30).

   a. **Superior laryngeal branch of the vagus.** Recall that the superior laryngeal nerve divided into internal and external branches (**ATLAS PLATES 480, 589**). The **internal laryngeal branch** was located penetrating the thyrohyoid membrane. The **external laryngeal branch** was followed downward behind the sternothyroid muscle on the side of the pharynx to the cricothyroid muscle, which it supplies.

   b. **Pharyngeal branch of the vagus.** The pharyngeal branch of the vagus nerve was located between the external and internal carotid arteries about 1 cm above the carotid bifurcation (Dissection 30). Near the middle constrictor muscle it joins branches from the glossopharyngeal and the sympathetic trunk to form the pharyngeal plexus (**ATLAS PLATE 589**). It is principally a motor nerve and supplies the pharyngeal constrictor muscles and all the soft palate muscles except the tensor palati.

B. Buccopharyngeal, Prevertebral, and Pharyngobasilar Fasciae. The so-called buccopharyngeal "fascia" is not a true fascial membrane but simply the

▶ Grant's 668, 723, 754
Netter's 31, 56, 59, 61
Rohen 174

◀ Grant's 768, 769, 819
Netter's 71, 76, 119, 120
Rohen 67, 161, 162, 165

◀ Grant's 739, 744, 745, 768
Netter's 28, 30, 65
Rohen 75, 183, 184

▶ Grant's 768, 769, 771
Netter's 59–61, 63, 69
Rohen 164, 165

▶ Grant's 769
Netter's 67, 119, 120, 124
Rohen 165

◀ Grant's 768, 769, 819
Netter's 76, 119, 124
Rohen 151, 162

▶ Grant's 768, 769
Netter's 63, 69
Rohen 167

◀ Grant's 769, 818, 819
Netter's 119, 124
Rohen 165

▶ Grant's 766–769, 776, 816, 817
Netter's 55, 61, 63, 64, 120
Rohen 67, 84, 167

▶ Grant's 766, 767, 816, 817
Netter's 119, 120
Rohen 67, 84

loose connective tissue epimysium that covers the posterior surface of the pharyngeal constrictor muscles. Within it can be found the pharyngeal venous plexus and the pharyngeal nerve plexus (**ATLAS PLATE 589**). The latter consists of **sensory fibers** to the mucous membrane of the nasopharynx (IX), **motor fibers** to the constrictor muscles (pharyngeal branch of the vagus; XI via X), and **postganglionic sympathetic fibers** (from the superior cervical ganglion). The **retropharyngeal space** is a fascial plane that separates the epimysium covering the constrictor muscles from the firm membranous **prevertebral fascia** that overlies the anterior vertebral muscles (**ATLAS PLATES 484 #484.3, 587**).

The **pharyngobasilar fascia** is a true fascial layer. It helps form a fibrous skeleton for the upper pharynx. Underlying the superior constrictor muscle, it is reinforced in the posterior midline by the pharyngeal ligament. This fascia closes the space between the upper border of the superior constrictor and the base of the skull medially and the pterygoid plates laterally (**ATLAS PLATE 588**). It forms a rigid wall for the nasopharynx, but it thins out inferior to the soft palate and allows the wall of the oropharynx and laryngopharynx to be soft and distensible for the act of swallowing.

Dissect the epimysium (buccopharyngeal "fascia") on the posterior wall of the pharynx, and note that delicate nerve branches from the Xth and IXth nerves and the sympathetic trunk form the **pharyngeal plexus.** Identify small branches derived from the **ascending pharyngeal artery** (from the external carotid) and the **ascending palatine artery** (from the facial) that ramify with the nerves (**ATLAS PLATE 589**).

Define the superior border of the superior constrictor muscle on both sides, and identify the fibrous **pharyngobasilar** fascia expanding from this border (**ATLAS PLATE 588**). Note that the inferior part of this fascia descends deep to the muscle fibers of the superior constrictor.

C. Stylopharyngeus Muscle and Glossopharyngeal Nerve. Descending from the styloid process to the pharynx is the important **stylopharyngeus muscle** (**ATLAS PLATES 586, 588**). During the reflexive stage of swallowing, the stylopharyngeus muscles (along with others) elevate the pharynx (and the attached larynx) so that the oropharynx receives the bolus of food from the oral cavity.

The stylopharyngeus is a slender muscle that descends to the pharynx and passes between the superior and middle constrictors (**ATLAS PLATE 576 #576.1,**

Figure 34-1). Many of its fibers blend with those of the constrictors, and others attach to the thyroid cartilage. The glossopharyngeal nerve descends posterior to the stylopharyngeus muscle and supplies it (**ATLAS PLATE 589**). The nerve also passes through the interval between the superior and middle constrictor muscles.

> Feel for the styloid process lateral to the pharynx and medial to the mandible. Identify the stylopharyngeus muscle coursing inferiorly to the lateral border of the pharynx. See how it penetrates through the interval between the superior and middle constrictor muscles (**ATLAS PLATE 588**). Using a probe, dissect the glossopharyngeal nerve as it courses along the posterior border of the stylopharyngeus muscle and supplies it. Follow the nerve to the pharynx, where it also courses between the superior and middle constrictor muscles to reach the base of the tongue (**ATLAS PLATE 589**).

◄
Grant's 766–769, 816
Netter's 63–66
Rohen 67, 167

►
Grant's 766–769
Netter's 63, 64, 71, 76, 230
Rohen 61, 164–167

II. Pharyngeal Constrictor Muscles (Figures 34-1, 34-2)

The pharyngeal wall consists of fibrous tissues around which are wrapped the three pharyngeal constrictor muscles: inferior, middle, and superior. The borders of the three muscles overlap so that the upper border of the inferior constrictor overlaps the lower border of the middle constrictor, and the upper border of the middle constrictor overlaps the lower border of the superior constrictor.

A. The Inferior Constrictor. The inferior constrictor is the thickest of the constrictors, and it consists of two parts, the **thyropharyngeus** and the **cricopharyngeus** (**ATLAS PLATE 588**). The thyropharyngeus arises from the thyroid cartilage, and its most inferior fibers are horizontal and blend in the fibrous raphe on the posterior pharynx. The middle and upper fibers sweep posteriorly and superiorly and overlap the lower border of the middle constrictor. They also

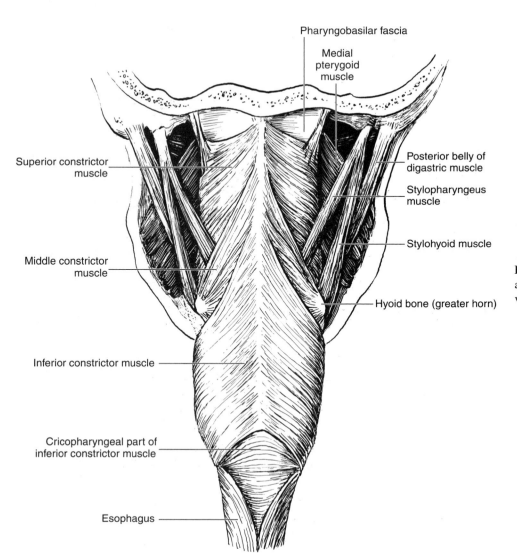

Pharyngobasilar fascia

Medial pterygoid muscle

Superior constrictor muscle

Posterior belly of digastric muscle

Stylopharyngeus muscle

Stylohyoid muscle

Middle constrictor muscle

Hyoid bone (greater horn)

Inferior constrictor muscle

Cricopharyngeal part of inferior constrictor muscle

Esophagus

Figure 34-1. Pharyngeal constrictor and stylopharyngeus muscles (posterior view).

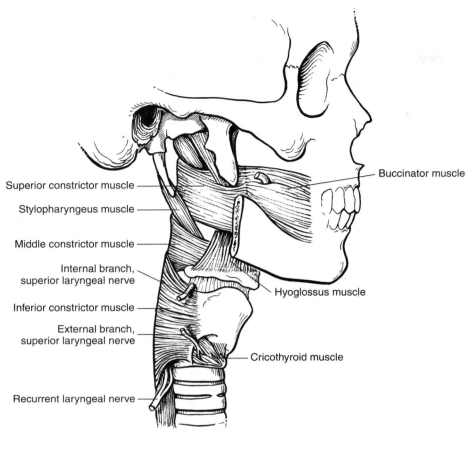

Superior constrictor muscle

Stylopharyngeus muscle

Middle constrictor muscle

Internal branch, superior laryngeal nerve

Inferior constrictor muscle

External branch, superior laryngeal nerve

Recurrent laryngeal nerve

Buccinator muscle

Hyoglossus muscle

Cricothyroid muscle

Figure 34-2. The pharynx, lateral view. Note the branches of the superior laryngeal nerve and the recurrent laryngeal nerve.

insert into the posterior raphe (**ATLAS PLATE 588**).

The cricopharyngeus part attaches to the side of the cricoid cartilage and **does not** end in a raphe posteriorly. Its fibers continue around the lowest part of the pharynx and attach on the opposite side of the cricoid cartilage. The cricopharyngeus is normally contracted and guards the entrance into the esophagus. Its fibers must relax briefly to allow a bolus of food to enter the esophagus.

B. The Middle Constrictor. The middle constrictor is fan shaped, and its fibers arise from the lesser horn of the hyoid bone, the stylohyoid ligament, and the greater horn of the hyoid bone (**ATLAS PLATES 576, 577**). It sweeps posteriorly and diverges widely before entering the midline raphe. Its inferior fibers descend deep to the inferior constrictor, its middle fibers pass posteriorly to the midline, and its superior fibers overlap the superior constrictor (**Figure 34-1**).

C. The Superior Constrictor. The superior constrictor attaches to the hamulus of the pterygoid plate, the pterygomandibular raphe (opposite the buccinator), the inner surface of the mandible, and the side of the tongue (**ATLAS PLATE 589**). It is quadrilateral, and its fibers course posteriorly to the median raphe,

▶
Grant's 769, 818, 819
Netter's 119, 120, 124
Rohen 165

◀
Grant's 766–769
Netter's 63, 64, 71
Rohen 164, 165, 167

▶
Grant's 766–768
Netter's 63, 64
Rohen 164, 165, 167

◀
Grant's 766, 769
Netter's 61, 63–65
Rohen 164–167

which is prolonged superiorly by an aponeurosis to the pharyngeal tubercle on the occipital bone.

The three pharyngeal constrictors are all supplied with motor fibers by the **pharyngeal branch of the vagus nerve (ATLAS PLATE 588**). The cricopharyngeus part of the inferior constrictor is innervated by the **recurrent laryngeal nerve**. The **maxillary nerve** supplies sensory innervation to part of the nasopharynx, the **glossopharyngeal nerve** supplies part of the nasopharynx and all of the oropharynx, and the **vagus nerve** supplies the mucosa of the laryngopharynx.

Define the borders of the constrictor muscles, and identify their attachments anteriorly and laterally (**Figure 34-2**). For the **superior constrictor,** identify its attachments to the pterygoid hamulus, the pterygomandibular raphe, and the inner surface of the mandible. You may not be able to see the fibers that arise from the tongue. Note the attachments of the **middle constrictor** to the hyoid bone and the stylohyoid ligament and that the **inferior constrictor** arises from the thyroid and cricoid cartilages.

Posteriorly on the pharynx, observe how the inferior constrictor overlaps the middle constrictor which, in turn, overlaps the superior constrictor (**ATLAS**

PLATE 588). Note that the most inferior fibers of the inferior constrictor (cricopharyngeus) form an incomplete ring from one side of the cricoid to the other and serve as a sphincter for entrance into the esophagus. Confirm the following:

1. That the **auditory (Eustachian) tube** enters the pharynx above the superior constrictor (**ATLAS PLATES 590, 591**).

2. That the **stylopharyngeus muscle** and the **glossopharyngeal nerve** enter the pharynx between the superior and middle constrictor muscles.

3. That the **thyrohyoid membrane** lies between the middle and inferior constrictors, and through this membrane pass the **internal laryngeal nerve** and **superior laryngeal artery** (**ATLAS PLATE 577 #577.1**).

4. That the **recurrent laryngeal nerve** enters the larynx just inferior to the cricopharyngeus part of the inferior constrictor, which it supplies (**Figure 34-3**).

III. Interior of the Pharynx (Figure 34-3)

The inner surface of the pharynx is lined with mucous membrane. Deep to the mucosa is a submucosal fascial layer that consists of the pharyngobasilar fascia around which spread the fibers of the pharyngeal constrictors. To study its internal anatomy, the pharynx must be opened posteriorly.

Cut the posterior wall of the pharynx vertically in the midline from the esophagus to the base of the skull (**ATLAS PLATE 590**). At both ends of the incision make lateral cuts so that the pharynx can be opened widely and its subdivisions identified. These are the nasopharynx, oropharynx, and laryngopharynx (**ATLAS PLATE 591**).

A. The Nasopharynx. The nasopharynx is the most superior part of the pharynx. It lies posterior to the nasal cavities and superior to the soft palate (**ATLAS PLATES 587, 590**). It is continuous inferiorly with the oropharynx by way of a narrow passage posterior to the uvula, called the **pharyngeal isthmus.** The nasal cavities communicate with the nasopharynx through two posterior apertures of the nose, called the **choanae** or **posterior nares** (**Figure 34-3**). The nasopharynx is an airway passage that is closed during swallowing by elevation and tensing of the soft palate. Simultaneously a band of muscle fibers contracts and

▶
Grant's 684, 697, 774, 775
Netter's 59–61
Rohen 86, 143–145

◀
Grant's 771, 774, 775
Rohen 58, 59, 61

◀
Grant's 776–769
Netter's 60, 67, 120, 124
Rohen 67, 167

◀
Grant's 755, 766, 767
Netter's 61, 64, 70, 73
Rohen 166

▶
Grant's 674, 770, 771
Netter's 8, 62, 63
Rohen 33, 143, 163

▶
Grant's 774, 775
Netter's 59, 60
Rohen 143, 145

◀
Grant's 770, 771
Netter's 62, 63
Rohen 163

▶
Grant's 770–776
Netter's 59–63, 231
Rohen 83, 145, 147, 150, 155

◀
Grant's 770, 771, 774, 775
Netter's 33, 58, 59, 62
Rohen 143, 145, 153, 155

acts as a palatopharyngeal sphincter of the pharyngeal wall (Passavant's muscle ridge).

The opening of the **auditory tube,** surrounded by an elevation of cartilage called the **torus tubarius,** is located in the lateral wall of the nasopharynx (**ATLAS PLATE 587**). Extending down from the torus is a vertical ridge of mucous membrane called the **salpingopharyngeal fold,** which overlies the delicate **salpingopharyngeus muscle** (**ATLAS PLATES 588 #588.2, 567 #567.2**). Posterior to the torus is a deep recess on the lateral wall called the **pharyngeal recess** and on the upper part of the posterior wall is located the **pharyngeal tonsil** (**ATLAS PLATE 567 #567.2**). This latter structure, best seen in children, is often called the **adenoid.**

Open the upper flaps of the pharyngeal wall and study the nasopharynx. Above the **uvula,** identify the two oblong posterior openings of the nasal cavity, the **choanae,** on the sides of the **nasal septum** (**ATLAS PLATE 590**). Look through the choanae, and identify the **middle and inferior conchae.** These curved projections extend from the lateral wall of the nasal cavity.

Locate the **pharyngeal opening of the auditory tube** by probing the lateral side of the nasopharynx about 2 cm posterior to the inferior concha (**ATLAS PLATE 591**). It can best be seen with a dental mirror if available. Posterior to this opening identify a rounded cartilaginous bulge, the **torus tubarius** (**ATLAS PLATE 588 #558.2**). Probe the **pharyngeal recess** in the lateral wall posterior to the torus. See if the **pharyngeal tonsil** is still present in the superior part of the posterior nasopharyngeal wall.

B. The Oropharynx. The oropharynx lies posterior to the oral cavity and the tongue, and it extends from the soft palate superiorly to the upper border of the epiglottis inferiorly (**Figure 34-3**). It communicates with the oral cavity anteriorly through the oropharyngeal isthmus formed by the **palatoglossal arches** (**ATLAS PLATES 566, 567**). On the lateral wall of the oropharynx are the **palatopharyngeal arches,** and between the two arches on each side is located the **palatine tonsil.** If the tonsil has been removed, identify the bed of the tonsil (**ATLAS PLATE 587**). The **pharyngoepiglottic folds** define the lateral borders of the oropharynx, and they extend from the soft palate to the lateral margin of the epiglottis (**ATLAS PLATE 591**). During swallowing, the pharynx is elevated, and the constrictor muscles close behind the bolus of food. At all other times the oropharynx is an open pathway for breathing.

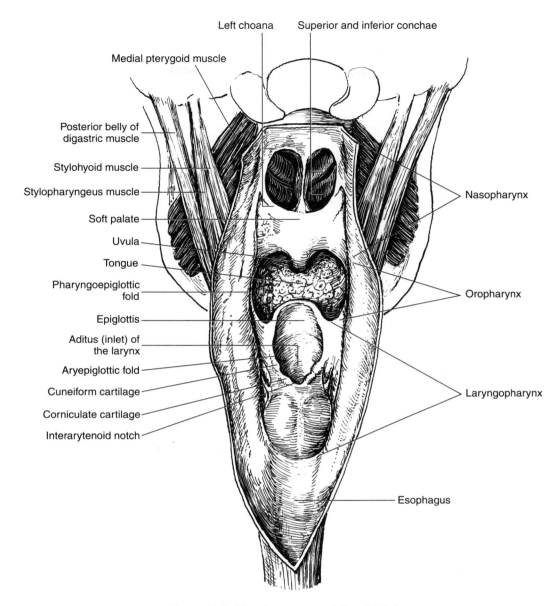

Figure 34-3. The pharynx, opened from behind.

Feel the pharyngeal surface of the posterior tongue, and note the many rounded lymphatic follicles of the **lingual tonsil (or follicles)** that cover its mucosal surface (**ATLAS PLATE 591**). Identify the **palatopharyngeal folds** (arches) descending to the pharynx from the soft palate. With fine scissors, remove some of the mucosa on the surface of the folds on one side, and identify strands of the palatopharyngeus muscle lying deep to the mucous membrane (**ATLAS PLATE 592**).

Anterior to the palatopharyngeal folds identify the **palatoglossal folds** (arches), and look for the palatine tonsil between the palatoglossal and palatopharyngeal folds (**ATLAS PLATE 590**). Identify the

◄
Grant's 666, 669
Netter's 54, 59, 60, 67
Rohen 150, 163

►
Grant's 770, 771, 784
Netter's 59, 62, 63
Rohen 155, 163, 165

◄
Grant's 771–774
Netter's 62, 63
Rohen 147, 163

smooth pharyngoepiglottic fold that descends from the soft palate to the lateral border of the epiglottis on each side. These folds define the lateral margins of the oropharynx posterior to the tongue (**ATLAS PLATE 591**).

C. The Laryngopharynx. The laryngopharynx extends from the superior border of the epiglottis to the inferior border of the cricoid cartilage, where it becomes the esophagus (**Figure 34-3**). Anteriorly are located the **epiglottis** and the **aditus** (or inlet) **of the larynx.** Extending inferiorly between the epiglottis and the notch between the two arytenoid cartilages of the larynx are the **aryepiglottic folds**

(ATLAS PLATES 590–592). They form the superior margins of the aditus. Lateral to the aditus on each side is a small fossa called the **piriform recess (ATLAS PLATE 591).**

Identify the epiglottis and run your finger along the edge of the **aryepiglottic fold** that forms the upper lateral margins of the **laryngeal inlet** or **aditus** (ATLAS PLATES 590, 591). Note that there are two small tubercles along this margin on each side. They are formed by small laryngeal cartilages deep to the mucosa (cuneiform and corniculate cartilages). Palpate the **piriform recesses.** These depressions are on both sides of the laryngopharynx, between the aryepiglottic folds and the lateral pharyngeal wall (ATLAS PLATE 591).

◄
Grant's 770
Netter's 62
Rohen 163

Probe the pharyngeal mucosa lateral to the epiglottis from the piriform recesses to the esophagus. Deep to the mucosa find the **internal branch of the superior laryngeal nerve** and the **superior laryngeal artery** as they enter the region through the thyrohyoid membrane (ATLAS PLATE 595). Inferiorly, identify branches of the **recurrent laryngeal nerve** ascending from the tracheoesophageal groove and coursing toward the larynx (ATLAS PLATE 595).

◄
Grant's 783–785
Netter's 63, 72, 76
Rohen 162, 163

Clinical Relevance

Pharyngotympanic tube. This tube interconnects the middle ear and the nasopharynx. It is important because air pressure in the pharynx is the same as air pressure on the outside of the tympanic membrane. This tube ensures that pressure in the middle ear (i.e., on the inside of the tympanic membrane) is maintained equal to atmospheric pressure on the outside of the tympanic membrane.

Swallowing. Once a bolus of food is pushed back in the oral cavity by the tongue, the palatoglossus and styloglossus muscles elevate the pharynx (and larynx) so that the food can enter the oropharynx. At this point the act of swallowing becomes involuntary. The nasopharynx is closed off from the oropharynx by the levator of the palate and palatopharyngeal muscles to prevent food from entering the nasal cavity. The pharynx (and larynx) is elevated by the stylopharyngeus muscles so that the oropharynx is now behind the oral cavity to receive the food. At the same time, the entrance into the larynx is closed by the epiglottis and food courses over the epiglottis into the laryngopharynx and then into the esophagus.

The nasopharyngeal tonsil. The nasopharyngeal tonsils, also called adenoids, are subject to infection and inflammation. In the past, these were frequently removed at the same time as the palatine tonsils. When the adenoids are especially enlarged, often in young children, they can obstruct the posterior nares (the choanae), requiring oral breathing. They can also obstruct the nasopharyngeal opening of the eustachian tube (the pharyngotympanic tube) and contribute to middle ear infections (otitis media), which can alter the ability to hear.

Tonsillitis. This is a frequently encountered condition (especially in children) in which there is an infection of the palatine tonsils in the oropharynx between the palatoglossal and palatopharyngeal arches. Earache is one of the symptoms of this condition, because the glossopharyngeal nerve that supplies the mucosa of the middle ear courses adjacent to the tonsillar bed and may be compressed by the inflammation. Additionally, painful oropharyngeal lymph nodes (such as the jugulodigastric node) may be secondarily infected because they drain the tonsillar region.

Esophageal cancer. Cancer of the esophagus often becomes recognized because the esophageal lumen is significantly reduced and swallowing becomes difficult and painful. It is thought that in some patients, consistent repetitive regurgitation of stomach contents into the esophagus may be related to the subsequent development of esophageal cancer. Enlarged deep paraesophageal lymph nodes often indicate esophageal cancer, and pressure on the adjacent recurrent laryngeal nerves may result in voice changes.

Gag reflex. The afferent limb of the gag reflex is the general sensory fibers of the glossopharyngeal nerve that supply the posterior one-third of the tongue and the mucosa or the oropharynx. The motor pathway involves the pharyngeal branch of the vagus nerve that supplies the levator of the palate and the pharyngeal constrictor muscles. Elicitation of this reflex tests the 9th, 10th, and 11th cranial nerves simultaneously during a physical examination. This is because the 9th nerve is the sensory limb of the reflex and the cranial root of the 11th nerve joins the vagus to supply palatal and pharyngeal muscles, which are the motor root.

Tonsillectomy. This procedure is performed to remove the palatine tonsil from the tonsillar bed in the oropharynx. The presence of a rich arterial blood supply and the presence of the tonsillar vein, however, make this procedure more than routine. Additionally, coursing across the tonsillar bed is the 9th cranial nerve (glossopharyngeal nerve) that supplies the posterior one-third of the tongue with general sensation and the special sense of taste. The presence of the internal carotid artery lateral to the tonsil must also be considered in this operation and care must be taken to avoid injuring it. Because of antibiotics, this operation is performed less frequently than it once was.

Foreign objects in the laryngopharynx. At times a person may inadvertently swallow a foreign body such as a chicken bone or fish bone that becomes lodged in the laryngopharynx (the lower part of the pharynx). This may cause the victim to gag strongly. If the foreign body is pointed or sharp, it may injure the laryngeal nerves or vessels. Removal of the foreign object requires a pharyngoscope to visualize the field directly.

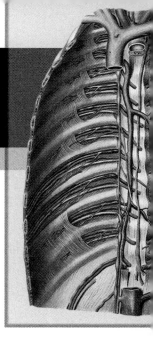

DISSECTION #35

The Nasal Cavity and Paranasal Sinuses in the Bisected Head

OBJECTIVES

1. Bisect the head and gain access to the nasal septum and the other walls of the nasal cavity.

2. Study the mucosa and skeletal framework of the nasal septum and dissect the structures traversing the incisive foramen.

3. Examine the roof and floor of the nasal cavity.

4. Dissect the lateral wall of the nasal cavity and see the openings of the paranasal sinuses and nasolacrimal duct.

5. Locate the pterygopalatine ganglion and dissect the vessels and nerves in the palatine canal.

6. Identify the paranasal sinuses, open the maxillary sinus, and visualize the maxillary nerve and pterygopalatine ganglion.

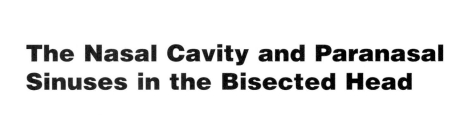

Atlas Key:

Clemente Atlas, 5th Edition = Atlas Plate #

Grant's Atlas, 11th Edition = Grant's Page #

Netter's Atlas, 3rd Edition = Netter's Plate #

Rohen Atlas, 6th Edition = Rohen Page #

I. Bisection of the Head (ATLAS PLATE 558 #558.2)

When the head was separated from the vertebral column, it gave access to the pharynx from behind, and it also now allows the head to be bisected for dissection of the nasal and oral cavities.

It is best to bisect the head 2 mm lateral to the midline. In this way the **nasal septum** and the **walls of the**

▶
Grant's 681–684, 788
Netter's 39, 59
Rohen 143–145

◀
Grant's 681–683, 693, 788
Netter's 35, 59
Rohen 143

nasal cavity become accessible for dissection. This procedure will also open the oral cavity for Dissection #36. The nasal cavity is divided into right and left halves by the nasal septum.

Inspect the nasal cavity, and determine whether the nasal septum is deviated from the midline. If so, bisect the head slightly away from the septum so that it will remain intact for dissection.

Start the bisection by cutting through the skin of the forehead, the lips, and the chin near the midline. Cut through the nostril and nasal cartilages slightly to one side of the septum so that the entire septum will be on one side of the bisected head (about 2.0 mm from the midline). Cut through the soft palate and the mucosa of the hard palate with a scalpel close to the midline.

Identify the nasal bones on the anterior aspect of the face (**ATLAS PLATE 588 #558.1**). Commence a saw cut along the base of the skull (slightly off the midline) through the body of the sphenoid bone and cribriform plate of the ethmoid bone. Make the saw cut in line with the left nasal bone so that the intact nasal septum remains within one-half of the head.

Bisect the skull until you reach the foramen magnum. Continue the bisection through the midline of the hard palate until the dorsum of the tongue and the oral cavity are exposed. **Do not bisect the tongue or mandible at this time.** Separate the two halves of the head and turn your attention to the nasal septum.

II. Nasal Septum

The nasal septum divides the nasal cavity into right and left halves. It is formed by two bones posteriorly and the septal cartilage anteriorly. These are covered on both sides by periosteum (or perichondrium) and lined by a mucous membrane (**ATLAS PLATE 560 #560.1**). Within the mucous membrane course the vessels and nerves that supply the septum.

The **bony part** of the septum consists of two midline structures, the **perpendicular plate of the ethmoid bone** that forms the superior, posterior part of the septum and the **vomer bone** that forms the inferior posterior part. The **septal cartilage** extends anteriorly from

◀ Grant's 589, 590, 640
Netter's 2, 32
Rohen 22, 144

▶ Grant's 681–683
Netter's 37, 38
Rohen 143, 146

▶ Grant's 682, 683
Netter's 37, 38
Rohen 143

▶ Grant's 681–683
Netter's 35
◀ Rohen 143
Grant's 681–683
Netter's 35
Rohen 49, 143

these bones and becomes continuous with the lateral nasal cartilage of the external nose (**Figure 35-1**).

The septal skeletal structures are covered by a mucosal–periosteal layer within which course the **anterior ethmoid** (V1) and **nasopalatine** (V2) **nerves and arteries** that form a rich anastomosis (**ATLAS PLATES 562, 563**). The vessels include branches of the **anterior** and **posterior ethmoid arteries** (ophthalmic), **septal branches** from the **sphenopalatine artery** (maxillary), **superior labial** (facial) arteries, and the terminal ascending branch of the **greater palatine artery** (**Figure 35-2**).

Identify the **nasopalatine nerve** coursing anteriorly and inferiorly to the floor of the nasal cavity on the deep surface of the septal mucosa. It is a branch of the maxillary nerve that traverses the **pterygopalatine ganglion** and carries both sensory and autonomic fibers. Confirm that it descends through the incisive foramen to enter the anterior part of the oral cavity (**Figure 35-3**). Identify the **anterior ethmoid nerve** that courses along the anterosuperior aspect of the septum. Try to find **posterior septal branches of the sphenopalatine artery** and the **anterior ethmoid artery** that usually accompany these nerves.

Remove the mucous membrane from the septum and identify the **vomer bone** posteroinferiorly, the **perpendicular plate of the ethmoid bone** posterosuperiorly, and the **septal cartilage** anteriorly (**Figure 35-1**).

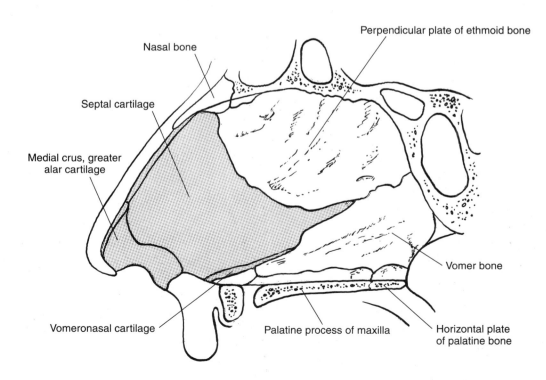

Figure 35-1. Bony and cartilaginous structure of the nasal septum.

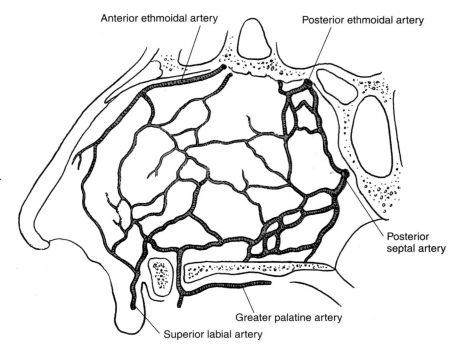

Figure 35-2. Blood supply of the nasal septum.

III. Roof and Floor of the Nasal Cavity

Each half of the nasal cavity is bounded **medially** by the nasal septum, **superiorly** by a bony roof, **inferiorly** by the hard palate, and **laterally** by an uneven and complex lateral wall. Study the bones that form the roof of the nasal cavity and the hard palate, which is its floor inferiorly (**ATLAS PLATE 559**).

◄
Grant's 681
Netter's 33, 34
Rohen 143–145

►
Grant's 681
Netter's 33, 34
Rohen 143–145

The bones and cartilage forming the skeleton of the septum are now to be removed with bone-cutting shears. This will allow the roof and floor of the nasal cavity to be studied and the lateral wall to be dissected.

Examine the bony roof, and identify the **sphenoid bone** most posteriorly, the **ethmoid bone** anterior to the sphenoid, and anterior to these, the **frontal** and **nasal bones** (**ATLAS PLATE 559**).

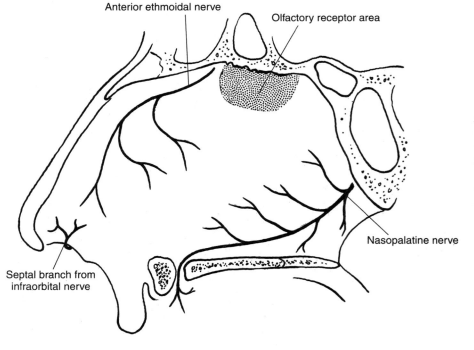

Figure 35-3. Sensory innervation of the mucosa of the nasal septum.

On a dried skull, identify the bones of the hard palate. These are the palatine processes of the two **maxillae** and the horizontal laminae of the **palatine bones** (**ATLAS PLATES 559, 582**). Note that the hard palate is 5 cm long and about 2 cm wide on each side. In the cadaver, probe the floor of the nasal cavity and remove the mucosa lining these bony structures on one side of the head. Anteriorly, find the incisive foramen (canal), which perforates the maxillae near the midline (**ATLAS PLATE 559**).

IV. Lateral Wall of the Nasal Cavity

A. The Conchae, Meatuses, and Openings of the Nasolacrimal Duct and Paranasal Sinuses. The lateral wall of the nasal cavity is marked by the projections of the **superior, middle,** and **inferior nasal conchae.** These are curved bony plates covered with mucosa that overhang nasal passages called meatuses (**Figures 35-4, 35-5**). The superior and middle nasal conchae are projections from the ethmoid bone, whereas the inferior nasal concha is a separate bone. Below each of the three conchae is its corresponding **meatus** (**ATLAS PLATES 559, 567**).

Anterior to the nasal conchae, the lateral wall is smooth and presents two smaller regions called the **atrium,** anterior to the middle meatus, and the **vestibule of the nose,** which lies anteriorly just above the nostril

◄
Grant's 672, 682, 683, 764
Netter's 8, 34, 52
Rohen 32, 33, 144

►
Grant's 684, 685
Netter's 33, 34
Rohen 144, 145

►
Grant's 685, 686
Netter's 33
Rohen 145

◄
Grant's 681–684
Netter's 33, 34
Rohen 34, 48, 144

►
Grant's 684
Netter's 33, 46, 78
Rohen 143, 145

(**Figure 35-5**). The lateral wall contains openings for all of the **paranasal sinuses** as well as the orifice of the **nasolacrimal duct** (**ATLAS PLATE 588 #558.2**). Most of these cannot be seen unless the nasal conchae are removed. An exception is the opening of the sphenoid sinus, which communicates with the **sphenoethmoidal recess** posteriorly **above the superior concha.** The **posterior ethmoid air cells** communicate with the superior meatus **below the superior concha** (**ATLAS PLATE 561 #561.2**).

The lateral wall of the **middle meatus,** hidden by the middle concha, contains a deep crescent-shaped groove, the **hiatus semilunaris,** above which is a bulge, the **bulla ethmoidalis,** formed by the middle ethmoid air cells (**Figure 35-7**). The **frontal sinus,** the **anterior and middle ethmoid air cells,** and the large **maxillary sinus** all open in proximity to the hiatus semilunaris and the bulla ethmoidalis. (**ATLAS PLATE 561 #561.2**). The anterior end of the hiatus semilunaris frequently leads superiorly into a passageway called the **infundibulum,** which communicates with the frontal air sinus. Near the posterior end of the hiatus is found the opening of the maxillary sinus (**Figure 35-7**). The anterior and middle ethmoid air cells usually open just above the bulla ethmoidalis.

The **inferior meatus** is a horizontal passage that lies inferior to the inferior concha. The **nasolacrimal duct** opens into the inferior meatus near the anterior attached site of the inferior concha (**ATLAS PLATES 558 #558.2, 561 #561.2, Figure 35-7**).

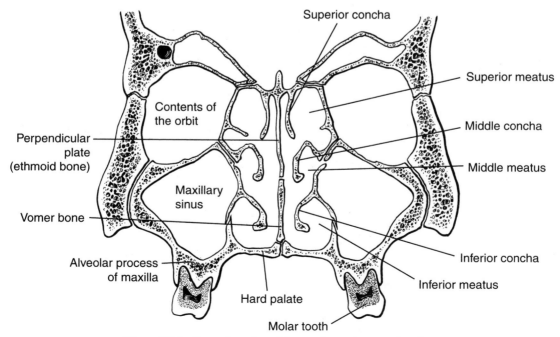

Figure 35-4. Coronal section of the nasal cavaties, anterior view.

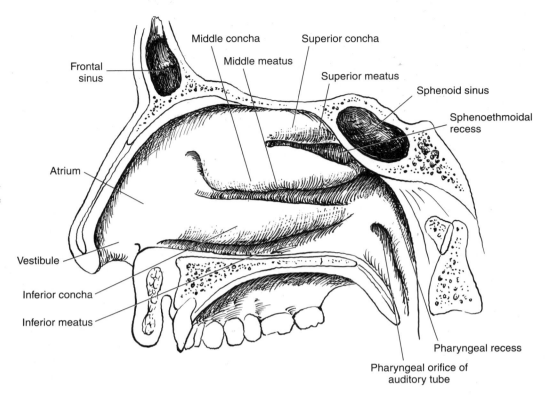

Figure 35-5. Conchae and meatuses of the lateral wall of the nasal cavity.

Frontal sinus

Middle concha

Middle meatus

Superior concha

Superior meatus

Sphenoid sinus

Sphenoethmoidal recess

Atrium

Vestibule

Inferior concha

Inferior meatus

Pharyngeal recess

Pharyngeal orifice of auditory tube

1. On the lateral wall of the nasal cavity identify the **inferior concha** and, below it, the **inferior meatus**, the **middle concha** and **middle meatus**, and the **superior concha** and **superior meatus** (**ATLAS PLATES 558, 561**). Identify the **vestibule of the nose** and, superior to it, the **atrium** (**Figure 35-5**). With scissors, cut away the inferior concha to find the opening of the **nasolacrimal duct** (**ATLAS PLATES 560 #560.2**). Look in the anterior part of the lateral wall of the inferior meatus 3 to 4 cm behind the nostril (**Figure 35-7**). Remove the mucosa in this region, and probe the bony nasolacrimal canal, which contains the nasolacrimal duct.

2. Cut away the middle concha, and identify the curved groove called the **hiatus semilunaris.** Above this groove see the rounded swelling called the **bulla ethmoidalis (Figure 35-7).** Identify the **frontal sinus** in the frontal bone. See if it opens directly by an orifice into the nasal cavity or by a **frontonasal duct** into the middle meatus (**ATLAS PLATE 561 #561.2**). Superior to the bulla probe the middle and anterior air cells. Find the opening of the **maxillary sinus** in the posterior part of the middle

◄
Grant's 630
Netter's 33, 34, 78
Rohen 36, 48, 144, 145

►
Grant's 685, 686
Netter's 33, 34
Rohen 144, 145

►
Grant's 685–687
Netter's 33, 34, 45
Rohen 47, 144, 149

◄
Grant's 685, 686
Netter's 33, 34
Rohen 145

meatus. Push your probe through the orifice into the large maxillary sinus (**Figure 35-7**).

3. Cut away the short **superior concha,** and visualize the narrow superior meatus. Probe the **posterior ethmoid air cells** and, posterior to these, the **sphenoid sinus** (**ATLAS PLATE 561 #561.2**). Note that the posterior ethmoid air cells open into the superior meatus. Identify the **sphenoethmoidal recess** as a vertical channel anterior to the sphenoid sinus and posterior to the superior meatus (**Figure 35-7**). Probe the anterior wall of the sphenoid sinus, find its orifice, and confirm that it opens into the sphenoethmoidal recess.

4. Return to the inferior meatus and remove the remaining mucosa posterior to the opening of the nasolacrimal duct. With bone forceps, open the large **maxillary sinus** (**ATLAS PLATES 540, 541**). Enlarge the opening and expose the entire sinus. With a probe, remove the mucosa along its roof, or orbital surface. Identify a longitudinal ridge formed by the **infraorbital canal.** Break through the bony ridge with a probe and find the **infraorbital nerve and vessels** coursing along this canal.

V. Pterygopalatine Ganglion; Greater and Lesser Palatine Nerves and Vessels (ATLAS PLATES 562, 563)

The **maxillary nerve** (V2) traverses the foramen rotundum, the infraorbital canal, and the infraorbital foramen before appearing on the anterior face inferior to the lower eyelid. Along this course it passes through the **pterygopalatine fossa,** where the **pterygopalatine ganglion** is attached to it (**ATLAS PLATE 563**). The ganglion contains **postganglionic parasympathetic neurons** that synapse with incoming preganglionic parasympathetic nerve fibers from the **nerve of the pterygoid canal.** These preganglionic parasympathetic fibers leave the brain in the facial nerve and then course along the **greater petrosal nerve** before helping to form the nerve of the pterygoid canal. Additionally, **through the ganglion without synapse course:**

1. **Postganglionic sympathetic nerve fibers** that originate from cells in the superior cervical ganglion, course along the internal carotid nerve, and join the nerve of the pterygoid canal by way of the **deep petrosal nerve.**

◀
Grant's 687, 688, 808, 809, 813
Netter's 38–41, 117, 126, 127
Rohen 72, 73, 146, 147

▶
Grant's 673, 686–688, 690
Netter's 38–41, 125, 127
Rohen 146, 147

◀
Grant's 813
Netter's 117

▶
Grant's 673, 686–688
Netter's 38, 41
Rohen 46, 147

2. **Sensory nerve fibers** from the nasal and palatal mucosa that enter the maxillary nerve after traversing the ganglion. These sensory fibers course in the posterior lateral nasal nerves, the greater and lesser palatine nerves, and the nasopalatine nerve.

The **greater** (anterior) **palatine nerve** carries sensory nerve fibers **from** the oral cavity and autonomic nerve fibers **to** the mucous glands of the hard palate. The nerve is accompanied by the **greater** (anterior) **palatine branch of the maxillary artery,** which descends to the hard palate in the oral cavity (**ATLAS PLATE 562 #562.2**). Within the palatine canal the greater palatine nerve and artery give off **lesser** (posterior) **palatine branches** that descend to the soft palate in the oral cavity.

Identify the pterygopalatine ganglion in the pterygopalatine fossa (**ATLAS PLATE 563 #563.1**). Find the **greater and lesser palatine nerves and vessels** by opening the greater palatine canal (**Figure 35-6**). Dissect as follows:

1. Strip the mucoperiosteum from the region anterior to the opening of the auditory tube and posterior to the ends of the cut conchae and the meatuses.

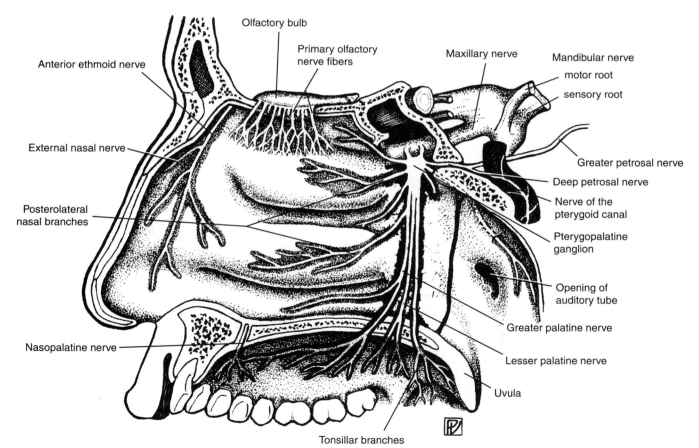

Figure 35-6. The pterygopalatine ganglion and its nasal and palatine branches and the nerve of the pterygoid canal.

2. The **palatine canal** may be visible through the perpendicular plate of the palatine bone. Break through the bone to expose the palatine nerve and vessels (**ATLAS PLATE 563 #563.2**).

3. Open the canal completely and dissect the connective tissue surrounding its neurovascular structures. With a probe, follow the greater palatine nerve superiorly to its junction with the **pterygopalatine ganglion (ATLAS PLATE 562 #562.2)**.

4. Dissect the greater palatine nerve and vessels to the hard palate. Note that the lesser palatine nerve branches from the greater and courses posteriorly to the soft palate through its own foramen.

VI. Paranasal Sinuses

The paranasal sinuses are air-filled spaces lined with mucosa, located within bones above and lateral to the nasal cavities. Superior to the nasal cavities are the **frontal, ethmoid,** and **sphenoid sinuses,** and more laterally is found the **maxillary sinus,** the largest of all the paranasal sinuses (**ATLAS PLATES 540 #540.2, 541 #541.2**).

The **frontal sinuses** are irregular cavities that usually are different sizes on the two sides. They lie between the inner and outer tables of the frontal bone above the medial third of the supraorbital ridges (**ATLAS PLATE 558–561**). Each frontal sinus opens into the anterior part

◄ Grant's 673, 682, 683, 813
Netter's 38–41, 125
Rohen 72, 73, 146, 147

◄ Grant's 673, 682, 809
Netter's 38, 39, 125
Rohen 73, 146, 147

► Grant's 687, 690, 694
Netter's 44, 45
Rohen 121, 144, 148

► Grant's 684–687
Netter's 6, 33, 34, 38
Rohen 48, 86, 90, 246

◄ Grant's 687
Netter's 45
Rohen 144, 145

► Grant's 688–692
Netter's 41, 44, 45
Rohen 46, 132, 149

◄ Grant's 684–687
Netter's 33, 34, 45
Rohen 145, 147

of the middle meatus in the nasal cavity by way of a **frontonasal duct** or drains directly through an ostium into the **ethmoidal infundibulum.**

The **ethmoid sinuses** are located within the labyrinth of the ethmoid bone, and their thin, irregular walls give the appearance of a honeycomb (**ATLAS PLATE 565 #565.1**). The air cells are frequently subdivided into anterior, middle, and posterior groups, and they are distinguished according to their site of drainage and their location in the ethmoid bone. The **anterior ethmoid air cells** (2 to 8 in number) usually open into a channel in the middle meatus called the ethmoidal infundibulum. The **middle ethmoid air cells** (sometimes called the bullar cells) are often three in number and open into the middle meatus on or above the ethmoidal bulla. The **posterior ethmoid air cells** (1 to 7 in number) are located posterior to the other ethmoid cells and open into the superior meatus.

The **sphenoid sinuses** are located posterior to the nasal cavity within the body of the sphenoid bone (**ATLAS PLATE 560–562, 564**). Separated by a thin, bony septum, the two sinuses often differ in size. The average diameter of the sphenoid sinus is 1.5 cm. Each sinus communicates with the **sphenoethmoidal recess** through a foramen on its anterior wall, the sphenoidal ostium (**ATLAS PLATE 561 #561.2, Figure 35-7**).

The **maxillary sinuses** are located in the body of the maxillae (**ATLAS PLATE 575**). Each sinus resembles a three-sided pyramid, with its apex directed laterally toward the zygomatic process of the maxilla and its base formed by the lateral wall of the nasal cavity. The roof of the sinus separates it from the orbit superiorly, and the floor of the sinus is the alveolar process of the max-

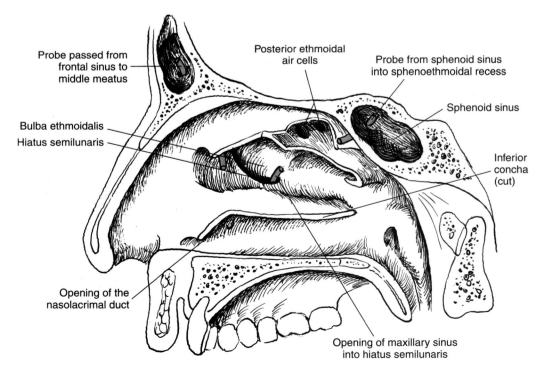

Figure 35-7. Openings of the nasal sinuses and nasolacrimal duct into the nasal cavity with the conchae removed.

Probe passed from frontal sinus to middle meatus

Posterior ethmoidal air cells

Probe from sphenoid sinus into sphenoethmoidal recess

Sphenoid sinus

Bulba ethmoidalis

Hiatus semilunaris

Inferior concha (cut)

Opening of the nasolacrimal duct

Opening of maxillary sinus into hiatus semilunaris

illa, with roots of the molar teeth often projecting into its mucosa (**ATLAS PLATES 540 #540.2, 563 #563.2**). The maxillary sinus has an average capacity of 15 cc, and it communicates **superiorly** with the hiatus semilunaris in the middle meatus of the nasal cavity (**Figure 35-7**).

The **frontal sinuses** were probably opened when the skullcap was removed. If they were not exposed, chip away the frontal bone near the midline above the supraorbital margin until the sinuses are opened. Probe the cavity to find its orifice into the frontonasal duct or directly into the ethmoidal infundibulum in the middle meatus.

Find the **ethmoid sinuses** deep to the anterior cranial fossa at the base of the skull. Remove 1 cm of bone on both sides of the cribriform plate of the ethmoid bone. Deep to the bone identify the ethmoid air cells as mucosa-lined sacs lying within thin bony compartments of the ethmoid bone (**ATLAS PLATE 565**). Probe the **anterior ethmoid cells** inferior and posterior to the frontal sinus. Probe the **posterior ethmoid air cells** located posteriorly and immediately anterior to the body of the sphenoid bone. Note that these lie anterior to the sphenoid sinus. The **middle ethmoid air cells** can be probed between the anterior and posterior cells. Realize that the anterior and middle cells open into the middle meatus, whereas the posterior cells open more superiorly in the superior meatus (**ATLAS PLATE 561 #561.2**).

The **sphenoid sinus** can be identified quickly within the body of the sphenoid bone (**ATLAS PLATES 558–561**). Look for its communication with the sphenoethmoidal recess through a foramen on its anterior surface (**Figure 35-7**).

The **maxillary sinus** is to be opened widely by cutting away its medial wall. Place a probe in the hiatus semilunaris (**ATLAS PLATES 558, 559**). Begin removing the lateral wall of the nasal cavity from the nasolacrimal duct anteriorly to the greater palatine canal posteriorly. Remove the mucoperiosteum from the inner surface of the maxillary sinus. Remove the posterior part of the roof of the maxillary sinus, and expose the **maxillary nerve** and **pterygopalatine ganglion** (**ATLAS PLATES 562 #562.2, 563**).

With bone cutters, remove a portion of the body of the sphenoid bone and identify the delicate **nerve of the pterygoid canal** as it joins the pterygopalatine ganglion (**ATLAS PLATE 563, Figure 35-6**).

▶
Grant's 688, 813
Netter's 41
Rohen 72, 73

◀
Grant's 684–687
Netter's 6, 33, 34, 45
Rohen 48, 145, 147

◀
Grant's 687, 690, 692, 694
Netter's 44, 45
Rohen 39, 48, 121, 148

◀
Grant's 684–690
Netter's 6, 33, 34
Rohen 48, 86, 88

◀
Grant's 688–690, 692
Netter's 41, 44, 45
Rohen 46, 144, 149

Continue removing bone from the **infraorbital canal** anteriorly, and follow the infraorbital nerve forward. Identify the **superior alveolar branches** of the infraorbital nerve that supply the upper teeth (**ATLAS PLATE 563 #563.2**).

Clinical Relevance

Sinusitis. This is an infection of one or more of the paranasal sinuses. It can be a complication from an upper respiratory or nasal infection. Because all the paranasal sinuses communicate with the nasal cavity, any one or more can become infected. Infections of the ethmoid sinuses can spread to the orbit by way of the delicate medial wall of the orbital cavity. This can give rise to inflammation around the optic nerve (optic neuritis) or the ophthalmic artery. More frequent, however, is the spread of nasal infections into the maxillary sinus. Because the opening into the maxillary sinus is high, it is difficult to drain when the person is upright. If necessary, the maxillary sinus can be drained with a cannula through the sinus orifice, or an opening can be surgically created near the floor of the sinus through the inferior meatus of the nose.

Deviation of the nasal septum. Deviation from the midline of the nasal septum is a common finding. In some instances it is caused by a birth trauma or by trauma sustained during childhood or adolescence from a fight with another child. If the deviation is severe and the septum contacts the lateral wall of the nasal cavity, it could make nasal breathing difficult, but this can be surgically remedied.

Rhinitis. This condition is an inflammation of the mucosa that lines the nasal cavity. It usually is caused by an upper respiratory infection or an allergic response to pollen or some other inhaled substance. Infections of the nasal cavity can spread to the nasopharynx, the middle ear (through the eustachion tube), the paranasal sinuses, and the intracranial meninges by way of the cribriform plate.

Primary sinusitis of the maxillary sinus. The roots of the three maxillary molar teeth are adjacent to the inferior wall of the maxillary sinus. Infections from these roots can spread to the mucosa of the maxillary sinus. When these molar teeth are extracted, a fistula between the oral cavity and the maxillary sinus can occur. If infection does not follow, this opening quickly heals. If, however, a root of one of the teeth is fractured, root can be displaced into the sinus. Subsequent procedures to retrieve the root must be followed, and if the mucosa does not become infected, the patient recovers without further problems.

Epistaxis. Nosebleeds usually develop from the richly supplied region in the anterior septum called Kiesselbach's anastomosis. Older patients with hypertension who perceive fear of illness may develop a nosebleed upon visiting a physician. The septum is supplied by branches from the ophthalmic, facial, and sphenopalatine arteries. Nosebleeds frequently occur from trauma that ruptures one of these vessels in the septum.

Fractures of the nose. Fractures of the nose usually involve the nasal bones. The walls of the nasal cavity are not fractured frequently with the possible exception of the cribriform plate of the ethmoid bone. Fractures can occur when there is direct trauma to the nose in sports events or in auto accidents. The interior of the nasal cavity can be visualized for injury by using a mirror inserted through the oral cavity to the oropharynx. Injury to the nasal septum or walls of the nasal cavity usually results in nosebleeds (epistaxis).

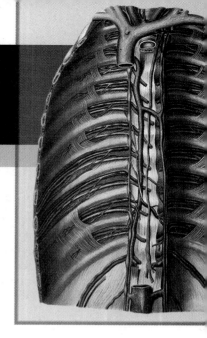

DISSECTION #36

Nasopharynx; Oropharynx (Inner Wall); Palate; Mouth and Tongue

OBJECTIVES

1 Visualize the internal structures of the nasopharynx and dissect its lateral wall.

2 Dissect the soft palate from the nasopharynx.

3 Visualize the internal structures of the oropharynx and dissect its folds and the palatine tonsil.

4 Dissect the hard palate from within the oral cavity.

5 Dissect the tongue and other structures in the oral cavity.

Atlas Key:

Clemente Atlas, 5th Edition = Atlas Plate #

Grant's Atlas, 11th Edition = Grant's Page #

Netter's Atlas, 3rd Edition = Netter's Plate #

Rohen Atlas, 6th Edition = Rohen Page #

Before the head was bisected, the pharynx was opened posteriorly, and its three parts briefly seen. In this dissection the wall of the nasopharynx and the oropharynx are studied on its internal surface and their parts related to the nasal cavity, oral cavity, and soft palate. The tongue and other structures in the mouth will then be dissected.

Posterior to the nasal cavities is located the **nasopharynx,** and posterior to the mouth is found the **oropharynx.** Separating the nasal and oral cavities is the **hard palate,** while the **soft palate** is interposed between the nasopharynx above and the oropharynx below (**ATLAS PLATE 587**). The mouth contains the **tongue, teeth,** and **salivary glands** and is the first part of the digestive tract. Solid and

▶
Grant's 770, 771, 774, 787–789
Netter's's 59–62
Rohen 143, 150, 155
◀
Grant's 770, 771, 774, 787, 789
Netter's 59, 62
Rohen 145, 150, 155
▶
Grant's 764, 770, 771, 774, 789
Netter's 8, 33, 35, 59, 60, 62, 63
Rohen 32, 33, 49, 144, 150, 162

liquid food passes from the posterior part of the oral cavity into the oropharynx.

I. Nasopharynx

The nasopharynx is the most superior part of the pharynx, and it is located above the soft palate and posterior to the nasal cavities (**ATLAS PLATE 591**). It communicates with the oropharynx by a narrow **pharyngeal isthmus that closes during swallowing, principally by the actions of muscles in the soft palate.** The nasopharynx is a passageway for air, and **closure of the isthmus prevents food from entering the nasopharynx and nasal cavities.**

The nasopharynx communicates **anteriorly** with the nasal cavities by way of the oblong **posterior nares** or **choanae** (**ATLAS PLATE 590**). The **roof** of the nasopharynx is formed by the body of the sphenoid bone and, posterior to this, the basilar part of the occipital bone. Located just below the roof on the posterior wall of the nasopharynx is the **pharyngeal tonsil** or adenoid (**ATLAS PLATES 558 #558.2, 587**). This mass of lymphoid tissue normally is enlarged in children and may impede the nasopharyngeal passageway. It often is surgically removed.

The **lateral wall** of the nasopharynx contains the **pharyngeal opening of the auditory tube.** Around this orifice is a rounded elevation, the **torus tubarius,** formed by the cartilaginous pharyngeal end of the auditory tube (**ATLAS PLATE 558 #558.2**). Descending to the pharynx from the lower end of the torus is a fold of mucosa, the **salpingopharyngeal fold,** which overlies a delicate muscle, the **salpingopharyngeus muscle.** Posterior to the torus is a cleft of variable depth called the **pharyngeal recess** (**ATLAS PLATE 587**).

Identify the **pharyngeal opening of the auditory tube (ATLAS PLATE 558 #558.2).** Probe the orifice and note that it is 1.5 cm posterior to the back end of the inferior concha. To see the delicate fibers of the salpingopharyngeus muscle, remove the mucosa from the cartilaginous **torus tubarius** and along the surface of the **salpingopharyngeal fold.**

Posterior to the torus, probe the **pharyngeal recess,** a deep cleft that extends laterally in the pharyngeal wall. Above the pharyngeal recess, probe the submucosa and determine if the pharyngeal tonsil (or adenoid) is still there.

II. Soft Palate From Above: Levator and Tensor Palati Muscles

The palate separates the oral cavity and oropharynx from the nasal cavity and nasopharynx. The anterior two-thirds of the palate has a bony substructure and is the **hard palate** (**ATLAS PLATE 536**). The posterior one-third is the **soft palate,** a fibromuscular structure suspended from the posterior border of the hard palate (**ATLAS PLATE 591**). There are five palatine muscles on each side. Two muscles, the levator and tensor palati muscles, descend to the soft palate from the base of the skull. They are best dissected at the posterior end of the nasal cavity in the nasopharynx (**ATLAS PLATE 586**).

The **levator palati muscle** (also called **levator veli palatini muscle**) is a rounded muscle that arises from the petrous part of temporal bone and from the auditory tube (**ATLAS PLATE 537**). As it descends, its fibers spread and blend with those from the opposite side. It inserts into the palatal aponeurosis and is innervated by the pharyngeal branch of the vagus nerve. Contraction of both levators elevates the soft palate.

▶ Grant's 766, 775
Netter's 59, 61, 64
Rohen 61, 62, 147

◀ Grant's 684, 771
Netter's 33, 34, 39, 45, 60, 61
Rohen 144, 145

▶ Grant's 775
Netter's 60, 61, 65
Rohen 61, 62, 143, 148

◀ Grant's 684, 685
Netter's 59–63
Rohen 144

◀ Grant's 774
Netter's 33
Rohen 143, 144

▶ Grant's 774, 775, 789
Netter's 51, 61, 64
Rohen 25

◀ Grant's 672–674, 770–775
Netter's 6, 8, 33, 59–62
Rohen 32, 45, 143, 144, 150

▶ Grant's 772–775
Netter's 59, 60, 62
Rohen 163

◀ Grant's 766, 767, 771, 775
Netter's 59, 61, 63
Rohen 145, 147, 167

▶ Grant's 774–776
Netter's 60

The **tensor palati** (or **tensor veli palatini**) is a thin muscle that arises from the scaphoid fossa of the sphenoid bone and also from the auditory tube. As it descends, its fibers become tendinous and then course medially around the hamulus of the pterygoid plate (**ATLAS PLATES 586, 591**). Its insertion helps form the aponeurosis of the soft palate. During swallowing, both tensors contract and tighten the soft palate until the bolus of food is in the oropharynx. Each tensor is supplied by the mandibular division of the trigeminal nerve.

Remove the mucoperiosteum from the region superior to the soft palate, **anterior to and just below** the opening of the auditory tube. Deep to the mucosa identify muscle fibers and some glistening tendinous fibers descending into the soft palate. With a probe, separate the more anterior **tensor palati muscle** that lies slightly lateral to the larger **levator palati muscle** (**ATLAS PLATES 586, 591**). Probe for the **ascending palatine artery** (from the facial artery) adjacent to the levator palati. Although other arteries supply the soft palate, this vessel is its chief artery.

Depress the soft palate manually, and separate the levator palati from the cartilaginous auditory tube. Sever the muscle superiorly and reflect it downward. Next, cut away the lower end of the auditory tube and expose the tensor palati. Follow the tensor muscle inferiorly and, with a finger, feel for the bony hamulus of the medial pterygoid plate (**ATLAS PLATE 569 #569.2**). Observe how the delicate tendon of the tensor courses around the hamulus to insert into the soft palate.

III. Internal Structure of the Oropharynx

The oropharynx extends down from the soft palate to the upper border of the epiglottis and lies posterior to the mouth and base of the tongue (**ATLAS PLATE 587**). It contains the **palatine tonsils.** These oblong lymphoid bodies are situated (one on each side of the lateral wall of the oropharynx) in a triangular tonsillar bed between the **palatoglossal** and **palatopharyngeal folds (Figure 36-1).** The lateral and posterior walls of the oropharynx are formed by the superior and middle constrictor muscles deep to the mucosa. Between these two muscles, the stylopharyngeus muscle inserts into the lateral pharyngeal wall (**ATLAS PLATE 586 #586.1**). Other important structures in the oropharynx include:

The **tonsillar branch of the facial artery,** which is the principal vessel supplying the tonsil

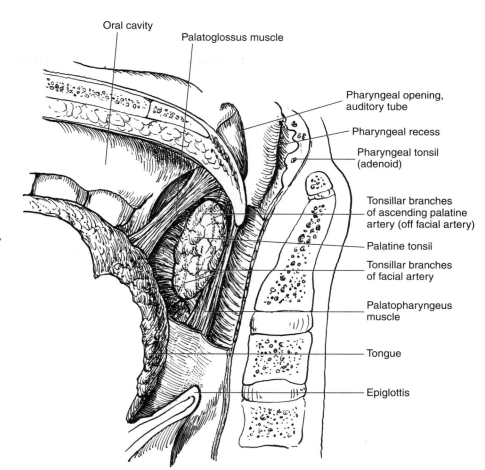

Oral cavity

Palatoglossus muscle

Pharyngeal opening, auditory tube

Pharyngeal recess

Pharyngeal tonsil (adenoid)

Tonsillar branches of ascending palatine artery (off facial artery)

Palatine tonsil

Tonsillar branches of facial artery

Palatopharyngeus muscle

Tongue

Epiglottis

Figure 36-1. Inner aspect of the oropharynx, the palatine, and pharyngeal tonsils.

The **glossopharyngeal nerve,** which is coursing to the posterior third of the tongue (**ATLAS PLATE 562 #562.1**)

The **lesser palatine nerves,** which descend to the oropharynx through the palatine canal (**ATLAS PLATE 567 #567.1**)

Identify the **palatoglossal** and **palatopharyngeal folds** by depressing the posterior part of the tongue and pulling it medially. Note that these folds extend from the inferior surface of the soft palate to the tongue anteriorly and to the pharynx posteriorly. With a probe, strip the thin mucous membrane from these folds and observe the delicate muscle fibers of the palatoglossus and palatopharyngeus muscles deep to the mucosa (**ATLAS PLATE 567 #567.1**).

Probe the fossa between the two folds and determine whether the palatine tonsil has been removed. If lymphoid tissue of the tonsil is still intact, probe deep to the mucosa in the tonsillar bed for the **tonsillar branch of the facial artery.** If, by chance, you probe

◄ Grant's 767, 769, 776, 816
Netter's 60, 67, 119, 129
Rohen 75, 151, 153

◄ Grant's 674, 772–774
Netter's 38, 39
Rohen 146, 147

◄ Grant's 770–776
Netter's 60–62
Rohen 147

► Grant's 766, 768, 776, 816, 817
Netter's 60, 67, 119, 129
Rohen 76, 151

◄ Grant's 766, 767, 775–777
Netter's 60, 61, 63, 64
Rohen 60, 61

too deeply and uncover the muscular floor of the tonsillar bed, realize that this is the **superior constrictor muscle.** Note that deep to the mucosa of the uvula are the muscle fibers of the small musculus uvulae (**ATLAS PLATE 591**).

Turn to the lateral wall of the oropharynx inferior to the tonsillar bed. To find the **glossopharyngeal nerve,** pull the base of the tongue forward and probe the mucosa obliquely in the interval between the superior and middle constrictor muscles. At this site the nerve enters the oropharynx on its course to the posterior tongue (**ATLAS PLATE 595**). Confirm that you have found the IXth nerve by gently pulling on it from the external surface of the pharynx. Recall that the IXth nerve descends in the neck from the jugular foramen. It supplies the stylopharyngeus muscle and then courses anteriorly between the internal and external carotid arteries to the interval between the superior and middle constrictor muscles. It supplies the posterior third of the tongue with both special (taste) and general sensation.

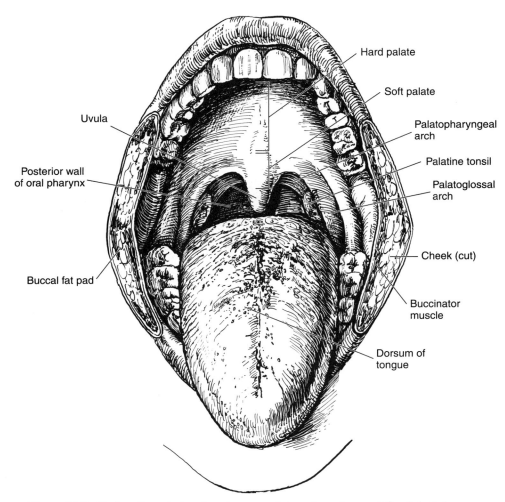

Hard palate

Soft palate

Palatopharyngeal arch

Palatine tonsil

Palatoglossal arch

Cheek (cut)

Buccinator muscle

Dorsum of tongue

Uvula

Posterior wall of oral pharynx

Buccal fat pad

Figure 36-2. Oral cavity, anterior view: tongue, palate, and oropharynx (after Sobotta).

IV. Hard Palate Dissected From Its Oral Surface

The roof of the oral cavity is formed by the hard palate anteriorly and the soft palate posteriorly (**Figure 36-2**). The hard palate has a bony substructure formed in front by the **premaxilla** and on each side by the palatine process of the maxilla and the horizontal plate of the palatine bone (**ATLAS PLATE 582 #582.2**). It is continuous anteriorly and laterally with the alveolar processes of the maxillae that contain the sockets of the upper teeth.

The oral surface of the hard palate is covered by a mucous membrane and periosteum. It contains many mucous glands and a **median palatine raphe** that ends anteriorly in a small **incisive papilla** (**ATLAS PLATE 582 #582.3**). The papilla, located between the two medial incisor teeth, overlies the **incisive canal.** The mucosa also presents three or four transverse folds or rugae, which are less distinct in older people.

▶
Grant's 673, 674, 682, 683
Netter's 48, 58, 60
Rohen 143, 146

◀
Grant's 672, 764, 765
Netter's 8, 52
Rohen 32, 33, 45, 165

◀
Grant's 672
Netter's 48

The hard palate is supplied by the **greater palatine artery and nerve,** which course forward in a groove adjacent to the lateral border of the hard palate (**ATLAS PLATE 567 #567.1**). Anteriorly, the artery **ascends** through the incisive canal and joins an anastomosis on the nasal septum. In contrast, **descending** through the incisive canal from the nasal septum is the **nasopalatine nerve.** It supplies sensory innervation to the anterior part of the hard palate beyond the sensory field of the greater palatine nerve (**ATLAS PLATE 526**).

Three cranial nerves supply sensory innervation to the mucosa of the palate (**Figure 36-3**). The hard palate is supplied by the greater palatine and nasopalatine branches of the trigeminal nerve (V2). The soft palate and oropharynx receive sensory innervation from the glossopharyngeal nerve (IX), and the bed of the palatine tonsil has some sensory fibers from the facial nerve (VII).

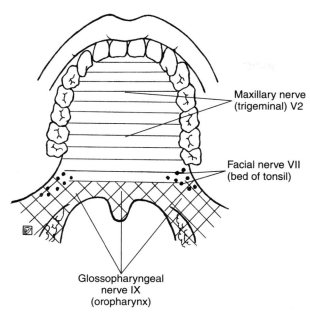

Maxillary nerve
(trigeminal) V2

Facial nerve VII
(bed of tonsil)

Glossopharyngeal
nerve IX
(oropharynx)

Figure 36-3. Sensory innervation of the palate: trigeminal, facial, and glossopharyngeal nerves.

Using a small mirror and a flashlight, inspect the hard palate on a lab partner. Note that it is concave from side to side and that the **incisive papilla** is a small elevation in the midline just posterior to the interval between the two medial incisors (**ATLAS PLATE 582 #582.1**). Realize that the papilla overlies the **incisive canal.** Observe the slight ridge crossing the roof of the mouth just anterior to the palatoglossal folds. This identified the posterior limit of the hard palate. Note many openings of underlying palatine mucous glands on the surface of the palate.

Look at the hard palate on a dried skull. Find the **greater palatine foramen** lateral and just posterior to the palatomaxillary suture. Note that the smaller **lesser palatine foramina** (usually two) perforate the palatine bone posterior to the greater foramen (**ATLAS PLATE 582 #582.3**). Observe the groove that courses anterior from the greater palatine foramen, along which travel the **greater palatine vessels and nerve.**

Palpate the oral surface of the palate in your cadaver to determine the border between the hard and soft palates. Posterior to the lateral angle of the hard palate (behind the 3rd molar tooth), feel for the delicate hamulus of the medial pterygoid plate, around which courses the tendon of the tensor palati muscle (**ATLAS PLATE 569 #569.1**).

▶
Grant's 673,
681–683, 772
Netter's 37–39
Rohen 143,
146, 147

▶
Grant's 666, 668
Netter's 47
Rohen 55

◀
Grant's 672
Netter's 48
Rohen 165

▶
Grant's 666, 670
Netter's 47, 49,
55–57
Rohen 153
▶
Grant's 670, 743,
746, 747
Netter's 42, 47, 57,
127
Rohen 149, 153

◀
Grant's 672, 772
Netter's 8, 34, 52
Rohen 45

▶
Grant's 772
Netter's 47, 48

◀
Grant's 772
Netter's 60
Rohen 144, 150

Laterally, 0.5 cm behind the maxillary dental arch, cut away the mucosa from the palate. With a probe, stroke longitudinally forward along the lateral edge of the hard palate and expose the **greater palatine vessels and nerve (ATLAS PLATE 563 #563.1).** Dissect forward and behind the two medial incisors to find the **incisive fossa.** Follow the greater palatine artery to the incisive foramen and find the **nasopalatine nerve** descending through the canal to the palate (**ATLAS PLATE 563 #563.1**).

Posterior to the greater palatine foramen try to find the **lesser palatine vessels and nerves** as they enter the soft palate.

V. Oral Cavity and Tongue

A. **Oral Cavity (ATLAS PLATES 566–569).** The oral cavity consists of a U-shaped arched cleft, called the **vestibule,** and the **oral cavity proper.** The slitlike vestibule lies between the lips and cheeks externally and the gums and teeth (**Figure 36-4**). The oral cavity proper is limited by the gums, teeth, and alveolar arches and communicates posteriorly with the oropharynx.

The palate forms the roof of the oral cavity, whereas the floor is principally the tongue and the mucous membrane that stretches laterally below the tongue to the mandibular arch. A fold in the midline that connects the inferior surface of the tongue to the floor of the mouth is called the **frenulum of the tongue (ATLAS PLATE 568 #568.1**). On both sides of the frenulum is located a small mound called the **sublingual papilla,** and at its apex is located the **opening of the submandibular duct.**

Deep to the mucosa laterally on both sides are located the **sublingual glands (ATLAS PLATE 573**). They form slight bulges, called the **sublingual folds,** along the lateral borders of the floor of the mouth (**ATLAS PLATE 568 #568.1**). Along each fold are located from 10 to 20 minute openings of the **sublingual ducts.**

1. **Inspection.** Inspect the oral cavity on a study partner or by looking at yourself in a mirror at home, using a flashlight. Observe the dorsum of the tongue and identify the **palatoglossal folds** and, posterior to them, the **palatopharyngeal folds (ATLAS PLATE 566 #566.1**). Elevate the tongue to the hard palate and look at the sublingual region. Identify the **frenulum of the tongue** attaching the inferior surface of the tongue to the floor of the mouth (**ATLAS PLATE 568 #568.1**).

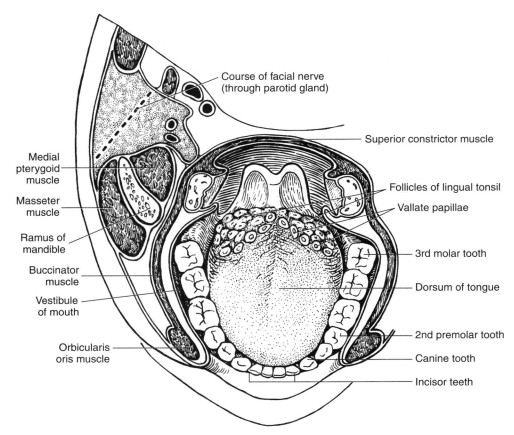

Figure 36-4. Oral cavity, showing the vestibule, tongue, and mandibular teeth.

Identify the *sublingual* **folds** formed by the sublingual glands deep to the mucosa (**ATLAS PLATE 568 #568.1**). These are slight longitudinal bulges on both sides of the frenulum. Note that the folds terminate anteriorly in slight elevations called the **sublingual papillae**. At this apex are the openings of the submandibular ducts (**Figure 36-5**).

Beneath the tongue identify the **deep lingual veins,** dark longitudinal vessels on each side of the frenulum (**ATLAS PLATE 570 #570.2, Figure 36-5**). The sublingual administration of drugs in pill form is a common practice when quick absorption into the bloodstream is required and intravenous administration is inconvenient or inappropriate.

2. **Dissection.** Bisect the dorsum of the tongue and the lower lip and saw through the mandible anteriorly in the midline. Carry the bisection inferiorly through the hyoid bone to the larynx. In the midline identify the **mylohyoid muscle** and, superior to this, the **geniohyoid muscle** that form the floor of the mouth (**ATLAS PLATE 571 #571.2**). Pull a bisected half of the tongue medially away from the mandibular

◄
Grant's 670, 743
Netter's 47, 57
Rohen 153

►
Grant's 666, 670,
743, 746
Netter's 42, 47,
49, 57
Rohen 149, 153

◄
Grant's 746
Netter's 55

◄
Grant's 666, 669,
670, 821
Netter's 55, 59
Rohen 150, 151,
155

►
Grant's 743–745,
812, 813
Netter's 42, 55, 57,
67, 125
Rohen 82, 84, 145,
149, 153

arch and remove the mucosa to expose the sublingual gland.

a. **Sublingual gland and submandibular duct (ATLAS PLATE 570 #570.2, 573).** With a probe, expose the **sublingual gland** and identify the delicate **submandibular duct** coursing anteriorly along the medial surface of the gland (**Figure 36-6**). Do not confuse the duct with the vein, artery, and nerves found more medially that serve the tongue. The submandibular duct can be identified with certainty by following it posteriorly to the deep part of the submandibular gland. Note its termination anteriorly behind the lower medial incisor tooth (**Figure 36-7**).

b. **Lingual nerve and submandibular ganglion.** Find the **lingual nerve** as it courses forward between the tongue and the sublingual gland, but close to the side of the tongue (**ATLAS PLATES 570 #570.2, 573**). Dissect initially in the region posterior and inferior to the last molar tooth. Identify the nerve as it travels anteriorly and is **crossed by the submandibular duct. To**

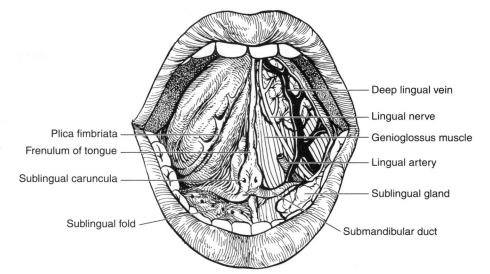

Figure 36-5. Sublingual region of the oral cavity. Note the frenulum, sublingual fold, caruncula and gland, submandibular duct, and lingual vessels.

Deep lingual vein

Lingual nerve

Genioglossus muscle

Lingual artery

Sublingual gland

Submandibular duct

Plica fimbriata

Frenulum of tongue

Sublingual caruncula

Sublingual fold

reach the tongue, the nerve crosses from lateral to medial under the duct (ATLAS PLATES 570 #570.2, 573). After finding the lingual nerve, identify the **submandibular ganglion** suspended from the nerve posteriorly in the mouth beyond the 3rd molar tooth (**ATLAS PLATES 513, 570 #570.2**). Note that two or more filaments attach the ganglion to the nerve. Other fibers course from the ganglion to the sublingual and submandibular glands.

c. Hypoglossal nerve and lingual artery. Reexamine the course of the hypoglossal nerve

▶
Grant's 666, 670, 741–746, 766
Netter's 30, 47, 55, 56, 57, 230
Rohen 81, 84, 151, 153

on the lateral side of the neck as it passes between the mylohyoid and hyoglossus muscles to enter the oral cavity (**ATLAS PLATE 492 #492.1**). Within the oral cavity identify and define the hyoglossus muscle extending between the hyoid bone and the posterior inferior surface of the tongue (**ATLAS PLATE 576 #576.1**). Find the hypoglossal nerve as it passes forward, **lateral to the hyoglossus muscle.** The position of this muscle is important in identifying the hypoglossal nerve in the oral cavity coursing anteriorly to the tongue (**ATLAS PLATE**

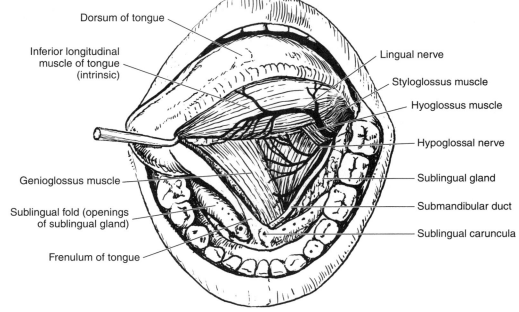

Figure 36-6. The lingual and hypoglossal nerves and submandibular duct dissected on one side of the mouth.

Dorsum of tongue

Inferior longitudinal muscle of tongue (intrinsic)

Genioglossus muscle

Sublingual fold (openings of sublingual gland)

Frenulum of tongue

Lingual nerve

Styloglossus muscle

Hyoglossus muscle

Hypoglossal nerve

Sublingual gland

Submandibular duct

Sublingual caruncula

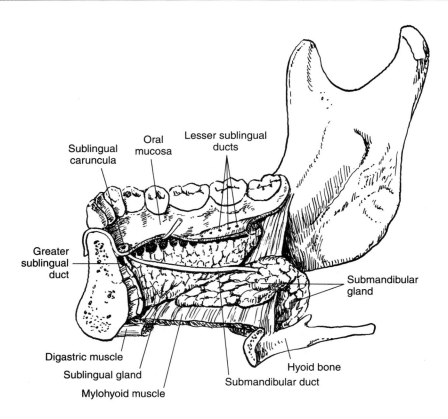

Sublingual caruncula

Oral mucosa

Lesser sublingual ducts

Greater sublingual duct

Submandibular gland

Digastric muscle

Sublingual gland

Hyoid bone

Mylohyoid muscle

Submandibular duct

Figure 36-7. The submandibular and sublingual glands in the oral cavity (after Sobotta).

570 #570.2). Probe the region between the hyoglossus muscle and the submandibular gland and find the **lingual artery.** It also enters the oral cavity from the neck, except that it courses **medial (or deep) to the hyoglossus muscle (Figure 36-8).** Follow the hypoglossal nerve to the tongue and note that it lies deep in the oral cavity, **significantly inferior to the lingual nerve (ATLAS PLATE 570 #570.2).**

B. The Tongue. The tongue is a muscular organ that is important for the functions of swallowing, taste, and speech. Although located in the floor of the oral cavity, its base extends posteriorly into the oropharynx. Its **extrinsic muscles (ATLAS PLATES 576, 577)** are attached to the hyoid bone **(hyoglossus),** mandible **(genioglossus),** styloid process **(styloglossus),** and soft palate **(palatoglossus).** The tongue also contains **intrinsic muscles** that form much of its bulk. These are arranged in **longitudinal, transverse,** and **vertical** bundles and can be identified by studying the bisected tongue and then cutting the tongue transversely.

The "dorsal surface" of the tongue is actually its superior surface on which is the V-shaped **sulcus terminalis** that divides the oral two-thirds (anterior) from the pharyngeal one-third (posterior). At the apex of the V is located a shallow pit called the **foramen cecum.**

► Grant's 666, 668
Netter's 54
Rohen 149

► Grant's 666, 668, 774
Netter's 54, 60
Rohen 149, 150

► Grant's 666
Netter's 58

◄ Grant's 666–668
Netter's 55–59
Rohen 151, 155

This marks the site where the thyroglossal diverticulum descended to give rise to the thyroid gland during development **(ATLAS PLATE 575 #575.1).**

The dorsal surface of the tongue contains many taste receptors; the largest are 8 to 10 **vallate papillae** arranged anterior to the V-shaped sulcus **(ATLAS PLATE 575 #575.1).** Other fungiform, filiform, and foliate taste receptors are distributed over the surface of the anterior part of the tongue. Lymphoid nodules (lingual tonsil) cover the posterior tongue surface **(Figures 36-9, 36-10).** The taste receptors and the lymphoid tissue give the mucous membrane of the tongue a roughened surface.

The tongue is supplied by five cranial nerves: **V, VII, IX, X, XII.**

1. **Motor nerve supply**
   a. All extrinsic and intrinsic muscles except the palatoglossus: **hypoglossal nerve (XII; ATLAS PLATE 570 #570.2)**
   b. Palatoglossus muscle: **pharyngeal branch of vagus (X; ATLAS PLATES 589, 634)**
2. **General sensation**
   a. Anterior two-thirds of the tongue: **lingual branch of trigeminal (V3; ATLAS PLATES 575 #575.3, 579, 622)**
   b. Posterior one-third of tongue: **glossopharyngeal nerve (IX; ATLAS PLATES 575, 579)**
   c. Small region on posterior one-third close to epiglottis: **superior laryngeal branch of vagus (X)**

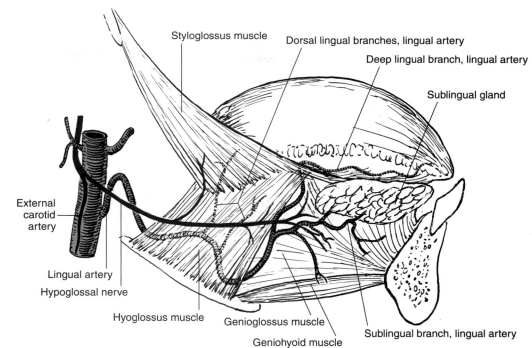

Figure 36-8. The lingual artery and hypoglossal nerve coursing from the neck to the oral cavity (after Grant).

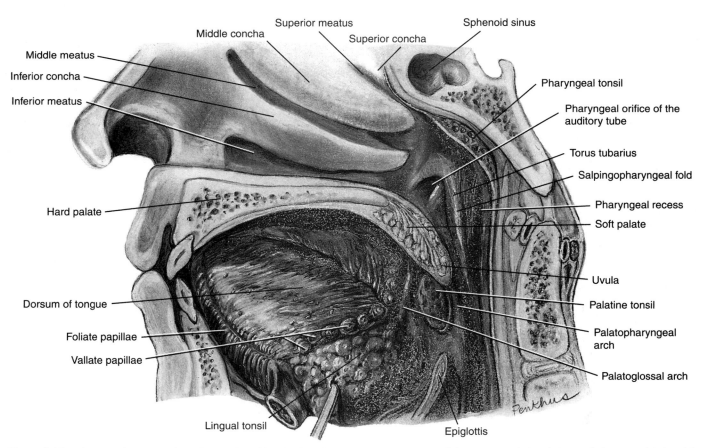

Figure 36-9. The nasopharnyx and oropharynx in midsagittal section showing the dorsum of the tongue and the platine and pharyngeal (adenoid) tonsils. (From Clemente CD. Gray's Anatomy. 30th American Edition. Philadelphia; Lea and Febiger, 1985.)

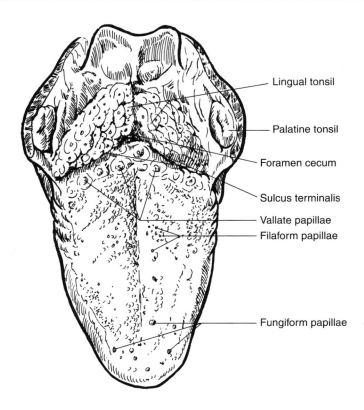

Lingual tonsil

Palatine tonsil

Foramen cecum

Sulcus terminalis

Vallate papillae
Filaform papillae

Fungiform papillae

Figure 36-10. Dorsal surface of the tongue, showing the various receptors, the sulcus terminalis, and the lingual tonsil.

3. **Special sense of taste (ATLAS PLATES 632, 633, #633.3)**
   a. Anterior two-thirds of the tongue: **chorda tympani branch of facial nerve (VII)**
   b. Posterior one-third of tongue: **glossopharyngeal nerve (IX)**
   c. Small region on posterior one-third close to epiglottis: **superior laryngeal branch of vagus (X)**

The principal vessel that supplies blood to the tongue is the **lingual artery,** a branch of the external carotid artery. It gives off dorsal and deep lingual branches as well as the sublingual artery to the sublingual gland (**Figure 36-8**).

Identify the extrinsic and intrinsic tongue muscles (**Figure 36-11**).

1. Find the **hyoglossus muscle** by locating it again on the lateral side of the neck. Trace the muscle from its attachment on the hyoid bone (deep to the mylohyoid muscle) superiorly to the side of the tongue (**ATLAS PLATE 576 #576.1**). Note that the hypoglossal nerve courses anteriorly along its outer surface, while the tortuous lingual artery lies deep to the muscle (**ATLAS PLATE 492 #492.1**).

2. Identify the **genioglossus muscle** on the hemisected tongue. Note that its fibers originate from the mental spine on the inner surface of

▶
Grant's 667, 669, 746, 821
Netter's 55, 59, 122
Rohen 86, 150, 166

▶
Grant's 744, 745, 766, 821
Netter's 55, 61, 62, 122
Rohen 60, 75, 151, 166

▶
Grant's 775, 776
Netter's 48, 55, 60
Rohen 147
◀
Grant's 741, 744, 776, 821
Netter's 49, 55, 64, 122
Rohen 63, 153, 166, 167
▶
Grant's 666
Rohen 55, 86, 149

▶
Grant's 744–746, 766, 776
Netter's 42, 55, 67, 119, 122
Rohen 75, 151, 153

the mandible behind the symphysis menti and spread superiorly and posteriorly into the tongue in a fanlike manner (**ATLAS PLATE 574 #574.2**).

3. Identify the **styloglossus** by pulling the tongue medially away from the mandible and probing through the mucosa at the upper lateral aspect of the tongue (**ATLAS PLATES 576 #576.1, 586 #586.1**). Feel for the styloid process located posterior and lateral to the superior constrictor muscle. Follow the styloglossus as it descends from the styloid process to the side of the tongue, where its fibers blend with those of the hyoglossus.

4. The delicate **palatoglossus** was uncovered earlier in this dissection when the oropharynx was dissected.

5. Identify the longitudinal and transverse intrinsic tongue muscles by observing the bisected tongue (**ATLAS PLATE 574 #574.2**). Cut the tongue transversely at about its middle and look for the transverse fibers.

6. Finally, review the locations in the oral cavity of the **lingual, hypoglossal,** and **glossopharyngeal nerves** that supply the tongue as well as the **lingual artery** and its branches.

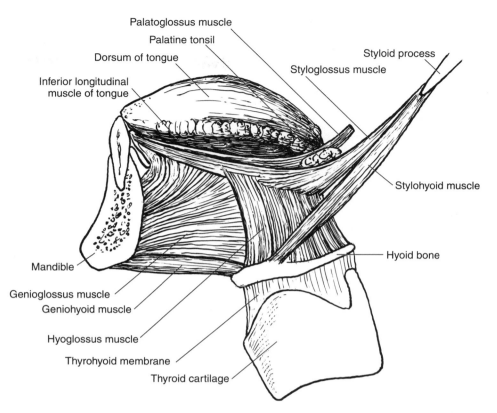

Figure 36-11. Extrinsic muscles of the tongue (after Sobotta).

Palatoglossus muscle
Palatine tonsil
Dorsum of tongue
Inferior longitudinal muscle of tongue
Styloid process
Styloglossus muscle
Stylohyoid muscle
Hyoid bone
Mandible
Genioglossus muscle
Geniohyoid muscle
Hyoglossus muscle
Thyrohyoid membrane
Thyroid cartilage

Clinical Relevance

Blockage of the pharyngotympanic tube. The pharyngotympanic tube connects the middle ear with the nasopharynx. It is therefore the means by which pressure in the middle ear is maintained equal to atmospheric pressure. Upper respiratory infections often block the lumen of this tube by swelling its mucous membrane. This tube is also the means by which upper pharyngeal infections spread to the tympanic cavity.

Lingual nerve injury. The lingual nerve within the oral cavity is closely related to the third molar tooth. Because of this, it is liable to be injured when the third molar tooth is extracted. If the nerve is severed, there is a total loss of general sensation, along with the special sense of taste, on the ipsilateral half of the anterior two-thirds of the tongue. Additionally, there is loss of sensation to much of the floor of the oral cavity on the same side—as a result, these patients inadvertently bite their tongue. Some sensory return may occur if the nerve is neurosurgically reunited successfully; however, sensation may never return.

The palatine tonsil. The palatine tonsil lies in the fossa between the palatoglossal and palatopharyngeal folds within the oropharynx. The medial surface of the tonsil contains 12 to 20 crypts, which in children with chronic tonsillitis may become inflamed and painful. Removal of the tonsils was a common practice before the development of antibiotics but is not routinely performed today. The tonsils can be seen through the mouth when the tongue is depressed. They are largest during childhood, but they become smaller during adolescence and early adulthood. They drain into cervical lymph nodes (especially into the jugulodigastric node) adjacent to the mandibular angle.

Cleft palate. More common in females than in males, this developmental defect can involve only the region of the uvula, but it can extend anteriorly through the soft palate and hard palate. This occurs because the tissue of the lateral palatine process fails to meet on the midline.

Cleft lip. This is more common in males than in females and can be either unilateral or bilateral. A cleft upper lip may involve only the lip, but, if more serious, it may extend more deeply and be continuous with a cleft palate. Although the anomaly is usually unilateral, it can be bilateral if both maxillary processes fail to meet with the medial nasal process. A cleft of the lower lip is less common and results because the mandibular processes do not fuse.

Cancer of the tongue. A lingual carcinoma in the posterior tongue is more serious than in the anterior tongue because posterior tongue tumors metastasize to deep cervical nodes relatively quickly. Tumor cells from the anterior tongue spread somewhat later. Because lingual cancer spreads to nodes in the upper neck and to the deep cervical nodes, these tumors can be exceedingly serious if not recognized early.

Hypoglossal nerve injury. Inadvertent injury to the hypoglossal nerve can occur when operations are performed in the suprahyoid region. This cranial nerve supplies all intrinsic and all extrinsic tongue muscles except the palatoglossus muscle. The ipsilateral half of the tongue becomes atrophied, and upon protrusion, the tongue deviates to the paralyzed side because the normal contralateral genioglossus muscle acts unopposed.

Anesthesia to the mandibular teeth. Dentists frequently anesthetize the inferior alveolar nerve when dental work must be done on the mandibular teeth. Once the medial side of the mandible is palpated for the region of the mandibular foramen, successful anesthesia is achieved by injecting the anesthetic adjacent to this foramen. The inferior alveolar nerve courses through this foramen on its way to innervat-ing all of the mandibular teeth. The region of the chin where the mental branch of the inferior alveolar nerve emerges is also anesthetized.

Gingivitis. This condition is an inflammation of the gum tissue that surrounds teeth, and it usually results from inadequate dental hygiene. If the condition is allowed to continue, the infection can lead to periodontal disease of structures surrounding the teeth in the dental sockets and in the mandibular bone itself.

Anesthesia of the nasopalatine or greater palatine nerve. Anesthesia of the nasopalatine nerves is achieved by injecting the anesthetic adjacent into the opening of the incisive canal at the anterior aspect of the hard palate where the nerve emerges into the oral cavity. The greater palatine nerve is anesthetized by injecting the anesthetic adjacent to the greater palatine foramen on the medial aspect of the mandibular dental arch between the second and third molar teeth.

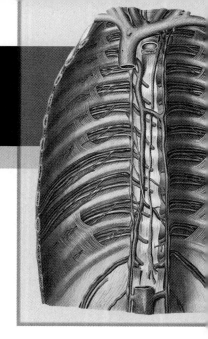

DISSECTION #37

The Larynx and Laryngopharynx

OBJECTIVES

1 Learn the skeleton of the larynx.

2 Learn the relationships of the larynx to other structures in the neck and identify anterior laryngeal structures.

3 Identify the posterior structures of the larynx, dissect the laryngeal part of the pharynx, expose the laryngeal vessels and nerves, and dissect the laryngeal muscles visible posteriorly and laterally.

4 Dissect the interior of the larynx and identify its components, fold, and membranes.

Atlas Key:

Clemente Atlas, 5th Edition = Atlas Plate #

Grant's Atlas, 11th Edition = Grant's Page #

Netter's Atlas, 3rd Edition = Netter's Plate #

Rohen Atlas, 6th Edition = Rohen Page #

The larynx lies superior to the trachea and serves as the organ of phonation. It also is an air passage capable of being closed if increased intra-abdominal pressure is required. The larynx lies anterior to the laryngeal part of the pharynx, and most of its neurovascular structures pass deep to pharyngeal mucosa to reach the larynx.

I. The Skeleton of the Larynx (ATLAS PLATES 596, 597)

The walls of the larynx are formed by cartilages interconnected by certain ligaments and membranes. Over these structures are draped the laryngeal muscles,

► Grant's 778, 779
Netter's 73
Rohen 158, 159

◄ Grant's 752, 766, 767
Netter's 64, 67, 70, 76
Rohen 156, 162

◄ Grant's 778, 779
Netter's 73
Rohen 158, 159

whereas the internal surface of the larynx is covered by a mucous membrane. Because the larynx is part of the airway and must remain open (except when it is voluntarily or reflexly closed), the skeleton supports its walls and prevents it from collapsing and inadvertently closing the respiratory passage.

The skeleton of the larynx consists of three unpaired cartilages and three smaller paired cartilages. The unpaired cartilages from superior to inferior are (a) the **epiglottis,** (b) the **thyroid cartilage,** and (c) the **cricoid cartilage**. Of the paired cartilages, the **arytenoid cartilages** are most important because their movements alter the tension of the vocal folds and the width of the rima glottidis (the space between the vocal folds). The paired **corniculate** and **cuneiform cartilages** are small and can be palpated as small nodules along the **aryepiglottic fold** that stretches between the apex of the arytenoid cartilage and the epiglottis.

Turn to **ATLAS PLATES 596** and **597.** Study the cartilages and the cricothyroid and thyrohyoid membranes.

A. The Epiglottis

1. Identify the epiglottis. It is a sheet of elastic fibrocartilage shaped somewhat like a leaf and located posterior to the tongue and hyoid bone (**ATLAS PLATE 595**).

2. Note that it extends superiorly in front of the laryngeal inlet and that its inferior pointed end attaches to the inner surface of the thyroid cartilage (**ATLAS PLATE 598 #598.2**).

3. Observe that the superior free border of the epiglottis attaches to the base of the tongue in the midline and laterally by the **median and lateral glossoepiglottic folds** (**ATLAS PLATE 575 #575.1**). Observe its attachment inferiorly to the arytenoid cartilages by the important **aryepiglottic folds.**

The aryepiglottic folds contain the aryepiglottis muscles that contract during swallowing and reduce the opening into the larynx (**ATLAS PLATE 596 #596.2**). Additionally, as the pharynx and larynx are elevated to receive a bolus of food, the epiglottic folds posteriorly over the laryngeal opening and helps to divert the food laterally through the piriform recesses away from the larynx.

B. The Thyroid Cartilage (Figures 37-1, 37-2)

1. Note that the thyroid cartilage is the largest of the laryngeal cartilages. It is formed of hyaline cartilage, which tends to ossify in the aged.

2. Observe that it consists of two broad laminae or fused wings anteriorly that are widely separate posteriorly (**ATLAS PLATE 598**). Note that the fused laminae end in a marked projection anteriorly, called the laryngeal prominence (or "Adam's apple").

3. Note that posteriorly the separated laminae end in two slender projections called the **superior and inferior horns.**

4. Identify the **thyrohyoid membrane,** which attaches the superior border of the thyroid cartilage with the inferior border of the hyoid bone.

C. The Cricoid Cartilage (Figures 37-1, 37-2)

1. Identify the cricoid cartilage. Note that, unlike the thyroid cartilage, it forms a complete arch around the larynx. Also note that it lies inferior to the thyroid cartilage and is interposed between it and the trachea.

2. Observe that anteriorly the cricoid is narrow (0.5 cm) and that it enlarges laterally to 1.0 cm.

◄
Grant's 770, 782, 784
Netter's 54, 62, 74
Rohen 158, 160, 163

►
Grant's 778, 783, 784
Netter's 73
Rohen 158

◄
Grant's 770, 781–783, 785
Netter's 62, 63, 73
Rohen 161, 163

►
Grant's 784, 785
Netter's 74, 75
Rohen 160

◄
Grant's 770, 781–783
Netter's 74
Rohen 160

►
Grant's 778–780, 782, 785
Netter's 73, 75
Rohen 158, 161

◄
Grant's 778, 779
Netter's 73
Rohen 158, 159

►
Grant's 778, 779, 782, 783, 785
Netter's 73, 75
Rohen 158, 160

►
Grant's 752, 755
Netter's 24, 25, 59, 64, 73
Rohen 156, 157, 162

◄
Grant's 778–780, 782
Netter's 73
Rohen 158

►
Grant's 752, 753
Netter's 25, 27
Rohen 156, 157

Note that posteriorly it expands vertically and horizontally to about 2.5 cm (**ATLAS PLATE 598**).

3. Identify the **median cricothyroid ligament** anteriorly. It attaches the cricoid cartilage to the thyroid cartilage. Note the **cricotracheal ligament** that attaches the cricoid cartilage to the first tracheal cartilage inferiorly (**Figure 37-1**).

4. Observe that the cricoid cartilage articulates posteriorly on both sides with the arytenoid cartilages at the cricoarytenoid synovial joints.

5. Observe on **ATLAS PLATE 596 #596.1** that the **straight** and **oblique heads** of the **cricothyroid muscle** attach to the anterior surface of the cricoid cartilage. Also, note on **ATLAS PLATE 597 #597.1** that the **posterior** and **lateral cricoarytenoid muscles** extend from the cricoid cartilage superiorly to the base of the arytenoid cartilage.

D. The Arytenoid Cartilages

1. On **ATLAS PLATES 598 #598.2** and **599** observe that the small arytenoid cartilages resemble three-sided pyramids. Observe that their bases are positioned on each side of the upper posterior border of the cricoid cartilage and that their apices support the small corniculate cartilages (**ATLAS PLATE 598 #598.2**).

2. Note on **ATLAS PLATE 599 #599.2** that the triangular base of the arytenoid cartilage has a lateral angle called the **muscular process** onto which attach both the **posterior and lateral cricoarytenoid muscles.** Also observe that the anterior angle of the base is pointed and called the **vocal process.** The vocal ligament attaches to it and extends forward horizontally to the inner surface of the thyroid cartilage.

II. Surface Anatomy of the Anterior Larynx

The larynx is an anterior cervical structure located in the midline, and it occupies the medial part of both anterior triangles. Its structures are easily palpated in living subjects but may be more difficult to feel in the embalmed cadaver.

1. Palpate the midline cervical structures on a laboratory partner. With your index finger start at the middle of the chin and progress down to the suprasternal notch (**ATLAS PLATE 470**).

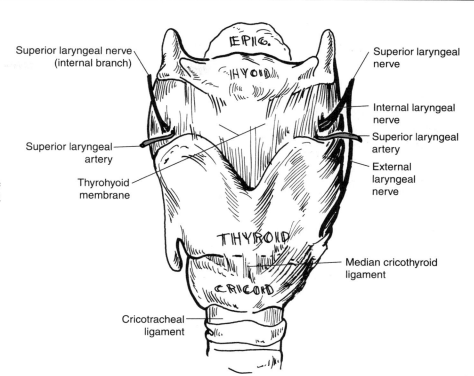

Figure 37-1. Anterior view of the larynx. Note that the thyroid cartilage is attached to the hyoid bone above and cricoid cartilage below.

2. Under the chin, in the upper neck, feel the body of the hyoid bone in the midline. With your thumb and index finger palpate the greater horns of the hyoid bone posteriorly nearly to the sternocleidomastoid muscle (**ATLAS PLATES 475, 586**).

3. Below the hyoid bone palpate the laryngeal prominence and the laminae of the thyroid cartilage that extend laterally from the prominence (**ATLAS PLATES 472, 473**). Have your lab partner swallow, and feel the entire larynx elevate 1 cm as the pharynx, attached posteriorly, is raised behind the oral cavity.

4. Feel the cricoid cartilage inferior to the thyroid cartilage and above the first tracheal ring. Below the cricoid, palpate about 5 cm of trachea above the jugular notch in the neck (**ATLAS PLATE 598 #598.1**).

5. On **ATLAS PLATE 587** observe that the hyoid bone lies at the level of the 3rd cervical vertebra, the thyroid cartilage at C4 and C5, and the cricoid cartilage at C6.

6. On yourself feel for the carotid pulse lateral to the hyoid bone and realize that the common carotid arteries (and their bifurcation), the internal jugular veins, and the vagus nerves extend through the carotid triangles lateral to the larynx (**ATLAS PLATES 479, 483**).

Study the anterior structures of the larynx on the cadaver. In addition to the hyoid bone and the thyroid and cricoid cartilages, dissect the thyrohyoid membrane, the superior laryngeal vessels and nerve, and the cricothyroid muscles.

► Grant's 752, 778, 779
Netter's 24, 64, 73
Rohen 156–160

► Grant's 787, 789
Netter's 59, 61

► Grant's's 739, 750–752
Netter's 27, 65, 67
Rohen 169, 183, 184

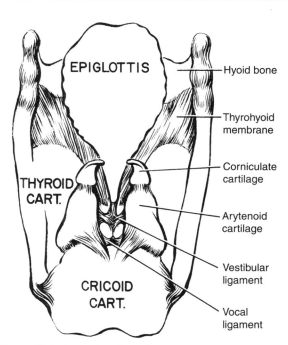

Figure 37-2. Posterior view of the laryngeal cartilages.

1. If the attachments of the omohyoid and sternohyoid muscles have not been severed from the hyoid bone, do that now. Identify the two thyrohyoid muscles (**ATLAS PLATES 576 #576.1, 586**). Deep to these lies the **thyrohyoid membrane,** which attaches the upper border of the thyroid cartilage to the hyoid bone (**Figure 37-3**).

   ◄
   Grant's 755, 756, 767
   Netter's 70, 72
   Rohen 158, 160

2. Along the lateral border of the thyrohyoid muscle again find the **internal laryngeal nerve** and **superior laryngeal artery** (**ATLAS PLATE 594**). Recall that the **superior laryngeal branch of the vagus** gives rise to both internal and external laryngeal branches and that the latter descends to supply the cricothyroid muscle.

   ►
   Grant's 783–785
   Netter's 75

   ◄
   Grant's 751, 783, 784
   Netter's 65–67, 70, 120
   Rohen 84, 151

3. Trace the **superior laryngeal artery** back to its source, the superior thyroid artery. Separate the nerve from the artery as both structures penetrate the thyrohyoid membrane to enter the larynx (**ATLAS PLATES 586, 594**). Note that the artery is slightly inferior to the nerve.

   ◄
   Grant's 741, 757
   Netter's 30, 65, 70, 130
   Rohen 84, 169

4. Dissect the **straight** and **oblique** parts of the **cricothyroid muscle** and confirm that the

   ◄
   Grant's 783–785
   Netter's 74, 75
   Rohen 160

slender external branch of the superior laryngeal nerve supplies it (**ATLAS PLATE 596 #596.1**). This delicate nerve courses inferiorly, lateral to the superior thyroid artery and deep to the sternohyoid muscle, to reach the cricothyroid.

Realize that the cricothyroid muscle tilts the cricoid cartilage superiorly, which results in pushing the arytenoid cartilages posteriorly. Simultaneously, the thyroid cartilage is pulled anteriorly and inferiorly (**ATLAS PLATE 596 #596.1**). These actions increase the distance between the arytenoid and thyroid cartilages, thereby lengthening the vocal folds and increasing their tension (**Figure 37-8A**).

III. The Posterior Larynx; the Laryngopharynx; the Lateral Laryngeal Muscles (ATLAS PLATE 595)

Of importance are the following structures visible posteriorly on the larynx: the **epiglottis** and its attachments to the tongue (median and lateral glossoepiglottic folds), the **aryepiglottic folds,** the **cuneiform** and **corniculate cartilages,** and the opening into the larynx, called the

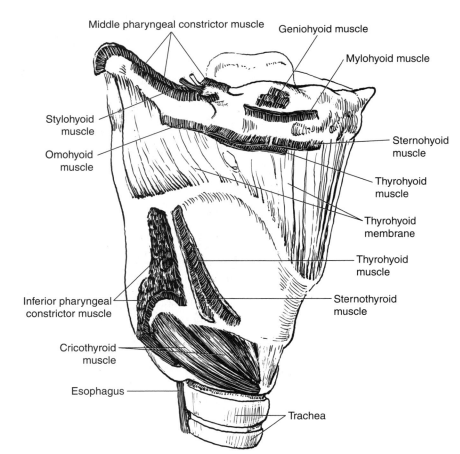

Figure 37-3. Muscle attachments onto the lateral surface of the larynx.

aditus (**ATLAS PLATE 592**). Also located posteriorly are the **piriform fossae,** which are two small recesses, one on each side of the laryngeal opening. These attach the larynx, located medially, to the walls of the laryngopharynx laterally.

Beneath the mucosa of the piriform fossa are found the **internal branch of the superior laryngeal nerve** and the **superior laryngeal vessels** that have penetrated the thyrohyoid membrane. The **recurrent laryngeal nerve,** accompanied by the **inferior laryngeal artery** (from the inferior thyroid artery), ascends in the groove between the trachea and esophagus to the larynx. These structures enter the larynx posteriorly behind the joint formed by the inferior horn of the thyroid cartilage and cricoid cartilage (**ATLAS PLATE 595**).

Posteriorly are located the following laryngeal muscles: posterior cricoarytenoid, the transverse and oblique arytenoid, and the aryepiglotticus.

◄
Grant's 770, 771, 784
Netter's 62
Rohen 160, 163

►
Grant's 770, 771, 784
Netter's 62, 63
Rohen 160, 163

◄
Grant's 741, 784, 785
Netter's 63, 76
Rohen 162, 163

A. The Epiglottis and Aryepiglottic Folds (ATLAS PLATE 596 #596.3). Turn the larynx and pharynx over so that their posterior surfaces can be visualized. Identify the following:

1. The **epiglottis,** located behind the base of the tongue. It forms the anterior boundary of the inlet (or aditus) of the larynx.

2. The **aryepiglottic folds** that bound the upper border of the inlet. Feel along the surface of these folds and detect the slight elevations in the mucous membrane made by the underlying **cuneiform** and **corniculate cartilages** (**ATLAS PLATE 597 #597.4**).

B. The Piriform Recess and the Laryngeal Vessels and Nerves (Figure 37-4)

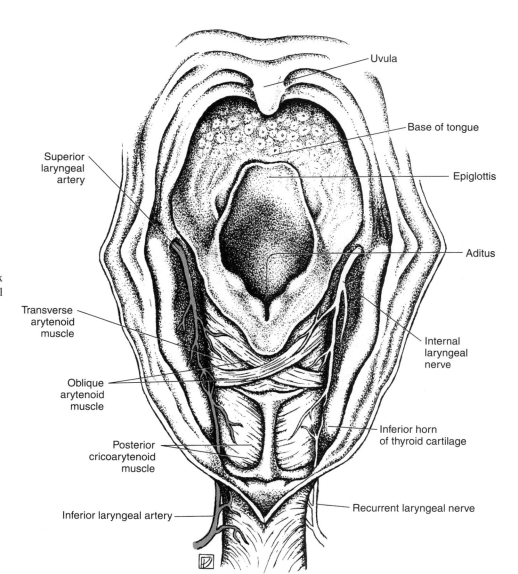

Figure 37-4. Posterior view of the larynx and laryngopharynx, showing laryngeal vessels and nerves.

1. Identify the **piriform recesses** (**ATLAS PLATES 590–592**). These longitudinal fossae in the laryngopharynx are located between the pharyngeal wall laterally and the sides of the inlet of the larynx medially.

2. Extend the exposure of the pharynx by cutting the upper part of the esophagus inferiorly about 5 cm. Remove the mucosa from the inner surface of the laryngopharynx, commencing superiorly, lateral to the epiglottis, and continue inferiorly to the esophagus. Identify the **superior laryngeal nerve and vessels** descending in the piriform recess lateral to the epiglottis (**ATLAS PLATE 495, Figure 37-4**).

3. Lower in the piriform recess identify the **recurrent laryngeal nerve** and the delicate inferior laryngeal vessels. Note that these laryngeal vessels and nerves course to the larynx deep to the mucosa lining the piriform recess (**ATLAS PLATE 595, Figure 37-4**).

C. **The Posterior Laryngeal Muscles**

1. Remove the connective tissue over the **posterior cricoarytenoid muscles** located on the posterior surface of the lamina of the larynx (**ATLAS PLATE 596 #596.3**).

The posterior cricoarytenoid muscles course superiorly and laterally to insert on the arytenoid cartilages. They pull the bases of the arytenoid cartilages medially and posteriorly and **serve as the only abductors of the vocal folds (Figure 37-5A)**.

2. Clean the **transverse and oblique parts of the arytenoid muscle** just superior to the cricoid cartilage posteriorly (**ATLAS PLATE 596 #596.3**). Follow the continuation of the oblique fibers superiorly to the epiglottis along the lateral surface of the aryepiglottic fold as the aryepiglottis muscle.

The aryepiglottic muscles course superiorly on both sides of the laryngeal inlet. Their contraction serves as a sphincter of the inlet by bringing the aryepiglottic folds closer together. The transverse and oblique arytenoid muscle approximates the arytenoid cartilages, and this **adducts the posterior part of the vocal folds (Figures 37-5B, 37-6)**.

D. **The Lateral Laryngeal Muscles.** Dissect the two muscles on the lateral aspect of the larynx. These are the **lateral cricoarytenoid** and the **thyroarytenoid muscles** (**ATLAS PLATE 597 #597.1**).

◀ Grant's 766, 767, 770, 771
Netter's 62
Rohen 160, 161, 163

◀ Grant's 741, 784, 785
Netter's 63, 76
Rohen 163

◀ Grant's 754, 783–785
Netter's 76
Rohen 162, 163

◀ Grant's 771, 784, 785
Netter's 62
Rohen 160, 163

◀ Grant's 783–785
Netter's 75

▶ Grant's 783–785
Netter's 74
Rohen 160

◀ Grant's 783–785
Netter's 74, 75
Rohen 160

◀ Grant's 783–785
Netter's 74, 75
Rohen 160, 163

▶ Grant's 783–785
Netter's 74, 75
Rohen 160

▶ Grant's 783–785
Netter's 74, 75
Rohen 160, 161

◀ Grant's 783–785
Netter's 74–76
Rohen 160

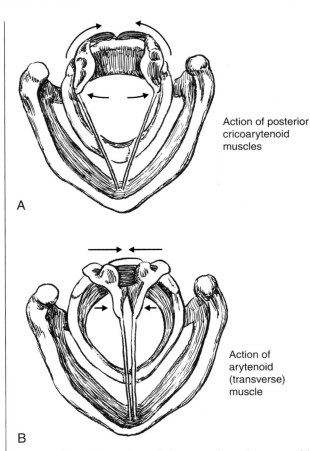

Action of posterior cricoarytenoid muscles

A

Action of arytenoid (transverse) muscle

B

Figure 37-5. A. Action of the posterior cricoarytenoid muscles (abduction of the vocal folds). **B.** Action of the transverse arytenoid muscle (adduction of the vocal folds).

1. In the following manner cut away the posterior half of one of the laminae of the thyroid cartilage (see **ATLAS PLATE 597**). Detach the lateral half of the thyrohyoid membrane from the hyoid bone. With scissors, cut the thyrohyoid membrane longitudinally, but leave the internal laryngeal nerve and superior laryngeal vessels intact. Continue the cut through the thyroid cartilage and cricothyroid muscle, and disarticulate the inferior horn from the cricoid cartilage (see **Figure 37-6**).

2. Clean the surface of the small **lateral cricoarytenoid muscle** and observe its oblique orientation (**ATLAS PLATE 597**). Note that it stretches superiorly and posteriorly from the arch of the cricoid cartilage to the muscular process of the arytenoid cartilage.

3. Define the **thyroarytenoid muscle.** Observe that this wide muscular sheet arises from the deep surface of the thyroid lamina and stretches posteriorly, superiorly, and laterally to insert onto the arytenoid cartilage (**ATLAS**

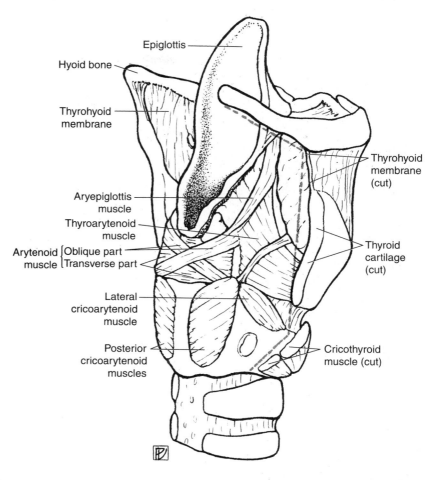

Figure 37-6. Line of incision through the thyrohyoid membrane, thyroid cartilage, cricoid cartilage, and cricothyroid muscle. This exposes the muscles on the lateral aspect of the larynx.

PLATE 597 #597.1). Note that its upper fibers (called the **thyroepiglottic muscle**) extend to the epiglottis and join the aryepiglottic fibers, while its most medial and deepest fibers form the **vocalis muscle (Figure 37-7)**. This latter muscle extends from the thyroid cartilage to the vocal process of the arytenoid cartilage along the lateral side of the vocal ligament (**ATLAS PLATE 601 #601.1**).

The lateral cricoarytenoid muscles act as **adductors of the vocal folds** and are the antagonists of the posterior cricoarytenoid muscles (**Figure 37-8B**). The thyroarytenoid muscles shorten or relax the vocal folds by pulling the arytenoid cartilages toward the thyroid cartilage. The vocalis muscles are thought to alter the pitch of the voice by both relaxing and tensing portions of the vocal ligaments (**Figure 37-8C**).

IV. The Interior of the Larynx (ATLAS PLATE 600)

The laryngeal cavity (**Figure 37-9**). The cavity within the larynx extends from the laryngeal inlet to

► Grant's 781–783 Netter's 589 Rohen 161

◄ Grant's 783–785 Netter's 75

► Netter's 59 Rohen 149

the lower border of the cricoid cartilage and becomes continuous with the trachea. Two pairs of membranous folds project into the laryngeal cavity from the sides of the larynx, and they divide the cavity into three parts. The more superior folds are called the **vestibular folds** (sometimes called false vocal folds), and the more inferior pair are important for voice production and are the true **vocal folds** (**ATLAS PLATE 600**). The opening between the vestibular folds is the **rima vestibuli,** and the opening between the true vocal folds is the **rima glottidis.** Thus, three compartments are found in the laryngeal cavity: the compartment superior to the vestibular folds is the **vestibule,** the small compartment between the vestibular and vocal folds is the **ventricle,** and the **infraglottic cavity** is that part of the cavity between the true vocal folds and the trachea (**ATLAS PLATE 600 #600.1**).

1. **The vestibule (ATLAS PLATE 600).** The vestibule of the laryngeal cavity lies between the laryngeal inlet and the vestibular folds. Wider superiorly than inferiorly, its anterior wall is the posterior surface of the epiglottis. The lateral walls are the mucous membrane covering the aryepiglottic folds, and the small posterior border is the mucosa covering the arytenoid cartilages.

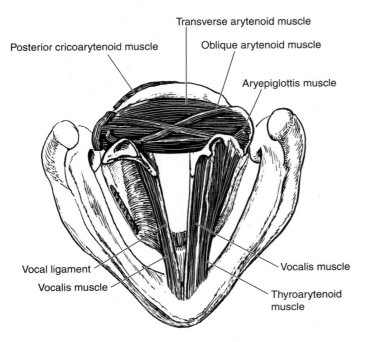

Posterior cricoarytenoid muscle
Transverse arytenoid muscle
Oblique arytenoid muscle
Aryepiglottis muscle
Vocal ligament
Vocalis muscle
Vocalis muscle
Thyroarytenoid muscle

Figure 37-7. The vocalis and thyroarytenoid muscles and the vocal ligament; also the transverse and oblique arytenoid muscles.

2. **The ventricle.** The ventricle is the smallest of the three parts of the cavity, and it is bounded above by the vestibular folds and below by the vocal folds (**ATLAS PLATE 597 #597.4**).

◄
Grant's 781–783
Netter's 59
Rohen 161

►
Grant's 781

The **vestibular folds** are soft and flaccid. They are formed by a band of fibroelastic tissue covered by a mucous membrane. The **rima vestibuli** between the two folds is wider than the rima glottidis. The vestibular folds have little to do with the production of voice, in contrast to the vocal folds (**ATLAS PLATE 600**).

The **vocal folds** are sharp, and the mucous membrane covering them is tightly bound to the underlying **vocal ligament** (**ATLAS PLATE 601**). They are white, and each extends from the vocal process of the arytenoid cartilage to the posterior surface of the thyroid cartilage. The vocal ligament is a continuation superiorly of the **conus elasticus** (see below). Lateral and parallel to the vocal ligament are fibers of the **vocalis muscle**. These are the deep lowermost fascicles of the thyroarytenoid muscle. The vocal folds are the important voice-producing structures in the larynx, and the **rima glottidis** is the elongated fissure between the folds (**Figure 37-10**).

◄
Grant's 783–785
Netter's 74, 75, 77
Rohen 158, 160, 161

►
Grant's 782
Netter's 74
Rohen 158

3. **The infraglottic cavity.** The laryngeal cavity, inferior to the rima glottidis and vocal folds, leads directly into the trachea (**ATLAS PLATE 600 #600.1**). Its walls are covered by mucous membrane. An emergency opening (laryngotomy) may be performed through its anterior aspect.

The quadrangular membrane and the conus elasticus. Deep to the mucosa covering the inner surface of the larynx is a layer of fibrous elastic tissue. **Above the vestibular folds** it is called the **quad-**

►
Grant's 781

rangular membrane, and **below the vocal folds** it is called the **conus elasticus (or cricovocal membrane).**

1. **The quadrangular membrane.** On each side, the quadrangular membrane extends from the lateral border of the epiglottis posteriorly to the corniculate and arytenoid cartilages (**ATLAS PLATE 600 #600.1**). Inferiorly, it reaches the vestibular folds. Along with the mucosa and muscle fibers, the two quadrangular membranes form the aryepiglottic folds between the piriform recesses and the aditus of the larynx.

2. **The conus elasticus (ATLAS PLATES 597 #597.4, 599 #599.3).** The conus elasticus (or cricovocal membrane) is a submucosal layer that contains a stronger elastic layer than the quadrangular membrane. It attaches to the upper border of the cricoid cartilage and extends medially and superiorly to the vocal ligament. The two sides of the conus elasticus join in the anterior midline just deep to the anterior cricothyroid ligament.

Look into the interior of the larynx through the aditus and identify the vestibular folds and, inferior to these, the vocal folds (**ATLAS PLATE 600**). Now open the larynx in the following manner so that the interior of the right and left halves are exposed.

With scissors, cut the trachea in the posterior midline about 2 cm inferior to the cricoid cartilage. Continue your cut superiorly through the lamina of the cricoid cartilage and then through the transverse arytenoideus muscle to the posterior notch of the

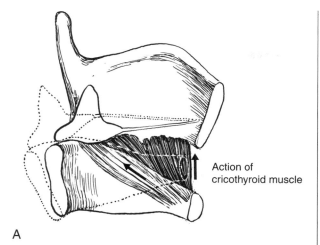

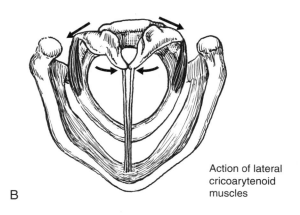

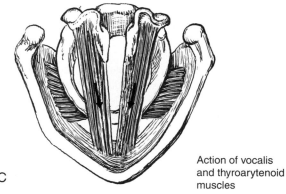

Figure 37-8. A. The action of the cricothyroid muscle (elongate and increase the tension of the vocal folds). **B.** The action of the lateral cricoarytenoid muscle (adduct the vocal ligaments). **C.** The action of the thyroarytenoid muscles and the vocalis muscles. The thyroarytenoid muscle shortens and relaxes the vocal fold. The vocalis muscle relaxes the posterior part of the vocal ligament, while the anterior part is tense, thereby raising the pitch of the voice.

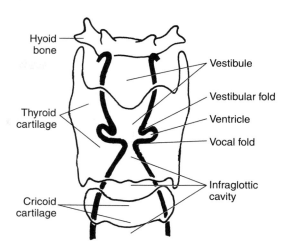

Figure 37-9. Cavity of the larynx.

▶
Grant's 781–785
Netter's 77
Rohen 160, 161

▶
Grant's 781

▶
Grant's 781–785
Netter's 74, 75
Rohen 158, 160, 161

▶
Grant's 781–785
Netter's 76
Rohen 162, 163

aditus. Next, cut the epiglottis in the midline and then the arch of the cricoid cartilage anteriorly in the midline. Open the larynx by unfolding it as if opening a book (see **ATLAS PLATE 600 #600.2**).

Identify the vestibular and vocal folds again, and probe the space called the **ventricle** between the folds. Note that the space superior to the ventricular folds is the **vestibule** and that the **infraglottic space** inferior to the vocal folds leads into the trachea (**ATLAS PLATE 600 #601.2**).

With forceps and a sharp scalpel, remove the mucosa from the inner surface of the aryepiglottic fold and uncover the **quadrangular membrane.** Observe that this membrane extends from the lateral border of the epiglottis to the arytenoid cartilage and that it becomes thickened inferiorly to help form the vestibular fold.

Remove the mucosa inferior to the vocal folds to the upper border of the cricoid cartilage, and expose the **conus elasticus** (cricovocal ligament). Note that it is triangular on each side and extends from the midline superiorly to the vocal folds (where it becomes the **vocal ligament**) and inferiorly to the upper border of the cricoid cartilage. Finally, remove the mucosa from the surface of the vocal fold, and identify the fibers of the **vocalis muscle.** These course anteroposteriorly, parallel to the vocal ligament (**ATLAS PLATE 601 #601.1**).

Sensory innervation to the mucosa that lines the interior of the larynx **below the vocal folds** is derived from the **recurrent laryngeal nerve,** whereas the mucosa **above the vocal folds** is supplied by the **internal laryngeal branch of the superior laryngeal nerve** (**ATLAS PLATE 595**). This latter nerve is important because it serves as the afferent limb of the cough reflex.

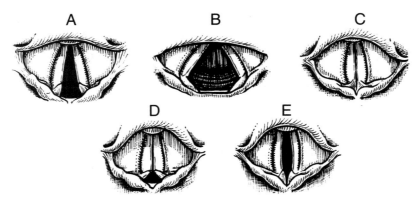

Figure 37-10. The rima glottidis during (**A**) normal breathing and resting; (**B**) deep or forced inspiration; (**C**) shrill tones; (**D**) whispering; (**E**) falsetto voice.

Clinical Relevance

Fractures of laryngeal cartilages. Fractures of the laryngeal cartilages usually are injuries to the thyroid or cricoid cartilages. These happen most often from sports injuries such as in boxing or football. The acute problems of such injuries include hemorrhage into the larynx and swelling (edema) of the laryngeal mucosa. These sequellae to laryngeal fractures can result not only in speech, but also potential obstruction of the airway.

Laryngoscopy. This is the procedure for examining the larynx either by laryngeal mirror (indirect laryngoscopy) or by laryngoscope (direct laryngoscopy). The tongue is pulled anteriorly to reveal the interior of the larynx, including the vestibular and vocal folds. The laryngoscope is a fiberoptic endoscope that has a light source and a cutting instrument for biopsy.

Internal laryngeal nerve block. Anesthesia of the internal branch of the superior laryngeal nerve is often necessary for an endotracheal intubation. This procedure is performed by inserting the anesthetic through the thyrohyoid membrane to the interior of the larynx superior to the vocal folds. The superior laryngeal nerve supplies sensory innervation to the mucosa of the larynx above the vocal folds, whereas the inferior laryngeal branch of the recurrent laryngeal nerve supplies the mucosa of the larynx from below the vocal folds to the trachea.

Cancer of the larynx. Cancer of the larynx occurs most frequently in persons who smoke cigarettes, and early signs include persistent hoarseness of speech and enlarged and palpable lymph nodes anterior to and along the borders of the trachea. This is a highly malignant cancer, and removal of the larynx may be performed followed by the use of several available speech prostheses.

Injury to the laryngeal nerves. The recurrent laryngeal nerves innervate all muscles in the larynx, except the cricothyroid muscle. The external branch of the superior laryngeal nerve supplies the cricothyroid, and denervation of this muscle results in weakness of the voice because tension of the vocal fold cannot occur. Severance of one recurrent laryngeal nerve (during thyroidectomy or because of esophageal cancer) is compensated for by the other nerve, but hoarseness is the result. Severance of both nerves results in loss of speech and breathing is affected, since the rima glottis is partially closed.

Mucosal edema of the vocal ligament. Edema of the mucous membrane superior to the rima glottidis can significantly reduce the airway passage. If this is severe, a cricothyroidotomy or a tracheostomy may be required.

Cricothyroidotomy. This procedure is used to insert an airway tube between the thyroid and cricoid cartilages, and it is often preferable to a tracheostomy. The latter, however, can be done when there has been severe trauma to the larynx. A transverse incision is made through the skin between the thyroid and cricoid cartilages and the fascia and strap muscles are separated. The larynx is also cut transversely through the cricothyroid ligament after which the tube is inserted.

Fracture of the hyoid bone. Trauma to the upper neck (such as in strangling) can fracture the greater horns of the hyoid bone. The remainder of the bone (the body and perhaps one still attached greater horn) descends over the larynx. The fractured hyoid is not able to be elevated, which makes swallowing difficult. Also there is a significantly increased possibility of food in the oropharynx entering the airway and causing pneumonia.

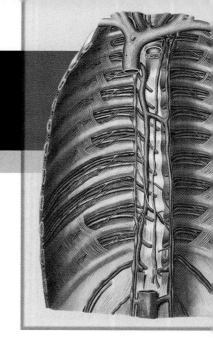

DISSECTION #38

The External and Middle Ear and the Semicircular Canals of the Inner Ear

OBJECTIVES

1 Dissect the auricle and the walls of the external acoustic meatus that together make up the external ear.

2 Expose the tympanic membrane, facial canal, and semicircular canals by a lateral or mastoid approach.

3 Open the middle ear cavity through the base of the skull, and expose the middle ear ossicles clearly.

Atlas Key:

Clemente Atlas, 5th Edition = Atlas Plate #

Grant's Atlas, 11th Edition = Grant's Page #

Netter's Atlas, 3rd Edition = Netter's Plate #

Rohen Atlas, 6th Edition = Rohen Page #

The ear consists of external, middle, and internal parts. It contains the **peripheral auditory apparatus** essential for the special sense of hearing and the **peripheral vestibular apparatus,** including the semicircular canals (**ATLAS PLATE 604 #604.1**). From this latter apparatus the brain receives a constant flow of impulses concerning the position and movements of the head in space, and it is essential for the maintenance of balance. This dissection focuses on the anatomy of the external and middle ear, although the semicircular canals will also be partially exposed.

◄
Grant's 696–698
Netter's 87
Rohen 122–124

I. The External Ear

The external ear consists of the auricle, the walls of the external acoustic meatus, and the lateral surface of

the tympanic membrane. These can be examined with an otoscope.

The Auricle (Figure 38-1). The **auricle** consists of an irregularly shaped single piece of elastic fibrocartilage that underlies the skin. Through its opening course the air vibrations that form the sound waves. The

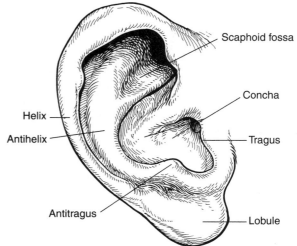

Figure 38-1. Right external ear (or auricle).

anatomic features of the auricle can be seen in **ATLAS PLATE 602.** The auricular muscles consist of three thin extrinsic muscles that connect the auricle to the scalp (**ATLAS PLATE 495**) and several smaller intrinsic muscles (**ATLAS PLATE 602**). These are of little functional significance in the human ear and will not be considered further. Sound waves are transmitted along the external acoustic meatus, a canal about 2.5 cm long, to the tympanic membrane. The latter separates the external ear from the cavity of the middle ear.

◄
Grant's 696
Netter's 88
Rohen 124

B. The External Acoustic Meatus (ATLAS PLATE 604, Figure 38-2). The external acoustic meatus is directed medially, and it inclines slightly anteriorly. It consists of a more lateral cartilaginous part (9 mm) and a more medial osseous part (16 mm). The subcutaneous tissue of the cartilaginous part contains glands and hairs. The glands secrete **cerumen,** a protective ear wax, and their coiled appearance resembles sweat glands. The external acoustic meatus is important clinically. Through it the tympanic membrane can be visualized with an otoscope. Its shape, slightly curved, must be considered when entrapped foreign objects within the canal require removal.

◄
Grant's 697, 698
Netter's 88
Rohen 122–124

C. The Tympanic Membrane (ATLAS PLATE 605). The tympanic membrane is an oval disc, 0.1 mm thick, which separates the external acoustic meatus and the tympanic cavity of the middle ear. Upon examination in the living patient, the lateral surface of the membrane appears concave. The deepest part of the concavity is called the **umbo,** and this corresponds to the lower part of the handle of the malleus (one of the middle ear ossicles) on the convex medial surface of the membrane. Most of

◄
Grant's 698, 699
Netter's 88
Rohen 126

the circumference of the membrane is thickened and forms a fibrocartilaginous ring (**Figure 38-3**).

Much of the tympanic membrane is tightly stretched and called the **pars tensa.** A small triangular area between two thickened folds, the **anterior** and **posterior malleolar folds,** is more lax and is called the **pars flaccida (ATLAS PLATE 605 #605.1).** The **external (lateral) surface** of the membrane is innervated by the auriculotemporal branch of the trigeminal nerve and several delicate auricular branches of the vagus nerve. It is supplied by the **deep auricular branch of the maxillary artery.**

The **medial (or internal) surface** of the tympanic membrane (**ATLAS PLATE 605 #605.1**) is supplied by the **tympanic branch of the glossopharyngeal nerve.** It receives blood from the **anterior tympanic branch of the maxillary artery** and the **stylomastoid branch of the posterior auricular artery.** These anastomose with the vessels supplying the external surface.

Examine the **auricle** or pinna and realize that it is attached to the lateral surface of the temporal bone by anterior and posterior ligaments. These ligaments are not to be dissected, nor are either the extrinsic or intrinsic muscles of the external ear.

Identify the **concha,** which is the deep cavity that occupies the middle of the auricle (**ATLAS PLATE 602**). Then identify the small curved flap called the **tragus,** located in front of the lower part of the concha (**Figure 38-1**). Cut the tragus away to expose the opening of the external acoustic meatus.

Gently probe the depth of the meatus. Remove the remainder of the cartilaginous wall and with a mallet

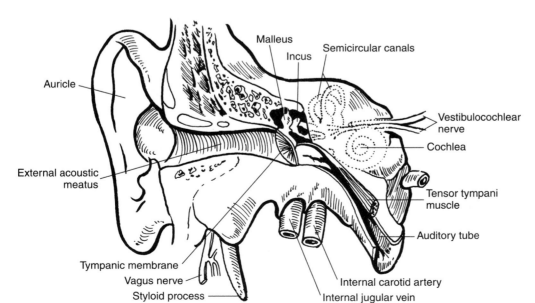

Figure 38-1.
Figure 38-2. External auditory canal (frontal view).

Malleus
Incus
Semicircular canals
Auricle
Vestibulocochlear nerve
Cochlea
External acoustic meatus
Tensor tympani muscle
Auditory tube
Tympanic membrane
Vagus nerve
Styloid process
Internal carotid artery
Internal jugular vein

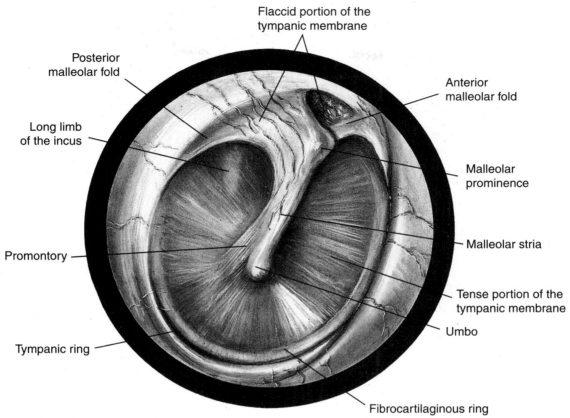

Flaccid portion of the
tympanic membrane

Posterior
malleolar fold

Anterior
malleolar fold

Long limb
of the incus

Malleolar
prominence

Malleolar stria

Promontory

Tense portion of the
tympanic membrane

Umbo

Tympanic ring

Fibrocartilaginous ring

Figure 38-3. The lateral surface of the tympanic membrane as seen with an otoscope. It measures 11 mm vertically and 9 mm across. (From Clemente CD. Gray's Anatomy. 30th American Edition. Philadelphia: Lea and Febiger, 1985.)

and chisel carefully remove the front of the osseous part of the meatus **without damaging the tympanic membrane (ATLAS PLATE 604).** When the membrane is exposed, use a small flashlight to examine its lateral surface. Identify the impression laterally made by the **handle of the malleus** on the medial surface of the membrane, and note the malleolar folds **(ATLAS PLATE 605).** Between the folds identify the flaccid part of the membrane **(pars flaccida).** Note that the remainder is called the **pars tensa.** Clinicians arbitrarily divide the latter into four quadrants by a line drawn along the handle of the malleus and another line drawn across the membrane just below the end of the malleus **(ATLAS PLATE 605).**

II. The Lateral (Mastoid) Approach to the Facial Nerve; Semicircular Canals; Tympanic Cavity (Figures 38-4, 38-5, 38-6, 38-8)

The tympanic cavity, its ossicles, and the facial nerve within the facial canal may all be seen by approaching the middle ear laterally. This is the "mastoid approach"

and requires dissection of the mastoid and petrous parts of the temporal bone posterior to the external ear **(ATLAS PLATES 609 #609.1, 611).**

A. **The Facial and Semicircular Canals.** The facial nerve initially traverses the **internal acoustic meatus** within the temporal bone from the middle cranial fossa **(ATLAS PLATES 611 #611.2, 628).** At the lateral end of this meatus the nerve becomes enlarged by the **geniculate ganglion,** and it enters the bony **facial canal** within the temporal bone **(Figure 38-4).** At this site it gives off the **greater petrosal nerve** and abruptly bends posteriorly and inferiorly to form the **genu of the facial nerve.** The facial nerve then descends posterior to the tympanic cavity to the stylomastoid foramen, where it leaves the facial canal medial and posterior to the earlobe **(ATLAS PLATE 611 #611.2).**

Medial to the tympanic cavity is located the **cochlea** of the internal ear, and posterior and superior to the genu of the facial nerve and canal are found the **lateral, posterior,** and **anterior semicircular canals (ATLAS PLATE 613).** Although the semicircular canals will not be specifically dissected, one or more will be opened as

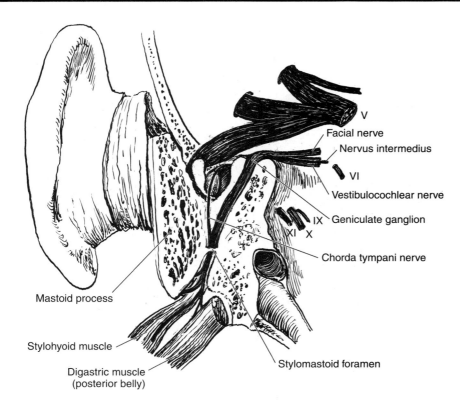

Figure 38-4. Course of the facial nerve in the facial canal.

bone is removed in this lateral approach. Situated in the bone posterior to the semicircular canals is a rounded bulge in the bone, formed by the sulcus in the floor of the cranial cavity that contains the sigmoid sinus.

B. The Tympanic Cavity. The **tympanic cavity** is an irregularly shaped air-filled space located medial to the tympanic membrane. It lies between the external and internal ear, and it is traversed by three small auditory bones, or ossicles: the **malleus, incus,** and **stapes** (**ATLAS PLATE 606**). These transmit vibrations from the tympanic membrane to the small **vestibular (oval) window.** The handle of the malleus is attached on the medial surface of the tympanic membrane, while the base of the stapes is planted medially in the oval window and contacts directly the perilymphatic fluid of the inner ear (**ATLAS PLATES 607, 608**).

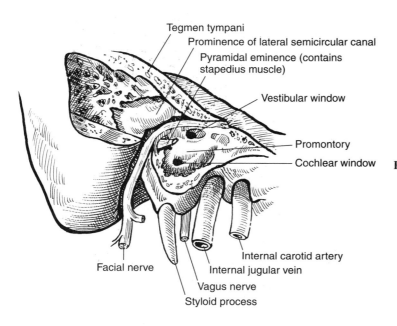

Figure 38-5. Bony medial wall of the tympanic cavity.

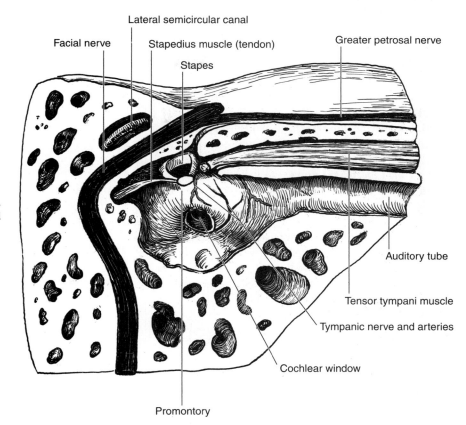

Figure 38-6. Medial wall of the tympanic cavity, showing the promontory and the stapedius and tensor tympani muscles.

The cavity of the middle ear is continuous posteriorly with the **aditus (or entrance) to the mastoid antrum,** the **mastoid antrum** itself, and the **mastoid air cells,** all located within the temporal bone (**ATLAS PLATE 603 #603.1**). Anteriorly, the tympanic cavity communicates with the nasopharynx by way of the auditory tube. Under normal conditions, therefore, the air pressure in the middle ear is the same as that in the nasopharynx.

This results in the same pressure on both sides of the tympanic membrane.

C. Boundaries of the Tympanic Cavity

Roof (the **tegmental wall**): a thin plate of bone that separates the tympanic cavity from the cranial cavity (**ATLAS PLATE 603 #603.2**).

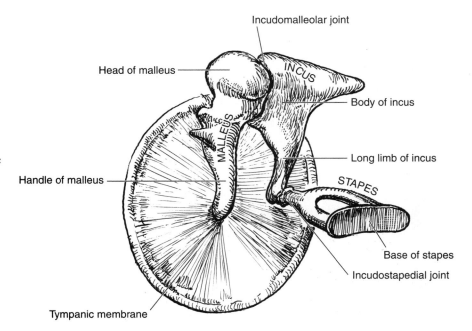

Figure 38-7. Medial surface of the tympanic membrane and the three middle ear ossicles.

Floor (the **jugular wall**): a narrow convex plate of bone that lies between the tympanic cavity and the bulb of the jugular vein.

Lateral wall (the **membranous wall**): formed by the tympanic membrane and the bony rim to which it is attached. It is crossed by the **chorda tympani nerve** (**ATLAS PLATE 607**).

Medial wall (the **labyrinthine wall**): separates the middle ear cavity from the internal ear (**ATLAS PLATES 608, 609**). It is marked by a rounded elevation called the **promontory** and the **prominence of the facial canal.** The medial wall contains the **vestibular** (oval) and **cochlear** (round) **windows** (**Figure 38-5**).

Posterior wall (the **mastoid wall**): contains the entrance to the tympanic antrum, which leads to the mastoid air cells. It also contains the **pyramidal eminence** within which is located the **stapedius muscle** (**ATLAS PLATES 608, 609**).

Anterior wall (the **carotid wall**): is bounded by a thin layer of bone that separates the tympanic cavity from the internal carotid artery. It also contains the canal for the **tensor tympani muscle** and the osseous part of the auditory tube (**ATLAS PLATES 607–609, Figure 38-6**).

1. **The Ossicles of the Tympanic Cavity.** The small bones of the middle ear form a chain of ossicles; from lateral to medial these are the **malleus,** the **incus,** and the **stapes.** The handle (or manubrium) of the malleus is attached to the medial surface of the tympanic membrane, and the posterior surface of its head articulates with the body of the incus (**ATLAS PLATE 606**). The long process of the incus articulates with the head of the **stapes,** and the flattened oval base of the stapes is bound to the **vestibular or oval window** (**Figure 38-7**).

On a dried skull, identify the suprameatal spine and suprameatal crest superior and posterior to the opening of the external acoustic meatus (**ATLAS PLATE 603 #603.1**). Find the suprameatal spine and crest on the cadaver by removing the remains of the cartilaginous auricle. Cut away all the soft tissue, including periosteum, from the lateral surface of the mastoid part of the temporal bone posterior to the auricle.

With a chisel and mallet or, if available, a pair of rongeurs (bone-cutting forceps), open the mastoid part of the temporal bone between the suprameatal spine and crest. This will expose some of the **mastoid air cells.** Continue removing the spongy mastoid bone carefully until the mastoid antrum is opened (**ATLAS PLATE 603 #603.2**) and the smoother, more compact bone located posteriorly becomes visible.

◄ Grant's 701–703, 705
Netter's 87
Rohen 127

◄ Grant's 699, 701, 703
Netter's 87–89
Rohen 126

► Grant's 701–703
Netter's 87, 89–91
Rohen 124–129

◄ Grant's 701, 654
Netter's 89
Rohen 126

◄ Grant's 701, 703
Netter's 89
Rohen 126, 127

► Grant's 697, 700–703
Netter's 87–89, 91
Rohen 122, 123, 126, 128

◄ Grant's 701–703
Netter's 89
Rohen 124, 125

◄ Grant's 698–701
Netter's 87, 88, 91
Rohen 128

► Grant's 700, 701, 707
Netter's 87
Rohen 122, 123

► Grant's 615, 706, 708
Netter's 9, 10
Rohen 30, 34, 37

◄ Grant's 608, 654

► Grant's 706–708, 814
Netter's 10, 92
Rohen 34, 130

► Grant's 701, 703, 705–707
Netter's 87, 91
Rohen 122, 123, 130

◄ Grant's 701–703
Netter's 88, 89
Rohen 122, 127

Identify the projection of the **canal for the facial nerve,** which curves inferiorly at almost 90°. Just superior, posterior, and medial to this **genu** of the facial canal (and nerve), locate the bulges of the **lateral, posterior,** and **anterior semicircular canals** (**ATLAS PLATES 612, 630**). Open the facial canal and expose the facial nerve. Identify the **chorda tympani branch** of the facial nerve as it courses anteriorly into the middle ear and along the medial surface of the tympanic membrane (**Figure 38-8**).

Posterior to the facial and semicircular canals identify a bulge in the bone made by the **sigmoid sinus** coursing superiorly in the cranial cavity. Remove more of the posterior and superior walls of the external acoustic meatus, and open the middle ear cavity to visualize the **malleus, incus,** and **stapes.** Identify the bulging **promontory** on the medial surface of the tympanic cavity. Realize that on its surface is the **tympanic plexus** of nerves and vessels. Medial to the promontory is located the basal turn of the **cochlea.** Finally, the base of the **stapes** is planted over the **vestibular (or oval) window,** situated superior and slightly posterior to the promontory.

III. The Superior (Cranial Cavity) Approach to the Middle Ear

The middle ear can also be approached superiorly through the petrous and mastoid parts of the temporal bone in the floor of the cranial cavity (**ATLAS PLATES 611, 612**).

Identify the **arcuate eminence** and the **internal auditory meatus** in the floor of the cranial cavity (**ATLAS PLATE 531**). Remove the dura covering the temporal bone, but do not destroy the facial and vestibulocochlear nerves within the internal auditory meatus (**ATLAS PLATES 532, 630, 631**).

To locate the internal ear beneath the surface of the temporal bone, visualize a line drawn at a 45° angle laterally from the middle of the posterior margin of the foramen magnum (**ATLAS PLATE 612**). This line should intersect the arcuate eminence near the location of the anterior semicircular canal (**Figure 38-9**).

With a mallet and chisel or with bone-cutting forceps (rongeurs), commence removing bone carefully from the **tegmen tympani located about 1 cm lateral to the line drawn from the foramen magnum to the arcuate eminence and the location of the anterior semicircular canal.** The tegmen tympani, or roof of the tympanic cavity, is a thin layer of bone separating the middle ear from the cranial cavity. By opening the tympanic cavity

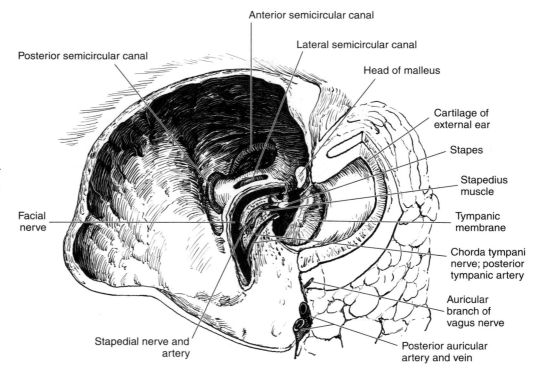

Figure 38-8. Lateral dissection of the right temporal bone (mastoid approach).

Anterior semicircular canal

Lateral semicircular canal

Posterior semicircular canal

Head of malleus

Cartilage of external ear

Stapes

Stapedius muscle

Tympanic membrane

Chorda tympani nerve; posterior tympanic artery

Auricular branch of vagus nerve

Posterior auricular artery and vein

Stapedial nerve and artery

Facial nerve

---

superiorly, the ossicles of the middle ear are exposed (**ATLAS PLATES 604, 606, 607**). Further anteriorly and laterally identify the tympanic membrane.

Identify the individual ossicles within the middle ear cavity. Observe the **handle of the malleus** attaching to the medial surface of the tympanic membrane and the **head of the malleus** articulating with the **incus**

▶
Grant's 700–703, 705
Netter's 87–89
Rohen 126, 128

▶
Grant's 702, 703
Netter's 88, 89
Rohen 122, 123

(**ATLAS PLATE 606**). Note that the **long process of the incus** articulates with the **head of the stapes** and that the **base of the stapes** fits into the **foramen vestibuli** (oval foramen; **ATLAS PLATE 608**).

With a sharp-pointed pair of forceps remove the incus and malleus. Remove more tegmen tympani anteriorly until the **auditory tube** and **tensor**

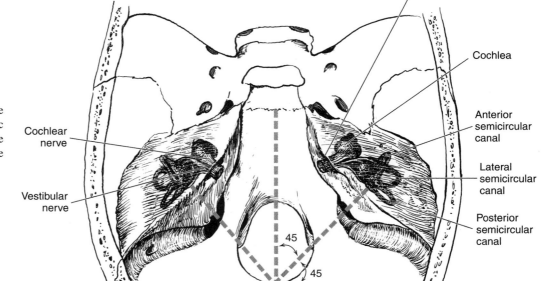

Figure 38-9. The appropriate angle for opening the tympanic cavity from above (i.e., from the inner surface of the base of the skull).

Internal acoustic meatus

Cochlea

Anterior semicircular canal

Lateral semicircular canal

Posterior semicircular canal

Cochlear nerve

Vestibular nerve

45

45

tympani muscle are exposed. Identify the **promontory** on the medial surface of the tympanic cavity (**ATLAS PLATES 608, 609**).

Open the internal auditory meatus by removing its bony roof with a pair of bone forceps, and identify the **facial nerve** laterally. Note that the **nervus intermedius** portion is located between the main part of the facial nerve and the **vestibulocochlear nerve** (**ATLAS PLATES 534, 563 #563.2**).

◄
Grant's 707, 813
Netter's 118
Rohen 64, 66, 74, 124

Identify the **geniculate ganglion.** It is an enlargement on the facial nerve (**ATLAS PLATES 563 #563.2, 628, 629**). This sensory ganglion contains the cell bodies for taste fibers in the facial nerve. Observe that the ganglion lies at the depth of the internal acoustic meatus, where the facial nerve bends sharply posteriorly (at the genu). Distal to the ganglion, the facial nerve enters the facial canal and descends posterior to the middle ear cavity to the stylomastoid foramen. Also, see the **greater petrosal nerve** that arises from the ganglion and courses anteriorly to the pterygopalatine ganglion (**ATLAS PLATES 563 #563.1, 626, 628**).

◄
Grant's 707
Netter's 89, 118
Rohen 124, 126

Follow the facial nerve inferiorly within the facial canal by continuing to remove bone posterior and inferior to the ganglion to the site where the **chorda tympani nerve** branches from the main trunk and enters the middle ear cavity (**ATLAS PLATES 605, 606, 629**). In the process you will probably open one or more of the semicircular canals located superior and posterior to the facial canal.

◄
Grant's 701–703, 705
Netter's 88, 89
Rohen 123, 126, 128

Clinical Relevance

Tympanic membrane perforation. Perforation of the tympanic membrane (eardrum) can occur from several causes, but the most common cause is middle ear infections. Other causes are perforation from foreign objects in the external acoustic canal and diving too deeply in water without adequate protection. Usually perforations heal spontaneously. If an incision is required to drain pus from a middle ear abscess, it should be made through the inferior part of the membrane to avoid injuring the chorda tympani nerve.

Mastoiditis. At one time, infection of the mastoid air cells was a common and difficult problem, but antibiotics have reduced the number of cases of spread to the mastoid region from middle ear infections. Drainage of an infected mastoid region (rarely done today) was important to prevent damage to the middle ear structures such as branches of the facial nerve (nerve to the stapedius, the chorda tympani nerve, etc.) or to prevent the spread of infection intracranially that could result in meningitis.

Otitis media. This condition is an infection in the middle ear and frequently results in an accumulation of pus in the tympanic cavity that causes pain and an inflamed eardrum. This usually develops from upper airway infections that spread to the middle ear by way of the eustachian (pharyngotympanic) tube. The inflammation is observable with the otoscope and should be treated to avoid injury to the delicate middle ear bones.

Stapedius muscle paralysis. The stapedius muscle is innervated by the facial nerve, and its function is to reduce the effects of loud noises on the tympanic membrane. It does this by inhibiting the movements of the stapes. Hyperacusis is an excessive acuteness in the sense of hearing that may be caused by the paralysis of the stapedius muscle (if there is a lesion of the facial nerve) such as may occur at times in Bell's palsy.

Meniere's syndrome. This condition is marked by tinnitus (ringing or buzzing in the ears), loss of hearing, and dizziness (vertigo). Its cause is thought to be a problem with the cochlear aqueduct and increased endolymphatic pressure. Hypersensitivity to noise and distortion of sound are also signs of this syndrome.

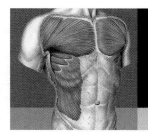

INDEX

Page numbers in *italics* denote figures.

A

Abdominal aorta, 149, 151, 161, 170–172
Abdominal cavity, 131–172
  bile passages, 147
  celiac artery, 141, 143, *143–144, 146*
  exposure to, 131–133
  gastrointestinal tract, development of,
    140–143
  greater curvature, 140, *141–142*
  greater omentum, 141
  hindgut, 142
  jejunum, 156–157
  large intestine, 157–160
  liver, 140, 145, *148*
  midgut, 141–142
  peritoneum, 133–137
  small intestine, 140
  spleen, 150
  stomach, 140, 143–151
Abdominal inguinal ring, 126
Abdominal skin incisions, 119, *120*
Abdominal viscera, 133–137, *134*
  topography, 131–139
Abdominal wall
  anterior, 118–130
    flat muscles, 122–124, *123*
    incisions through, 131, *132*
    inner surface of, 132, *133*
    nerves of, 122–124, *123,* 124
    surface anatomy, 118–119
  inner surface, 131–133
  posterior, 161–172
    muscles of, 165–169, *166*
Abducens nerve, 361, 370
Abductor digiti minimi, 254
Abductor hallucis, 253–254
Abductor pollicis brevis, 53
Abductor pollicis longus, 57, 60–61
Accessory hemiazygos vein, 111–112
Accessory left/right hepatic arteries, 144
Accessory obturator nerve, 167, 169, 230
Accessory pancreatic duct, 149
Acetabular labrum, 264, 266, *267*
Acetabulum, 264
Achilles tendon, 250
Acromioclavicular joint, 5, 65
Acromioclavicular ligament, 66, 73
Acromion, 5, 9, 24
Acute margin of heart, 99
Adductor brevis muscle, 230–232
Adductor canal, 226–228
Adductor hallucis, 257–258
Adductor hiatus, 228
Adductor longus, 227, 230–231

Adductor magnus, 216, 230–232
Adductor minimus, 231
Adductor pollicis, 54–55
Adductor region, thigh, *230,* 230–233
Adductors longus, 223
Aditus of larynx, 391
Adrenal cortex, 165
Adrenal glands, 164
Adrenal medulla, 165
Alar folds, 268
Alar ligament, 381
Alveolar nerves, 304
Ampulla of Vater, 149
Anal orifice, 194
Anal sphincter muscle, 194
Anal triangle, 192, 194–197
Anatomic planes, 2, *4*
  coronal planes, 2
  horizontal plane, 2
  midsagittal plane, 2
  parasagittal planes, 2
  transverse plane, 2
Anatomic position, 1–2, *3*
Anatomic snuff box, 51
Anconeus muscle, 31, 56
Angina pectoris, 108
Angle of Louis, 2
Ankle, 236–239, 243–246, *244*
  joints, 243, 260, 272–275, *273–274*
Annular ligament, 69
Annulus tendinous, 368
Anococcygeal raphe, 174, 194
Ansa cervicalis, 341–343, *343*
Anterior abdominal wall, 118–130
  flat muscles, 122–124, *123*
  incisions through, 131, *132*
  inner surface, 132, *133*
  nerves, 122–124, *123,* 124
  surface anatomy, 118–119
Anterior cardiac veins, 100
Anterior cecal artery, 153
Anterior chest wall
  auscultation, 95
  percussion, 95
Anterior compartment muscles, 223
Anterior compartment syndrome, 247
Anterior cranial fossa, 360
Anterior cruciate ligament, 268, 270
  ruptured, 279
Anterior cutaneous nerves, 121
Anterior esophageal surface, 145
Anterior ethmoid vessel, 370
Anterior forearm, 34–45, *43*
  muscles, 40–44, *43*
  nerves, 40–44, *43*

Anterior forearm muscles, 41
  superficial layer, 40
Anterior forehead skin flaps, 305
Anterior gastric nerves, 111
Anterior humeral circumflex artery, 19
Anterior inferior tibiofibular ligament, 272
Anterior intercavernous sinus, 361
Anterior internal jugular vein, 339
Anterior interosseous artery, 41, 43, 63
Anterior interosseous nerve, 41, 43
Anterior interventricular sulcus, 100
Anterior jugular vein, 340
Anterior larynx, surface anatomy, 416–418
Anterior left vagus nerve, 145
Anterior malleolar fold, 426
Anterior mediastinum, 88–96
Anterior meniscofemoral ligament, 270
Anterior nasal aperture, 303
Anterior orbital region, 307–308
Anterior primary ramus, 82, 281
Anterior sacroiliac ligament, 260–261
Anterior segmental bronchus, 93
Anterior semicircular canal, 427, 430
Anterior shoulder, 4
Anterior superior iliac spine, 119, 210, 223
Anterior surface of kidney, 163
Anterior talofibular ligament, 274
Anterior thigh, 223–233
  superficial nerves, 225, *226*
Anterior thoracic wall, 82–84
  muscles, 82
  removal, 84–85, *85*
Anterior thorax, 2
  surface anatomy, 2–7
Anterior tibial artery, 221, 234, 240, 245, 251
Anterior tibial-dorsalis pedis artery, 245
Anterior tibial vein, 221
Anterior tibiotalar part, 274
Anterior tubercle, 298
Anterior vagal trunk, 111
Anterior wrist
  nerves, 44–45
  vessels, 44–45
Anterior thoracic wall, 76–87
Aorta, 95, 97, 165, 169–170
  abdominal, 170
  arch, 92, 113–114
  coarctation, 117
  descending thoracic, 109
Aortic bruits, 172
Aortic hiatus, 169
Aortic orifice, 104–105, *105–106*
Aortic sinuses, 99
Aortic valve, 104, *105*
  cusps, 105, *106*

Apex of heart, 80, 98
Apex of lung, 87
Apical axillary nodes, 12
Apicoposterior segmental bronchus, 93
Appendices epiploicae, 157
Appendicular artery, 153
Appendix, 136
Arachnoid granulations, 357
Arachnoid mater, 292
Arch of foot, 275
    lateral longitudinal, 244
    longitudinal, 275
    medial longitudinal, 244, *245*
    transverse, 275
Arcuate eminence, 360, 430
Arcuate ligaments, 113
Arcuate line, 125, 173
Arcuate pubic ligament, 263
Areola, 9
Arm, 5
    anterior compartment, 37–40
    extensor compartment, 30–33
    posterior compartment, 23–33
    surface anatomy, 34
Arterial occlusive disease, 259
Arteries. *See* specific artery
Arthroscopy of knee, 279
Articular capsule, 278
Articular processes, 291
Aryepiglottic folds, 419
Arytenoid cartilages, 416
Arytenoid muscle, transverse, 420
Ascending colon, 136, 157–159
Ascending lumbar veins, 171
Ascending pharyngeal artery, 347
Asterion, 298
Atlantooccipital joint, 381–384
Atlas, 298, *299*, 380–381
    anterior arch, 381
    dislocation, 302, 385
    transverse ligament, 381
Atlas plates, 106–107, *107*
Atria, 97
Atrial septal defects, 107
Atrioventricular bundle, 103, 106
Atrioventricular node, 106
Atrioventricular orifice, 102
Atrioventricular valve, 105
Auditory tube, 390, 431
Auricle, 425–426
Auriculotemporal nerve, 354
Autonomic nerve fibers, 129
Avulsion of greater tubercle, 75
Axilla, 2–7, 16–22
Axillary fossa, 5
Axillary nerve, 19, 22, 27–29
Axillary vein, 16–17, *17,* 35
Axis, 380–381
    dislocation, 302
    transverse ligament, 381
Azygos vein, 76, 90, 109, 111, *111,* 112, 169

B

Back
    cutaneous nerves, 24, *25*
    deep, 280–296

    deep muscles, 287–290
    intermediate muscles, 286
    midportion, 81
    spinal cord, 290–295
    superficial, 280–296
    vertebral canal, 290–295
Baker's cyst, 222
Bartholin glands, 205
Basal segmental bronchi, posterior, 93
Base of heart, 98, *98*
Base of skull, 360–362, *362*
Baseball finger, 51
Basilic vein, 35, 58
Benign prostate enlargement, 191
Bennett's fracture, 64
Biceps, 216
Biceps brachii, 6, 34, 68
    short head, 18
Biceps femoris, 216
Biceps muscle
    long head, 68
    short head, 67
Bicipital aponeurosis, 6, 35, 37, 40
Bicipital sulcus, 5, 34
Bicipital tendinitis, 45
Bicuspid valve, 104
Bifurcated ligament, 278
    calcaneocuboid part, 277
Bile passages, 147
Bladder. *See* Urinary bladder
Blood circulation, 97–108
Bone marrow biopsy, 15
Bony orbit, 303, 366–367
Bony pelvis, 190
Brachial artery, 35, 39–40
Brachial plexus, 20, *21–22,* 332, 334–335
Brachialis muscle, 37, 69
Brachii artery, 39
Brachii vessels, 35
Brachiocephalic, 113
Brachiocephalic artery, 114
Brachiocephalic veins, 113
Brachioradialis, 40, 56, 58–59, 69
Brain
    arterial blood supply, 362–364, *363*
    base, 353–365
    removal, 357–360
Bregma, 355
Broad ligament, 177–178
Bronchi, 76, 113, 115, *116–117*
    lobar, 90
Bronchopulmonary segments, 92
    left lung, 93
Bronchoscopic examination, 95
Bronchus, 90
    eparterial, 90
    hyparterial, 90
    left, 92
    right, 90
Buccinator muscle, 306
Buccopharyngeal fascia, 387
Buck's fascia, 199
Bulb of penis, artery to, 200
Bulbar fascia, 374, *374*
Bulbocavernosus, 198, 205
Bulbospongiosus, 198–199, 205
Bulbourethral glands, 202

Bunions, 259
Bursae, 268
Bursitis at olecranon, 64

C

Cadaver care, 1
Calcaneal bursitis, 259
Calcaneal tendon, ruptured, 259
Calcaneocuboid joint, 276–278
Calcaneofibular ligament, 272, 274
Calcaneus, 234, 275
    fracture, 259
    tubercles, 249
Calcaneus tendon, 248
Camper's fascia, 120
Canaliculi, 147
Cancer
    of bladder, 190
    of colon, 190
    of kidney, 172
    of lung, 96
    of prostate, 191
    of rectum, 190
Canine eminence, 304
Capitate, 72, 74
Capitulum of humerus, 68
Cardiac branches, 115
Cardiac dullness, superficial, 81
Cardiac nerves, 113
Cardiac orifice, 145
Cardiac plexus, 115
Carina, 116
Carotid arteries, 387
Carotid sinus nerve, 347
Carotid triangle, 339, 345–348
Carotid wall, *429,* 430
Carpal bones, 7
Carpal tunnel, 46
Carpometacarpal joint, 72
Caruncula, 375
Cauda equina, 295
Caudal anesthesia, 191
Cavernous sinus, 361
Cecum, 136, 155, 157, *158*
Celiac, 141, 143, *143–144, 146*
Celiac plexus, 171
Celiac trunk, 143, 171
Central artery, 372, *373*
Central tendinous point, perineum, 195
Central venous line, 22
Cephalic vein, 13–14, 35, 45, 58
Cerebrospinal fluid, 294
Cerumen, 426
Cervical canal, 184
Cervical nerves, dorsal rami, 298–300, *299–300*
Cervical pleura, 85, 89
Cervical plexus, cutaneous branches, 328
Cervical ribs, 22
Cervical vertebra, 291, 297–298, *298*
    spinous process, 23
Cervix, 184
Chambers of heart, 101–106
Check ligament, 373–374, *374*
Chest wall, anterior
    auscultation, 95
    percussion of, 95

Chorda tympani nerve, 430, 432
Chordae tendinae, 103, 105
Ciliary ganglion, 371
Circulation
  blood, 97
  pulmonary, 97
  systemic, 97
Circumflex scapular artery, 28
Cirrhosis of liver, 151
Cisterna chyli, 159
Clavicle, 3, 5, 9, 332
Clavipectoral fascia, 14, *15*
Clinoid processes, 360
Clitoris, 183, 194, 204, 206
Club feet, 279
Coarctation of aorta, 117
Coccygeal nerve, 185
Coccygeus muscle, 174, 189, 197
Coccyx, 174, 192, 194, 291
  fractures, 190
  injury, 295
Cochlea, 427, 430
  window, 430
Collateral ligaments, 74, 278
Colles' fascia, 121, 128, 197
Colles' fracture, 64
Colliculus seminalis, 181–182
Colon, cancer, 190
Common bile duct, 137–138, 144, 147, 149–150
Common carotid artery, bifurcation, 347
Common digital arteries, 258
Common fibular nerve, 221, 234, 237
  injury, 246
Common hepatic artery, 144
Common hepatic duct, 144, 147, 149
Common iliac artery, 187
Common interosseous artery, 43, 60
Common plantar digital nerves, 253, 256
Compression of sciatic nerve, 222
Concha, 397, 426
Condyles of tibia, 237
Congenital anomalies of kidney, 172
Conjunctiva, 374, *374*
Conjunctival fornix, 308
Conoid ligament, 66
Constriction of ureter, 190
Conus arteriosus, 102–104
Conus elasticus, 422
Conus medullaris, 294, *294*, 295
Coracoacromial ligament, 66
Coracobrachialis, 18, 37, 67
Coracoclavicular joint, 65–66, *66*
Coracohumeral ligament, 67
Coracoid process, 5, *6*, 34
Cornea, 371
Corniculate cartilage, 419
Corona of glans, 201
Coronal planes, 2
Coronal suture, 355
Coronary angioplasty, 108
Coronary bypass operation, 108
Coronary ligament, 135, 146
  anterior leaf, 147
  posterior leaf, 147
Coronary sinus, 97, 100
  orifice, 101
  valve, 101

Coronary sulcus, 98
Coronoid process, 37
Corpora cavernosa penis, 199
Corpus spongiosum penis, 199
Corrugator supercilii muscle, 311
Costal facets, 291
Costal pleura, 85, 89
Costochondritis, 87
Costodiaphragmatic recesses, 86, 113
Costomediastinal recesses, 86
Costotransverse joints, 78
Costovertebral joints, 78
Cowper glands, 202
Cranial cavity, floor, 353–365
Craniovertebral joints, 380–385
Cremaster muscle, 123
Cremasteric artery, 129
Cremasteric fascia, 128
Cremasteric reflex, 123
Cribriform fascia, 225
Cricoid cartilage, 338, 416
Crista galli, 358, 360
Crista terminalis, 101
Cruciate anastomosis, 219, 227
Cruciate ligaments, 268–269, *270*
Crura, 166
Crural fascia, 238–239
Crural interosseous membrane, 271
Cubital fossa, 6, 34–45, *40*
Cuboid bone, 234, 244, 275
Cuneiform bone, 234, 244, 275
Cuneiform cartilage, 415
Cupula of pleura, 80
Cusps of aortic valve, 105, *106*
Cysterna chyli, 111
Cystic artery, 144
Cystic duct, 144, 147, 149
Cystitis, 191

D

Dartos, 121, 128, 197
Deep artery of clitoris, 205–206
Deep artery of penis, 200
Deep cardiac plexus, 115
Deep dorsal vein, 200
Deep femoral artery, 231
Deep fibular nerve, 236, 238–240, 245
  entrapment, 246
Deep iliac circumflex artery, 123
Deep infrapatellar bursa, 268
Deep inguinal ring, 126
Deep palmar arch, 49, 54–55, 64
Deep pectoral region, 16–22
Deep perineal compartment, 192, 197, 203
Deep plantar artery, 246
Deep plantar venous arch, 251
Deep radial nerve, 40
Deep transverse metacarpal ligament, 74
Deep transverse metatarsal ligament, 259, 278
Deep transverse perineal muscle, 206
Deep vein thrombosis, 233
Deferential artery, 181
Deltoid, 5, 24–27, *26*, 67, 272
Deltoid region, posterior compartment of arm, 23–33
Deltopectoral triangle, 13

Dens, apical ligament, 381, *383*
Dental probe, 1
Denticulate ligaments, 294–295
Depressor anguli oris, 305
DeQuervain's disease, 64
Dermal papillae, 9
Descending aorta, 112
Descending colon, 157–159
Descending genicular artery, 221
Detrusor muscle, 183
Diaphragm, 109–117, 161, 163, 166
  from abdominal aspect, *169,* 169–170, *170*
  crura, 113, 167
Diaphragma sellae, 357, 362
Diaphragmatic pain, 172
Diaphragmatic pleura, 85, 89
Diaphragmatic surface, 150
Digital nerves, 46–49
Digital vessels, 46–49, 256
Digitorum superficialis, 69
Direct inguinal hernia, 126, 130
Dislocation
  elbow, 75
  lunate bone, 75
  patella, 279
  ribs, 86–87
  sternoclavicular joint, 75
Dissection instruments, 1, *2*
  dental probe, 1
  grease marking pencil, 1
  scalpel handle, 1
  scissors, 1
  tissue forceps, 1
Distal radio-ulnar joint, 71, *71,* 71–72
Distal thumb, 53–54
Dorsal artery of clitoris, 205–206
Dorsal artery of penis, 200
Dorsal carpal arch, 63
Dorsal carpal network, 63
Dorsal digital arteries, 63
Dorsal digital expansions, 59, 278
Dorsal digital nerves, 58
Dorsal interossei, 55, 57, 63–64, 258
Dorsal metacarpal arteries, 63
Dorsal metatarsal, 246
Dorsal nerve to clitoris, 205
Dorsal nerves of penis, 200
Dorsal primary rami, spinal nerves, 281, *283*
Dorsal radiocarpal ligament, 72
Dorsal root ganglion, 295
Dorsal scapular nerve, 286, 335
Dorsal tubercles, 74
Dorsal vein of clitoris, 206
Dorsalis pedis artery, 240, 246, 258
Dorsum of foot, 234–247, *244,* 245
Dorsum of hand, *62,* 63, *63*
Dorsum of penis, 199
Ductus deferens, 128, 177, 179–182, *181,* 182
  artery, 128–129
Ductus venosus, 132, 147
Duodenal fossae, 160
Duodenojejunal flexure, 149
Duodenojejunal junction, 136, 153, 160
Duodenum, 140–151, *148,* 149, 151, 163
Dupuytren's contracture, 51
Dura mater, 292, 357
Dural folds, 357

E

Ectopic pregnancy, 191
Efferent ductules, 129
Ejaculatory duct, 180–181
  openings, 182
Elbow
  dislocation, 75
  fractured, 75
Elbow joint, 68–71, *69–70*
Elevate scapula, 282
Emphysema, 96
Epididymis
  head, 129
  tail, 129
Epidural space, 292
Epigastric anastomosis, 124–126, *125,* 130
Epigastric region, 119
Epigastric vessels, 177
Epiglottis, 416, 419
Epiploic foramen of Winslow, 137
Episiotomy, 208
Erb-Duchenne paralysis, 22
Erector spinae, 262, 288
Esophageal arteries, 111
Esophageal cancer, 351, 392
Esophageal hiatus, 169
Esophageal plexus, 111
Esophageal varicosities, 116
Esophagus, 76, 109, *110,* 113, 115, *116–117,*
  169–170
  cancer, 351, 392
Ethmoid bone, cribriform plate, 360
Ethmoid sinus, 400
Eustachian tube, 390
Extensor carpi radialis, 40, 58
Extensor carpi ulnaris, 59, *60,* 69
Extensor digiti minimi, 59, *60*
Extensor digitorum brevis, 59, *60,* 69, 245–246
Extensor digitorum longus, 239–240, 246
Extensor hallucis brevis, 246
Extensor hallucis longus, 237, 239–240, 246
Extensor indicis, 58, 60–61
Extensor pollicis brevis, 57
Extensor pollicis longus, 61
Extensor retinaculum, 59, 61–63, *62*
Extensor synovial sheaths, 61–63, *62*
Extensors carpi radialis brevis, 59, 69
Extensors carpi radialis longus, 59, 69
Extensors digitorum longus, 245
Extensors pollicis brevis, 60
Extensors pollicis longus, 60
External acoustic meatus, 426, *426*
External anal sphincter, 194, 196–197
External carotid artery, 338, 387
  branches, 316, 347, *348*
External ear, *425,* 425–432
External genitalia, 192
External iliac artery, 187
External intercostal membrane, 82
External intercostal muscles, 82
External jugular vein, 330, 354
External nasal nerve, 310
External oblique muscle, 122
External occipital protuberance, 297
External opening, 194

External ostium, 184
External pudendal artery, 121
External rotators, 214
External spermatic fascia, 128–129
Extraocular muscles, 375, *375–377*
Eyelids, 307

F

Face
  bony landmarks, 303–304
  infratemporal regions, 316–327
  nerves, *309,* 309–312, *311*
  superficial, 303–315
  superficial structures on, 312–313
  superficial vessels, *309,* 309–312, *311*
  temporal region, 316–327
Facial artery, 309, 347
  tonsillar branch, 404–405
Facial canal, 427
  prominence, 430
  promontory, 430
Facial nerve, 313, 359, 427–430, *428,* 432
  canal, 430
  cervical branch, 339, 349
  chorda tympani branch, 412
  genu, 427
  mastoid approach, 427–430, *428*
Falciform ligament, 131–134, 140, 146
Falciform margin, 225
False pelvis, 173–174
Falx cerebelli, 357
Falx cerebri, 357, *358,* 359
Falx inguinalis, 122–123
Fascia lata, 120, 210, 225–226
Fascia transversalis, 167, 226
Female inguinal canal, 129–130
Female pelvic organs, 182–185
Female pelvis, clinical relevance, 191
Female perineum, 208
Female rectum, 184
Female superficial perineal compartment, muscles
  in, *202–203,* 205
Female urethra, 208
Female urogenital diaphragm, deep perineal com-
  partment, 206, *207*
Female urogenital region, fascial reflections in, 203
Female urogenital triangle, 203–206, *204*
Femoral, obturator, accessory obturator, 265
Femoral artery, 223–224, 226–227
Femoral canal, 226
Femoral hernia, 130, 226, 233
Femoral nerve, 167–168, 223–224, 226–228, *228*
  anterior cutaneous branch, 225
  posterior branches, 228
  surface projection, 224
Femoral sheath, 226
Femoral triangle, 226–228
Femoral vein, 121, 223–224, 226–227
Femoral vessels, 226–228
  surface projection, 224
Femoris, 216
Femur
  fracture, 233
  head, 264
  ligament, 264

Fibrocartilaginous disc, 72
Fibrous capsule, 264
Fibrous renal capsule, 165
Fibula, 234, 237, 271
Fibular artery, 234, 243, 251
Fibular collateral ligament, 268
Fibular fractures, 246
Fibular retinacula, 238–239
Fibularis brevis, 243, 246
Fibularis longus, 243, 246, 275–276
Fibularis tertius, 239–240
Filum terminale, 294–295
Fistulae involving vagina, 208
Flail chest, 87
Flat feet, 279
Flex metatarsophalangeal joints, 258
Flexor carpi radialis, 41, 45, 69
Flexor carpi ulnaris, 41, 44, 69
Flexor digiti minimi brevis, 255, 257, *257,* 258
Flexor digitorum brevis, 254–256
Flexor digitorum longus, 251, 253, 255–256
Flexor digitorum profundus, 41, 43
Flexor digitorum superficialis, 41, *43,* 45
Flexor hallucis brevis, 254, 257–258
Flexor hallucis longus, 251–253, 255–256
Flexor pollicis brevis, 53
Flexor pollicis longus, 41, 43
Flexor-pronator muscles, 40
Flexor retinaculum, 46, 50–53
Flexor tendon, 50–53
  fibrous sheaths, 51, *52–53*
Floor of pelvis, 173, *174–176,* 185–190
Foot
  arch, 244, *245,* 275
  bones, 243
  dorsum, 234–247, *244, 245*
    nerves, 245
  joints, *275,* 275–278, *276*
  lateral longitudinal arch, 244
  longitudinal arch, 275
  medial longitudinal arch, 244, *245*
  nerves on dorsum, 245
  plantar aspect, *253,* 253–259, *254*
  plantarflex, 248
  sole, 248–259
  transverse arch, 275
Foramen lacerum, 360
Foramen magnum, 360, 380, 430
Foramen ovale, 360
Foramen rotundum, 360
Foramen spinosum, 360, 362
Foramen vestibuli, 431
Foramina, 360–362, *362,* 367, *367*
Forearm, 5–6
  anterior, 34–45, *43*
  anterior muscles, 41
  biceps brachii muscle, 6
  extensor compartment, 58–61
  flexion, 6
  posterior compartment, 56–64
  posterior cutaneous nerve, 31
  superficial extensor, 58, *59*
  superficial layer, 40
  supination, 6
  surface anatomy, 34
Foregut, 140

Forehead
   bony landmarks, 303–304
   surface anatomy, 303–304
Foreign objects, swallowing, 95
Foreskin, 194
Fossa ovalis, 101
Frenulum, 194
Frenulum clitoridis, 206
Frenulum of labia minora, 206
Frontal crest, 357
Frontal nerve, 369
Fundiform ligament, 121
Fundus, 147, 184
Furrow, 6

G

Gallbladder, 119, 135, 143–151, *148*
   surface projection, 139
Gallstones, 151
Ganglion, short ciliary nerves from, 371
Gastric vessels, 169
Gastrocnemius, 221, 250, 269
Gastroduodenal artery, 149
Gastroesophageal reflux, 116
Gastrointestinal tract, development, 140–143
Gastrosplenic ligament, 134–135, 150
Gemellus, 212, 265
Genicular veins, 221
Geniculate ganglion, 427, 432
Genioglossus muscle, 412
Genitofemoral nerve, 167
   femoral branch, 225
   genital branch, 124
Glans of clitoris, 203
Glans of penis, 194, 199
Glenohumeral joint, 67, *67–68*
Glenohumeral ligaments, 67
Glenoid labrum, 68
Glossopharyngeal nerve, 386–388, *388,*
      410, 412
   tympanic branch, 426
Gluteal nerve, 209
Gluteal region, 209–222, *213*
Gluteal sulcus, 210
Gluteal vessels, 209
Gluteus maximus, 197, 210, 212
Gluteus medius, 214, *215–217*
Gluteus minimus, 214, 265
Gonadal arteries, 171
Gonadal vessels, 161–165, *162*
Gracilis muscle, 223, 230–231
Gray rami communicantes, 112, 171
Grease marking pencil, 1
Great auricular nerve, 330–331, 340
Great cardiac vein, 98–100
Great saphenous vein, 224, 226, 237–238, 247
Great toe, 256
Great vessels, 76, 80, 94
   projections onto anterior thoracic wall, 80, *80*
Greater omentum, 134–135, 140–141
Greater palatine nerve, 399–400
Greater pelvis, 173–174
Greater peritoneal sac, *137,* 137–139
Greater petrosal nerve, 427, 432
Greater sciatic foramina, 174–175, 212, 262

Greater splanchnic nerve, 113, 170–171
Greater trochanter, 210
Greater tubercle, 5, 34
   avulsion, 75
Greater vestibular glands, 203, 205, 208
Groin fold, 223
Groin injury, 233
Gubernaculum testis, 129
Guyon's canal syndrome, 55

H

Hallucis longus, 245
Hamate, 72, 74
Hammer toe, 247
Hamstring injury, 222
Hamstring muscles, tendons, 237
Hand, 7
   arteries, 63–64
   digital nerves, 46–49
   digital vessels, 46–49
   dorsum, 56–64
   fascial spaces, 49–50, *50*
   nerves, 63–64
   palmar aponeurosis, 46–49
   palmar aspect, 46–55
   skin incisions, 46–49
   surface anatomy, 46–49
Hard palate, 405–407, *406–407*
Haustrae coli, 157
Head, bisection, 394–395
Heart, 76, 80, 94, 97–108
   acute margin, 99
   apex, 80, 98
   arteries, *99,* 99–100, *100*
   base, 80, 98, *98*
   chambers, 101–106
   conducting system, 97–108, *107*
   diaphragmatic surface, 98
   diaphragmatic surface of, 98
   inferior margin, 99
   left margin, 99
   lower border, 80
   outer surface, 94
   projection, 76–81, *77, 80, 80*
   removal, 88–96
   right margin, 80, 99
   sternocostal surface, 98, *98*
   surface anatomy, 97–108
   veins, *99,* 99–100, *100*
   venous drainage, 100, *100*
Heart sounds, 107
Heel, ball, 249
Hemiazygos, 76, 111–112, 169
Hemorrhoids, 196, 207
Hepatic artery, 137–138, 143–144, 146
Hepatic duct, 146
Hepatic flexure, 136
Hepatic veins, 145–147, 171
Hepatoduodenal ligament, 132, 135
Hepatogastric ligament, 132, 135
Hepatopancreatic ampulla, 149
Hernia
   congenital inguinal, 126
   femoral, 130
   hiatus, 116

   indirect, 126
   inguinal
      direct, 126, 130
      indirect, 130
      paraumbilical, 130
      spigelian, 130
      umbilical, 130
Herniated disc, 296
Hesselbach's triangle, 126
Hiatus hernia, 116
Hiatus semilunaris, 398
Hindgut, 142
Hip, 260
   fracture, 279
Hip joint, 264–267, *265–266*
   congenital dislocation, 279
   stability, 279
Horizontal fissure, 89
Horizontal plane, 2
Humerus
   capitulum, 68
   supracondylar fracture, 45
   trochlea, 68
Hyoglossus muscle, 412
Hyoid bone, 338
Hyparterial bronchus, 90, 93
Hypochondriac regions, 119
Hypogastric regions, 119
Hypoglossal canal, 360
Hypoglossal nerve, 346, 362, 412
Hypothenar eminence, 46, 54
Hypothenar muscles, 53–54
Hypothenar space, 50
Hysterectomy, 191

I

Ileocecal junction, 154
Ileocecal valve, 157
Ileocolic artery, 152–153, *154*
Ileum, 136, 154, 156–157
Iliac, 167
Iliac crest, 24, 119, 166, 174
Iliac fossa, 167
Iliacus, 265
   psoas major, 227
Iliacus muscle, 166–167
Iliocostalis, 289
Iliocostalis cervicis, 289
Iliocostalis column, 289
Iliocostalis lumborum, 289
Iliocostalis thoracis, 289
Iliococcygeus, 174, 189
Iliofemoral ligament, 264, 266
Iliohypogastric nerve, 122, 167, 225
Ilioinguinal nerve, 122, 167, 225
Iliolumbar artery, 186–187
Iliolumbar ligament, 166
Iliopsoas muscle, 166, 223, 226, 232
Iliopubic eminence, 174
Iliotibial tract, 226
Ilium, 175
   auricular surface of, 260
   crest, 210
Incisura angularis, 145
Incontinence of urine, 208

Incus, 428, 430–431
  long process, 431
Indirect congenital inguinal hernia, 126
Indirect hernia, 126
Indirect inguinal hernias, 130
Inferior alveolar nerve, 322
  mylohyoid branch, 324
Inferior articular facet, 298
Inferior cluneal nerves, 211–212
Inferior clunial, 197
Inferior concha, 390, 398
Inferior constrictor, 388
Inferior duodenal recess, 153
Inferior epigastric artery, 121, 126
Inferior epigastric vessels, 126, 128
Inferior extensor retinacula, 239, 245
Inferior femoris, 212
Inferior fibular retinaculum, 239
Inferior gemellus, 214–215
Inferior genicular, 221
Inferior glenohumeral ligament, 68
Inferior gluteal artery, 186, 188, 227
Inferior gluteal vein, 214
Inferior hypogastric plexus, 188–189
Inferior ileocecal fold, 155
Inferior ileocecal recess, 155
Inferior lateral genicular, 222
Inferior lingular segmental bronchus, 93
Inferior lobar bronchus, 93
Inferior margin of heart, 99
Inferior medial genicular, 222
Inferior mediastinum, 93
Inferior nasal concha, 397
Inferior oblique muscle, 372
Inferior orbital fissure, 367
Inferior pancreaticoduodenal artery, 150, 152, 154
Inferior pancreaticoduodenal vessel, 149
Inferior phrenic artery, 143, 165, 167, 171
Inferior rectal nerve, 195, *195,* 197
Inferior rectal vessels, 195, *195,* 197
Inferior thyroid artery, 343–345
Inferior tibiofibular joint, 272
Inferior transverse ligament, 272
Inferior vena cava, 99, 145–147, 161, 169–172
  compression, 172
  opening, 101, *102*
Inferior vesical artery, 180, 187–188
Infraclavicular fossa, 34
Infraglottic cavity, 422
Infrahyoid muscles, 82, 341, *342*
Infrahyoid strap muscles, 341–343
Infraorbital margin, 303
Infraorbital nerve, 311, *313,* 372
Infrapatellar bursa, 236
Infrapatellar synovial fold, 268
Infrapubic angle, 175
Infraspinatus, 25, 37, 67
Infraspinatus fossa, 25
Infraspinous fossa, 24–27
Infrasternal angle, 3
Infratemporal fossa, 304, 319–325, *320*
Infratrochlear nerve, 370–371
Infundibulum, 103, 184
Inguinal falx, 126
Inguinal ligament, 119, 121, 126, 128, 223, 227
Inguinal region, 119, 126–128, *127*

Inguinal ring, 139
Inguinal triangle, 126
Inion, 23
Inlet of larynx, 391
Inner ear, 425–432
Interphalangeal joint, *74,* 74–75
Interatrial septum, 04
Intercarpal joint, 72
Intercostal artery, 10, 82
Intercostal muscles, 82, *83–84*
Intercostal nerve, 82
Intercostal space, 77
  relationships, 87
Intercostal vein, 82
Intercostobrachial nerve, 12, 21, 31
Intercrural fibers, 122
Interlobular ductules, 147
Intermediate tarsometatarsal joint, 278
Intermetatarsal joint, 260, 275, 278
Internal acoustic meatus, 360, 427
Internal anal sphincter, 196
Internal auditory meatus, 430
Internal carotid artery, 346, 359, 387
Internal iliac artery, 187
  anterior trunk, 186
  posterior trunk, 186
Internal iliac vessels, 185
Internal intercostal membranes, 82
Internal intercostal muscle, 82
Internal jugular vein, 114, 345, 386
Internal laryngeal nerve, 418
Internal oblique muscle, 122, *124*
Internal pudendal artery, 187–188, 215
Internal pudendal vessels, 194–195, 215
Internal spermatic fascia, 128
Internal thoracic artery, 10, 83
Internal thoracic nodes, 12
Internal thoracic vein, 10, 83, 114
Internal thoracic vessels, 83
Interosseous ligament, *72,* 272
Interosseous metatarsal ligaments, 278
Interosseous muscle, 54–55, *55,* 258
Interosseous sacroiliac ligament, 260–262
Interosseous talocalcaneal ligament, 277–278
Interphalangeal creases, 46
Interphalangeal joint, 74, 260, 275, 278
Interpubic disc, 264
Interpubic fibrocartilaginous disc, 263
Interspinous ligaments, 292
Interspinous muscle, 290
Intertarsal joint, 260, 275–276
Intertransverse muscle, 290
Intertubercular line, 157, 210
Intertubercular sulcus, 5, 34, 37
Interventricular septum, 105
Intervertebral discs, 292
Intervertebral foramina, 292
Intestinal arteries, 152
Intestine. *See* Large intestine; Small intestine
Intramuscular injections, 222
Iris, 308, 371
Ischia, rami, 192
Ischial spines, 174
Ischial tuberosity, 174, 192, 194, 197, 203, 210
Ischiocavernosus muscle, 198–199, 205
Ischiococcygeus, 174

Ischiofemoral ligament, 265–266
Ischiorectal fossa, 194
  abscesses in, 207
Ischiorectal fossae, 194
Ischium, 175
Isthmus, 184

J

Jejunum, 136, 149, 156, 163
Joint. *See* specific joint
Jugular foramen, 360, 362
Jugular notch, 2, 338
Jugular wall, 430

K

Kidneys, 149–150, 161–165
  anterior relationships, 163, *163*
  cancer, 172
  posterior relationships, 163
Klumpke's paralysis, 21
Knee, 260
  joint, 268–271
  lateral aspect, 268
  medial aspect, 268
  posterior aspect, 268
Kyphosis, 295

L

Labia majora, 129–130, 194, 203
Labia minora, 194, 203, 206
Labyrinthine wall, 430
Lacrimal apparatus, 375, *375,* 376, *376–377*
Lacrimal canaliculi, 375
Lacrimal caruncle, 308
Lacrimal nerve, 369
Lactiferous ducts, 9
Lactiferous sinuses, 9
Lacunar ligament, 126
Lambda, 297, 355
Lambdoid suture, 355
Laminae, 298
Laminectomy, 295
Large intestine, 157–160
Laryngeal muscle, 418–421
Laryngeal nerve, 115
  injury, recurrent, 117
Laryngeal prominence, 338
Laryngeal vessels, 419, *419*
Laryngopharynx, 391, 415–424
Larynx, 338, 415–424
  cancer, 424
  interior, 421–424, *423*
  skeleton, 415–416
Lateral antebrachial cutaneous nerve, 35, 37, 56
Lateral arcuate ligament, 163, 166–167, 169
Lateral atlantoaxial joint, 381–384
Lateral atlantoaxial joints, 382
Lateral check ligament, 374
Lateral condyle, 234
Lateral cricoarytenoid muscle, 416, 420
Lateral cutaneous nerves, 122
Lateral dorsal cutaneous nerve, 238, 245
Lateral epicondyle, 6, 35

Lateral femoral circumflex, 227, 265
Lateral femoral cutaneous nerve, 167–168, 225
Lateral glossoepiglottic fold, 416
Lateral intermuscular septa, 37
Lateral laryngeal muscles, 420
Lateral longitudinal arch, 244, 275
Lateral meniscus, 268, 270–271
Lateral palpebral ligament, 308
Lateral pectoral nerve, 13–14, 20
Lateral pelvic floor, 185–190
Lateral pelvic wall, 185–190
Lateral plantar artery, 256
Lateral plantar nerve, 255–256, 258
    deep branch, 256–258
    superficial branch, 256
Lateral plantar nerves, 255
Lateral plantar vein, 251
Lateral popliteal nerve, 220
Lateral pterygoid, 304, 318
Lateral puboprostatic ligament, 182
Lateral rectus muscle, 370
Lateral sacral arteries, 186, 188
Lateral segmental bronchi, 93
Lateral semicircular canal, 427, 430
Lateral shoulder, 4
Lateral sural cutaneous nerve, 221, 238
Lateral tarsometatarsal joint, 278
Lateral thoracic artery, 19
Lateral umbilical folds, 132
Lateral umbilical ligaments, 177
Latissimus dorsi, 18, 37, 280–285
Latissimus dorsi muscle, 24, 27, 283
Least splanchnic nerve, 113
LeFort fractures, 327
Left atrioventricular opening, 104
Left atrium, 104
    smooth-walled cavity, 104
Left brachiocephalic veins, 113
Left bronchus, 92
Left colic artery, 156
Left colic flexure, 136, 157–158
Left common carotid artery, 113–114
Left common iliac vein, 171
Left coronary artery, 98, 100
    circumflex branch, 99
Left gastric artery, 143
Left gastric vein, 143
Left gastric vessel, 170
Left gastroepiploic artery, 145, 151
Left gonadal vein, 165
Left hepatic duct, 144, 149
Left inferior phrenic artery, 110, 169
Left inferior phrenic vein, 165
Left internal jugular vein, 111
Left lung, 90, *91*
    bronchopulmonary segments, 93
Left phrenic nerve, 115
Left posterior pulmonary plexus, 115
Left primary bronchus, 115
Left recurrent laryngeal, 115
Left renal vein, 171
Left renal vessels, 149
Left subclavian arteries, 113
Left subclavian artery, 114
Left superior intercostal vein, 111–114
Left suprarenal gland, 163

Left suprarenal vein, 165
Left testicular vein, 162
Left triangular ligament, 135, *136,* 147
Left umbilical vein, 132, 147
Left vagus nerve, 115, 141
Left ventricle, 104, *105*
Left vitelline vein, 147
Leg, 216
    anterior, 234–247, *240–242*
        deep fascia of, 238
        muscles, 239
        nerves, 240
        vessels, 240
    lateral, 234–247
        muscles, 243
        nerves, 243
        vessels, 243
    posterior, 248–259, *249,* 249–253
        incisions, 249, *249*
        superficial dissection, 249, *249*
Lesser curvature of stomach, 135
Lesser occipital nerve, 331, 340
Lesser omentum, 132, 134, 140
Lesser palatine nerve, 399–400
Lesser pelvis, 173–174
Lesser peritoneal sac, *137,* 137–139
Lesser sciatic foramina, 174–175, 212
Lesser splanchnic nerve, 113, 170–171
Lesser supraclavicular fossa, 338
Lesser tubercle, 5, 34
Levator anguli oris, 306
Levator ani muscle, 174, 182, 189, 194, 197
Levator labii superioris, 305–306
Levator muscle, 404
Levator palati muscle, 404
Levator palpebrae superioris, 369, *369,* 374, *374,*
    375
Levator scapulae, 280–285, *285–286*
Lienorenal ligament, 135, 150
Ligament of Treitz, 160
Ligamenta flava, 292
Ligamentum arteriosum, 115
Ligamentum nuchae, 24
Ligamentum teres hepatis, 132
Ligamentum venosum, 147
Limbus fossae ovalis, 101
Linea alba, 118
Linea semilunaris, 118
Lingual artery, 347, 409, *411*
Lingual nerve, 412
Lingual thyroid, 345
    vein, 345
Liver, 140–151, *148,* 151
    bare area, 135
    inferior border, 135
    right lobe, 163
    round ligament, 132
Lobar bronchi, 90
Lobar bronchus, 93
Long ciliary vessels, 371
Long plantar ligament, 275–278
Long thoracic nerve, 18, 335
Longissimus capitis, 289
Longissimus cervicis, 289
Longissimus thoracis, 289
Longitudinal arch, foot, 275

Lower lateral brachial cutaneous nerve, 31
Lower limb joints, 260–279
    ankle joint, 272–275, *273–274*
    foot joints, 275, 275–278, *276*
    hip joint, 264–267, *265–266*
    joints within foot, *275,* 275–278, *276*
    knee joint, 268–271
    sacroiliac joint, 260–263, *261–263*
    symphysis pubis, 263–264, *264*
    tibiofibular joints, *271,* 271–272
Lumbar arteries, 171
Lumbar ganglia, 172
Lumbar part of sympathetic trunks, 171
Lumbar plexus, 161, 165–169, *166,* 167, *168*
Lumbar spinal puncture, 295
Lumbar splanchnic nerves, 171
Lumbar sympathectomy, 172
Lumbar sympathetic chain, 161, 170–172
Lumbar triangle, 281–282
Lumbar veins, 169, 171
Lumbar vertebra, 291
Lumbosacral trunk, 167, 169, 185
Lumbrical muscles, 48, 51, 255–256
Lumbricals, 256
Lunate bone, 72
    dislocation, 75
    surface, 267
Lung, 81, 86, 88–96, 336
    apex, 87
    cancer, 96
    left, 90, *91,* 93
    lesion, resection, 95
    projection, 80, *81*
        onto anterior thoracic wall, 80, *80*
        onto thoracic wall, 76–81, *77*
    removal, 85–87, *86*
    right, 89, *90–91,* 92
Lymphatic vessels, 12, 129

M

Mackenrodt, 184
Main pancreatic duct, 149–150
Major calyx, 165
Major duodenal papilla, 149–150
Male ejaculation, 207
Male pelvis
    clinical relevance, 191
    viscera, 179–182
Male perineum, 207
Male superficial perineal compartment, muscles
    in, 198, *199*
Male urogenital diaphragm, 201, *201*
Male urogenital region, fascial reflections, 197
Male urogenital triangle, 197–203
Malleoli, 243
Mallet finger, 51
Malleus, 428, 430
    handle, 427, 431
    head, 431
Mammary gland, 8–15, *10–11*
    apical axillary nodes, 12
    areola, 9
    arteries, 10
    intercostal arteries, 10
    internal thoracic artery, 10

Mammary gland, *(continued)*
  internal thoracic vein, 10
  lactiferous ducts, 9
  lactiferous sinuses, 9
  lymphatic vessels, 12
  parasternal thoracic nodes, 12
  pectoral nodes, 12
  venous channels, 10
Mandible, 303–304
  angles, 304
Mandibular foramen, 304
Mandibular nerve, 319
  auriculotemporal branch, 313
  buccal branch, 322
Mandibular ramus, 304
Mandibular skin flaps, 305
Manubrium, 8
Marginal artery, 153, *155*
Masseter muscle, 312, 318, *318,* 318–319
Mastoid air cells, 429–430
Mastoid antrum, 429
Mastoid process, 304
Mastoid wall, 430
Mastoiditis, 432
Maxillary artery, 320, *321, 322, 322,* 324
  anterior tympanic branch, 426
  deep auricular branch, 426
  greater palatine branch, 399
Maxillary sinus, 367, 398
Maxillary skin flaps, 305
McBurney's point, 139
Meckel's diverticulum, 159
Medial antebrachial cutaneous nerve, 21, 35, 56
Medial arcuate ligament, 163, 166–167, 169
Medial brachial cutaneous nerve, 21, 36
Medial cluneal, 211
Medial condyle, 234
Medial crus, 122
Medial cubital vein, 35
Medial epicondyle, 6, 35
Medial femoral circumflex artery, 227, 231, 265
Medial intermuscular septa, 37
Medial longitudinal arch, 275
Medial malleolus, 234, 237
Medial meniscus, 268, 270–271
Medial metatarsals, 275
Medial pectoral nerve, 13, 21
Medial plantar arteries, 256
Medial plantar artery, 256
Medial plantar nerve, 255–256
  entrapment, 259
Medial plantar nerves, 255
Medial plantar vein, 251
Medial popliteal nerve, 220
Medial pterygoid muscle, 319
Medial puboprostatic ligament, 182
Medial segmental bronchi, 93
Medial sural cutaneous nerve, 221
Medial tarsometatarsal joint, 278
Medial thigh, 223–233, *230,* 230–233
Medial umbilical folds, 132
Medial umbilical ligament, 177–178, 180, 188
Median atlantoaxial joint, 381–384
Median cricothyroid ligament, 416
Median cubital vein, 6, 35
Median glossoepiglottic fold, 416

Median nerve, 35, 40–41, *43,* 45, 50, 56
  lesions, 45
  recurrent branch, 47, 50, 53
Median plane, 2
Median sacral artery, 171, 186
Median umbilical fold, 132
Median umbilical ligament, 176, 178
Mediastina, anterior, 93
Mediastinal lymph nodes, 109
Mediastinal pleura, 85, 89, 109
Mediastinum, 76, 85, 93
  anterior, 93–94
  inferior, 93
  middle, 94
  posterior, 94
  subdivisions, 93–94
  superior, 93
Ménière's syndrome, 432
Meninges, 357–360
  spinal cord, 292, *293*
Menisci, 270
  injuries to, 279
Mental nerve, 312
Mesoappendix, 153
Mesocolon, 149
Mesogastria, 132
Mesosalpinx, 178–179
Mesovarium, 183
Metacarpal bone, 7, 57
  fracture, 64
Metacarpophalangeal crease, 46
Metacarpophalangeal joints, 74, *74,* 74–75
Metatarsal bone, 249, 275
  fracture, 246
  heads, 249
Metatarsals, 234
Metatarsophalangeal joint, 260, 275, 278
Midaxillary line, 81
Midcarpal joint, 72
Midclavicular line, 81
Middle cardiac vein, 99–100
Middle colic artery, 152–153
Middle constrictor, 389
Middle cranial fossa, 360, 362
Middle ear, 425–432, *431*
Middle ethmoid air cells, 397
Middle finger, 50–53, *52–53*
Middle genicular, 221–222
Middle geniculate artery, 270
Middle glenohumeral ligament, 68
Middle mediastinum, 80, 88–96
Middle nasal concha, 397
Middle palmar space, 50
Middle posterior cranial fossae, 360
Middle radio-ulnar joint, 71–72
Middle rectal artery, 187–188
Middle scalene muscle, 332
Midgut, 141
  rotation, 142
Midsagittal plane, 2
Minor alar cartilage, 307
Minor calyces, 165
Minor pelvis, 173
Mitral valve, 104–105
Mixed spinal nerve, 281

Mons pubis, 194, 203
Monteggia's fracture, 75
Motor nerve supply, 410
Mouth, 305–306, *306–307,* 403–414
Multifidus, 290
Muscle. *See* specific muscle
Muscular triangle, 339
Musculi pectinati, 101
Musculocutaneous nerve, 18
Musculophrenic epigastric artery, 83
Myocardial infarct, 108

N

Nasal bone, 396
Nasal cavity, 394–402
  floor, 396–397
  lateral wall, *397,* 397–398, *398*
  roof, 396–397
Nasal septum, *395,* 395–396, *396*
Nasalis muscle
  alar part, 307
  transverse part, 307
Nasociliary nerve, 370–371
Nasolacrimal duct, 397
Nasopalatine artery, 395
Nasopharynx, 390, 403–414
Navicular, 234, 275
Navicular bone, tuberosity, 249
Neck
  anterior triangle, 337–352
  back, 297–302
  brachial plexus, 334
  posterior triangle, 328–336
  root, 349–350, *350*
  superficial vessels, nerves, *330,* 330–331, *331*
  surface landmarks, 338
  triangles, 338, *339*
Nephrectomy, 172
Nerve. *See* Specific nerve
Nervus intermedius, 432
Nipple, 4, *5,* 9
Nose, 306–307

O

Oblique fissure, 89
Oblique pericardial sinus, 95
Oblique popliteal ligament, 218, 220, 269
Obturator artery, 186, 188
Obturator externus, 214–216, 232, 265
Obturator internus, 174, 194, 197, 212, 214–215, 265
Obturator membranes, 173
Obturator muscles, 173
Obturator nerve, 167, 169, 188, 225, 230–231, *231*
Occipital artery, 347, 354
Occipital bone, 380
  basilar part, 380–381
  wedge removal, 356, *356,* 356–357
Occipital nerve, 299, 354
Occipitofrontalis muscle, 311
Oculomotor nerve, 370
  inferior division, 372
  superior division, 371

Odontoid process, 298
Olecranon, 6, 31, 35
  bursitis, 64
Olfactory nerve, 362
Omental bursa, 136–138, 141
Omental foramen, 137–138, *138,* 143
Omohyoid muscle, 332, 342
Ophthalmic artery, 370, *371*
Opponens digiti minimi, 54
Opponens pollicis, 53
Optic canal, 367
Optic foramen, 360
Optic nerve, 359, 362, 370–371
Oral cavity, 407–413, *408*
Orbicularis oris muscle, 305
Orbit, 366–379
  from above, 367–373
    anterior approach, 373–378
    anterior rim, 366
    bones, 366
    floor, 366
    medial wall, 367
    roof, 366
    superficial muscles, 308, *310*
Orbital septum, 373
Orbital vessels, 310, *311*
Oropharynx, 390, 403–414
  internal structure, 404–405, *405*
Otitis media, 432
Oval window, 428, 430
Ovarian artery, 162, 183, 186
Ovarian vein, 183
Ovarian vessels, 178
Ovary, 177–178, 182–185
  ligament, 179, 183–184

P

Palate, 403–414
Palatine canal, 400
Palatoglossus, 412
Palatopharyngeal fold, 404
Palm, surface anatomy, 46
Palmar aponeurosis, 46–49, *48–49*
Palmar digital arteries, 54
Palmar digital nerves, 54
Palmar interossei, 55
Palmar metacarpal arteries, 54
Palmar radiocarpal ligament, 72
Palmar ulnocarpal ligament, 72
Palmaris brevis muscle, 49
Palmaris longus, 41, 45, 69
Palpebral conjunctiva, 374
Palpebral fissure, 307
Palpebral ligaments, 373
Pampiniform plexus, 129
Pancreas, 140–151, 163
  body, 149
  carcinoma, 151
  head, 149
Pap smear test, 208
Papillary muscles, 103
Paraduodenal recess, 154
Paralysis of quadriceps, 233
Paramedium plane, 2
Paranasal sinus, 394–402, *400,* 400–401

Pararectal fossae, 177
Pararenal fat, 163, 165
Parasagittal plane, 2
Parasternal thoracic nodes, 12
Parathyroid glands, 343–345
Paraumbilical hernias, 130
Paravesical fossae, 177–178
Parietal pleura, 85, 89
  projection, 80, *81*
Parotid duct, 312
Pars flaccida, 426–427
Pars tensa, 426–427
Patella, 229, 236, 268, *269*
  fracture, 246
Patellar ligament, 229–230, 268
Patellar reflex, 279
Patent ductus arteriosus, 117
Pectineal ligament of Cooper, 126
Pectineal line, 126
Pectineus muscle, 223, 227, 230–231, 265
  nerve to, 228
Pectoral girdle, 65
Pectoral muscle, 13–15, *14*
Pectoral nodes, 12
Pectoral region, 8–15
Pectoralis major, 13, 18, 37, 82
Pectoralis minor, 14, 17, *17,* 18, 82
Pedicles, 291, 298
  to transverse processes, 78
Pelvic diaphragm, 174
Pelvic measurements, 191
Pelvic nerves, 188, *189*
Pelvic splanchnic nerves, 188, 207
Pelvic vessels, 186
Pelvis
  female, 173–192
  fractures, 190–191
  male, 173–192
  walls, 173, *174–176*
Penis, 199, *200*
  body, 194
  fascia, 197, 199
Perforating arteries, 218–219, 227
Pericardiacophrenic vessels, 94, *94*
Pericardial sac, opening, 94, *95*
Pericardiacophrenic vessels, 86
Pericardium, 88–96
Perineal body, 194–195
Perineal membrane, 173, 198
Perineal vessels, posterior scrotal branches, 198
Perineum, 192–208
  central tendinous point, 195
Peripheral auditory apparatus, 425
Peripheral vestibular apparatus, 425
Perirenal fat, 162
Peristaltic waves, ureter, 172
Peritoneal cavity, 134, 137, *137,* 137–139
Peritoneum, 133–137
  reflections, 131–139
Peritoneum overlying pelvic organs, 176
Pes anserina, 218
Peyer's patches, 156
Phalanges, 7, *7,* 234
Pharyngeal artery, 347
Pharyngeal constrictor muscles, 388–390
Pharyngobasilar fascia, 387

Pharynx, 386–393
  interior, 390–392
  structure, 386–388
Phrenic nerve, 86, 94, *94,* 113, 115, 335
Phrenic vagus, 115
Phrenicocolic ligament, 159
Pia mater, 292, 294
Piriform recess, 419, *419,* 420
Piriformis, 174, 189, *190,* 212, 214, 265
Pisiform-triquetral joint, 72
Pituitary stalk, 359
Plantar aponeurosis, 249, 253, 275
Plantar arch, 256–258
Plantar aspect, foot, *253,* 253–259, *254*
Plantar calcaneocuboid ligament, 275, 277–278
Plantar calcaneonavicular ligament, 275–278
Plantar fasciitis, 259
Plantar interossei, 258
Plantar metatarsal arteries, 256, 258
Plantar metatarsal vessels, 253
Plantar muscles, 253, 255, *255,* 257–258, *258*
Plantar vessels, 255
Plantarflex foot, 248
Plantaris muscle, 221, 250–251, 269
Pleura, 76, 85–87, *86,* 88–96
  cupula, 80
  in place, 85–87, *86*
  projections, 80, *80*
Pleural cavity, 87, 89
Pleural reflections, 88–89, *89*
Pleural tap, 87
Plicae circulares, 157
Popliteal abscesses, 222
Popliteal aneurysm, 222
Popliteal artery, 220
Popliteal fossa, 209–222, *220,* 220–222, 268
Popliteal vein, 221
Popliteal vessels, 220
Popliteus, 221–222, 251, 269–270
Porta hepatis, 143, *143–144,* 146, *146*
Portal vein, 138, 144–146, 149–150, 152
Posterior abdominal wall, 161–172, *166*
Posterior antebrachial cutaneous nerve, 58–59
Posterior arch, 298
Posterior atlantooccipital membrane, 383
Posterior auricular artery, 304, 347, 426
Posterior axillary fold, 5
Posterior basal bronchopulmonary segments, 93
Posterior basal segmental bronchi, 93
Posterior cecal artery, 153, 155
Posterior cranial fossa, 360, 362
Posterior cricoarytenoid muscles, 420
Posterior cruciate ligament, 268, 271
Posterior cutaneous nerve of forearm, 31
Posterior esophageal surface, 145
Posterior ethmoid artery, 395
Posterior ethmoid vessel, 370
Posterior femoral cutaneous nerve, 197–198, 209,
  211–212, 214
Posterior forearm, deep muscles, 60, *60–61*
Posterior formix, 178
Posterior gastric nerves, 111
Posterior humeral circumflex artery, 19, 28–29
Posterior inferior tibiofibular ligament, 272
Posterior intercavernous sinus, 361
Posterior intercostal arteries, 112

Posterior interosseous artery, 41, 56, 63
Posterior interosseous nerve, 60
Posterior interosseous vessels, 72
Posterior interventricular artery, 100
Posterior interventricular sulcus, 99–100
Posterior laryngeal muscles, 420, *420*
Posterior larynx, 418–421
Posterior layer of rectus sheath, 125
Posterior ligament, 271
Posterior malleolar fold, 426
Posterior mediastinum, 93–94, 109–117
Posterior meniscofemoral ligament, 270
Posterior primary rami, 24, 280–285, *283*
Posterior primary ramus, 82, 281
Posterior right vagus nerve, 145
Posterior sacroiliac ligament, 260–261
Posterior scrotal nerve, 198
Posterior semicircular canal, 427
Posterior skull, 297–298, *298*
Posterior superior iliac spine, 24, 210
Posterior surface of kidneys, 163
Posterior talofibular ligament, 274
Posterior temporal vein, 317
Posterior thigh, 209–222, *217–218*
    cutaneous nerves, 211
    muscles, 216
    perforating arteries in, 218
    sciatic nerve, 218
Posterior tibial artery, 221, 251
Posterior tibial vein, 221, 251
Posterior tibial vessels, 250–251, *252*
Posterior tibiotalar fibers, 274
Posterior triangle, 332
    boundaries, 328–329, *329*
Posterior tubercle, 298
Posterior vagal trunk, 111
Postganglionic fibers, 112
Postganglionic parasympathetic fibers, 372
Postganglionic sympathetic fibers, 372, 399,
    399
Potts ankle fractures, 279
Prepatellar bursa, 236, 268
Prepuce of clitoris, 194
Prevertebral fascia, 387
Prevertebral region, 380–385
Primary bronchi, 93, 109
Princeps pollicis, 54, 64
Processus vaginalis, 126, 128
Profunda brachii artery, 30
Profunda brachii vessel, 31, *32*
Profunda femoris artery, 227, 229, 232
Prolapse
    of rectum, 2097
    of uterus, 191
Promontory, 430, 432
    facial canal, 430
Pronator quadratus muscle, 43
Pronator teres, 40–41, 69
Proper digital branch, 256
Proper plantar digital arteries, 258
Prostate, 177, 179–182, 263
    cancer, 191
    transurethral resection, 191
Prostatic ducts, openings, 182
Prostatic sinus, 181–182
Prostatic urethra, 179–182

Prostatic utricle, 181–182
Proximal radio-ulnar joint, 71, *71*
Psoas fascia, 167
Psoas major, 149, 163, 166
    tendon, 265
Psoas minor, 166
Psoas sign, 172
Pterion, skull fracture at, 327
Pterygopalatine fossa, 324
Pterygopalatine ganglion, 399–401
Pubic bones, rami, 192
Pubic crest, 119
Pubic tubercle, 119, 223
Pubis, 175
Pubococcygeus, 174, 189
Pubofemoral ligament, 264, 266
Puborectalis, 174, 189
Pudendal canal, 195, 215
Pudendal nerve, 188, 194–195
    perineal branch, 205
Pudendal vessels, 209
Pulmonary artery, 90, 92, 95, 97, 114
Pulmonary branches, 115
Pulmonary circulation, 97
Pulmonary embolism, 96
Pulmonary ligament, 86
Pulmonary orifice, 102, *103*
Pulmonary sinuses, 104
Pulmonary valve, 104
Pulmonary veins, 90, 92, 95, 97
    symmetrical orifices, 104
Pulp space infection, 51
Pump handle respiratory movement, 78
Pupil, dilator, 372
Purkinje fibers, 106
Pyloric antrum, 145
Pylorus, 145
Pyramidal eminence, 430

Q

Quadrangular membrane, 422
Quadrangular space, 19, 28, *28*
Quadratus femoris, 212, 214–215, 265
    nerve to, 265
Quadratus lumborum, 113, 163, 166, 287
    fascia, 287
Quadratus plantae, 255–256
Quadriceps, paralysis, 233
Quadriceps femoris, 223, 228–230
    parts, 228, *229*
Quadriceps tendon, 268

R

Radial artery, 35, 41, *42,* 45, 57
    dorsal carpal branches, 63
    superficial branch, 50
Radial collateral ligament, 69, 72
Radial indices artery, 54
Radial nerve, 22, 30–31, *32,* 40, 56, 60
    deep branch, 56
    injury, 33
    superficial branch, 41, *42,* 45
Radiate carpal ligament, 74
Radio-ulnar joint

distal, 71, *71,* 71–72
    middle, 71–72
    proximal, 71, *71*
Radiocarpal joint, 72
Radius
    fracture of head, 45
    head, 35
    styloid process, 35
    tuberosity, 37
Rectouterine folds, 179
Rectouterine pouch, 177–178
Rectovesical fossa, 177
Rectum, 157, 159, 177, 179–182, *182,* 182–185
    cancer, 190
Rectus abdominis, 119, 122, 124–126, *125,* 126
    sheath, 124–126, *125*
Rectus femoris, 223, 228
    nerve to, 229
    reflected head, 265
    straight head, 265
Rectus sheath, 122
    anterior layer, 125
Recurrent laryngeal nerve, 115, 343–345, 390,
    420
Reflection of skin, 8–9, *9,* 47, *47*
Reflex inguinal ligament, 126
Renal artery, 163, 165, 171
Renal biopsy, 172
Renal columns of Bertin, 165
Renal cortex, 165
Renal fascia, 162, 164
Renal hilum, 162–163, 165
Renal medulla, 165
Renal pelvis, 163, 165
Renal pyramids, 165
Renal veins, 163, 165
Respiratory movements, 76–81, *77, 78, 79*
Rete testis, 129
Reticular fibers, 264
Retinacula, 58, 239
Retroduodenal artery, 150
Retroduodenal recess, 154
Retromandibular region, veins, 316–318, *317*
Retromandibular vein
    anterior branch, 316
    posterior branch, 316
Retropubic space, 183, 263
Retrovesical pouch, 179
Rhomboid major, 286
Rhomboid minor, 286
Rhomboid muscle, 284, *285–286*
Rhomboids, 280–285
Ribs, 22, 76–81, *77, 78,* 80–81, 166, 385
    dislocation, 86–87
    fracture, 87
Right atrioventricular orifice, 103
Right atrioventricular valve, 102
Right atrium, 101, *101*
Right bronchus, 90, 115
Right colic artery, 152–153
Right colic flexure, 136, 157, 163
Right common carotid, 114
Right common iliac vein, 171
Right coronary artery, 99
Right gastric artery, 143
Right gastric vein, 143

Right gastroepiploic artery, 145
Right hepatic duct, 144, 149
Right inferior phrenic artery, 169
Right kidney, 163
Right lung, 89, *90–91, 92*
    bronchopulmonary segments, 92, *92*
Right margin of heart, 99
Right ovarian vein, 162
Right phrenic nerve, 114–115
Right posterior intercostal veins, 112
Right posterior pulmonary plexus, 115
Right psoas major muscle, 149
Right subclavian arteries, 114
Right superior intercostal veins, 111
Right suprarenal gland, 163
Right testicular vein, 161
Right triangular ligament, 135, *136,* 147
Right ureter, 149
Right vagus nerve, 115, 141
Right ventricle, 102, *103*
Risorius muscle, 306
Rotation of gut, 140–151
Rotator cuff, 32
Rotatores, 290
Round ligament
    of liver, 131–133, 147
    of uterus, 129–130, 179
Round window, 430

S

Sacral plexus, 167, 185, 188
Sacral vertebra, 291
Sacrococcygeal plexus, 188
Sacroiliac joint, 260–263, *261–263*
Sacroiliac ligaments, 261–262
Sacrospinalis muscle, 289
Sacrospinous ligament, 174–175, 212, 261
Sacrotuberous ligament, 174–175, 192, 212,
    260–262
Sacrum, 174, 260–261
    fractures, 190
Sagittal suture, 355
Salivary gland, 403
Saphenous nerve, 226, 228, 237–238
Saphenous vein, 121
Sartorius muscle, 221, 223
    nerve to, 228
Scalene, 82
Scalp, 353–365, *354*
    anterior, 303–315
    nerves, 354, *355*
    vessels, 354
Scalpel handle, 1
Scaphoid bone
    fracture, 75
    tubercle, 47
Scaphoid triquetral bone, 72
Scapula, 24, 27–29, 37
    anastomoses around, *29,* 29–30
    lateral border, 27
    spine, 24
Scapular region, 23–33
Scarpa's fascia, 120, 197
Sciatic nerve, 169, 188, 209, 214, 216, 218, *219*
Scissors, 1

Sclera, 308
Scoliosis, 295
Scrotal sac, 194
Scrotal surface, 194
Scrotum, 128–129
Second digit, 259
Segmental bronchus, 92
    superior, 93
Segmental pulmonary arteries, 92
Semen, 180
Semicircular canal, 425–432, *428*
Semimembranosus muscle, 218, 237
Seminal vesicles, 177, 179–182, *181*
Seminiferous tubules, 129
Semispinalis capitis, 290
Semispinalis cervicis, 290
Semispinalis thoracis, 290
Semitendinosus muscle, 218, 221, 237
Sensory fibers, 371–372
Sensory innervation of scrotum, 207
Sensory nerve fibers, 399
Septal cartilage, 307
Septomarginal trabecula, 103
Serratus anterior, 18, *18*
Serratus posterior inferior, 284, 286
Serratus posterior superior, 286
Shaft of penis, 199
Short ciliary nerves, 371–372
Shoulder
    joint, 65–68, *66,* 67, *67–68*
    separation, 75
    surface anatomy, 1–7
Sigmoid arteries, 156, *156*
Sigmoid colon, 137, 157–159
Sigmoid mesocolon, 134, 137, 140, 142, 159
Sigmoid sinus, 361, 430
Sigmoidoscopy, 190
Sinoatrial node, 99, 106
Sinus of epididymis, 129
Sinus tarsi, 277
Sinus venarum, 101
Skin, reflection, 8–9, *9,* 47, *47*
Skull
    front, 303
    internal surface, 360
    lateral aspect, 304
Skull cap, removal, 356–357
Small accessory spleen, 150
Small cardiac vein, 100
Small intestine
    herniation, 154
    lymphoid tissue, 159
Small oblique vein, 100
Small saphenous vein, 221, 237–238, 249
Soft palate, 404
Soft tissue injuries in knee, 279
Sole of foot, 248–259
Soleal line, 251
Soleus muscle, 221, 250
Spermatic cord, 122, 128–129
Sphenoid bone
    greater wings, 360
    lesser wings, 360
Sphenoid sinus, 400
Sphenopalatine artery, posterior septal branches,
    395

Sphincter of Oddi, 149
Sphincter of pupil, 308
Sphincter urethrae, 183, 206
Spigelian hernias, 130
Spina bifida, 295
Spinal accessory nerve, 330
Spinal cord, 280–296
Spinal nerve, 295
Spinal roots, 294
Spinalis capitis, 290
Spinalis cervicis, 290
Spinalis thoracis, 290
Spine. *See* Vertebrae
Spinoglenoid notch, 26
Spinous process, 23, 78, 291
Spiral valves, 147
Splanchnic nerves, 109, 112–113, 169
Spleen, 139–151, 163
    enlargement, 151
    ligaments of, 140
Splenic artery, 143, 145, 150
Splenic flexure, 136, 158
Splenic vein, 145, 150, 152
Splenius capitis, 287–288, *288*
Splenius cervicis muscle, 287, *288*
Sprained ankle, 279
Spring ligament, 277
Squamosal suture, 355
Stapedius muscle, 430
    paralysis, 432
Stapes, 428, 430
    base, 431
    head, 431
Sternal angle, 2, 9, 78
Sternoclavicular joint, 3, 5
    dislocation, 75
    midaxillary line, 4
    midclavicular, 4
    midsternal line, 3
    parasternal line, 3
Sternocleidomastoid, 82
Sternocostal surface of heart, 98, *98*
Sternohyoid muscle, 341
Sternothyroid muscle, 342
Sternum
    body, 3
    left margin, 80
    manubrium, 3
    right margin, 80
Stomach, 135, 140–151, 163
    rotation, 140
Straight sinus, 360
Strangulation, loop of small intestine, 154
Styloglossus, 412
Styloid process, 7, 35, 57
Stylomastoid foramen, 304
Stylopharyngeus muscle, 387, *388,* 390
Subacromial bursa, 25
Subarachnoid space, 292–294
Subclavian artery, 332, *334*
Subclavian vein, 114, 332
Subclavian vessels, 332–334, *333*
Subclavius muscle, 82, 335
Subcostal arteries, 112
Subcostal nerve, 82, 124, 165, 167–168
Subcutaneous infrapatellar bursa, 268

Subcutaneous prepatella bursa, 268
Subdural space, 292
Sublingual gland, 408, *409–410*
Submandibular duct, 408, *409–410*
Submandibular ganglion, 408
Submandibular triangle, 339
Submental triangle, 339
Suboccipital region, 297–302
Suboccipital triangle, 300, *301*
Subsartorial canal, 228
Subscapular artery, 19, 28–29, 284
Subscapularis, 18, 37, 67
Subtalar joint, 243, 276–277
Sulcus terminalis, 101
Superficial anterior cervical structures, 339–341, *340–341*
Superficial cervical artery, 282
Superficial circumflex iliac artery, 121, 225
Superficial dorsal vein, 201
Superficial epigastric arteries, 121, 225, 227
Superficial extensor forearm muscles, 59, *60*
Superficial external pudendal area, 201, 224–225
Superficial fibular nerve, 236, 238, 243
Superficial iliac circumflex, 224, 227
Superficial inguinal ring, 122, 126
Superficial palmar arch, 49
Superficial perineal compartment, 192, 197, 203–204
Superficial perineal pouch, 207
Superficial radial nerve, 63
Superficial temporal artery, 313
Superficial transverse perineal muscles, 198–199, 205
Superior aperture, thorax, 77
Superior cluneal nerves, 211–212
Superior concha, 398
Superior constrictor, 389, *389*
Superior duodenal recess, 153
Superior epigastric artery, 83, 121, 126
Superior extensor retinaculum, 239
Superior fibular retinaculum, 239
Superior gemellus, 214–215
Superior genicular, 221
Superior glenohumeral ligament, 68
Superior gluteal artery, 186, *187,* 188, 214, 227, 265
Superior gluteal nerve injury, 222
Superior hypogastric plexus, 172, 188–189
Superior ileocecal recess, 155
Superior laryngeal artery, 418
Superior laryngeal nerve, 420
   internal branch, 392, 419
   internal laryngeal branch, 423
Superior lateral genicular, 222
Superior lingular segmental bronchus, 93
Superior mediastinum, 85, 93, 109–117
   blood vessels, 113
Superior oblique muscle, 372
Superior ophthalmic vein, 370, *371*
Superior orbital fissure, 360, 367
Superior pancreaticoduodenal artery, 145
Superior pancreaticoduodenal vessel, 149
Superior petrosal sinus, 361, *361*
Superior phrenic artery, 112
Superior pubic ligament, 263–264
Superior rectal artery, 156, 182, 185–186

Superior rectus muscle, 370
Superior sagittal sinus, 357–358, *359,* 360
Superior segmental bronchus, 93
Superior thoracic artery, 19
Superior thyroid artery, 343–345, 347
Superior thyroid vein, 345
Superior tibiofibular joint, 271
Superior transverse scapular ligament, 25
Superior ulnar collateral artery, 40
Superior vena cava, 95, 99, 113–114
   orifice, 101
Superior vesical arteries, 177, 187–188
Supinating forearm, 61
Supinator, 40, 56, 60, 69
Supraclavicular fossa, 338
Supraclavicular nerve, 12, 330–331, 341
Supracondylar ridge, 59
Supraduodenal artery, 150
Supraglenoid tubercle, scapula, 37
Suprahyoid region, 348–349, *349*
Supraorbital artery, 369
Supraorbital foramen, 303
Suprapatellar bursa, 268
Suprapleural membrane, 89
Suprarenal artery, 171
Suprarenal glands, 161–165, *164–165,* 172
Suprarenal vein, 164–165
Suprascapular artery, 29, 333
Suprascapular nerve, 25, 334
   injury, 30
Suprascapular vessels, 25
Supraspinatus fossa, 25, *27*
Supraspinatus, 25, 37, 67
Supraspinous fossa, 24–27
Supraspinous ligaments, 292
Suprasternal notch, 2, 338
Supratrochlear artery, 354
Supratrochlear nerve, 311
Supratrochlear vessel, 310
Sural nerve, 221, 238, 245, 249
Suspensory ligaments, 201, 374, *374*
   clitoris, 263
   ovary, 183–184
   penis, 263
Sustentaculum tali, 237, 244, 252
Swallowing of foreign objects, 95
Sympathetic nerve trunk, 82
Symphysis pubis, 119, 179, 192, 194, 197, 203, 260, 263–264, *264*
Syndesmosis, 66
Synovial cysts, at wrist, 64
Synovial joint, cavity of, 262
Synovial membranes, 72
Synovial sheath, 51
Systemic circulation, 97

T

Taenia libera, 157
Taenia omentalis, 157
Taeniae coli, 157
Tail of pancreas, 150
Talocalcaneonavicular joint, 244, 276–277
Talus, 234, 275
   fracture, 247
Tarsal plate, 373–374

Tarsometatarsal joint, 260, 275, 278
Tarsometatarsal ligaments, 275
Tarsus, 308
Taste, sense, 412, *413*
Tectorial membrane, 381, *382*
Teeth, 403
Tegmen tympani, 430
Tegmental wall, 429
Temporal fascia, 319
Temporal fossa, 304, 360
Temporal lobe, 360
Temporal region, veins, 316–318, *317*
Temporal vessels, 319
Temporalis muscle, *318,* 318–319
Temporomandibular joint, 304, *325,* 325–327, *326*
   closing, 326
   movements at, 325
   opening, 326
   protraction, 326
   retraction, 326
   side-to-side movements, 326
   structure, 325
Tendinous arch, 189
Tendo calcaneus, medial border, 251
Tendocalcaneus, 250
Tennis elbow, 64
Tensor fasciae, 223, 226
Tensor palati muscle, 404
Tensor tympani muscle, 430, 432
Tentorium cerebelli, 357
Teres major, 18, 27, 37
Teres minor, 25, 27, 37, 67
Testicular arteries, 128–129, 161
Testis, 128–129
Tetralogy of Fallot, 107
Thenar eminence, 46
Thenar muscles, 53, *53,* 53–54
Thenar palmar crease, 46
Thenar space, 50
Thesinoatrial node, artery, 99
Thigh, 216
   adductor region, *230,* 230–233
   anterior, 223–233
      superficial nerves of, 225, *226*
   medial, 223–233, *230,* 230–233
      muscles of, 230
   posterior, 209–222, *217–218*
      cutaneous nerves of, 211
      muscles, 216
      perforating arteries in, 218
      sciatic nerve, 218
      sciatic nerve in, 218, *219*
Thoracic duct, 76, 109, 111, *111,* 113, 115, *116–117,* 169–170
   severance, 116
Thoracic outlet syndrome, 21
Thoracic region, 287
Thoracic skeleton, anterior, 76
Thoracic splanchnic nerves, 112
Thoracic vertebra, 76–81, *77, 78,* 291
Thoracic viscera, in place, 85–87, *86*
Thoracic wall, anterior, 76–87
   removal of, 84–85, *85*
Thoracoacromial artery, 13–14, 19
Thoracoacromial vein, 13
Thoracocentesis, 87

Thoracodorsal artery, 19
Thoracodorsal nerve, 19, 284
Thoracoepigastric vein, 121, 224
Thoracolumbar fascia, 286–287, *287*
Thoracostomy, 15
Thorax, 2, 76–117
    superior aperture, 77
    surface anatomy, 1–7
Thumb
    abduction, 54
    adduction, 54
    carpometacarpal joint, 72
    extension-flexion, 53
    flexion, 54
    movements, 53–54
    opposition, 54
Thymic veins, 94
Thymus, 85, 94, 96, 113
Thyroarytenoid muscle, 420, *421–423*
Thyrocervical trunk, inferior thyroid branch, 110
Thyrohyoid membrane, 390, 416, 418, *418*
Thyrohyoid muscle, 342
Thyroid cartilage, 416, *417*
Thyroid gland, 114, 338, 343–345, *344–345*
Tibia, 234, *235*
    condyles, 237
Tibial collateral ligament, 216, 268
Tibial fractures, 246
Tibial nerve, 221, 250–251, *252*
    injury, 259
    lateral plantar branch, 253
    medial plantar branch, 253
Tibial shaft, anterior border, 237
Tibial tuberosity, 234, 236, *236*
Tibial vessels, 251
Tibialis anterior, 245
    tendon, 237
Tibialis anterior muscle, 239–240
Tibialis posterior, 251–253
Tibiocalcaneo fibers, 272
Tibiofibular joints, 260, *271*, 271–272
Tibionavicular fibers, 272
Tissue forceps, 1
TMJ. *See* Temporomandibular joint
Toe, 248–249, 258
Tongue, 403–414, *408*, 410, *411–412*
    cancer, 413
Trabeculae carnae, 103, *103*
Trachea, 76, 93, 109, 113, 115, *116–117*, 338
Tragus, 426
Transplantation of gracilis muscle, 233
Transpyloric line, 139
Transpyloric plane, 119
Transtubercular plane, 119
Transverse abdominis muscle, 122
Transverse arch, foot, 275
Transverse cervical artery, 29, 334
    dorsal scapular branch, 286
    superficial branch, 282
Transverse cervical ligaments, 184
Transverse cervical nerve, 330–331, 341
Transverse colon, 135, 149, 157–158
Transverse ligament of acetabulum, 264, 267
Transverse mesocolon, 134, 136–137, 140
Transverse palmar creases, 46, *46*
Transverse pericardial sinuses, 95

Transverse plane, 2
Transverse processes, 291
Transverse sinuses, grooves for, 357
Transverse tarsal joint, 260, 276
Transverse thoracic muscle, 82, 84
Transversospinalis, 290
Transversus abdominis muscles, 122, 163
Trapezium, 72, 74
Trapezius, 24, 282, *284*
Trapezoid, 66, 72, 74
Trendelenburg sign, 279
Triangle of auscultation, 281
Triangles of neck, 338, *339*
Triangular ligaments, 135
Triangular space, 28, *28*
Triceps, 30–31, *31*, 69
    long head, 28, 67
Tricuspid valve, 103
    cusps, 103
Trigeminal cave, 361
Trigeminal nerve, 362
    lingual branch, 410
Trigone, 183
Triquetral bone, 72
Trochanteric anastomosis, 227
Trochanteric bursa, 213
Trochanteric bursitis, 222
Trochlea of humerus, 68
Trochlear nerve, 361, 368–369
Trochlear notch of ulna, 68
True pelvis, 174
Tubal ligation, 191
Tubal pole, 183
Tubercle of iliac crest, 119
Tuberosity of navicular, 237
Tuberosity of tibia, 229
Tunica albuginea, 129
Tunica vaginalis, 126, 128–129
Tympanic cavity, 427–430, *428–429*, 430, *431*
    boundaries, 429
    ossicles, *429*, 430, *431*
Tympanic membrane, 426–427, *427*
    perforation, 432
Tympanic plexus, 430

U

Ulna, 31
    shaft, 35
    styloid process, 35
    trochlear notch, 68
    tuberosity, 37
Ulnar artery, 39, 41, *42*, 45, 49–50
    common interosseous branch, 41
    dorsal carpal branch, 63
Ulnar collateral ligament, 69
Ulnar nerve, 6, 20, 35, 39–41, *42*, 44, 49–50, 54–56
    common digital branch, 48
    deep branch, 54
    dorsal cutaneous branch, 63
Ulnar notch, 72
Umbilical arteries, 132, 177–178, 180, 188
Umbilical hernias, 130
Umbilical region, 119
Uncinate process, 150

Upper extremity, joints, 65–75
Upper lateral brachial cutaneous nerve, 31
Upper limb, surface anatomy, 1–7
Upper lateral brachial cutaneous nerve, 28
Urachus, 176, 178, 183
Ureters, 149, 161–165, 177, 179–182, *180*, 182–185
    constriction, 190
    peristaltic waves, 172
Urethra, 182–185, 194
    penile part, 199
Urethral crest, 181–182
Urethral orifice, 194, 203
Urethral sphincter, 202
Urethral surface, 194, 199
Urinary bladder, 163, 177, 179–182, *180*, 182–185, 263
    cancer, 190
    ruptured, 190
Urogenital diaphragm, 173, 195, 197, 263
Urogenital muscle, motor branch, 205
Urogenital triangle, 192, 197
    female, 203–206, *204*
    male, 197–203
Uterine arteries, 182–183, 187–188
Uterine body, cavity, 184
Uterine ligaments, 184, *185–186*
Uterine pole, 183
Uterine tube, 177–178, 182–185
    openings, 184
Uterine vessels, 178
Uterosacral ligaments, 179, 184
Uterus, 177, 182–185, *185–186*
    body, 184
    round ligament, 129–130

V

Vagina, 182–185, *185–186*, 194
Vaginal artery, 187
Vaginal fornix, 184
Vaginal orifice, 203
Vagus nerve, 76, 109, 113, 115, 145, 170, 346, 386–388
    pharyngeal branch, 345–346, 387, 389, 410
    recurrent laryngeal branch, 113
    superior laryngeal branch, 345–346, 387, 410, 412, 418
Varicose veins, 224, 233
Vas deferens, 128
Vasa rectae, 154
Vasectomy, 207
Vastus intermedius, 228–229
    nerve to, 229
Vastus lateralis, 223, 228
    nerve to, 229
Vastus medialis, 223, 226, 228–229
    nerve to, 228–229
Veins. *See* specific vein
Vena cava, 95
Venae cava, 97
Venae cordis minimae, 100
Venous drainage of heart, 100, *100*
Ventral mesogastrium, 132, 135, 140
Ventricles, 97, 422
Ventricular septal defects, 107

Vermiform appendix, 153–155, 157, *158*
  location, 139
Vertebra prominens, 23
Vertebrae, fractures, 295
Vertebral arch, 78, 291
Vertebral artery, 300–302, 362
Vertebral canal, 290–295
Vertebral column, 80, 291, *291,* 292
  separation of head, cervical viscera from, 384
Vertebral veins, internal plexus, 292
Vertebral venous plexus, 296
Vertical plane, 119
Vesicouterine pouch, 177–178
Vestibular bulb, 205
  artery to, 205

Vestibular window, 428, 430
Vestibulocochlear nerve, 359, 432
Vincula, 52
Visceral pleura, 85, 88
Vitelline duct, 142

W

White rami communicantes, 112, 171
Winged scapula, 22
Wrist, 7, 34–45, 61–63, *62*
  bones, 7
  distal crease, 46
  joints, 72–74
  nerves, 44–45

synovial cysts, 64
tendons, 44–45
Wrist drop, 64

X

Xiphoid process, 3, 8–9

Z

Zona orbicularis, 264
Zygomatic bone, 304
Zygomaticofacial nerve, 310
Zygomaticus major, 305